Advanced Assessment: Interpreting Findings and Formulating Differential Diagnoses

Mary Jo Goolsby, EdD, MSN, ANP-C, FAANP
Director of Research and Education
American Academy of Nurse Practitioners
Austin, Texas

Laurie Grubbs, PhD, MSN, ANP-C
Professor
Florida State University
School of Nursing
Tallahassee, Florida

F.A. Davis Company • Philadelphia

F. A. Davis Company
1915 Arch Street
Philadelphia, PA 19103
www.fadavis.com

Printed in the United States of America

Last digit indicates print number: 10 9 8 7 6 5

Acquisitions Editor: Joanne P. DaCunha, RN, MSN
Developmental Editor: Alan Sorkowitz
Project Editor: Ilysa Richman
Design Manager: Carolyn O'Brien

As new scientific information becomes available through basic and clinical research, recommended treatments and drug therapies undergo changes. The author and publisher have done everything possible to make this book accurate, up to date, and in accord with accepted standards at the time of publication. The author, editors, and publisher are not responsible for errors or omissions or for consequences from application of the book, and make no warranty, expressed or implied, in regard to the contents of the book. Any practice described in this book should be applied by the reader in accordance with the professional standards of care used in regard to the unique circumstances that may apply in each situation. The reader is advised always to check product information (package inserts) for changes and new information regarding dose and contraindications before administering any drug. Caution is especially urged when using new or infrequently ordered drugs.

Library of Congress Cataloging-in-Publication Data

Advanced Assessment: Interpreting Findings and Formulating Differential
  Diagnoses / [edited by] Mary Jo Goolsby Laurie Grubbs.
     p. ; cm.
  Includes bibliographical references and index.
  ISBN 10: 0-8036-1363-6 (alk. paper)   ISBN 13: 978-0-8036-1363-8
  1. Diagnosis, Differential. 2. Nursing assessment. 3. Nurse practitioners.
I. Goolsby, Mary Jo. II. Grubbs, Laurie, 1951-
  [DNLM: 1. Nursing Assessment—methods. 2. Diagnosis, Differential.
3. Nurse Practitioners.   WY 100.4 F931 2006]
RC71.5.F76 2006
616.07¢5—dc22   2005013575

Preface

The idea for this book evolved over several years, while teaching an advanced health assessment course designed primarily for nurse practitioner (NP) students. Although many health assessment texts have been available, they have lacked an essential component—the information needed to arrive at a reasonably narrow differential diagnosis of a patient who presents with one of the almost endless possible complaints. We hope that this book will be helpful to advanced practice students, new practitioners, and experienced practitioners faced with new presentations.

As NPs increasingly become the providers of choice for individuals seeking primary and specialty care, the need for expertise in the assessment and diagnostic processes remains essential. In spite of the growth in available technology and diagnostic studies, performing assessment skills correctly, obtaining valid data, and interpreting the findings accurately are necessary for the safe, high-quality, and cost-effective practice for which NPs are known.

Even once these skills are accomplished, accurate diagnosis remains a difficult aspect of practice. However, we noticed that students and practicing clinicians rarely referred to their health assessment book after completing their assessment course. Instead, they tended to turn to clinical management texts, which focus on what to do once the diagnosis is known. This supported our belief that although assessment texts cover common findings for a limited range of disorders, they are not perceived as helpful in guiding the diagnostic process. Novice practitioners often spend much energy, expense, and time narrowing their differential diagnosis when they have no clear guidance that is driven by the patient and/or complaint. For this reason, our aim has been to develop a text that serves as a guide in the assessment and diagnostic process, is broad in content, and is suitable for use in varied settings.

From Advanced Assessment to Differential Diagnosis has been designed to serve as a textbook during advanced health assessment course work, and as a quick reference for practicing clinicians. We believe that studying the text will help students develop proficiency in performing assessment and interpreting findings, and to recognize the range of conditions that can be indicated by specific findings. Once in practice, we believe that the text will be an aide to guide the assessment and the narrowing of differential diagnosis.

The book consists of three parts. Part 1 provides a summary discussion of assessment and some matters related to clinical decision-making. In addition to discussing the behaviors involved in arriving at a definitive diagnosis, the chapter discusses some pitfalls that clinicians often experience and the types of evidence-based resources that are available to assist in the diagnostic process.

Part 2 serves as the core of the book and addresses assessment and diagnosis using a system and body region approach. Each chapter in this part begins with an overview of the comprehensive history and physical examination of a specific system, as well as a discussion of common diagnostic studies. The remainder of the chapter

Preface

is then categorized by chief complaints commonly associated with that system. For each complaint, there is a description of the focused assessment relative to that complaint, followed by a list of the conditions that should be considered in the differential diagnosis, along with the symptoms, signs, and/or diagnostic findings that would support each condition.

Finally, Part 3 addresses the assessment and diagnosis of specific populations: those at either extreme of age (young and old) and pregnant women. This part is designed to include a heavy emphasis on the assessments that allow clinicians to evaluate the special needs of individuals in these populations, such as growth and development in children and functionality in older patients.

To aid the reader, we have tried to follow a consistent format in the presentation of content so that information can be readily located. This format is admittedly grounded on the sequence we have found successful as we presented this content to our students. However, we have a great appreciation for the expertise of the contributors in this edited work, and some of the content they recommended could not consistently fit our "formula." We hope that the organization of this text will be helpful to all readers.

Acknowledgments

We want to express our sincere appreciation for the support and assistance provided by so many in the development of this book. Their contributions have made the work much richer.

Particular mention goes to all at F.A. Davis for their enthusiasm, support, and patience during the process. Most specifically, we acknowledge the invaluable assistance of Joanne DaCunha, our publisher. Joanne's belief in the concept and in our ability to develop the content was a vital factor in our work and she was always available to guide us throughout the process. We also want to express our gratitude to Alan Sorkowitz, our development editor, for being so patient and supportive as we struggled to complete the final tasks associated with this work and to Ilysa Richman, our project editor, for coordinating so many tasks.

We are immensely grateful to our contributors, who shared their expertise and knowledge to enhance the content. They were a pleasure to work with. In addition to the contributors, we also want to thank the many reviewers for their timely and thoughtful feedback.

Personal acknowledgments from Laurie Grubbs
Most of all, I would like to thank my friend and co-author, Mary Jo, for providing the impetus to write this book—an often talked about aspiration that became a reality; and to F.A. Davis for their enthusiasm, support, and patience during the process.

I would like to thank my children, Jennifer and Ashley, for their support and for being themselves—intelligent, talented, beautiful daughters.

Personal acknowledgments from Mary Jo Goolsby
I must also express thanks to my dear friend and colleague, Laurie. Throughout the majority of my time in academia, I had the pleasure and honor of being "tied at the hip" with Laurie, from whom I learned so much.

Above all else, I also thank my husband, H. G. Goolsby. Without his constant support and encouragement, this would not have been possible.

Contributors

Sara F. Barber, MSN, ARNP
Professional Park Pediatrics
Tallahassee, Florida

Deborah Blackwell, PhD, RNC,
  WHCNP
Dean
Carolinas College of Health Sciences—
  School of Nursing
and
Mercy School of Nursing
Charlotte, North Carolina

James Blackwell, MS, APRN, BC
Nurse Practitioner
Department of Internal Medicine
Carolinas HealthCare System
Charlotte, North Carolina

Valerie A Hart, EdD, APRN, CS
Associate Professor of Nursing
College of Nursing and Health Professions
University of Southern Maine
Private Practice
Portland, Maine

Patricia Hentz, EdD, CS, PMH/NP-BC
Associate Professor
College of Nursing and Health Professions
University of Southern Maine
Portland, Maine

Diane Mueller, ND, RN, CFNP
Doctor of Nursing, Neurosurgery Nurse
  Practitioner
Division of Neurological Surgery
University Health Care
Columbia, Missouri

Karen Koozer Olson, PhD, FNP-C
Professor of Nursing, Texas A&M
  University
Faculty, University of Phoenix Online
Corpus Christi, Texas

Charon A. Pierson, PhD, RN, GNP, BC,
  FAANP
Assistant Professor, Department of
  Geriatric Medicine
University of Hawaii, John A. Burns
  School of Medicine
Editor-in-Chief, Journal of the American
  Academy of Nurse Practitioners
Honolulu, Hawaii

Susanne Quallich, APRN, BC, NP-C,
  CUNP
Nurse Practitioner, Division of Andrology
  and Microsurgery
Michigan Urology Center
University of Michigan Health System
Ann Arbor, Michigan

Randolph F. R. Rasch, PhD, RN, FNP,
  FAANP
Professor and Director
Family Nurse Practitioner Specialty
Vanderbilt University School of Nursing
Nashville, Tennessee

Phillip R. Rupp, MS, APRN, BC
Nurse Practitioner
University of Michigan Urology Center
Ann Arbor, Michigan

Saundra Turner, EdD, RN, BC-FNP
Associate Professor, Chair
Biobehavioral Nursing and
Acting Director of Faculty Practice
School of Nursing
Assistant Professor, Family Medicine
Medical College of Georgia,
Augusta, Georgia

Reviewers

Karen Chamberlain, RN, MSN
Milwaukee Area Technical College
Milwaukee, Wisconsin

Sharon Ewing, PhD, FNP, RN, CS
University of Arizona, College of
  Nursing
Tucson, Arizona

Nicole Harder, RN, MPA
University of Manitoba
Winnipeg, Manitoba, Canada

Janet Ihlenfeld, RN, PhD
D'Youville College
Buffalo, New York

Clair Kaplan, RN/MSN, APRN
  (WHNP), MHS, MT (ASCP)
Yale School of Nursing
New Haven, Connecticut

Joyce Kunzelman, RN, BScN, GNC(C)
Interior Health Authority of British
  Columbia
Vernon, British Columbia, Canada

Jocelyn Loftus, MSN, APRN, BC
Simmons College
Boston, Massachusetts

Maureen McDonald, M.S., R.N.
Massasoit Community College
Brockton, Massachusetts

Kelly McManigle, RN, BSN
Manatee Technical Institute
Bradenton, Florida

Jo Ann Nicoteri, PhD(c), MS, CS,
  CRNP, BC
University of Scranton
Scranton, Pennsylvania

Michael Rackover, PA-C, M.S.
Philadelphia University
Philadelphia, Pennsylvania

Nancy Watts, RN, MN, PNC
London Health Sciences Centre
London, Ontario, Canada

Sally Weiss, RN, MSN, EdD
Nova Southeastern University
Fort Lauderdale, Florida

Jennifer Whitley, RN, MSN, CNOR
Huntsville Hospital
Huntsville, Alabama

Contents

Contents

Contents

Contents

Contents

Contents

Contents

Contents

Contents

Contents

Contents

PART 1

The Art of Assessment and Clinical Decision-Making

Chapter 1

Assessment and Clinical Decision-Making: An Overview

Mary Jo Goolsby & Laurie Grubbs

C linical decision-making is often fraught with uncertainties. However, expert diagnosticians are able to maintain a degree of suspicion throughout the assessment process, to consider a range of potential explanations, and then to generate and narrow their differential diagnosis, based on their previous experience, familiarity with the evidence related to various diagnoses, and understanding of their individual patient. Through the process, they perform assessment techniques involved in both the history and physical examination in an effective and reliable manner and select appropriate diagnostic studies to support their assessment.

HISTORY

Among the assessment techniques that are essential to valid diagnosis is the performance of a "fact-finding" history. To obtain adequate history, providers must be well organized, attentive to the patient's verbal and nonverbal language, and be able to accurately interpret the patient's responses to questions. Rather than reading into the patient's statements, they clarify any areas of uncertainty. The expert history, like the expert physical examination, is informed by the knowledge of a wide range of conditions, their physiologic basis, and their associated signs and symptoms.

The ability to draw out descriptions of the patient's symptoms and experiences is important, as only the patient can tell his or her story. To assist the patient in describing a complaint, a skillful interviewer knows how to ask salient questions to draw out necessary information without straying. A shotgun approach, with lack of focus, is not recommended and the provider should know, based on the chief complaint and any preceding information, what other questions are essential to the history. It is important to determine the capacity of the symptom to bring the patient to the office, that is, the significance of this symptom to the patient. This may uncover anxiety that the patient has about a certain symptom and why. It may also help to determine severity in a stoic patient who may underestimate or underreport symptoms.

Throughout the history, interviewers recognize that patients may forget details, so probing questions may become necessary. Moreover, patients sometimes have trouble finding the precise words to describe their complaint. However, good descriptors are necessary to isolate the cause, source, and location of symptoms. Often, the patient must be encouraged to use common language and terminology, to tie a symptom to something common. For instance, encourage the patient to describe the problem to you just as he or she would describe it to a relative or neighbor.

The history should include specific components, to ensure that the problem is comprehensively evaluated. These components are summarized in Table 1-1, and the specific questions to include in each section are described in detail in subsequent chapters.

PHYSICAL EXAMINATION

The expert diagnostician must also be able to perform a physical assessment accurately. This requires extensive practice with all components of the physical examination and keen

Table 1-1. ■ Components of History

Component	Purpose
Chief Complaint	To determine the reason patient seeks care. Important to consider using the patient's terminology. Provides "title" for the encounter.
History of Present Illness	To provide a thorough description of the chief complaint and current problem. Suggested format: P-Q-R-S-T.
P: precipitating and palliative factors	To identify factors that make symptom worse and/or better; any previous self-treatment or prescribed treatment, and response.
Q: quality and quantity descriptors	To identify patient's rating of symptom (e.g., pain on a 1–10 scale) and descriptors (e.g., numbness, burning, stabbing).
R: region and radiation	To identify the exact location of the symptom and any area of radiation.
S: severity and associated symptoms	To identify the symptom's severity (e.g., how bad at its worst) and any associated symptoms (e.g., presence or absence of nausea and vomiting associated with chest pain).
T: timing and temporal descriptions	To identify when complaint was first noticed; how it has changed/progressed since onset (e.g., remained the same or worsened/improved); whether onset was acute or chronic; whether it has been constant, intermittent, or recurrent.
Past Medical History	To identify past diagnoses, surgeries, hospitalizations, injuries, allergies, immunizations, current medications.
Habits	To describe any use of tobacco, alcohol, drugs, and to identify patterns of sleep, exercise, etc.
Sociocultural	To identify occupational and recreational activities and experiences, living environment, financial status/support as related to health care needs, travel, lifestyle, etc.
Family History	To identify potential sources of hereditary diseases; a genogram is helpful; the minimum includes 1st-degree relatives (parents, siblings, children), although 2–3 orders are helpful.
Review of Systems	To review a list of possible symptoms that the patient may have noted in each of the body systems.

observation skills. Extensive, repetitive practice is required to develop physical examination skills, with exposure to a range of normal variants and abnormal findings. Each component of the physical examination must be performed correctly to ensure that findings are as valid and reliable as possible. While performing the physical examination, the examiner must be able to

- differentiate between normal and abnormal findings
- recall knowledge of a range of conditions, including their associated signs and symptoms
- recognize how certain conditions affect the response to other conditions in ways that are not entirely predictable
- differentiate between the importance of varied abnormal findings

The aspects of physical examination are summarized in each of the following chapters, using a systems approach. Each of the subsequent chapters also reviews the relevant examination for varied complaints. In addition to the specific skills, it is crucial that vital signs and the patient's general appearance/condition always be considered in the decision-making.

DIAGNOSTIC STUDIES

In addition to deciding which questions and physical assessment techniques to implement, the decision-making also guides the selection of any diagnostic studies. Diagnostic studies should be considered if a patient's diagnosis remains in doubt following the history and physical. Additionally, they are often helpful to establish the severity of the diagnosed condition or to rule out conditions included in the early differential diagnosis. Just as the history should not be performed using a shot-gun approach, the selection of diagnostic studies should be judicious and directed toward specific conditions under consideration. Moreover, the clinician should select the study(ies) with the highest degree of sensitivity and specificity for the target condition, while also considering the available options' cost-effectiveness, safety, and degree of invasiveness. Thus, selection of diagnostics requires a range of knowledge specific to various studies, as well as the ability to interpret the study's results. There are some resources that assist clinicians in the selection of diagnostic studies. For imaging, the American College of Radiology's Appropriateness Criteria Web pages provide materials to guide the practitioner on which imaging studies are warranted (see www.acr.org/s_acr/sec.asp?CID=1845&DID=16050). There are a number of texts that review variables relative to the selection of laboratory studies. Subsequent chapters identify specific studies that should be considered for varied complaints, depending on the conditions included in the differential diagnosis.

DIAGNOSTIC STATISTICS

In the selection and interpretation of assessment techniques and diagnostic studies, providers must understand and apply some basic statistical concepts. These concepts include the tests' sensitivity and specificity, the pretest probability, and the likelihood ratio. These characteristics are based on population studies involving the various tests, and they provide a general appreciation of how helpful a diagnostic study will be in arriving at a definitive diagnosis. Each concept is briefly described in Table 1-2; detailed discussions of these and other diagnostic statistics can be found in numerous reference texts.

Table 1-2. ■ Clinical Statistics

Statistic	Description
Sensitivity	The percentage of individuals with the target condition who would have an abnormal, or positive, result. Because a high sensitivity indicates that a greater percentage of persons with the given condition will have an abnormal result, a test with a high sensitivity can be used to rule out the condition for those who do not have an abnormal result. For example, if redness of the conjunctiva is 100% sensitive for bacterial conjunctivitis, then conjunctivitis could be ruled out in a patient who did not have redness on exam. However, the presence of redness could indicate several conditions, including bacterial conjunctivitis, viral conjunctivitis, corneal abrasion, or allergies.
Specificity	The percentage of healthy individuals who would have a normal result. The greater the specificity, the greater the percentage of individuals who will have negative, or normal, results if they do not have the target condition. If a test has a high level of specificity so that a significant percentage of healthy individuals are expected to have a negative result, then a positive result would be used to "rule-in" the condition. For example, if a rapid strep screen test is 98% specific for streptococcal pharyngitis and the person has a positive result, then they have "strep throat." However, if that patient has a negative result, there is a 2% chance that that patient's result is falsely negative, so that the condition cannot be entirely ruled out.
Pretest Probability	Based on evidence from a population with specific findings, this probability specifies the prevalence of the condition in that population, or the probability that the patient has the condition based on those findings.
Likelihood Ratio	This is the probability that a positive test result will be associated with a person who has the target condition and a negative result will be associated with a healthy person. A likelihood ratio above 1.0 indicates that a positive result is associated with the disease; a likelihood ratio less than 1.0 indicates that a negative result is associated with an absence of the disease. Likelihood ratios that approximate 1.0 provide weak evidence for a test's ability to identify individuals with or without a condition. Likelihood ratios above 10 or below 0.1 provide stronger evidence relative to the test's predictive value. The ratio is used to determine the degree to which a test result will increase or decrease (from the pretest probability) the likelihood that an individual has a condition.

Bayes's theorem is frequently cited as the standard for basing a clinical decision on available evidence. The Bayesian process involves using knowledge of the pretest probability and the likelihood ratio to determine the probability that a particular condition exists. Given knowledge of the pretest probability and a particular test's associated likelihood ratio, providers are able to estimate posttest probability of a condition, based on a population of patients with the same characteristics. Posttest probability is the product of the pretest probability and the likelihood ratio. Nomograms are available to assist in applying the theorem to clinical reasoning. Of course, the process becomes increasingly more complex as multiple signs, symptoms, and diagnostic results are incorporated.

In addition to the complexity that exists in patient-based presentations, there are other issues related to the quality of available statistics. Reliable and valid basic statistics needed for evidence-based clinical reasoning are not always readily available. When available, they may not provide a valid representation of the situation at hand. Sources for the statistics include textbooks, primary reports of research, and published meta-analyses. Another source of statistics and the one that has been most widely used and available for application to the reasoning process includes the recall or estimation based on a provider's experience, although these are rarely accurate. Over the past decade, the availability of evidence on which to base clinical reasoning is improving and there is an increasing expectation that clinical reasoning be based on scientific evidence. Evidence-based statistics are also increasingly being used to develop resources to facilitate clinical decision-making.

CLINICAL DECISION-MAKING RESOURCES

Clinical decision-making begins when the patient first voices the reason for seeking care. Expert clinicians immediately compare their patients' complaints with the "catalog" of knowledge that they have stored about a range of clinical conditions and then determine the direction of their initial history and symptom analysis. It is crucial that the provider not jump to conclusions or be biased by one particular finding; information is continually processed to inform decisions that guide further data collection and to begin to detect patterns in the data.

Depending on the amount of experience in assessing other patients with the presenting complaint, a diagnostician uses varied systems through which information is processed and decisions are made. Through experience, it is possible to see clusters or patterns in complaints and findings, and compare against what is known of the potential common and urgent explanations for the findings. Experience and knowledge also provide specifics regarding the statistics associated with the various diagnostic options. However, experience is not always adequate to support accurate clinical decision-making, and memory is not perfect. To assist in clinical decision-making, a number of evidence-based resources have been developed to assist the clinician. Resources such as algorithms and clinical practice guidelines assist in clinical reasoning when properly applied.

Algorithms are formulas or procedures for problem solving and include both decision trees and clinical prediction rules. Decision trees provide a graphic depiction of the decision-making process, showing the pathway based on findings at various steps in the process. A decision tree begins with a chief complaint or physical finding and then leads the diagnostician through a series of decision nodes. Each decision node or decision point provides a question or statement regarding the presence or absence of some clinical finding. The response to each of these decision points determines the next step. In this book, an example of a decision tree is Figure 12-5, which illustrates a decision-making process for amenorrhea. These devices are helpful in identifying a logical sequence for the decisions involved in narrowing the differential diagnosis and also provide cues to recommended questions/tests that should be answered through the diagnostic process. A decision tree should be accompanied by a description of the strength of the evidence on which it has been developed, as well as a description of the settings and/or patient population to which it relates.

Clinical decision (or prediction) rules provide another support for clinical reasoning. Clinical decision rules are evidence-based resources, which provide probabilistic statements regarding the likelihood that a condition exists if certain variables are met and/or the prognosis of patients with specific findings. Decision rules use mathematical models and are

---

Box 1-1

Online Sources of Medical Calculators

Emergency Medicine on the Web: www.ncemi.org
Med Students: Online Clinical Calculators: www.medstudents.com.br/calculat/index2.htm
Medical Algorithms Project: www.medalreg.com
Mount Sinai School of Medicine: www.mssm.edu/medicine/general-medicine/ebm
National Center for Emergency Medicine Informatics:
www.med.emory.edu/emac/curriculum/informatics.html
NIH: www.nih.gov
Sites active as of February 9, 2005. Other subscription-based sites are also available.

---

specific to certain situations, settings, and/or patient characteristics. They are used to express the diagnostic statistics described earlier. The number of decision, or predictive, rules is growing, and select examples have been included in the text. For instance, the Ottawa ankle and foot rules are described in the discussion of musculoskeletal pain in Chapter 13. The Gail model, a well-established rule relevant to screening for breast cancer is discussed in Chapter 8. Many of the rules involve complex mathematical calculations, but others are simple. In addition to discussions of tools in the text, there are several sources of electronic "calculators," based on rules. Box 1-1 includes a limited list of sites with clinical prediction calculators. These resources should be accompanied with information describing the methods by which the rule was validated.

Clinical practice guidelines have also been developed for the assessment and diagnosis of various conditions. They are typically developed by national advisory panels of clinical experts who base the guidelines on the best available evidence. An easily accessible source of evidence-based guidelines is the National Guideline Clearinghouse, which provides summaries of individual guidelines, as well as syntheses and comparisons on topics if multiple guidelines are available. Like decision trees and diagnostic rules, guidelines should be accompanied by a description of their supporting evidence and the situations in which they should be applied.

These resources are not without limitations, and it is essential that they be applied in the situations for which they were intended. In applying these to clinical situations, it is essential that the diagnostician determine the population in which the tool was developed and that it is applicable to the case at hand, as well as have accurate data to consider in their application. For instance, a clinical prediction rule based on a population of young adult college students is not valid if applied to an elderly patient. The provider must also recognize that these resources are intended to assist in the interpretation of a range of clinical evidence relevant to a particular problem, but that they are not intended to take the place of clinical judgment, which rests with the provider.

THE DIAGNOSTIC PROCESS

As noted earlier, the process of diagnostic reasoning begins when the patient is first encountered. As data is collected through the history and physical examination, providers tailor their approach to subsequent data collection. They begin to detect patterns that guide the development of a differential diagnosis that is based on an understanding of probability and prognosis. This means that conditions considered are those that most commonly cause the perceived cluster of data (probability), as well as conditions that may be less common, but would require urgent detection and action (prognosis).

Several adages are frequently used when teaching health assessment, to encourage novice diagnosticians to always consider clinical explanations that are most likely to explain a patient's situation. For instance, students often hear that, "Common diseases occur commonly." Most clinicians learn to use the term "zebra" to refer to less likely (and more rare) explanations for a presentations, using the adage, "When you hear hooves in Central Park, don't look for zebras." Both adages direct novices to consider the most likely explanation for a set of findings. This text describes common conditions that should be considered in the differential diagnosis of common complaints, as well as some of the less common possibilities. With the emergence of conditions, zebras may well be responsible for findings and providers must always maintain some level of suspicion for these less common explanations.

Moreover, even though it is definitely appropriate that conditions with high probabilities be considered in the differential diagnosis, it is also vital that those conditions that put the patient at the highest risk also be considered in the diagnostic process. To do otherwise places the patient in jeopardy of life-threatening or disabling complications. These life-threatening situations are often referred to as "red flags," which are clues signaling a high likelihood of an urgent situation, requiring immediate identification and management. This text also includes red flags for the various systems to promote their recognition in clinical practice.

As the potential list of conditions in the differential diagnosis develops, the provider determines what, if any, diagnostic studies are warranted to confirm or rule out specific diagnoses. A knowledge of the tests' specificity and sensitivity is helpful in the selection process. The diagnostician then combines the knowledge gained through the history and physical with the findings from any diagnostic studies to assess the probability for the conditions remaining in the differential diagnosis.

There are times when a definitive diagnosis is not identified, yet urgent explanations have been ruled out. In this situation, options include moving forward with further diagnostic measures, including further history, physical examination, diagnostic studies, and/or referral or consultation. Another option involves waiting briefly before further diagnostic studies are performed, in order to see whether or not the condition declares itself. In this case, serial assessments should be scheduled over a period of days or weeks, in order to arrive at a diagnosis. An important factor involved in the decision to wait is the patient's ability, willingness, and likelihood of returning for follow-up at the specified intervals. In certain situations, for instance, emergency rooms or urgent care centers, the clinician has no long-term relationship with the patient and the likelihood of the patient returning for follow-up is greatly decreased. In any event, there should be a plan in place to complete the assessment and diagnosis, and the patient should be informed of and should verbalize his or her understanding of the plan, as well as what symptoms would warrant reconsideration. Missed diagnosis and delayed diagnosis are among the most common causes of malpractice complaints, particularly the failure to diagnose myocardial infarctions and breast cancer.

Box 1-2

Common Diagnostic Errors

Jumping to conclusion, being biased by an early finding (e.g., something in the patient's past medical history or recheck from a previous visit).

Accepting previous diagnosis/explanation without exploring other possible explanations (e.g., diagnosis of chronic bronchitis as explanation of chronic cough in patient on ACE inhibitor).

Using a shotgun approach to assessment, without adequate focus.

Focusing solely on the most obvious or likely explanation.

Failure of memory, so only recognize what is memorized or recalled.

Using the wrong rule, decision tree, or other resource to guide analysis or using the correct device incorrectly.

Performing skills improperly.

Misinterpreting or using wrong data.

Allowing the patient to make diagnosis for you (e.g., "I had sinusitis last year and the symptoms are exactly the same.").

Allowing other health care professionals to lead you down the wrong diagnosis path.

Accepting the "horses" without even contemplating the "zebras"; contemplating "zebras" without adequately pursuing the possibility of a more common condition.

Accommodating patient wishes against clinician judgment.

Ignoring basic findings, such as vital signs.

Failing to consider medical conditions as the source of "psychiatric" symptoms and psychiatric conditions as the source of "medical" symptoms.

Although not always to the patient's advantage, patient expectations often play a part in clinical decision-making. Some patients are less willing to wait; others are less willing to be treated. This can be the cause for errors, and clinicians should be aware that they should try to accommodate patients' wishes without putting them at risk.

Box 1-2 includes a list of common diagnostic errors. Although the list is far from exhaustive, avoidance of these errors will improve clinical decision-making.

SUMMARY

The content of this textbook is directed toward assisting clinicians to adequately assess presenting complaints and then to consider reasonable explanations for the complaint and findings. For each complaint, a summary of the relevant history and physical assessment is provided, along with a list of conditions that should be considered in the differential diagnosis. The lists of conditions are not exhaustive. However, by considering the possibility of those included, clinicians will consider various potential etiologies and, by weighing the likelihood of these options, begin to develop critical-thinking skills necessary for clinical decision-making. The authors have provided very brief descriptions of the possible findings for each of the conditions listed, with the hope that this will guide the reader in recognizing definitive clusters of signs and symptoms.

Above all, practice and experience provide the skills necessary for accurate diagnosis. These skills are supported by life-long learning, through which clinicians maintain an awareness of the highest level of evidence relative to assessment and diagnosis.

SUGGESTED READINGS

Center, R. M. (2001). *Clinical Prediction Rules for Dummies.* Accessed online at URL www-cme.erep.uab.edu/onlineCourses/ClinPredictRules/ID0058.html on February 9, 2005.

Ebell, M.H. (2001). *Evidence-Based Diagnosis: A Handbook of Clinical Prediction Rules.* New York: Springer.

Elstein, A.S., & Schwarz, A. (2002). Evidence base of clinical diagnosis: Clinical problem solving and diagnostic decision making: Selective review of the cognitive literature. *BMJ,* 324: 729–732.

Gross, R. (2001). *Decisions and Evidence in Medical Practice: Applying Evidence-Based Medicine to Clinical Decision Making.* St. Louis: Mosby.

Guyatt, G., & Ronnei, D. (Ed.) (2002). *Users' Guides to the Medical Literature: A Manual for Evidence-Based Clinical Practice.* Chicago, IL: AMA Press.

PART 2

Advanced Assessment and Differential Diagnosis by Body Regions and Systems

Chapter 2
Skin

Mary Jo Goolsby

The skin is the largest of all organs. In addition to the obvious protective functions, the skin serves to regulate body heat and moisture, and it is a major sensory organ. Even though many skin disorders are self-limiting, almost any skin condition can be extremely distressing for an individual. Not only is a large portion of the skin clearly visible, so that all can see any abnormality, but the skin is also an extremely sensitive organ and its disorders invoke a wide range of symptoms, including pruritus, pain, burning, and stinging. However, in addition to minor, self-limited conditions, the skin serves as a barometer for overall health because it often exhibits changes occurring in response to serious systemic problems. Moreover, there are dermatologically specific conditions, such as skin cancer, that present significant risks to a patient's health.

Because the skin is such a large organ and exhibits changes in response to so many elements in the internal and external environments, the list of skin disorders is extensive. For this reason, this chapter is organized to provide information to assist providers in making a definitive diagnosis for most common conditions. Information is provided on these common conditions and on some less-common mimics, to assist the reader in applying the content in a practical manner.

HISTORY
General Integumentary History
When patients present with complaints related to the skin, there is an inclination to immediately examine the skin, as the lesion or change is often so readily observable. However, it is crucial that clinicians obtain a history before proceeding to the exam, so that they understand the background of the problem. A thorough symptom analysis is essential and should include details regarding the onset and progression of the skin change; anything the patient believes may trigger, exacerbate, or relieve the problem; how it has changed since first noticed; and all associated symptoms, such as itching, malaise, and so on. When a patient has a skin complaint, it is important to

include a wide range of other integumentary symptoms in the review of systems. For instance, ask whether the patient has recently experienced any of the following: dryness, pruritus, sores, rashes, lumps, unusual odor or perspiration, changes in warts or moles, lesions that do not heal, or areas of chronic irritation. Establish whether the patient has noticed any changes in the skin's coloration or texture. Determine what the patient believes caused or contributed to the problem, any self-treatment and the response, and any distress caused by the complaint. Even minor and self-limited skin problems can cause a great amount of anxiety owing to their visibility and their uncomfortable symptoms, such as burning, oozing, or itching.

Past Medical History

The past medical history should include details on any previous dermatologic illnesses. Ask about infectious diseases associated with skin changes, such as chicken pox, measles, impetigo, pityriasis rosea, and others. Identify chronic skin problems, such as acne vulgaris or rosacea, psoriasis, and eczema. Ask patients about prior diagnoses of skin cancer. Determine the history of any previous skin treatments, biopsies, or procedures, as well as general surgical history. Because disorders in other systems frequently affect the skin, ask about the history of cardiovascular, respiratory, hepatic, immunologic, and endocrine disorders. Identify any recent exposures to others who have been ill and/or who have had obvious skin problems that might have been contracted. Many medications affect the skin, and a list of all prescribed and over-the-counter agents should be obtained, including herbal and nutritional supplements. Table 2-1 includes a nonexhaustive list of medications with potential adverse skin effects. Finally, ask the patient how he or she generally tolerates exposure to the elements, such as heat, cold, and sun, to determine whether environmental exposure is responsible for or may contribute to the patient's complaint.

Family History

The family history should include the occurrence of such skin diseases as eczema, psoriasis, and skin cancer, as well as other disorders commonly associated with skin problems, such as cardiovascular, respiratory, hepatic, immunologic, and endocrine disorders.

Habits

Investigate habits related to skin, hair, and nail care. Identify any chemicals used in grooming, as well as potential exposures encountered through work and recreational activities. Identify occupational, daily living, and recreational activities that could be responsible for lesions resulting from friction, infestations, environmental extremes (heat/cold/sun), and other variables. Dietary history is helpful for identifying the potential sources of atopic reactions.

PHYSICAL EXAMINATION
Order of the Exam

During the general examination of the skin, compare side to side for symmetry of color, texture, temperature, and so on. Then look more closely at specific areas. Good lighting is essential. There are many situations in which additional equipment, such as a magnifier,

Table 2-1. ■ Medications Affecting Skin

Classification	Agent	Possible Adverse Effects
Adrenocorticosteroids	Methylprednisolone, prednisone, corticotropin (ACTH)	Urticaria, atrophy/thinning, acne, facial erythema, allergic dermatitis, petechiae, ecchymoses
Anticonvulsants	Carbamazepine, lamotrigine	Pruritic rash, toxic epidermal necrolysis, Stevens-Johnson syndrome
	Valproate	Alopecia
	Phenytoin sodium	Morbilliform (measleslike) rash, excessive hair growth
	Ethosuximide	Urticaria, pruritic and erythematous rashes
Antimalarial	Chloroquine phosphate	Pruritis, pigmentary changes, lichen planus–like eruptions,
Antineoplastic	Neomycin sulfate	Hypoesthesia, hyperesthesia, urticaria, erythematous swelling, hyperpigmentation, patchy hyperkeratosis, alopecia
	Busulfan	Cheilosis, melanoderma, urticaria, dry skin, alopecia, anhidrosis
	Cyclophosphamide	Pigmentary changes (skin/nails), alopecia
Barbiturates	Pentobarbital sodium, phenobarbital	Urticaria, varied rashes
Cephalosporins	Variety	Rash, pruritus, urticaria, erythema multiforme
Gold salts	Auranofin, gold sodium thiomalate	Rash, pruritus, photosensitivity, urticaria
Nonsteroidal anti-inflammatory agents (NSAIDs)	Variety	Rash, pruritus, erythema multiforme, Stevens-Johnson syndrome, photosensitivity
Oral antidiabetics	Variety	Photosensitivity, varied eruptions
Penicillins	Variety	Urticaria, erythema, maculopapular rash, pruritus
Phenothiazines	Chlorpromazine hydrochloride, thioridazine hydrochloride, trifuoperazine hydrochloride	Urticaria, pruritus, dermatoses, photosensitivity, erythema, eczema, exfoliative dermatitis
Sulfonamides	Co-trimoxazole, sulfamethoxazole, sulfasalazine, sulfisoxazole	Rash, pruritus, erythema nodosum, erythema multiforme, Stevens-Johnson syndrome, exfoliative dermatitis, photosensitivity
Tetracyclines	Demeclocycline hydrochloride, doxycycline hydrate, tetracycline hydrochloride	Photosensitivity
Miscellaneous	Allopurinal	Pruritis, maculopapular rash, exfoliative dermatitis, urticaria, erythematous dermatitis
	Captopril	Maculopapular rash, pruritus, erythema
	Oral contraceptives	Chloasma/melasma, rash, urticaria, erythema
	Thiazide diuretics	Photosensitivity
	Lithium	Acne
	Warfarin	Skin necrosis

Adapted with permission from Dillon, P (2003) Nursing health assessment: A critical thinking, case studies approach. Philadelphia: F.A. Davis, pp 147–148.

measuring device, flashlight/transilluminator, and Wood's (ultraviolet) lamp, are helpful. The progression for the skin exam can be completed in a systematic head-to-toe fashion, or by region as other systems are being examined and are uncovered. Regardless of the sequencing or system chosen, the exam of the skin consists of both inspection and palpation. Privacy is an important consideration because any area being examined must be completely bared. As the skin is examined, it is important to keep in mind the structures underlying the skin and the amount of exposure a particular area is likely to receive. This can help to explain any particular "wear and tear" patterns, scars, calluses, stains, and/or bruises. For instance, an eczematous rash on the area of the nipple and/or areola should always trigger consideration of Paget's disease, a malignant breast condition (see Plate 20).

As the history is obtained, a general survey is performed to determine the patient's general status. Notice the posture, body habitus, obvious respiratory status, and whether the patient is guarding or protecting any area of the skin. The general survey should provide an indication of the patient's overall skin condition, including color, visible lesions, moisture, and perspiration.

As each section of skin is inspected and palpated, there are basic considerations. These include the skin's color, moisture, texture, turgor, and any lesions.

Color

Color is highly variable among individuals of all racial and ethnic backgrounds. Color variation is even found among an individual's own various body regions, depending on several factors, including general exposure to the elements. For instance, coloring is typically darker in exposed areas and calluses may be slightly darkened or have a yellow hue. Some patients develop a vascular flush over their face, neck, chest, and extremity flexor surfaces when they are exposed to warm environments or emotional disturbances.

Changes in color can also indicate a systemic disorder. Cyanosis, caused by decreased oxyhemoglobin binding, may indicate pulmonary or heart disease, a hemoglobin abnormality, or merely that the patient is cold. Observe for cyanosis in the nail beds, lips, and oral mucosa. Jaundice indicates an elevation in bilirubin and often is evident in the sclera and mucous membranes before obvious in the skin. Pallor can indicate decreased circulation to an area or a decrease in hemoglobin. Like cyanosis, pallor is frequently first noticed in the face, conjunctiva, oral mucosa, and/or nail beds. Redness of the skin may indicate a generalized problem associated with a fever or localized problems, such as sunburn, infection, or allergic response. Table 2-2 depicts a number of alterations in coloring that are associated with specific conditions.

Temperature

As each area is observed for visible changes, palpation helps to further explore the findings. Through palpation, alterations in temperature, moisture, texture, and turgor are detected and assessed. The temperature of the skin is best assessed by the dorsal aspects of the hand and fingers. Several situations increase skin temperature, including increased blood flow to the skin or underlying structures; thermal or chemical burns; local infections; and generalized, systemic infections and fever. Decreased skin temperature may occur as a result of atherosclerosis and shock.

Table 2-2. ■ Pigmentary Variations Associated with Systemic Conditions

Pigmentary Change	Associated Conditions
Bronze	Addison's disease (adrenal insufficiency)
	Hemochromatosis
Tan	Chloasma (pregnancy)
	Lupus
	Scleroderma
	Ichthyosis
	Sprue
	Tinea versicolor
Yellow	Uremia
	Jaundice, hepatic diseases
	Carotenemia
Dusky blue	Arsenic poisoning
	Cyanosis
Red	Polycythemia
Pallor	Anemia
	Vitiligo
	Albinism

Moisture

The moisture of the skin varies among body parts and with changes in the environmental temperature, activity level, or body temperature. Skin is typically more dry during winter months and more moist in the warm months. Dehydration, myxedema, and chronic nephritis can all cause skin to be dry. Older patients tend to have drier skin than those who are young.

Texture

The texture of the skin is an important consideration. Coarseness may be a sign of chronic or acute irritation, as well as hypothyroidism. Texture that is extremely fine or smooth may indicate hyperthyroidism.

Turgor

Finally, skin turgor and elasticity are indications of several variables, including the level of hydration and aging. Some disorders, such as scleroderma, are associated with increases in skin turgor. The skin should feel resilient, move easily, and return to place quickly after a fold is lifted. The skin overlying the forehead or dorsal hand is more likely to provide a false impression of tenting or decreased elasticity; therefore, turgor should be tested by gently pinching a fold of skin over the abdomen, forearm, or sternum.

Assessing Skin Lesions

Any lesion identified must be assessed in detail. The characteristics to note include the size, shape, configuration, color, and texture. There should be a determination of whether the lesion is elevated, depressed, or pedunculated. The color, odor, amount, and consistency of any exudate should be determined. If multiple lesions are present, the pattern, location, and distribution must be determined. All of theses variables, along with information obtained during the history and findings related to other systems, are important to making an accurate diagnosis.

The color atlas (see Plates 1–4) includes photographs of specialized techniques that are helpful in assessing skin lesions: magnification, diascopy, skin scrapings, and the use of Wood's lamp.

DIFFERENTIAL DIAGNOSIS OF COMMON CHIEF COMPLAINTS

Note: The color atlas (see Plates 5–32) includes photographs, in alphabetical order, of many of the conditions described in the following section.

Vesicles (Blisters)

Vesicles (blisters) are small, fluid-filled lesions. They may erupt at a site that initially appears inflamed, with a macule or papule. A wide range of conditions can cause vesicles, including infectious and atopic disorders, as well as trauma. The history is very helpful in narrowing the differential diagnosis.

HERPES SIMPLEX (PLATE 15)

Herpes simplex is a viral infection that involves the skin and mucous membranes. It is transmitted via direct contact between a susceptible person and one who is shedding virus. The infection can cause significant systemic symptoms. Orolabial lesions are typically caused by HSV-1 and genital lesions by HSV-2.

Signs and Symptoms.

There may be a history of recurrent lesions in the same location. Herpes simplex is often associated with lymphadenopathy. The skin lesions consist of multiple vesicles, which cluster and are usually preceded by an area of tender erythema. The vesicles erode, forming ulcerations. The lesions can occur anywhere on the body, although common sites include perioral and perigenital regions.

Diagnostic Studies.

Diagnostic studies are typically not warranted or ordered. Definitive diagnosis can be made by viral culture of the lesion and Tzanck smear.

VARICELLA (PLATE 29)

The varicella-zoster virus causes chickenpox, which is considered a common childhood disease. Owing to the recent introduction of chickenpox vaccine, the incidence of chickenpox/varicella is decreasing.

Signs and Symptoms.

The onset of the condition often is evident only when the characteristic skin lesions appear, although some patients describe a brief prodromal period of malaise and fever. The prodromal period is more common in adults with the disease than in children. The skin lesions appear first randomly scattered on the trunk and then extend to the extremities. Lesions may also appear on the mucosal surfaces. Similar to other herpes lesions, the lesions progress from area of redness, to form a vesicle, then become pustular, and, finally, ulcerate. The vesicles look like a dew drop on a rose petal. New vesicles continue to appear while older lesions ulcerate and crust over, so that there is a range of lesion types at a given time.

The lesions are intensely pruritic. The systemic symptoms may become severe, and complications include pneumonia and encephalitis.
Diagnostic Studies.
 None indicated.

HERPES ZOSTER (SHINGLES) (PLATE 30)

Herpes zoster is caused by the varicella-zoster virus. Patients who have circulating antibodies to the virus, usually adults, develop zoster with later exposure.
Signs and Symptoms.

The skin lesions associated with herpes zoster are usually preceded by a period of regional neuralgia and discomfort, as well as a period of malaise. Skin lesions appear as reddened macules, which later develop as clusters of vesicles, and then ulcerate, crusting over. There is lymphadenopathy in the region of the skin lesions. The distribution lies along a dermatome and is typically unilateral. There are many variations of the condition, depending on the affected dermatome. The healing of the lesions is frequently followed by development of postherpetic neuralgia. In patients who are immunocompromised, the condition may be disseminated.
Diagnostic Studies.

A Tzanck smear taken from the base of a vesicle is positive.

TINEA PEDIS

Tinea pedis is caused by a number of dermatophytes. The fungi invade the skin, and the infection is limited to the keratin layer.
Signs and Symptoms.

There is often complaint of pruritus over scaling areas and pain at any developing fissures. The condition usually involves the interdigital areas, causing maceration, inflammation, and fissures. However, the plantar areas of the feet are prone to developing painful blisters in response to the infection. The vesicles often erode and the patient is then prone to secondary infection.
Diagnostic Studies.

None needed. Scraping will reveal hyphae.

CONTACT DERMATITIS (PLATE 10)

Contact dermatitis is an inflammatory response to contact with some chemical or other agent. The range of potential contactants is immense and includes agents that are used in grooming, recreation, and occupation, as well as medications.
Signs and Symptoms.

The patient presents with complaints of pruritic dermatitis. The history assists the patient in identifying the offending agent. The dermatitis appears within days following the contact or exposure. The first exposure usually results in a delayed response, whereas reactions to subsequent exposures develop more rapidly, commonly within 1–2 days. The distribution and configuration of skin lesions associated with contact dermatitis is determined by the exposure. The lesions can range in appearance; they emerge as reddened papules, which form vesicles and which later erode and encrust. The area is usually intensely pruritic. Any area of skin can be affected. As lesions erupt, the skin is at risk for developing secondary infection.
Diagnostic Studies.

None needed. Patch test will be positive.

DYSHIDROSIS (PLATE 11)

The cause of dyshidrosis is not clear, but it is often attributed to some abnormality in the sweating of the hands and feet.

Signs and Symptoms.

Dyshidrosis affects the hands and feet. Lesions are often first evident along the lateral aspects of the digits and later involve the palms and/or soles. In very mild cases, patients may notice only a recurrent scaling or peeling of affected areas. However, the condition usually involves the appearance of small vesicles that itch and burn. With time, the vesicles open and crust. If secondary infection is present, the area will be come inflamed. The distribution is usually symmetrical and there are often recurrences.

Diagnostic Studies.

None needed.

SCABIES

The mite *Sarcoptes scabiei* is responsible for this condition. Individuals are infected through direct contact. After the mites mate on the skin surface, the females burrow beneath the skin and the infected person develops a delayed sensitivity reaction to the mite, larvae, and fecal material.

Signs and Symptoms.

The patient complains of intense pruritus, often worst at night. There is frequently a history of similar symptoms in other family members or contacts. The initial lesions of scabies are small red papules, which often form vesicles, erode, and crust. The distribution depends on the area of infestation. However, the most common areas involve the hands, finger webs, wrists, axillae, and pubic areas. The affected areas continue to be intensely pruritic, and there can be secondary lesions related to the person's scratching the primary site. The lesions' configuration is typically linear, as the larvae burrow beneath the skin. Lesions become painful and reddened if secondary infection is present.

Diagnostic Studies.

There is generally no reason to perform diagnostic tests, as the diagnosis is made based on history and physical. However, skin scraping from a burrow viewed microscopically will often reveal the mite, egg, and/or fecal packet.

DERMATITIS HERPETIFORMIS

Dermatitis herpetiformis is an autoimmune skin disorder, associated with a number of other conditions, including gluten enteropathy, diabetes, rheumatoid arthritis, and lupus.

Signs and Symptoms.

Preceding the development of a skin lesion, the patient experiences pruritus, burning, or stinging at the site. The lesions are clustered vesicles on a reddened base. The lesions have a herpetiform configuration, and the distribution is symmetrical. The extensor surfaces of the knees and elbows are often affected, as well as the posterior scalp, neck, back, and thighs. The condition is chronic. The oral mucosa is rarely involved, and the palms and soles are not affected.

Diagnostic Studies.

Biopsy with characteristic findings.

Bullae (Large Blisters)

Bullae are the fluid-filled lesions that are greater than 1 cm in diameter. They can be caused by thermal trauma, as well as by infectious or atopic disorders.

ERYTHEMA MULTIFORME (PLATE 13)

Erythema multiforme is usually a self-limited skin condition that results from exposure to a medication or infection. This condition occurs in varying grades and is commonly classified as erythema multiforme minor, erythema multiforme major, and Stevens-Johnson syndrome. Erythema multiforme minor is caused by the herpes virus. Erythema multiforme major usually occurs in association with herpes or mycoplasma infection or in response to medications, although a range of infections are implicated. Stevens-Johnson syndrome is usually associated with medications.

Signs and Symptoms.

The patient with erythema multiforme often provides the history of having recently taken a drug that has caused the disorder, or it may have been caused by a range of other diseases, including autoimmune disorders, malignancies, and infections. The lesions are nonraised, reddened papules, and/or plaques. The lesions may have a "target" appearance, such that the outer rim and center are deep red, separated by a pale area. The lesions may progress to form vesicles and/or bullae that lie over the reddened base. As the lesions erode, they form crusts. Although the lesions are generalized, they are usually most prominent over the limbs. The mouth, trunk, and soles of the feet are frequently involved.

Diagnostic Studies.

Associated with erythema multiforme, there may be decreased white blood count and red blood cells, and increased erythrocyte sedimentation rate (ESR) and increased blood urea nitrogen/creatinine in severe cases. In severe cases of Stevens-Johnson syndrome, the patient may be at risk for septicemia, particularly if immunocompromised, and therefore require hospitalization for isolation.

Contact Dermatitis

See p. 18.

BULLOUS IMPETIGO (PLATE 9)

Bullous impetigo is caused by *Staphylococcus aureus* and is less common than the non-bullous form. Although it can occur at any age, it is most common in children younger than 6 years old.

Signs and Symptoms.

The patient or parent may recall being exposed to another person with similar lesions. The bullae progress rapidly, have a thin surface that bursts easily, and subsequently erode. A honey-colored crust is characteristic of impetigo, and smaller lesions may develop near the first. If the crust is removed, there is a reddened base visible. Lesions can occur anywhere. There is no associated lymphadenopathy.

Diagnostic Studies.

None needed. Culture may be performed.

Pustules

Pustules are lesions that are filled with purulent fluid. The cause is typically infectious.

ACNE VULGARIS
Acne vulgaris affects most people at some time during their life. The multifactorial condition affects the sebaceous follicles.
Signs and Symptoms.
The lesions may be tender. The areas most frequently involved include the face and the upper trunk. Patients with moderate acne commonly exhibit a range of lesions, including pustules. Other lesions include comedones, papules, and nodules.
Diagnostic Studies.
None needed.

ACNE ROSACEA (PLATE 5)
Although there are many theories, the cause of rosacea is not clear. It is a condition affecting adults, with varying degrees of sebaceous hyperplasia.
Signs and Symptoms.
The patients relate a history of facial flushing, which becomes more permanent over time. There is often some degree of facial edema. The central third of the face is most often involved. The lesions vary and include erythema, telangiectasia, hyperplastic sebaceous glands, and rhinophyma. Inflammatory papules and/or pustules are often present on the face, neck, and upper trunk.
Diagnostic Studies.
None needed.

BACTERIAL FOLLICULITIS
Folliculitis is an inflammation of the hair follicles and is typically associated with staphylococci. Other microorganisms and causes include pseudomonas (associated with hot tubs), candida (tinea barbae), and herpes.
Signs and Symptoms.
The patient complains of reddened areas of swelling often associated with a mild discomfort from pruritus. Folliculitis lesions often develop as red papules and then progress to form pustules. Lesions are located in the areas with greater hair growth, including the face, scalp, neck, upper trunk, axillae, and inguinal areas. When the lesions erode, crusting occurs. Scarring often develops as the lesions heal. The site of previously healed lesions often have a keloid scar or atrophic scar with no hair growth.
Diagnostic Studies.
None generally needed, although a gram stain and/or culture may be performed.

Keratotic Lesions
Keratotic lesions are rough and generally raised. As the name implies, they contain a high amount of keratin.

WARTS
Warts are harmless skin tumors caused by the human papilloma virus.
Signs and Symptoms.
Warts are raised lesions with no significant pigmentation, often paler than surrounding skin. The surface is irregular and may be stippled. If the surface is scraped or pared, minute bleeding points appear. The most common sites include the hands and feet, face, and genitalia. They are frequently found in clusters.

Diagnostic Studies.

None needed. However, biopsy will reveal characteristic features.

ACTINIC KERATOSES (PLATE 6)

Actinic keratoses, also called solar keratoses, are premalignant lesions that appear in sun-exposed areas of skin. They typically are found in individuals with fair skin and who have a history of developing sun burns without tanning.

Signs and Symptoms.

Typical sites include the face and hands, although any area of chronic sun exposure is at risk. The margins are irregular, as is the surface, which has slight scale and which can be removed to reveal bleeding. The lesions vary in color and may be hypo- or hyperpigmented.

Diagnostic Studies.

Biopsy will reveal features characteristic of this premalignant lesion.

CORNS AND CALLUSES

A callus is an area of skin thickening at a site exposed to repetitive force and wear and tear. With time, a callus may develop a central area of dead cells, which is the "corn."

Signs and Symptoms.

Although calluses are generally painless, corns do become painful. Calluses have rather indistinct borders, yet corns have very distinct borders. The coloring varies. The sites include area exposed to wear-and-tear pressures, often against bony prominences, such as on the hands and feet. Unlike warts, these lesions will not reveal pin-point black dots and bleeding if pared or scraped.

Diagnostic Studies.

None needed.

Raised, Skin-Colored Lesions

BASAL CELL CARCINOMA (PLATE 8)

Basal cell carcinoma is the most common form of human malignancy and involves sun-exposed skin. This malignancy is generally very slow growing. However, it can become quite destructive and invasive if not diagnosed and treated in a timely manner.

Signs and Symptoms.

The typical complaint is of a nonhealing sore that is located on the face, ear, or other sun-exposed area. The patient may complain that the lesion is nonhealing because of repeated trauma. The history often includes previous incidences of basal cell or other skin cancers. Although the lesions can vary, the typical lesion has a waxy/pearly appearance, with a central indentation. The surface often reveals telangiectasia. Over time, the central area erodes and becomes crusty. The border of the lesion typically has a "rolled" appearance. However, basal cell carcinoma appears in several variants and can be flat, hyperpigmented, and/or have very indistinct margins.

Diagnostic Studies.

The diagnosis is made by biopsy.

SQUAMOUS CELL CARCINOMA (PLATE 26)

Squamous cell carcinoma is second in prevalence only to basal cell carcinoma and also involves sun-exposed areas of skin. These carcinomas are more rapidly growing and can become invasive over time.

Signs and Symptoms.

The patient complains of a nonhealing lesion that is growing in size. The lesion is often tender. There is frequently also a history of a lesion consistent with actinic keratosis that progressed into the offending lesion. The appearance of squamous cell carcinoma varies. The lesion may have a warty appearance, a pink-colored plaque, a nodule, or a papule with eroded surface. The size is usually between 0.5 and 1.5 cm in diameter, although the size can be much larger.

Diagnostic Studies.

Diagnosis is made by biopsy.

EPIDERMAL INCLUSION CYST

Also called *epidermoid cysts*, these are formed of epidermal hyperplasia. The cause is unknown. Some epidermal inclusion cysts develop malignancy.

Signs and Symptoms.

The patient complains of a cystic lesion that produces cheesy discharge, with foul odor. The lesion is sometimes tender or painful. The lesion is nodular, round and firm, and subcutaneous; thus, it is flesh colored. The most common sites include the face, scalp, neck, upper trunk, and extremities. However, epidermoid cysts can involve the oral mucosa, breasts, and perineum.

Diagnostic Studies.

Usually none are necessary. However, the contents can be cultured and the lesion can be biopsied.

MOLLUSCUM CONTAGIOSUM (PLATE 19)

Molluscum contagiosum is a skin lesion caused by the DNA poxvirus. It affects persons of all ages.

Signs and Symptoms.

On occasion, patients present with the complaint of burning or pruritus at the site of lesion, although they are usually asymptomatic. The lesion has a smooth surface, with exception of a central indentation. Although the lesion is skin-colored or pink, the area immediately surrounding the lesion may be red. If the surface over the center of the lesion is broken, pressure may express keratotic material. The skin over trunk and extremities is most often the site, although it can affect oral mucosa and the inguinal area.

Diagnostic Studies.

Studies are not generally necessary because diagnosis is made based on findings. Biopsy will reveal characteristic features.

XANTHOMAS (PLATE 32)

Xanthomas are reflective of lipid metabolism and are caused by accumulations of lipid-laden macrophages in the skin.

Signs and Symptoms.

There may be a family history of similar lesions and/or a history of hyperlipidemia or heart, thyroid, or liver disorders. The lesion is asymptomatic. The color ranges from flesh to yellow. The distribution includes the area surrounding the eyes, including the eyelids, and the extensor areas of the elbows, knees, and elbows.

Diagnostic Studies.

None warranted specific to the skin lesion. Lipid studies will reveal elevations.

White Lesions

PITYRIASIS ALBA

The cause of pityriasis alba is unknown. It is very common in children and young adults.
Signs and Symptoms.

There are usually no symptoms associated with the lesions, although patients complain of mild pruritus on occasion. There is commonly a family history of atopic diseases, such as asthma and eczema. Occurrence often has a seasonal pattern. The lesions consist of areas of hypopigmentation, usually covered with a very fine scale. The hypopigmented area is poorly defined and often dry. Over time, the dryness and/or scaling resolves to leave a smooth area of hypopigmentation. The lesions sometimes arise from an initial area of mild erythema. Common sites include the face and arms.
Diagnostic Studies.

None warranted.

TINEA VERSICOLOR (PLATE 27)

Caused by *Malassezia furfur* (formerly named *Pityrosporum orbiculare*), a yeastlike organism that is not contagious.
Signs and Symptoms.

Tinea versicolor, also know as *pityriasis versicolor*, consists of scaly patches of hyper- or hypopigmented skin. The color can range from paler than the surrounding skin to dark brown. An individual's multiple lesions are similar in color. The margins are well discriminated. Itching is often present. It usually occurs in the warm months and in adolescents and young adults. Size ranges widely.
Diagnostic Studies.

Skin scrapings with potassium hydroxide solution reveal hyphae and spores.

MILIA

Milia occur in infants and are similar to epidermal inclusion cysts.
Signs and Symptoms.

Milia consist of 1–2-mm pearl-colored lesions scattered over a newborn infant's face. They may involve the oral mucosa over the palate (Epstein's pearls).
Diagnostic Studies.

None warranted.

VITILIGO (PLATE 31)

Vitiligo is a progressive loss of pigmentation. The average age of onset is 20 years.
Signs and Symptoms.

The patient often describes a history of the progressive development of small, multiple areas of depigmentation that, over time, become larger and confluent. The lesions are well demarcated. There is no overlying scale or vesicle development. Any area of skin can be involved. The hair in the affected area may also lose pigmentation. There is a higher incidence of vitiligo in patients with autoimmune disorders, particularly those affecting the endocrine system, including hypothyroidism, diabetes mellitus, and Addison's disease.
Diagnostic Studies.

None warranted, except to rule out other causes of hypopigmented lesions. Thyroid studies and/or blood glucose should be considered.

Brown Lesions

FRECKLES

Freckles are usually benign lesions. They are responsive to sun exposure, usually becoming more evident in response to sun. Found in most individuals.

Signs and Symptoms.

Asymptomatic. Tan to brown macules ranging 1–5 mm in diameter. The color is consistent on an individual.

NEVI

Melanocytic nevi are extremely common and have genetic predetermination for the number, distribution, and coloring among individuals. Nevi reflect "nests" of melanocytes with hyperpigmentation.

Signs and Symptoms.

The lesions are less than 1 cm in diameter and are evenly pigmented. The margins are well demarcated, and the shape is round. The patient reports that the nevus has existed for a long period without change. The distribution is random.

Diagnostic Studies.

None necessary. Biopsy can be performed to rule out malignancy.

SEBORRHEIC KERATOSIS (PLATE 25)

Seborrheic keratoses are common, benign skin changes found in older adults. The cause is unknown, although they do appear most commonly on sun-exposed areas.

Signs and Symptoms.

Usually asymptomatic. If the keratoses are subjected to frequent trauma, by location and exposure, patients may complain of itching, tenderness, or irritation at their site. Seborrheic keratoses start as flat, light tan lesions and then evolve to become raised and have keratotic surfaces, often with increased pigmentation. The mature lesion has a "stuck-on" appearance and the keratotic cover can be scraped off. Although they can occur anywhere, the most common sites include the trunk, face, and arms.

Diagnostic Studies.

None are warranted.

MELANOMA (PLATE 18)

Malignant melanomas are responsible for most skin cancer–related deaths each year. Most arise in sites without prior hyperpigmentation, but some do arise from previously pigmented sites. The risk is increased among fair-skinned persons with extensive sun exposure, persons with a family history of melanoma, and persons who have had previous changes in moles.

Signs and Symptoms.

Usually patients present with a history of a changing mole or other area of hyperpigmentation. The lesion is usually greater than 0.5 cm in diameter, has notched or irregular edges, irregular pigmentation, and asymmetry of shape. Like other skin disorders, there are variants in appearance, and there should be a high suspicion for melanoma in any changing pigmented skin lesion.

Diagnostic Studies.

Diagnosis is made by biopsy of the lesion.

CAFÉ AU LAIT

Café au lait spots are caused by increased melanin content and are associated with neurofibromatosis. The lesions vary in appearance and size, with coloring ranging from tan to brown.

Signs and Symptoms.

There frequently is a history of a variety of developmental and congenital conditions. The lesions are asymptomatic. They range in size from millimeters to over 10 cm and are usually flat macules or patches. Although the color varies, the most common coloring is that of coffee. Physical findings include signs of accompanying conditions.

Diagnostic Studies.

Biopsy reveals specific characteristics.

GIANT HAIRY PIGMENTED NEVUS

These are congenital lesions. Hairy pigmented lesions vary in size. The ones classified as "giant" are over 20 cm in diameter in adults and adolescents. In infants and children, giant lesions cover at least 5% of the body surface area. The lesions have a high likelihood of becoming malignant.

Signs and Symptoms.

The lesions are quite large, as noted. They are typically round or oval in shape and have an irregular surface, with coarse hairs in approximately 50% of cases. They are usual single lesions and the color ranges from light to dark brown. The coloring may be speckled.

Diagnostic Studies.

Biopsy reveals specific features.

Inflammatory or Red Lesions

CHERRY HEMANGIOMAS

Cherry hemangiomas, or angiomas, arise from dilated venules. They are more common with advancing age. The cause is unknown, and they are not inflammatory lesions.

Signs and Symptoms.

The patient may describe onset after age 30, with number and size increasing over time. The lesions are asymptomatic. The color is typically bright red, though they may be darker, including purple to black in coloring. They do not blanch.

Diagnostic Studies.

None warranted.

PYOGENIC GRANULOMAS (PLATE 23)

Pyogenic granulomas are benign lesions that stem from vascular proliferation. These hemangiomas often occur after a minor skin injury, but also occur spontaneously. While the cause is not known, they are not caused by infection, as the name would imply.

Signs and Symptoms.

The 1–10-mm lesion initially appears as a bright-red papule, which consists of capillaries and collagen, and quickly evolves over a period of a few weeks to become a more dull shade of red with a roughened and friable surface. They open and bleed with mild trauma. While the lesion may become a pale, flesh-colored chronic lesion, they rarely resolve spontaneously. It is important to diagnose these early so that they can be treated at a more manageable stage.

ASSESSMENT TECHNIQUES

Plate 1. ■ Magnifying lesion for inspection. (From Goldsmith, LA, Lazarus, GS, & Tharp, MD. Adult and pediatric dermatology: A color guide to diagnosis and treatment. Philadelphia: F.A. Davis, 1997. Reprinted with permission.)

Plate 2. ■ Diascopy (compression). (From Goldsmith, LA, Lazarus, GS, & Tharp, MD. Adult and pediatric dermatology: A color guide to diagnosis and treatment. Philadelphia: F.A. Davis, 1997. Reprinted with permission.)

Plate 3. ■ Skin scraping. (From Goldsmith, LA, Lazarus, GS, & Tharp, MD. Adult and pediatric dermatology: A color guide to diagnosis and treatment. Philadelphia: F.A. Davis, 1997. Reprinted with permission.)

Plate 4. ■ Wood's lamp. (From Goldsmith, LA, Lazarus, GS, & Tharp, MD. Adult and pediatric dermatology: A color guide to diagnosis and treatment. Philadelphia: F.A. Davis, 1997. Reprinted with permission.)

SKIN CONDITIONS

Plate 5. ■ Acne rosacea. (From Goldsmith, LA, Lazarus, GS, & Tharp, MD. Adult and pediatric dermatology: A color guide to diagnosis and treatment. Philadelphia: F.A. Davis, 1997. Reprinted with permission.)

Plate 6. ■ Actinic keratosis. (From Goldsmith, LA, Lazarus, GS, & Tharp, MD. Adult and pediatric dermatology: A color guide to diagnosis and treatment. Philadelphia: F.A. Davis, 1997. Reprinted with permission.)

Plate 7. ■ Atopic dermatitis. (From Goldsmith, LA, Lazarus, GS, & Tharp, MD. Adult and pediatric dermatology: A color guide to diagnosis and treatment. Philadelphia: F.A. Davis, 1997. Reprinted with permission.)

Plate 8. ■ Basal cell carcinoma. (From Goldsmith, LA, Lazarus, GS, & Tharp, MD. Adult and pediatric dermatology: A color guide to diagnosis and treatment. Philadelphia: F.A. Davis, 1997. Reprinted with permission.)

Plate 9. ■ Bullous impetigo. (From Goldsmith, LA, Lazarus, GS, & Tharp, MD. Adult and pediatric dermatology: A color guide to diagnosis and treatment. Philadelphia: F.A. Davis, 1997. Reprinted with permission.)

Plate 10. ■ Contact dermatitis. (From Goldsmith, LA, Lazarus, GS, & Tharp, MD. Adult and pediatric dermatology: A color guide to diagnosis and treatment. Philadelphia: F.A. Davis, 1997. Reprinted with permission.)

Plate 11. ■ Dyshidrosis. (From Goldsmith, LA, Lazarus, GS, & Tharp, MD. Adult and pediatric dermatology: A color guide to diagnosis and treatment. Philadelphia: F.A. Davis, 1997. Reprinted with permission.)

Plate 12. ■ Eczematous dermatitis. (From Goldsmith, LA, Lazarus, GS, & Tharp, MD. Adult and pediatric dermatology: A color guide to diagnosis and treatment. Philadelphia: F.A. Davis, 1997. Reprinted with permission.)

Plate 13. ■ Erythema multiforme. (From Reeves, JRT, & Maibach, HI. Clinical dermatology illustrated: A regional approach, 3rd ed. Philadelphia: F.A. Davis, 1998. Reprinted with permission.)

Plate 14. ■ Furuncle. (From Goldsmith, LA, Lazarus, GS, & Tharp, MD. Adult and pediatric dermatology: A color guide to diagnosis and treatment. Philadelphia: F.A. Davis, 1997. Reprinted with permission.)

Plate 15. ■ Herpes simplex. (From Goldsmith, LA, Lazarus, GS, & Tharp, MD. Adult and pediatric dermatology: A color guide to diagnosis and treatment. Philadelphia: F.A. Davis, 1997. Reprinted with permission.)

Plate 16. ■ Hidradenitis suppurativa. (From Goldsmith, LA, Lazarus, GS, & Tharp, MD. Adult and pediatric dermatology: A color guide to diagnosis and treatment. Philadelphia: F.A. Davis, 1997. Reprinted with permission.)

Plate 17. ■ Lupus erythematosis. (From Goldsmith, LA, Lazarus, GS, & Tharp, MD. Adult and pediatric dermatology: A color guide to diagnosis and treatment. Philadelphia: F.A. Davis, 1997. Reprinted with permission.)

Plate 18. ■ Malignant melanoma. (From Goldsmith, LA, Lazarus, GS, & Tharp, MD. Adult and pediatric dermatology: A color guide to diagnosis and treatment. Philadelphia: F.A. Davis, 1997. Reprinted with permission.)

Plate 19. ■ Molluscum contagiosum. (From Goldsmith, LA, Lazarus, GS, & Tharp, MD. Adult and pediatric dermatology: A color guide to diagnosis and treatment. Philadelphia: F.A. Davis, 1997. Reprinted with permission.)

Plate 20. ■ Paget's disease. (From Goldsmith, LA, Lazarus, GS, & Tharp, MD. Adult and pediatric dermatology: A color guide to diagnosis and treatment. Philadelphia: F.A. Davis, 1997. Reprinted with permission.)

Plate 22. ■ Psoriasis. (From Reeves, JRT, & Maibach, HI. Clinical dermatology illustrated: A regional approach, 3rd ed. Philadelphia: F.A. Davis, 1998. Reprinted with permission.)

Plate 21. ■ Pityriasis rosea. (From Reeves, JRT, & Maibach, HI. Clinical dermatology illustrated: A regional approach, 3rd ed. Philadelphia: F.A. Davis, 1998. Reprinted with permission.)

Plate 23. ■ Pyogenic granuloma. (From Goldsmith, LA, Lazarus, GS, & Tharp, MD. Adult and pediatric dermatology: A color guide to diagnosis and treatment. Philadelphia: F.A. Davis, 1997. Reprinted with permission.)

Plate 24. ■ Seborrheic dermatitis. (From Goldsmith, LA, Lazarus, GS, & Tharp, MD. Adult and pediatric dermatology: A color guide to diagnosis and treatment. Philadelphia: F.A. Davis, 1997. Reprinted with permission.)

Plate 25. ■ Seborrheic keratoses. (From Goldsmith, LA, Lazarus, GS, & Tharp, MD. Adult and pediatric dermatology: A color guide to diagnosis and treatment. Philadelphia: F.A. Davis, 1997. Reprinted with permission.)

Plate 26. ■ Squamous cell carcinoma. (From Goldsmith, LA, Lazarus, GS, & Tharp, MD. Adult and pediatric dermatology: A color guide to diagnosis and treatment. Philadelphia: F.A. Davis, 1997. Reprinted with permission.)

Plate 27. ■ Tinea versicolor. (From Goldsmith, LA, Lazarus, GS, & Tharp, MD. Adult and pediatric dermatology: A color guide to diagnosis and treatment. Philadelphia: F.A. Davis, 1997. Reprinted with permission.)

Plate 28. ■ Urticaria. (From Goldsmith, LA, Lazarus, GS, & Tharp, MD. Adult and pediatric dermatology: A color guide to diagnosis and treatment. Philadelphia: F.A. Davis, 1997. Reprinted with permission.)

Plate 29. ■ Varicella (chickenpox). (From Venes, D. Taber's cyclopedic medical dictionary, 19th ed. Philadelphia: F.A. Davis, 2001. Reprinted with permission.)

Plate 30. ■ Varicella zoster (shingles) . (From Goldsmith, LA, Lazarus, GS, & Tharp, MD. Adult and pediatric dermatology: A color guide to diagnosis and treatment. Philadelphia: F.A. Davis, 1997. Reprinted with permission.)

Plate 31. ■ Vitiligo. (From Dillon, PM. Nursing health assessment: A critical thinking, case studies approach. Philadelphia: F.A. Davis, 2003. Reprinted with permission.)

Plate 32. ■ Xanthomas. (From Goldsmith, LA, Lazarus, GS, & Tharp, MD. Adult and pediatric dermatology: A color guide to diagnosis and treatment. Philadelphia: F.A. Davis, 1997. Reprinted with permission.)

Diagnostic Studies.

Biopsy will reveal specific histopathologic findings, if performed.

FURUNCLES (PLATE 14)

Furuncles are also commonly called "boils." These lesions are staphylococcal infections of hair follicles or sebaceous glands. Multiple or clustered furuncles are called carbuncles.

Signs and Symptoms.

Patients complain of pain, redness, and swelling at the affected site. The lesion may ooze pus. The most common sites are the axillae and groin. The temperature may be elevated and there is often lymphadenopathy. The size of lesion varies. There is significant tenderness.

Diagnostic Studies.

None generally indicated. Cultures can be performed.

CELLULITIS

Cellulitis is an infection of the skin and subcutaneous tissue. The causative organism varies, although staphylococcal and streptococcal infections are common. Superficial cellulitis, erysipelas, is associated with streptococcal infections.

Signs and Symptoms.

The patient often describes a skin injury preceding the onset of redness, swelling, and pain at the site. The affected area is tender, swollen, reddened, and warm. There is regional lymphadenopathy. When streptococcal infection is involved, bullae may form on the surface.

Diagnostic Studies.

Typically none are indicated unless the condition is severe; if so, CBC and cultures may be warranted.

HIDRADENITIS SUPPURATIVA (PLATE 16)

Hidradenitis suppurativa involves occlusions of hair follicles. The site is commonly the axillae or groin. The cause or trigger of the occlusion is unknown.

Signs and Symptoms.

The patient complains of pain at the site of swelling and redness. The lesions range from papules to nodules and are red, warm, and tender. There are usually multiple lesions present. The lesions often become infected, drain, and/or may form abscesses. Lymphadenopathy is absent. Without treatment, the lesions can become chronic, with prolonged drainage, and/or scarring.

Diagnostic Studies.

None are usually indicated, but CBC and blood chemistries and blood glucose may be ordered to assess contributing factors.

URTICARIA (PLATE 28)

Urticaria, also commonly called "hives," involves a histamine-mediated response that can be either acute or chronic. A wide range of situations are known to be associated with hives, including a variety of infections, foods, and medications.

Signs and Symptoms.

The patient may be able to identify a potential trigger based on experience. The complaint may include a recurrence of the pink or red wheals. The lesions are usually very pruritic and, depending on the severity, may cause localized pain and/or burning. The lesions are nonblanching and vary in size. There are often lesions of various stages, as they emerge from pink to red and then gradually fade before disappearing. New lesions appear as others resolve. The lesions are palpable, with a nonpalpable area of peripheral erythema. There may be associated signs of anaphylaxis and/or angioedema. Dermographism is frequently positive.

Diagnostic Studies.

Performed only based on recurrence and/or severity. These include skin tests for allergen identification, CBC, and other studies specific to presentation.

ERYTHEMA NODOSUM

Erythema nodosum is not well understood, but it is believed to be an antigen-related reaction. The condition can be acute and isolated, or chronic. Erythema nodosum is associated with the use of certain medications (sulfa drugs and oral contraceptives), chronic conditions (sarcoidosis), streptococcal infections, and pregnancy.

Signs and Symptoms.

The patient may have experienced a period of arthralgia and malaise preceding the development of the skin lesion. The lesion is usually isolated, although multiple sites are possible. The lesion emerges as a firm, tender, reddened nodule, usually along the anterior aspect of the leg, although other sites can be involved. Over a period of up to 2 weeks, the lesion fades in color and the degree of firmness decreases.

Diagnostic Studies.

The ESR is often elevated. Chest x-ray may reveal findings consistent with sarcoidosis or another chronic condition (performed only after pregnancy is excluded).

PSORIASIS (PLATE 22)

Psoriasis is a chronic condition that affects the skin and is associated with arthritis. There is a genetic predisposition.

Signs and Symptoms.

The patient often provides the history of recurrent and/or chronic skin changes that most frequently involve the extensor surfaces of extremities and scalp, although other regions are frequently involved. The lesions are described often described as itchy, although this is highly variable. There may be associated concurrent arthralgia. The typical psoriasis lesion has a well-demarcated border, with a silvery colored scale overlying an area of obvious erythema. If the scale is removed, the erythemic base reveals minute bleeding points. The shape of most lesions is oval, and several often coalesce to form one larger lesion. Patients frequently exhibit nail pitting and oncholysis.

Diagnostic Studies.

Diagnosis is typically made on physical findings. However, biopsy will reveal specific histopathologic features.

LUPUS ERYTHEMATOSUS (PLATE 17)

Lupus is described in more detail in Chapter 13, on the musculoskeletal system. However, this chronic connective tissue disorder does have specific dermatological findings.

Signs and Symptoms.

The patient will have a range of symptoms relevant to the diagnosis, depending on the affected organs. There is often coexisting arthralgia and malaise. The rash is macular and erythematous. It is described as a "butterfly rash" because the distribution resembles a but-

terfly's wings, as it overlies the forehead and cheeks. Other skin manifestations include discoid plaques, generalized photosensitivity, and lesions of erythema nodosum.
Diagnostic Studies.
    See Chapter 13.

LICHEN PLANUS

Lichen planus is believed to be a cell-mediated response. The highest incidence occurs in the winter months.
Signs and Symptoms.
    The lesions emerge initially on the extremities and then become generalized over a period of days to weeks. The lesions then persist for months and may involve the skin overlying all body parts. The lesions are red papules of 1 cm or greater in diameter. They can occur individually or in clusters. The presence and severity of pruritus is variable.
Diagnostic Studies.
    If performed, specific histopathologic features identified.

SECONDARY SYPHILIS

Secondary syphilis is commonly referred to as the "great imitator" because the associated skin lesions can have a variety of presentations and appearances. The condition is caused by infection with *Treponema pallidum*. The onset of the rash associated with secondary syphilis occurs weeks to months following the primary lesion.
Signs and Symptoms.
    The patient may provide the history of a more generalized rash developing two or more weeks following the primary lesion. The primary lesion may still be evident. The primary lesion is usually an isolated, single red lesion, which ultimately ulcerates, forming a nontender chancre. There may be a period of malaise preceding the eruption of secondary lesions. These lesions vary in appearance and distribution, but the typical finding is of red maculopapular lesions smaller than 1 cm in diameter. Any portion of skin can be involved, including the scalp, mucous membranes, perineum, and the soles and palms. There is generalized lymphadenopathy. Depending on the involvement of other organs, there may be findings consistent with meningitis, hepatitis, iritis, and arthritis.
Diagnostic Studies.
    The diagnosis is confirmed by positive serology.

TINEA CORPORIS

Tinea corporis is caused by a dermatophyte infection. Depending on the site of the lesion, the condition is referred to differently: tinea capitis (scalp), tinea cruris (groin), and so on. The disorder is commonly called "ringworm."
Signs and Symptoms.
    The patient may recall exposure to another individual with similar lesions or exposure to the dermatophyte through such circumstances as gardening or handling animals. The lesion is pruritic. It begins as a small, annular, erythemic, and scaling lesion that develops a central area of clearing as it grows in diameter. The edge may develop vesicles, is typically scaling, and remains palpable and reddened, so that it presents as a ring.
Diagnostic Studies.
    The diagnosis is typically evident based on the appearance of the lesion and history. However, skin scraping will reveal the hyphae.

PITYRIASIS ROSEA (PLATE 21)

Pityriasis rosea is believed to be caused by a virus. It is most common in the spring and autumn.

Signs and Symptoms.

The patient is usually asymptomatic, although some complain of a prodromal period of malaise preceding the emergence of the rash. The rash is often pruritic. The first sign is typically a "herald patch," which is an annular pink patch that, similar to tinea, has an area of central clearing with a fine scale. The herald patch is most commonly located on the trunk. The herald patch is followed several days later by a more diffuse set of smaller pink, salmon, or fawn-colored lesions, which, at 0.5–1.5 cm, are much smaller than the herald patch, which is typically between 2 and 10 cm in diameter. The distribution of the smaller lesions is described as "Christmas tree distribution" because the lesions have a slightly diagonal axis and are distributed along the skin tension lines.

Diagnostic Studies.

The diagnosis is made on history and physical findings. Skin scraping will differentiate the condition from tinea, by the absence of hyphae.

Eczematous Lesions with Excoriations

ATOPIC DERMATITIS (PLATE 7)

Atopic dermatitis, commonly called eczema, is an atopic condition. The term eczematous dermatitis encompasses a broad set of conditions that include atopic dermatitis, contact dermatitis, and others (see Plate 12). Atopic dermatitis, however, is differentiated in often having onset in infancy or early childhood, as well as being associated with other atopic diseases, including asthma and rhinitis/hayfever.

Signs and Symptoms.

The patient presents with complaint of recurrent, itchy skin rash. The most common sites involve the flexor surfaces of extremities, neck, and face, although the condition is certainly not limited to these areas. The patient may provide a personal or family history of other atopic conditions. The lesions are erythematous, exudative eruptions that can be intensely pruritic. The lesions often progress to form areas of lichenification, which may become chronic. The sites are prone to secondary infections.

Diagnostic Studies.

The diagnosis is typically based on history and physical findings. However, eosinophilia and/or IgE elevations are present on laboratory testing.

Dyshidrosis

See p. 19.

STASIS DERMATITIS

Statis dermatitis is a condition affecting the skin in areas with vascular compromise. It affects the lower extremities.

Signs and Symptoms.

There is typically a gradual emergence of patches of erythemic scaling, associated with pruritus. Edema is often present. The most frequent site is the medial ankle. Over time, the lesions enlarge and become eczematous, so that they weep and/or form crusting. If the site heals, there is a residual area of discoloration, caused by leaking of hemosiderin into the tissues.

Diagnostic Studies.

Deep venous thrombosis may be revealed through Doppler studies. Biopsy reveals characteristic features.

SEBORRHEIC DERMATITIS (PLATE 24)

The cause of seborrheic dermatitis is believed to be immunologic. It is more common in males than females.

Signs and Symptoms.

The patient typically presents with complaints of itching and/or burning associated with scaling lesions on the hairy parts of body, such as scalp, central face, and presternal areas. The lesion consists of a greasy scale lying over an erythematous patch. The problem is recurrent. It can become eczematous, allowing for secondary infection.

Diagnostic Studies.

None necessary; diagnosis is made based on the distribution and appearance of lesion, and the history.

Contact Dermatitis

See p. 18.

 SUGGESTED READINGS

Bickley, L.S., & Szilagyi, P.G. (2003). *Bates' Guide to Physical Examination and History Taking.* Philadelphia: Lippincott, Williams, and Wilkins.

Dillon, P. (2003). *Nursing Health Assessment: A Critical Thinking, Case Studies Approach.* Philadelphia: F.A. Davis.

Goldsmith, L.A., Lazarus, G.S., & Tharp, M.D. (1997). *Adult and Pediatric Dermatology: A Color Guide to Diagnosis and Treatment.* Philadelphia: F.A. Davis.

Swartz, M.H. (2002). *Textbook of Physical Examination: History and Examination.* Philadelphia: Saunders.

Chapter 3
Head, Face, and Neck

Laurie Grubbs

In the United States, malignancies of the head and neck are responsible for 2%–5% of the cancers. People with a history of tobacco and alcohol (EtOH) abuse are particularly susceptible. Other systemic diseases, such as thyroid, kidney, neurologic, heart, skin, and autoimmune diseases, may manifest themselves as alterations in the appearance of the neck and face and may be detectable upon physical examination. This chapter focuses on causes of head, jaw, and facial pain; facial swelling; facial numbness; neck pain or neck mass; and dysphagia. Owing to the complexity of the head and neck exam, subsequent chapters pertain to the Eye (Chapter 4) and the Ear, Nose, Mouth, and Throat (Chapter 5).

HISTORY
General History
The origins of head, face, and neck disorders vary. A history of acute trauma or injury to the head may require x-ray, computed tomographic (CT), or magnetic resonance imaging (MRI) technologies, depending on the location and extent of the injury. Chronic headaches need investigation, and CT scanning or referral to a neurologist may be warranted. A complaint of syncope or dizziness would alert you to the possibility of decreased cerebral blood flow. A complaint of enlarged lymph nodes or masses, in the absence of infection, alerts you to the possibility of a malignant process. Any changes in taste, dysphagia, frequent sore throats, mouth sores that do not heal, hoarseness, or voice changes may indicate oral or throat cancer. Ask about tobacco and alcohol use or abuse because those are the biggest risk factors for malignancies of the head and neck. Ask about dental disease and dental practices. A complaint of swelling or fullness in the neck may be related to thyroid disease. A psychosocial and mental health history should be done, especially for any complaints of chronic pain, to determine any relation to stress, anxiety, or other mental health problems. Other, more specific histories should be undertaken according to the chief complaint.

Past Medical History

Of course, prior history of the disorders of the head, face, and neck should be thoroughly reviewed. A history of head trauma in the presence of chronic headaches is a difficult management issue and should be thoroughly investigated. There is an increased risk of medication overuse in these patients. Prior histories containing syncopal episodes, transient ischemic attacks (TIAs), or cerebrovascular accidents (CVAs) are red flags and should be referred. A past history of malignancies of the head, face, or neck raises a high index of suspicion for recurrence. Any past radiation administered to the head and neck may cause long-term side effects, such as mouth sores, dysphagia, dry mouth, excessive salivation, or hoarseness. Past radiation to the thyroid may cause secondary malignancies.

Family History

A positive family history of cerebrovascular disease, thyroid disease, or migraine creates some increased risk in family members depending on the age and general health of the patient. Malignancies of any kind should be reviewed. A family history of smoking raises the risk of second-hand smoke exposure in the patient.

Habits

As previously mentioned, alcohol and tobacco use are significant risk factors for malignancies of the head and neck. Environmental exposures may also cause malignancies, and a thorough occupational and social history should be obtained.

PHYSICAL EXAMINATION

The physical exam includes inspection of the face for symmetry, sensation (cranial nerves [CNs] V and VII), color, lesions, edema, or masses. Palpate the head and neck for tenderness, paying particular attention to the sinuses, temporal areas, temporomandibular joints (TMJs), and lymph nodes. The mouth, ears, eyes, and nose (covering all the CNs) are included. See Eye (Chapter 4) or Ear, Nose, Mouth, and Throat (Chapter 5), and chief complaints in this chapter for more detail.

DIFFERENTIAL DIAGNOSIS OF CHIEF COMPLAINTS
Head Pain and Headache

History

The history is a very important element of head pain assessment and is often more telling than the physical examination. Inquire about head trauma, recent fever, history of migraines or temporal arteritis in the patient or family members, lung disease, or sleep disorders.

The information gathered during the history that should alert you to the need for an immediate referral includes headache described as "the worst headache I've ever had" in a patient who has no history of headache; headache accompanied by nausea and vomiting without a history of migraines; headache not relieved by standard medication; and headache associated with fever or stiff neck. Headache is covered in detail in the Neurological System (Chapter 14).

Physical Examination

Patients whose headache is prolonged or severe enough to cause them to seek medical attention warrant a complete neurological examination, including CNs; mental status exam; deep tendon reflexes (DTRs); and motor, sensory, and coordination tests. Pay particular attention to the fundoscopic exam, which can give you information about increased intracranial pressure; neck range of motion, which may be decreased in meningitis; and throat, sinuses, and nose, which can cause headache when infection is present. Check vital signs for elevated blood pressure or heart rate, which may indicate a vascular component, and fever, which may indicate inflammation or infection. Palpate the head and temporal arteries for tenderness or any gross abnormalities.

Tension Headache

See Neurological System (Chapter 14).

Migraine Headache

See Neurological System (Chapter 14).

Meningitis

See Neurological System (Chapter 14).

TRAUMA

Blunt trauma to the head can result in acute or chronic headache, regardless of whether there was loss of consciousness or traumatic brain injury (TBI). Generally, the severity of the trauma is correlated with the duration of the headache, but that is not always the case. Certainly, an acute head injury with complaint of severe headache warrants an emergency CT scan, MRI, and/or skull x-ray to rule out a cerebral contusion, subdural or intracerebral hematoma or hemorrhage, or skull fracture. Also see Neurological System (Chapter 14).

Signs and Symptoms.

The headache related to trauma is highly variable in frequency, intensity, and duration and can be difficult to manage. The pain may be localized to the site of the injury or generalized. The patient may be irritable and/or may complain of dizziness, difficulty with concentration, and difficulty sleeping owing to the pain. Stress and/or depression may play a role.

Diagnostic Studies.

In addition to the history and physical, labs should include a complete blood count (CBC), a serologic test for syphilis (STS), chemistries, and possibly a lumbar puncture. A thorough eye exam is also recommended.

CEREBRAL HYPOXIA/EDEMA

Cerebral hypoxia results in edema and can occur in TBI, chronic obstructive pulmonary disease (COPD), and sleep disorders, specifically sleep apnea.

Signs and Symptoms.

In TBI, the hypoxia can be severe and neurological injury significant, ranging from temporary loss of consciousness to a vegetative state. In chronic, low-level hypoxia—as seen in COPD and sleep apnea—the headache is dull and persistent. Hypertension may also be present in these individuals.

Diagnostic Studies.

The diagnosis for TBI is usually obvious from the history of trauma. For chronic hypoxemia, arterial blood gases, oxygen saturation readings, pulmonary function tests, CBC results, and sleep studies can help in determining the cause.

Temporal Arteritis

See Neurological System (Chapter 14).

Jaw Pain and Facial Pain

Jaw pain or facial pain is often a manifestation of a problem in another area of the head and neck, such as ear infection, dental disease, or sinusitis, or from an unrelated system, as is the case with angina.

History

A logical place to start is with any past history of disorders of the jaw, mouth, ear, or nose. You should inquire about psychosocial problems because bruxism and TMJ are often associated with increased stress. Recent trauma is a red flag and should alert you to a possible facial or mandibular fracture. A history of smoking could indicate a neoplasm of the mouth and its associated structures or of the neck. Characteristics of the pain are important—nerve pain is qualitatively different from the pain of soft-tissue, musculoskeletal, or cardiac origin. Nerve pain is usually described as burning or tingling. Pain of cardiac origin is more likely to occur with activity. Inquire about the timing of the pain because pain associated with TMJ syndrome or bruxism may be worse in the morning; pain with trigeminal neuralgia is usually paroxysmal. Pain in the frontal or maxillary area is often caused by sinus congestion/infection, and a history of allergies or a recent upper respiratory infection assists in identifying sinusitis as the cause.

Physical Examination

It is important to examine the entire head and neck, paying particular attention to the jaw, ears, mouth, sinuses, and lymph system. Be sure to include CNs V and VII, which govern jaw clench, facial sensation, and facial movement. If other systems are suspected, such as cardiac or musculoskeletal, those systems should be thoroughly examined.

TEMPOROMANDIBULAR JOINT (TMJ) SYNDROME

Temporomandibular joint syndrome, more appropriately called myofacial pain dysfunction (MPD) syndrome, is a common syndrome with several causes, the most common being a psychosomatic response to stress. Such stress responses may be jaw clenching or bruxism, resulting in fatigue or spasm of the masticatory muscles and, in turn, TMJ pain. Other causes include malocclusion, dental disease, disease of the TMJ tissues, and poorly fitting dentures. The pain can be severe and debilitating and can interfere with daily activities, particularly eating.

True TMJ syndrome is a more serious condition resulting from congenital anomalies, fractures and dislocations, intra-articular disk disease, arthritis, ankylosis, and neoplasias but can have symptoms similar to those of MPD.

Signs and Symptoms.

The signs and symptoms range from mild aching to severe, sharp pain in and around the TMJs. Typically, there is pain with movement of the joint, particularly with chewing, and a clicking sound may be heard on movement. Although often present in TMJ syndrome, jaw clicking is not pathognomonic since many people who have jaw clicking are asymptomatic. There is tenderness of the masticatory muscles. The pain is often referred to the ear, causing pain, tinnitus, and hearing difficulties.

Diagnostic Studies.

Clinical findings are most helpful for ruling in MPD, but x-rays of the TMJ can assist in ruling out degenerative arthritic or possible neoplastic causes. Generally, treatment is supportive and a referral to a dentist or maxillofacial specialist is recommended.

TRIGEMINAL NEURALGIA

The jaw pain associated with this condition is caused by inflammation, degeneration, or pressure on the trigeminal nerve, CN V.

Signs and Symptoms.

The pain of trigeminal neuralgia is usually sharp and paroxysmal, lasting from seconds to minutes, but with recurrent paroxysms that may continue for hours. Bouts of neuralgia are recurrent and may be triggered by movement, but they may subside for weeks and months without an exacerbation. Because there are three branches to this nerve (ophthalmic, maxillary, and mandibular), the pain radiates from the angle of the jaw to one or more of the three places innervated: the forehead and eye area, the cheek and nose area, or the tongue, lower lip, and jaw area (Figure 3-1).

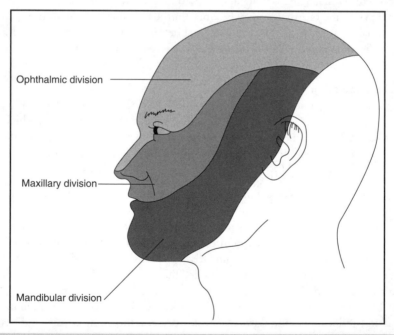

Figure 3-1. ■ Branches of the trigeminal nerve (Cranial Nerve V). (From Swartz, M. Textbook of Physical Diagnosis, 3rd ed. Philadelphia: WB Saunders, 1998, p. 509. Reprinted with permission.)

Diagnostic Studies.

The history is most helpful in the diagnosis of trigeminal neuralgia because no clinical or pathologic signs are present. Sensory changes or abnormalities in the function of CN V suggest a more serious cause, such as a neoplasm, brainstem lesion, cerebrovascular insult, multiple sclerosis, Sjögren's syndrome, rheumatoid arthritis, or migraine, although there are generally other defining symptoms with the systemic diseases.

ANGINA

The pain from myocardial ischemia can often be referred to the neck and jaw areas, and these can occasionally be the only areas of pain. The examiner should retain an index of suspicion for angina being the cause of jaw pain in order to elicit a proper history and physical.

Signs and Symptoms.

A thorough history should lead the examiner in the right direction. Middle-age males with a history of cardiovascular disease in themselves or family members should raise the index of suspicion. The red flag complaints that should alert the examiner to the possibility of a cardiac origin are accompanying chest pain, pain with exertion, dyspnea, nausea, or diaphoresis.

Diagnostic Studies.

The diagnosis can be made with electrocardiogram if it is obtained while the patient is having pain, or with a graded exercise test.

DENTAL PAIN

The most common causes of dental-related jaw pain are the eruption of wisdom teeth and tooth decay or abscess, particularly in the molars. Wisdom teeth generally erupt in the late teens or early twenties, so they should be part of the differential diagnosis in patients of that age. In patients with obviously poor dental hygiene, decay should be included in the differential diagnosis at any age. There are several other periodontal diseases that can cause jaw pain, and these are more prevalent with aging and poor dental hygiene.

Signs and Symptoms.

Jaw pain that is constant and throbbing in nature is typical when dental decay or abscess is the cause. The pain can be quite severe and requires analgesics and, if infection is present, antibiotics, until dental referral can be made. With the eruption of wisdom teeth, the pain is milder and generally not constant.

Diagnostic Studies.

Diagnosis can be made with dental exam. Decay and abscess are quite obvious with a simple oral exam, whereas other forms of dental disease require in-depth dental evaluation. In any case, dental referral is necessary.

BRUXISM

The term is used to define the clenching or grinding of teeth during sleep. The most common causes are malocclusion or tension and stress.

Signs and Symptoms.

Over the long term, bruxism can cause the teeth to wear down, erode, and loosen. Patients are usually not aware of the problem because it occurs during sleep, but they may experience TMJ pain.

Diagnostic Studies.

The diagnosis is usually made via the report of family members or through a routine dental exam. Occlusal guards for the teeth are helpful to prevent dental injury. Fixing the underlying cause is most helpful.

PAROTITIS

There are two types of parotid infection, suppurative (usually caused by *Staphylococcus aureus*) and epidemic, more commonly called mumps (caused by a paramyxovirus). In developed countries, mumps is rarely seen because children are immunized against it within the first 2 years of life. Patients with Sjögren's syndrome are also predisposed to inflammation of the salivary glands (Figure 3-2)—parotid or submandibular—termed sialadenitis.

Signs and Symptoms.

In bacterial parotitis, the symptoms include fever, chills, rapid onset of pain, and swelling, usually in the preauricular area of the jaw. The gland is firm on palpation, with tenderness and erythema overlying the gland. Symptoms are similar to those of mumps, with both glands usually being affected.

Diagnostic Studies.

Clinical signs and symptoms most often make the diagnosis of infectious parotitis. The examiner should attempt to express pus from Stensen's duct, which helps to make the diagnosis of infection. The pus will most often show gram-positive cocci. Treatment includes antibiotic therapy and massage of the gland to promote drainage. Surgery is rarely necessary in infectious parotitis.

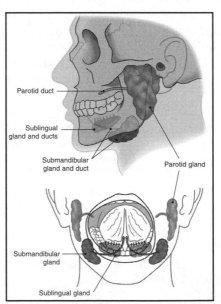

Figure 3-2. ■ Parotid and salivary glands. (From Dillon, PM: Nursing Health Assessment: A Critical Thinking, Case Studies Approach. Philadelphia: FA Davis, 2003, p. 199. Reprinted with permission.)

SALIVARY GLAND TUMORS

The majority of these tumors occur in the parotid gland, and over 80% are benign. Those occurring in the submandibular gland are more likely to be malignant (about 50%). **Signs and Symptoms.**

Salivary gland tumors are often painless and may go unnoticed for months. If malignancy is present, the facial nerve is often affected. *Diagnostic Studies.*

Magnetic resonance imaging or a CT scan is recommended once a mass is found. Fine needle aspiration is necessary for diagnosis and treatment. Surgical excision is necessary and radiation is warranted for large tumors.

SALIVARY DUCT STONE (SIALOLITHIASIS)

The submandibular glands are most often affected rather than the parotid. Often these patients have a history of recurrent sialadenitis, and the stones are composed of calcium phosphate as a result of the pH of the saliva. **Signs and Symptoms.**

Anything that causes the affected salivary gland to be stimulated, usually related to eating, will elicit pain. Swelling also may be apparent over the affected gland. *Diagnostic Studies.*

Clinical diagnosis is made by inspection and palpation. The stones are expressed by manipulation or excision.

TRAUMA

A history of trauma to the jaw alerts the examiner to the need for x-ray to evaluate the presence of a fracture or dislocation of the mandible. Fist fighting and boxing are the most common causes, as well as other sources of trauma, such as motor vehicle accidents. **Signs and Symptoms.**

Pain over a TMJ and difficulty with opening and closing of the jaw are the hallmark symptoms. *Diagnostic Studies.*

The definitive diagnosis is made by x-ray.

Sinusitis

An infection in the sinuses can cause referred pain to the jaw, especially if the middle ear is also involved and/or there is preauricular, tonsillar, or mandibular lymphadenopathy. Sinusitis is covered in Ear, Nose, Mouth, and Throat (Chapter 5).

Facial Swelling

Facial swelling is most often due to an allergic reaction, but systemic diseases can also be associated with facial swelling, as is the case with hypothyroidism, Cushing's disease, or hepatic disease.

History

Inquire about environmental allergies to plants, animals, or chemicals. A medication history is particularly important because facial swelling can be a sign of a medication allergy or a side effect of certain medications, particularly steroids. Ask about a history of thyroid disorders, which can be a cause of myxedematous facies. Ask the patient about any history of adrenal or renal disease, which can cause generalized edema and facial swelling. Inquire about any recent fever, although facial swelling related to infection is usually accompanied by redness and increased skin temperature, which will be evident on physical exam.

Physical Examination

The physical exam is straightforward in determining whether the swelling is localized, which may be caused by a problem or infection in the underlying tissues, or generalized, which would suggest an allergic reaction or systemic disease. Look for any redness, skin changes, tenderness, and lymphadenopathy that would indicate infection.

ANGIOEDEMA

Angioedema is basically anaphylaxis that is restricted to the skin and is generally benign and self-limiting. The causes are numerous and include insect stings; atopic conditions; food allergies (typically nuts, eggs, shellfish, fruit, sulfites); drug allergies; allergy desensitization injections; a reaction to blood products; a response to exercise, cold, or pressure; heredity; and vasculitis.

Signs and Symptoms.

The edema is often accompanied by urticaria, which presents as wheals and is usually seen around the mouth, nose, eyes, mucous membranes, and hands and feet. It can be accompanied by a systemic reaction, and, therefore, the patient should be watched and questioned about any dyspnea or shortness of breath. Angioedema is usually self-limiting and lasts 1–7 days, but can be a chronic, recurring condition depending on the cause.

Diagnostic Studies.

The diagnosis is usually made by history. Allergy testing may give information if the cause is related to food or drug allergies.

CELLULITIS

Cellulitis is defined as an acute inflammation of cellular or connective tissue, usually confined to the skin and subcutaneous tissue, but that may extend beyond to deeper tissues. Group A β-hemolytic streptococcus is the most common organism responsible for superficial cellulitis. It can occur from a wound or bite or as a complication of infections of the eyes, ears, mouth, or nose.

Signs and Symptoms.

The symptoms include redness, warmth, edema, leukocyte infiltration, tenderness, and regional lymphadenopathy. The skin may have a thick, orange peel appearance, and the borders are usually indistinct. Systemic symptoms may be present, such as fever, tachycardia, and headache. Tissue necrosis and suppuration may ensue.

Diagnostic Studies.

The diagnosis can be made solely by history and physical exam, but wound or tissue cultures will help to identify the causative organism. Cellulitis in the head and face should be treated promptly and can usually be accomplished with outpatient antimicrobials.

Cushing's Disease

See Nonspecific Complaints (Chapter 15), under Fatigue.

LONG-TERM USE OF STEROIDS

A cushingoid look can occur in patients who take long-term steroids for chronic diseases, including respiratory, hematologic, and autoimmune.

Signs and Symptoms.

The typical symptoms are those of Cushing's disease, with a rounded "moon face" appearance and truncal obesity.

Diagnostic Studies.

In the case of steroid use, the diagnosis is made by history.

Myxedema

Myxedema is related to hypothyroidism. See Neck Fullness/Mass or Pain in this chapter.

Nephrotic Syndrome

See Nonspecific Complaints (Chapter 15) under Fatigue.

Facial Numbness

A sensation of numbness, tingling, or hypersensitivity in the face should be taken seriously because the causative conditions can be grave neurological diseases.

History

Inquire about the presence of other neurological symptoms, such as weakness, unsteadiness, hemiparesis, disequilibrium, diplopia or other visual changes, which are possible indications of either CVA or multiple sclerosis (MS). Bell's palsy can occur at any age and is often a sequela of a viral illness. Multiple sclerosis occurs more in the young adult population, whereas CVA occurs more in the older population, especially in those with hypertension or diabetes. A thorough family history may disclose a predisposition to CVA, hypertension, diabetes, and other neurological diseases. Twin studies show a genetic susceptibility for MS.

Physical Examination

The physical exam should include testing facial sensation on each side of the face (CN V), as well as movement by having the patient perform certain facial expressions (CN VII). Symptoms are almost always unilateral. Diagnostic imaging can be helpful to rule in CVA or MS.

BELL'S PALSY

Bell's palsy is a unilateral paralysis of the face. The etiology is uncertain but the paralysis is thought to be due to an inflammation of CN VII, secondary to a viral infection.

Signs and Symptoms.

The onset of Bell's palsy is sudden, and the symptoms are unilateral. The affected side of the face droops with asymmetrical facial movement; there is excessive lacrimation and salivation, and inability to close the eye. The result may be partial or complete paralysis. No sensory loss is demonstrable. The affected eye must be kept moist and patched to avoid excessive dryness.

Diagnostic Studies.

The diagnosis is made by physical examination. There are no diagnostic tests for initial diagnosis, but an electromyogram can be helpful to determine the extent of the nerve damage. Recovery from partial paralysis occurs in 2–6 months; complete recovery from total paralysis varies from 20%–90%. Corticosteroids and antivirals may hasten recovery.

MULTIPLE SCLEROSIS

Multiple sclerosis is a progressive disease of the central nervous system, resulting in a variety of neurological symptoms affecting the motor, sensory, mental, CNs and the autonomic nervous system. See Neurological System (Chapter 14).

Signs and Symptoms.

The onset is insidious and may go undiagnosed for months or years. Unilateral facial paresthesia or pain is seen occasionally early in the disease process, although most of the symptoms involve the eye.

Diagnostic Studies.

A good history—especially one that describes remissions and exacerbations of the symptoms—can raise an index of suspicion. Computed tomography, MRI, lumbar puncture, and evoked potentials are all part of the diagnostic workup.

Cerebrovascular Accident

Although it would be unusual for facial numbness to be the presenting complaint for stroke, it should be considered in the differential diagnosis. Age and past medical history are very helpful in raising the index of suspicion for CVA. A thorough physical exam and diagnostic imaging are definitive. See Neurological System (Chapter 14).

Scalp and Face Pruritus

History

It would be unusual for pruritus in the head and neck to indicate anything except a skin condition/disease or infestation. If the patient is a school-age child, pediculosis is an obvious choice and the child's friends and school administrators should be questioned about recent outbreaks. You should ask about sun exposure and blistering sunburns. A history of other skin cancers in the patient or family is important to determine.

Physical Examination

The physical exam includes careful inspection of the head and scalp for nits or actual lice. Nits are fixed to the hair shaft and are grayish-white in appearance. Unlike the flakiness of seborrhea, nits cannot be easily dislodged. The skin of the head and face should be inspected for lesions, color changes, new or changing moles, crusting, scaling, ulceration, or bleeding, which might be indicative of cancer or psoriasis.

Pediculosis (Head Lice)

See Pediatric Patients (Chapter 17).

Seborrhea

See Skin (Chapter 2).

Tinea Capitus

Tinea capitus is a fungal infection of the scalp seen mainly in children. It is characterized by scaly patches, sometimes annular, and often accompanied by hair loss in the area. Topical and oral treatments are available. See Pediatric Patients (Chapter 17).

Psoriasis

See Skin (Chapter 2).

Neck Fullness/Mass or Pain

History

Start with a thorough history, including a past medical history for cancer or exposure to environmental toxins. Ask about frequent infections; allergies; chronic ear, nose, and throat problems; or surgeries. Ask about living arrangements because close quarters, such as classrooms and college dormitories, can predispose the patient to a variety of infections. Ask about sexual practices. Inquire about family history, especially thyroid disease.

The symptoms will vary depending on the underlying cause. In thyroid disease, patients may describe a feeling of having something in their throat. The complaint is more likely to be one of fullness rather than of pain or dysphagia. The history should inquire about signs and symptoms of hyper- or hypothyroidism, such as weight loss or gain, nervousness or fatigue, diarrhea or constipation, intolerance to heat or cold, insomnia or lethargy, menstrual irregularities, and skin or hair changes. Laboratory studies and thyroid scanning can diagnose most problems.

Lymphadenopathy has numerous causes but can generally be placed into two categories: infection or malignancy. Infection often presents with fever, sore throat, runny nose, cough, and malaise. A history of an upper respiratory infection is common.

Symptoms of malignancies are more likely to be fatigue, weakness, anorexia, weight loss, fever, night sweats, bleeding, and easy bruisability. A history of tobacco and/or EtOH abuse may be present in neoplasms of the head and neck.

Physical Examination

The physical exam includes palpation of the thyroid for enlargement, asymmetry, or nodules. Inspect the skin and hair for moistness or dryness. Look for periorbital edema, which may be present in hypothyroidism. Check the vital signs for hyper- or hypotension, tachy- or bradycardia, and fever or subnormal temperature. Notice any tremor. Check the DTRs for hyper- or hyporeflexia. Abnormalities in any of these areas would indicate the need for further thyroid studies, including thyroid-stimulating hormone (TSH), T_3, T_4, and possibly a thyroid scan.

A complete examination of the mouth, throat, nose, ears, and eyes should be performed as you look for infection. Palpate for lymphadenopathy in other areas of the body, which might be present in malignancies. Laboratory studies for a CBC might be warranted to check for leukocytosis or leukopenia. A "mono spot" would definitively diagnose mononucleosis. If that is suspected, palpate for splenomegaly. A chest x-ray may be necessary to look for mediastinal lymphadenopathy, indicating Hodgkin's or other malignancy. Depending on sexual practices, a *Neisseria gonorrhoeae* (GC) or *Chlamydia trachomatis* culture of the throat may be necessary, or blood studies for rapid plasma reagin (RPR) or human immunodeficiency virus (HIV).

Goiter

A deficiency in thyroid hormone can result from thyroid failure, likely autoimmune in etiology (primary hypothyroidism), or failure of the hypothalamic-pituitary axis (secondary hypothyroidism). Goiter, an enlargement of the thyroid gland, may be associated with hypothyroidism or hyperthyroidism, but patients with goiter also may be euthyroid, a condition termed nontoxic goiter.

Hypothyroidism   There are numerous causes of hypothyroidism, including Hashimoto's thyroiditis; iodine deficiency; genetic thyroid enzyme defects; iodine deficiency; medications (amiodarone, iodine-containing contrast media, lithium, methimazole, phenylbutazone, sulfonamides, aminoglutethimide, interferon-α); thyroid cancer; and infiltrative disorders, such as sarcoidosis, amyloidosis, scleroderma, cystinosis, and hemochromatosis. Thyroid diseases, in general, are more common in women.

Signs and Symptoms.

The severity of symptoms ranges from unrecognized states found only by TSH screening to striking myxedema. Symptoms include fatigue, cold intolerance, constipation, weight gain, depression, menorrhagia, hoarseness, dry skin and hair, cool skin with slow capillary refill, paresthesias of the hands and feet, bradycardia, delayed DTRs, periorbital edema, anemia, and hyponatremia. The thyroid may be of normal size or enlarged and nodular, depending on the cause. In rare and extreme cases, myxedematous coma may ensue, with severe hypothermia, hypoventilation, hyponatremia, hypoxia, hypercapnia, hypotension, and seizures.

Diagnostic Studies.

Diagnosis is made by measurement of TSH, T_4, and radioiodine uptake. Because it is a feedback system, the TSH is elevated and the T_4 and radioiodine uptake are low. A thyroid ultrasound is helpful for determining the size and differentiation of nodules.

Hyperthyroidism   Graves' disease is the most common cause of hyperthyroidism, except in patients over 55, in whom multinodular goiter is a more common etiology. Onset of this condition can occur at any age, but it is most common between the ages of 20 and 40 years. Often patients have a family history of Graves' disease or other autoimmune thyroid diseases, such as Hashimoto's disease. See Box 3-1 for predisposing factors for hyperthyroidism.

Signs and Symptoms.

Clinical manifestations include diffuse goiter, nervousness, irritability, tremor, heat intolerance, weakness, tachycardia, palpitations, widened pulse pressure, increased sweating, weight loss, insomnia, frequent bowel movements, menstrual irregularities, exophthalmos, and infiltrative dermopathy. Patients older than 50 years often present with cardiac symptoms, such as hypertension, atrial fibrillation, or heart failure.

Box 3-1
Predisposing Factors for Hyperthyroidism

- Heredity
- Female gender
- Recent adverse life events causing psychological stress
- Smoking
- Pregnancy
- Parity
- Viral and bacterial infections that cause subacute thyroiditis
- Iodine supplementation or exposure to an iodine load
- Lithium, amiodarone, or antiretroviral therapy
- Type I diabetes

Diagnostic Studies.

A decreased TSH and elevated free T_4 and T_3 will generally make the diagnosis. Also consider the erythrocyte sedimentation rate, which can be elevated in Graves' disease; the CBC, to rule out anemia or an elevated white blood cell count; and the metabolic profile, with special attention to calcium, glucose, and potassium, to rule out pheochromocytoma or adrenal disease. Thyroid autoantibodies will be elevated in Graves' disease and Hashimoto's thyroiditis. Radioactive iodine (RAI) imaging should be performed to look for increased uptake and the presence of hot or cold nodules. Fine needle aspiration is recommended. Most can be managed medically or with RAI ablation.

Euthyroid Goiter Simple, endemic, nontoxic diffuse, and nontoxic nodular goiter indicate an enlargement of the thyroid gland with diminished thyroid hormone production, but without clinical thyroid disease. Euthyroid goiter is the most common type of goiter and commonly occurs during puberty, pregnancy, or at menopause. Endemic goiter is caused by an inadequate intake of dietary iodine. Other causes of goiter include foods containing goitrogens (e.g., turnips) and such medicines as sulfonylureas, lithium, iodine, and aminosalicylic acid.

Signs and Symptoms.

In the early stages, the thyroid becomes symmetrically enlarged and smooth. Later, multiple nodules and cysts may develop.

Diagnostic Studies.

An RAI uptake test may be normal or may show high uptake, and a normal thyroid scan. The serum T_4 and thyroid hormone–binding ratio are usually normal.

Thyroid Cancer Patients are often asymptomatic with thyroid cancer, and it is commonly found, by the patient or practitioner, as a non-tender nodule. Most thyroid nodules are benign adenomas, but evaluation is necessary. Predisposing factors include young age; female gender; family history; and a history of radiation exposure to the head, neck, or chest. There are four main types: papillary, follicular, medullary, and anaplastic, and the papillary type accounts for 60%–70% of all thyroid cancers.

Signs and Symptoms.

Clinical signs are usually absent, except for a painless enlargement of the thyroid gland. Anterior cervical lymph nodes may be enlarged. A history of rapid enlargement and a hard consistency should raise the index of suspicion for carcinoma. Radiographic evidence of a stippled calcification or a dense, homogeneous calcification warrants a fine needle aspiration. Thyroid function tests are usually normal.

Diagnostic Studies.

A thyroid scan is necessary to differentiate "cold" nodules from "hot" nodules. A solitary cold nodule on RAI uptake scanning is suspicious of carcinoma. Ultrasound of the neck is helpful to determine size, location, and metastases. Fine needle aspiration with histologic or cytologic tissue examination is necessary to confirm the diagnosis.

Lymphadenopathy

Lymphadenopathy in the head and neck has numerous causes but is, in general, caused by either infection or malignancy (Figure 3-3). Lymphadenopathy resulting from infection produces enlarged, tender, smooth, mobile lymph nodes, whereas lymphadenopathy resulting from malignancy produces enlarged, non-tender, irregular, fixed nodes. The most common causes are the following.

Posterior auricular
Occipital
Superficial
Posterior cervical
Preauricular
Tonsillar
Submental
Superclavicular   Deep mandibular   Submandibular

Figure 3-3. ■ Cervical lymph nodes. (From Dillon, PM: Nursing Health Assessment: A Critical Thinking, Case Studies Approach. Philadelphia: FA Davis, 2003, p. 199. Reprinted with permission.)

- Pharyngitis/tonsillitis—Both viral and bacterial pharyngitis can cause lymphadenopathy in the head and neck region, with streptococcal infections being the most common. Throat cultures may be necessary for definitive diagnosis, including viral cultures if herpes simplex is suspected, or chlamydia if this sexually transmitted disease is suspected.
- Mononucleosis—The lymphadenopathy is usually dramatic in mononucleosis. The most common cause of mononucleosis is the Epstein-Barr virus, with cytomegalovirus being second. The diagnosis is made with CBC and serologic testing for heterophil antibodies (the test is commonly referred to as a "mono spot"). Treatment is supportive, and the patient should be cautioned against contact sports because splenomegaly may accompany mononucleosis.
- Infections of the head, eyes, ears, nose, mouth, and throat—The head and cervical lymph nodes typically drain more than one area, and any infection in the area has the ability to cause lymphadenopathy. Fever may or may not be present. It is necessary for the health care provider to determine the origin of the infection in order to treat effectively.
- Dental problems—Abscessed teeth are likely to cause lymphadenopathy of the tonsillar, maxillary, mandibular, or cervical nodes. Rarely do other diseases of the teeth and gums cause lymphadenopathy.
- Neoplasms of the head and neck—The most common malignancies of the head and neck are squamous cell carcinomas of the larynx, palatine tonsil, and hypopharynx. Over 80% of patients with these cancers have a history of tobacco and/or EtOH abuse. Other causes include a history of radiation to the area, Epstein-Barr virus, poor dental

hygiene or poorly fitting dental appliances, and dipping snuff. Symptoms include a palpable mass, ulcerated lesion, edema, or pain at the primary site. Biopsy is necessary for diagnosis, and referral to an ear, nose, and throat physician is warranted.

- Leukemia—This disease is a malignant neoplasm of the blood-forming cells in the bone marrow. Besides being acute or chronic, leukemias are classified according to cell type, lymphoblastic or myeloid. Lymphadenopathy may be present, although other symptoms are more common, including fatigue, weakness, anorexia, weight loss, fever, night sweats, bleeding, and easy bruisability. Diagnosis is made through hematologic studies and bone marrow biopsy. Prompt referral to a hematologist and/or oncologist is warranted.
- Lymphomas—This group of neoplasms arise from the lymphatic system and lymphoid tissues. The most common types are Hodgkin's lymphoma, which occurs more often in younger patients, and non-Hodgkin's lymphoma, which occurs more in the older population. Burkitt's lymphoma and mycosis fungoides are rare types. Cervical and mediastinal lymphadenopathy are often the presenting complaints and generally precede systemic symptoms, which include fever, night sweats, weight loss, and fatigue. Diagnosis is made through hematologic studies and bone marrow biopsy. If lymphoma is suspected, prompt referral to a hematologist and/or oncologist is warranted.

Difficulty Swallowing

Dysphagia is characterized as an esophageal transport disorder and is caused by lesions of the pharynx and esophagus or by neuromuscular disorders that cause functional limitations. It is important to differentiate between pre-esophageal dysphagia, which occurs mostly in patients with neuromuscular disorders, and esophageal disorders, which can include obstructive or motor disorders. Neuromuscular disorders include myasthenia gravis, muscular dystrophy, dermatomyositis, and poliomyelitis. The obstructive disorders include cancer, peptic stricture secondary to gastroesophageal reflux disease (GERD), and esophageal rings. The obstructive esophageal disorders are often limited to solid food. Motor disorders can affect both solid and liquid intake and are caused by impaired esophageal peristalsis, which occurs with such conditions as achalasia and scleroderma.

History

The history is particularly important in these patients because physical examination is of little value in diagnosing dysphagia. Ask whether there is difficulty swallowing only with liquids or with both solids and liquids. Discern whether it is constant or intermittent. Ask about a past history of cancer, neuromuscular or autoimmune diseases, or GERD. If the patient is elderly, inquire whether there have been frequent bouts of pneumonia, which might alert you to aspiration as a cause. Inquire as to all medications. The bisphosphonates, a drug class used for treating osteoporosis, can cause esophagitis if not taken with a full glass of water. Ask about habits, such as smoking and EtOH intake, because cancers of the head and neck are more common in these individuals.

Physical Examination

Physical examination is not helpful other than as an observation of patient discomfort when swallowing or a regurgitation or cough following attempted swallowing. Definitive diagnosis will require swallow studies and/or endoscopy to determine the exact cause of the problem.

ACHALASIA

The term achalasia refers to diffuse esophageal spasm involving the smooth muscle of the esophagus and is the most common cause of motor dysphagia. It occurs with both liquid and solid foods. It occurs more frequently in the geriatric client and is the most likely cause of aspiration pneumonia. In addition, GERD, strictures, and neoplasms are more common in the elderly, which also contribute to aspiration prevalence in this population.

Signs and Symptoms.

With achalasia, the patient will complain of discomfort or fullness in the throat, with difficulty swallowing. In the elderly client who is nonverbal, aspiration may be the first sign.

Diagnostic Studies.

The diagnosis of achalasia is made with endoscopy. Having the client take small amounts of food, a soft diet, and sitting while eating are helpful preventive measures.

ESOPHAGITIS

Esophagitis is a general term referring to an inflammation of the esophagus that can occur with GERD, certain medicines (especially when not taken with enough fluid), the ingestion of caustic substances, neoplasms, chemotherapy, or radiation.

Signs and Symptoms.

The patient with esophagitis describes burning and pain in the esophagus with or without dysphagia. The symptoms may occur more with eating or drinking and at night when the patient is recumbent.

Diagnostic Studies.

The diagnosis of esophagitis is made with endoscopy. Removal of the causative agent, if possible, helps toward healing. Medicines such as H_2 blockers and proton pump inhibitors may be necessary.

BARRETT'S ESOPHAGUS

This condition is typically associated with GERD or with mucosal damage secondary to chemotherapy or radiation; it is characterized by inflammation of the lower esophagus with possible ulceration.

Signs and Symptoms.

As with esophagitis, patients may describe a burning sensation in the throat or difficulty swallowing.

Diagnostic Studies.

The diagnosis is made via endoscopy with a biopsy of the mucosal tissue. Barrett's esophagus is associated with an increased frequency of squamous cell carcinoma, and, therefore, regular follow-up is necessary.

SCHATZKI'S RING

Schatzki's ring is a mucosal narrowing of the distal esophagus at the squamocolumnar junction. It is thought to be congenital but may not manifest itself until later in life.

Signs and Symptoms.

Dysphagia is the presenting symptom in patients with Schatzki's ring, especially with ingestion of solid foods.

Diagnostic Studies.

The diagnosis is made via endoscopy, and the stretching of the stricture alleviates the symptoms. Recurrence is common and repeat dilations or resection may be necessary.

SCLERODERMA

Scleroderma is a chronic disease of unknown etiology characterized by a progressive systemic fibrosis of the skin, joints, and internal organs, especially the esophagus, gastrointestinal (GI) tract, heart, lung, and kidney.

Signs and Symptoms.

There is a wide range in the severity of the symptoms and the prognosis. It may affect only the skin and manifest as generalized thickening, or it may be systemic, involving the vital organs and resulting in death. The initial symptoms usually involve GI complaints, such as dysphagia or reflux; shortness of breath; polyarthralgia; or Raynaud's disease, causing a thickening and stiffening of the skin on the hands and feet. The symptoms may worsen with time and involve numerous systems— skin, musculoskeletal , GI tract, cardiorespiratory , and kidneys. It may take several years for these manifestations to occur, and the constellation of symptoms are often referred to by the acronym CREST (Calcinosis, Raynaud's, Esophageal dysfunction, Sclerodactyly, and Telangiectasias).

Diagnostic Studies.

A positive ANA is present in over 90% of patients. An anticentromere antibody (ACA) is present in a high portion of patients who progress to CREST syndrome.

NEUROMUSCULAR DISEASES

There are several neuromuscular disorders that can cause pre-esophageal dysphagia, including myasthenia gravis, muscular dystrophy, dermatomyositis, and poliomyelitis.

Signs and Symptoms.

Dysphagia is one of the common presenting symptoms in these neuromuscular diseases. Other symptoms vary according to the underlying disease but include proximal limb weakness, general muscle fatigability, ocular muscle weakness, quadriparesis, polyarthralgias, skin eruptions, muscle spasms, and loss of DTRs, to name only a few. Aspiration can be a risk in these patients.

Diagnostic Studies.

Diagnosis depends on the underlying disease, which is beyond the scope of this text. These patients need to be immediately referred to a neurologist for diagnosis and follow-up.

 SUGGESTED READINGS

Beers, M., Berkow, R., & Burs, M. (Eds.). (1999). *Merck Manual of Medical Therapeutics* (17th ed.). Rahway, NJ: Merck & Co., Inc.

Braunwald, E., Fauci, A.S., Kasper, D.L., Hauser, S.L., Longo, D.L., & Jameson, J.L. (Eds.). (2001). *Harrison's Manual of Medicine* (15th ed.). New York: McGraw-Hill.

Fitzgerald, P.A. (2004). Endocrinology. In Tierney, L.M., McPhee, S.J., & Papadakis, M.A. (Eds.), *CURRENT: Medical Diagnosis & Treatment* (43rd ed.). Stamford CT: Appleton & Lange Medical Books.

Swartz, M.H. (2001). *Textbook of Physical Diagnosis: History and Examination* (4th ed). Philadelphia: W.B. Saunders & Co.

Taber's Cyclopedic Medical Dictionary (2002). (19th ed.). Philadelphia: F.A. Davis.

Chapter 4
The Eye

Mary Jo Goolsby

E ye disorders are common in all age groups, although the nature of the problems varies across the life span. Of all eye disorders, those resulting in visual impairment are the source of greatest disability. The incidence of vision loss is rising, in spite of the fact that much blindness can be prevented. The most common forms of visual impairment are refractive errors. In fact, over 150 million Americans are reported to use corrective lenses for refractive errors.

Another extremely common cause of visual disturbance in adults is cataract. Over 20 million adults over 40 years of age are afflicted with cataracts and the majority of Americans over 80 years of age have cataracts. Other less prevalent but relatively common causes of visual impairment include macular degeneration associated with age (1.6 million), diabetic retinopathy (over 5 million), and glaucoma (approximately 4 million, almost one-half of which are undiagnosed). Figure 4-1 illustrates basic eye anatomy.

HISTORY
General Eye History
When a patient complains of some concern related to the eye(s) and/or vision, it is necessary to obtain a thorough analysis of that symptom, as well as a general history related to the eyes. Ask about symptoms such as scotoma; floaters; decreased, blurred, or double vision; eye pain, discharge, and redness; lid weakness, masses, or changes. It is important to ask about eye disorders during the past medical history.

Past Medical History
Determine whether the patient has been prescribed corrective lenses and, if so, how they are worn and whether they successfully correct the vision. The past medical history should include disorders specific to the eyes, such as glaucoma, strabismus, amblyopia, cataracts, retinopathy, and macular degeneration, as well as a prior history of eye surgery. Any current or previous diagnoses of systemic disorders

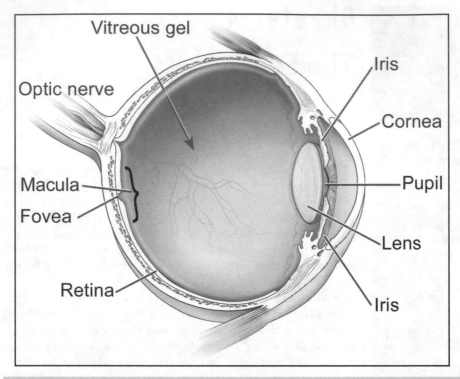

Figure 4-1. ■ Basic eye anatomy. (From National Eye Institute, National Institutes of Health.)

that affect the eyes should be determined, including diabetes, hypertension, vascular disorders, infections, and neuromuscular disorders. A history of all diagnostic procedures related to the eye and surrounding structures should be determined, as well as responses or findings.

All medications should be identified. In addition to identifying drugs that are prescribed or used to control diseases of the eyes or surrounding structures, the medication history also identifies varied agents that can alter vision. Box 4-1 includes a list of commonly prescribed drugs that affect the eyes or vision. Finally, knowing what medications the patient routinely takes may suggest the need for a more detailed medical history if it is found that the patient is taking drugs for disorders that were not disclosed earlier.

Family History

Identify the family history of eye disorders, including those conditions mentioned in the preceding paragraphs. Determine whether immediate relatives have refractive errors requiring correction.

Habits

Obtain a history of any recreational or occupational activities that expose the patient to trauma or to other contact that might place the eyes at risk, as well as the use of protec-

---

Box 4-1

Examples of Drugs with Oculotoxic Effects

Amiodarone	Gold salts
Anticholinergic agents	Hydroxychloroquine
Antihistamines	Isoniazid
Chloramphenicol	Phenothiazines
Chloroquine	Quinine
Contraceptives (oral)	Rifampin
Corticosteroids	Sympathomimetics
Digitalis	Tamoxifen
Ethambutol	

---

tive equipment. If the patient wears contact lenses, determine how long the lenses are worn and when they are changed, as well as how they are cleansed and stored between wearings.

PHYSICAL EXAMINATION
Order of the Examination
The eye examination begins with determination of the patient's visual acuity. Next, it is typical for the examiner to inspect the external and accessory structures and then move inward to include the eye. Inspection is the primary technique used in the eye exam. However, when a mass or lesion is discovered, palpation of the area is indicated. If the patient has complained of discharge, palpation of the punctum, lids overlying meibomian glands, and in the region of the medial canthus may express the discharge. The globe also can be palpated gently to determine tone. If the patient has experienced sudden onset of eye pain, it is important not to dilate the eyes before determining whether acute angle glaucoma is present because dilating the eye may increase the intraocular pressure.

Visual Acuity
Visual acuity should, at a minimum, be measured, with the patient's corrective lenses in place, if corrective lenses are used, and in a well-lighted area. Testing the visual acuity assesses a patient's central vision and should be performed one eye at a time and then with both eyes simultaneously. Visual acuity is typically assessed with a Snellen chart, with the patient standing 20 feet from the chart. There are times when the patient cannot read even the top line of the Snellen chart from 20 feet. In this case, you may have the patient move progressively closer to the chart and record the distance at which the top line can be read, if needed. If the patient cannot read the chart at a near distance, record whether the patient can count fingers, identify gross hand motion, or detect light. Near vision is tested using a hand-held chart, such as a Rosenbaum chart, typically held 14 inches from the eyes. Color vision can be grossly tested using the color strips (green and red) on the Snellen chart or by asking the patient to identify the colors of other objects. Ishihara plates can be used for a more thorough assessment of color vision. Peripheral vision is tested separately.

Peripheral Vision

Peripheral vision is tested very grossly through confrontation with the examiner. Carefully identify the location of any visual defects. Alternatively, peripheral vision can be measured much more objectively using equipment designed specifically for this purpose. There are several screening devices available.

Alignment

Observe the position of the eyes as the patient follows an object as it is moved smoothly through the six cardinal positions, approximately 12 inches in front of the face. Perform the cover/uncover test observing for movement as an eye is covered and uncovered. Ask the patient to focus on a distant object and observe one eye, as the opposite eye is covered. If the visible eye, which is uncovered, moves as it fixates on the distant object as the opposite eye is covered, this is an abnormal finding, indicating that the eye was not aligned prior to the opposite eye being covered. Next, uncover the opposite eye, as the patient continues to focus on the distant object. If this eye moves as it is uncovered, it indicates that the eye did not maintain alignment as it was covered and unable to focus on an object. Repeat the same process, as you cover and uncover the opposite eye. Later, as pupillary responses are assessed, alignment can be further evaluated as a penlight beam is directed toward the bridge of the nose as the patient looks straight ahead and the examiner observes for symmetry of light reflex.

Accessory Structures

Inspect the eyebrows and lashes for symmetry and orientation. Inspect for symmetry and placement; palpate the lids for masses or tenderness, observe for ptosis. Observe for areas of discoloration, masses, and xanthomas.

External Eye Structures

Inspect the conjunctiva, cornea, and sclera, noting the condition of the surface, clarity, color, and vascularity. Examples of several abnormalities are identified in Table 4-1. Box 4-2 reviews the procedure for performing a fluorescein stain, to assess for potential corneal lesions.

Pupils

Observe the shape and symmetry of the pupils, including the response to light and accommodation. The pupils provide important indications of the cause for vision change. Examples of abnormal findings and causes are noted in Table 4-2. The cornea is also assessed during the pupil examination. Box 4-3 describes assessment of the pupils.

Anterior Chamber and Lens

Determine the approximate depth and clarity of the anterior chamber using oblique lighting. Also with the oblique lighting, assess the clarity of the lens. During the funduscopic exam, the clarity of the lens is also identified when the red reflex is noted.

Cranial Nerves

The eye examination includes an assessment of cranial nerves II, III, IV, and VI, which is accomplished during assessment of visual acuity, accessory structures, and pupils. The optic nerve is finally directly observed during the funduscopic examination.

Table 4-1. ■ External Eye Abnormalities

Finding	Photograph/Example	
Ciliary flush		(From Dillon, P.M. *Nursing health assessment: A critical thinking, case studies approach.* Philadelphia: F.A. Davis. 2003. Reprinted with permission.)
Episcleritis		(From Dillon, P.M. *Nursing health assessment: A critical thinking, case studies approach.* Philadelphia: F.A. Davis, 2003. Reprinted with permission.)
Corneal arcus		(From Dillon, P.M. *Nursing health assessment: A critical thinking, case studies approach.* Philadelphia: F.A. Davis, 2003. Reprinted with permission.)
Corneal ulceration		(From Dillon, P.M. *Nursing health assessment: A critical thinking, case studies approach.* Philadelphia: F.A. Davis, 2003. Reprinted with permission.)
Pterygium		(From Dillon, P.M. *Nursing health assessment: A critical thinking, case studies approach.* Philadelphia: F.A. Davis, 2003. Reprinted with permission.)
Subconjunctival hemorrhage		(From Dillon, P.M. *Nursing health assessment: A critical thinking, case studies approach.* Philadelphia: F.A. Davis, 2003. Reprinted with permission.)

Box 4-2

Special Procedure: Fluorescein Stain Technique to Assess Corneal Integrity

After determining that the patient has no relevant allergies, inspect the cornea and sclera without staining, if tolerated. Instillation of a topical ocular anesthetic will improve tolerance of further examination. Approximately 1 minute following installation of topical anesthetic, moisten the tip of a fluorescein stain strip with sterile saline. Holding the lids open with thumb and index finger, apply the stain by touching the moistened strip to the lower conjunctiva. Ask patient to blink to disperse the stain. If both eyes are being stained, use a separate strip for each eye to avoid cross-contamination.

Once the stain has been distributed by blinking, inspect the cornea and conjunctiva beneath the upper and lower lids using a cobalt blue light source, held oblique to the structure being examined. Areas of stain uptake, indicating abrasion to the cornea, will fluoresce bright green. Any visible and superficial foreign body should be removed, if possible.

Following inspection, flush the stain with sterile saline solution.

Funduscopic Examination

In a darkened room, the funduscopic examination of each eye is performed. The sequence may vary, but this portion of the exam includes the identification of the red reflex and inspection of the lens, retinal background and vessels, the optic disk, and the anterior and posterior chambers. (Box 4-4.) The background and vessels should be assessed in four quadrants in each eye. It is important to recognize that there are limitations in the portion of the eye that is seen through an undilated pupil, as is performed in the typical primary care setting. Table 4-3 lists several abnormalities, with the related significance for each. Figures 4-2 through 4-5 illustrate the normal fundus and selected abnormal findings.

Box 4-3

Special Procedure: Pupil Testing

The assessment of pupil shape, size, and reactivity provides much data. It is important to always assess direct and consensual papillary response. If these are abnormal, you should then also assess for accommodation. By using the "swinging penlight" test in assessing the response to light, afferent defects—in which the consensual response is more pronounced than the direct response—are more easily detected. This method is performed by holding the light source in front of the patient, so that it is directed toward one eye. At this point, observe both pupils, noting the direct response of the eye receiving the direct light and the consensual response in the opposite eye. Leave your attention on the opposite eye, continuing to note the consensual response as you briskly swing the light source in the direction of this eye. Note whether the pupil response is a slight constriction, slightly more pronounced with direct light as is normal, or the pupil slightly relaxes, so that the response is slightly less pronounced with direct light, which is an abnormal, Marcus Gunn effect. Then observe the opposite eye, swinging the light back to that eye as you note any change between the indirect and direct responses. In some optic nerve disorders, such as ischemic optic neuropathy or optic neuritis, as well as other conditions that affect the pathway anterior to the optic chiasm, this afferent defect may be the only objective finding.

Table 4-2. ■ Pupil Abnormalities

Horner's syndrome	Miosis is present unilaterally. Pupillary responses intact. Associated with ptosis, and appearance that eye is "sunken" on affected side, with lack of sweating on opposite side. Cause by sympathetic lesion.
Benign anisocoria	Some asymmetry of the pupil size is considered normal if the difference is <0.5 mm.
Argyll Robertson pupils	The pupil is small and may have an abnormal shape. Although the pupil does not respond to light, it exhibits a brisk response to accommodation (near vision). Usually bilateral involvement. Associated with neurosyphilis.
Tonic pupil	No response to light (direct or consensual). Accommodation usually also affected. Most common in females. Unilateral. Caused by denervation of the ciliary muscle and sphincter.

DIFFERENTIAL DIAGNOSIS OF CHIEF COMPLAINTS
Visual Disturbances

Visual disturbances include a wide range of complaints, including blurred vision, loss of vision, blind spots, and altered color perception. When the patient presents with altered vision as the chief complaint, it is crucial to be alert for indications of potential irreversible loss of vision. Most important is the complaint of a sudden loss of vision, regardless of whether the disturbance is partial or complete and whether or not it is accompanied by pain.

Altered vision can refer to decreased vision where there is a decreased visual acuity, without loss of partial or full visual field. This is a common complaint and, with age, is associated with the development of cataracts. It can also be associated with relatively benign refractive errors or with hyperglycemia and diabetes, macular degeneration, or glaucoma. In contrast, the loss of vision—whether limited to a specific visual field or area, one eye, or both eyes—is typically indicative of a very significant health problem and one that may result in permanent visual loss and disability.

Box 4-4

Special Procedure: Funduscopic Examination

Successful use of the ophthalmoscope takes much practice and patience. The ophthalmoscope provides the ability to directly visualize both the external and internal structures of the eye. It is important that the examiner be familiar with adjusting the intensity of the light source, vary the apertures, and understand how to adjust the diopters to best visualize the target structures. As the dial on the ophthalmoscope is moved counterclockwise, the diopters shift from positive to negative. Because the more negative diopters direct the focus posteriorly, by moving from the positive to negative diopters, your focus will shift from the anterior eye to the posterior eye, retina, and optic disc. Adjustment of the ophthalmoscope while inspecting the eye takes considerable practice and coordination. The newer panoptic ophthalmoscope provides a magnified view and is easier to manipulate during the exam than traditional equipment.

Table 4-3. ■ Retinal/Background Abnormalities

Finding	Significance
Flame hemorrhages (superficial)	Linear hemorrhages, often associated with extreme elevation of blood pressure
Preretinal hemorrhages	Superficial hemorrhage, often characterized by a rounded inferior margin and a linear upper visible margin. Associated with both diabetic and hypertensive retinopathy and retinal tears
Microaneurysms	Tiny rounded dilations of retinal arteries, frequently associated with hypertension
Neovascularization	Proliferation of new, fragile vessels on the surface of retina, which have increased likelihood of bleeding. Associated with diabetes
Dot/Blot hemorrhages (deep)	Deeper, rounded and/or irregularly shaped hemorrhages associated with diabetes
Cotton wool exudate	Yellow to white "fluffy" areas of ischemia. Associated with both diabetic and hypertensive retinopathy
Hard exudate	Very discrete yellow-to-white lesions, often distributed in a circular pattern. Associated with leakage of fluids into retinal tissue. Associated with both diabetic and hypertensive retinopathy

History

When patients complain of altered vision, it is important to obtain a history of any other eye symptoms or disease, in addition to exploring the altered vision. Determine when the patient first noticed the altered vision and how, if at all, it has progressed since onset, as well as whether it has been transient or persistent. Ask whether the visual disturbance has affected the patient's ability to perform any normal activities, in addition to whether the patient has participated in any activities that have included exposure to chemicals or trauma. Always determine what the patient means if he or she complains of decreased or blurred vision; discriminate between decreased visual acuity and any episodes of actual visual loss. Ask whether the alteration involves one or both eyes and is limited to central, peripheral, near, and/or distant vision. Figures 4-6 through 4-9 illustrate examples of normal versus select types of altered vision. Establish the date and results of the patient's last visual exam and whether corrective lenses are prescribed and used. Find out whether there is history of systemic diseases, such as diabetes, and what medications the patient has recently taken. The family history of eye disease and other chronic diseases is important.

Physical Examination

The physical examination for altered vision starts with determination of visual acuity, testing both far and near vision in each eye alone and in combination, making adaptations for very low vision. Whenever possible, vision should be tested with the patient wearing any prescribed corrective lenses. Although it is tempting to go directly from testing visual acuity to the funduscopic exam, the assessment should next include inspection of the external structures, eye movement, peripheral vision/visual fields, and pupil reactions. It is important to assess the appearance of the cornea and anterior chamber, as well as to determine the quality of the red reflex. A funduscopic examination should be performed, although there may be certain conditions in which the funduscopic examination may not be possible. Examples include situations in which the patient is experiencing severe eye pain and photophobia, as occurs with acute angle-closure glaucoma, or when visualization of the retina is obscured owing to clouding of the lens in advanced cataract. The decision to examine other systems should be determined in the context of the patient's history and general survey. For instance, if eye movement or pupil reaction is asymmetrical, a neurological examination will be warranted. With a history of diabetes, blood glucose should be determined, as well as other signs of diabetes control. As necessary, the physical examination should include careful assessment of the cardiovascular and neurologic systems.

Figure 4-2. ■ Normal fundus. (From Dillon, P.M. *Nursing health assessment: A critical thinking, case studies approach.* Philadelphia: F.A. Davis, 2003. Reprinted with permission.)

Figure 4-3. ■ Diabetic retinopathy. (From Dillon, P.M. *Nursing health assessment: A critical thinking, case studies approach.* Philadelphia: F.A. Davis, 2003. Reprinted with permission.)

Figure 4-4. ■ Hypertensive changes. (From Dillon, P.M. *Nursing health assessment: A critical thinking, case studies approach.* Philadelphia: F.A. Davis, 2003. Reprinted with permission.)

Figure 4-5. ■ Optic nerve pallor. (From Dillon, P.M. *Nursing health assessment: A critical thinking, case studies approach.* Philadelphia: F.A. Davis, 2003. Reprinted with permission.)

Figure 4-6. ■ Normal vision. (From National Eye Institute, National Institutes of Health.)

Figure 4-7. ■ Scene as it might be viewed by person with glaucoma. (From National Eye Institute, National Institutes of Health.)

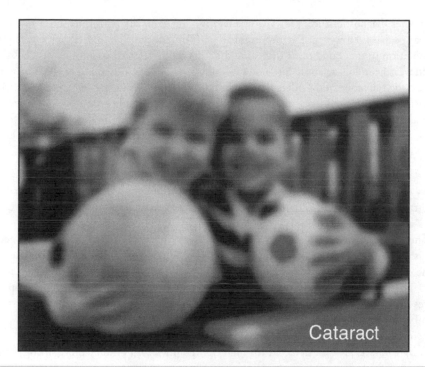

Figure 4-8. ■ Scene as it might be viewed by person with cataract. (From National Eye Institute, National Institutes of Health.)

Figure 4-9. ■ Scene as it might be viewed by person with diabetic retinopathy. (From National Eye Institute, National Institutes of Health.)

Further diagnostic studies for vision alteration are generally performed after referral to an eye specialist. However, it is important to perform adequate history taking and physical examination so that conditions that should be promptly referred to another specialist, for instance, a neurologist, are identified. Although it is beyond the scope of this chapter to address the full scope of disorders that could result in visual disturbance, many of the characteristic disorders are identified. The definitive diagnostic studies are not performed at a general practice site, but rather are performed by a specialist to whom the patient is referred. These include dilation of the eye, intraocular pressure measurement, magnification, etc.

CATARACTS

Cataracts are opacities of the optic lens and most typically occur as a disease of aging. However, cataracts can be caused or accelerated by certain conditions, including exposure to ultraviolet light and to certain drugs as well as by such systemic diseases as diabetes.

Signs and Symptoms.

The patient with cataract generally complains of a progressive decrease in visual acuity that is painless. The altered vision includes general blurring and haziness of vision, as well as the development of halos and glares in response to bright lights, as when driving in the dark. The opacities may be visible as gray or whitening areas over the pupil. The opacity makes ophthalmologic examination difficult, obscuring the visualization of the posterior chamber and retinal structures.

Diagnostic Studies.

Early cataracts are best detected through ophthalmic exam of dilated eye, using magnification.

CHRONIC OPEN-ANGLE GLAUCOMA

Glaucoma is the condition in which an increased intraocular pressure results in neuropathy of the optic nerve. This most common form of glaucoma results in a gradual and progressive altered vision. Certain individuals have a higher incidence of chronic glaucoma, among them, African Americans, diabetics, and those over 35 years of age, particularly if they have a positive family history.

Signs and Symptoms.

Patients with chronic open-angle glaucoma generally have no complaints other than altered vision. The disease may progress before the patient perceives the decreased vision. The visual disturbance progresses from blurring to complete vision loss, if not recognized and treated. The patient may have required frequent corrective prescription changes up until definitive diagnosis. The vision loss begins peripherally, so that central vision is not lost until late in the disorder. The physical examination identifies an increased cup-to-disk ratio. The intraocular pressure is elevated.

Diagnostic Studies.

A normal tonometric value is under 21, although the value can vary or fluctuate. Tonometry must be considered in combination with retinal signs of glaucoma and visual fields. Ophthalmologists can perform additional tests, including gonioscopy, which assesses the drainage angle, to determine whether it is open or closed.

ACUTE CLOSED-ANGLE GLAUCOMA

This less-common form of glaucoma results in acute visual disturbance. The increased intraocular pressure may be transient, triggered by conditions that cause pupillary dilatation, such as darkened rooms. As the intraocular pressure acutely increases, the patient typically experiences considerable symptoms, although they may resolve before the patient arrives for evaluation. It is very important that the examiner *not* dilate the eyes when a patient presents with a history of unilateral eye pain and visual disturbance because the dilation may further exacerbate the intraocular pressure increase.

Signs and Symptoms.

During an episode of acute closed-angle glaucoma, the patient usually experiences severe, unilateral eye pain. Accompanying symptoms may include photophobia, headache, and nausea. The vision blurs, and the patient may perceive halos around lights. The eye reddens, with a ciliary flush, and the pupil may become fixed and mid-dilated. The cornea may become edematous, causing it to appear "hazy" and may develop a "dew drop" appearance.

Diagnostic Studies.

Whenever acute angle-closure glaucoma is suspected, the patient must be immediately referred to an ophthalmologist, who can complete tonometry and further diagnosis, in order to provide definitive treatment and to preserve the vision.

AMAUROSIS FUGAX

Amaurosis fugax is a monocular, transient loss of vision. It stems from transient ischemia of the retina and presents an important warning sign for impending stroke. Depending on the circumstances reported, the patient should be immediately referred to either a cardiovascular or neurological specialist. Four broad causes of amaurosis fugax include emboli, retinal vascular insufficiency, arterial spasms, and idiopathy.

Signs and Symptoms.

An episode of the vision loss that accompanies amaurosis fugax may last from only seconds to minutes. The patient often describes the episode as vision loss that is as if a shade were being pulled over one eye in a descending fashion and then, a short time later, the shade is raised. Unlike acute glaucoma, there is no associated pain during the episode. Depending on the duration of the episode, the funduscopic examination may reveal the retina as whitened, with a bright red fovea. If the occlusion is of the carotid, the patient may report or exhibit transient sensorimotor deficits. The funduscopic exam may reveal emboli, altered vessels, microaneurysms, and blot hemorrhages. Carotid bruit(s) may be present.

Diagnostic Studies.

Depending on the setting, a primary care provider can obtain carotid studies before the patient is actually seen by the physician. If valvular embolus has caused the disorder, the embolus may be visible.

RETINAL DETACHMENT

Retinal detachments are caused by trauma or by the traction caused by diabetic retinal disease. Regardless of the cause, patients suspected of having a retinal detachment should be immediately referred to an ophthalmologist.

Signs and Symptoms.

The patient usually provides a history of some trauma, followed by a sudden visual disturbance, such as flashing light, floaters, or scotoma. The visual defect may advance or progress, as the retinal detachment enlarges. Depending on the size of the defect, the patient may exhibit an afferent pupil defect. The affected retina appears wrinkled and gray.

ISCHEMIC OCULAR NEUROPATHY

Unlike the transient ischemia that is associated with amaurosis fugax, the visual disturbances of ischemic ocular neuropathy stem from chronic ischemia. The resulting vision loss is irreversible. However, unilateral loss of vision in patients over 65 years of age may be caused by temporal arteritis; in this case, the patient is at risk for losing vision in the alternate eye.

Signs and Symptoms.

The visual loss is unilateral and may be limited to either the upper or lower visual field. There is no associated pain of the eye. However, patients with temporal arteritis will have previously experienced pain of the head, temple, or face, as well as more generalized symptoms of polymyalgia rheumatica, including joint pain, malaise, weakness, fatigue, and even weight loss.

Diagnostic Studies.

With temporal arteritis, the sedimentation rate will often be elevated. A temporal artery biopsy is diagnostic, although treatment must not be withheld pending the biopsy.

MACULAR DEGENERATION

Most commonly, macular degeneration is associated with aging and results either from atrophy of the macula or exudation and hemorrhage of the vessels in the macular region.

Signs and Symptoms.

Visual alterations associated with macular degeneration are typically unilateral, vary from gradual to sudden in onset, and can range from blurring to complete blindness. The retina may show altered pigmentation, hemorrhage, or hard and soft exudates. In diabetics, neovascularization and microaneurysms may be visible.

Diagnostic Studies.

An ophthalmologist will further evaluate the patient's central vision and perform fluorescein angiography. A commonly used test is called the Amsler grid, which assesses the patient's ability to accurately see a set of grids.

Trauma

Blunt trauma to the eye or orbit can be associated with altered vision. Depending on the type of trauma, the history should provide details of the event and the physical examination may allow detection of other signs of trauma.

Differentiating the Causes of Vision Changes

Table 4-4 provides a summary of characteristics that help differentiate among the causes of visual change.

Reddened Eye

Eye redness can be caused by a wide range of disorders, ranging from conjunctivitis to acute closed-angle glaucoma. Eye redness may herald a disorder that has no associated visual impairment or others associated with complete loss of vision. Although the majority of causes of eye redness are self-limiting, it is essential to perform a complete assessment when this is the presenting complaint.

Table 4-4. ■ Differentiating Among the Causes of Vision Changes

	Cataracts	Chronic Open-Angle Glaucoma	Acute Closed-Angle Glaucoma	Amaurosis fugax	Retinal Detachment	Ischemic Ocular Neuropathy	Macular Degeneration
Onset	Gradual	Gradual	Sudden	Sudden	Sudden	Sudden	Gradual to Sudden
Associated Symptoms			Head/eye pain, nausea, eye redness	Neurological deficits possible	Possible signs of trauma	Head, jaw, temple pain or soreness	
Severity of Vision Change	Ranges from cloudy, hazy to vision loss	Gradual darkening may range to complete vision loss	Blurring, halos; can range to total vision loss	Complete, but transient loss initially; may lead to complete vision loss	Flash of light, darkened areas; may progress to complete loss	Affected portion lost	Blurring may progress to complete loss
Portion of Vision Affected	Unilateral or bilateral	Unilateral or bilateral; peripheral vision lost first	Unilateral	Unilateral	Unilateral, often specific fields affected; can be complete loss	Unilateral; may affect only portion but progress to complete loss	Unilateral or bilateral; starts centrally
Inspection	Clouding; loss of red reflex	Cup/disk ratio change; late afferent effect possible	Red eye, ciliary flush, fixed pupil, corneal edema	Pale retina with red fovea, embolus	Wrinkling/graying of retina, afferent pupil defect		Altered pigmentation; hemorrhage, exudates, microaneurysms, and/or neovascular

History

When patients complain of a reddened eye, first determine whether they have experienced eye trauma or whether there is any associated vision loss. Obtain a history of the redness and its progression, then ask about other symptoms, including eye itching, pain, swelling, or discharge and visual disturbance or photophobia. Ask about exposures to chemical agents. Establish whether the patient wears contact lenses and, if so, what type and how they are cared for. It is important that other systemic symptoms be explored, such as general malaise, skin rashes, and cold or allergy symptoms. Ascertain whether the patient's history includes previous episodes of eye disorders or systemic problems, such as atopic or rheumatologic disorders. It is very important to identify any drugs or other products that have been used around or on the eyes. Old mascara has been shown to be full of bacteria. Determine also whether there is a family history of eye conditions, such as glaucoma, iritis, or allergic conjunctivitis, and ask about the family history of systemic disorders. Autoimmune disorders and HIV are associated with certain eye diseases that may cause redness. If the patient has had eye trauma and/or corneal abrasion, determine their tetanus status.

Physical Examination

The physical examination must begin by determining the patient's corrected visual acuity, then proceed by observing the general characteristics of the redness, and finish by doing a rapid assessment to rule out signs of trauma. Determine whether there is any photophobia and adjust the light to the patient's comfort, if possible. Note the condition of the outer and appendage structures, looking for swelling, redness, discharge, or lesions. Next, focus on the eye itself, observing the cornea and conjunctiva for redness and noting the degree, pattern, and location of the redness. Identify any shadowing as oblique lighting is passed over the anterior chamber. Assess the conjunctiva beneath the upper and lower lids; observe for foreign bodies or lesions. Assess the size, shape, and responsiveness of the pupils. If tolerated, perform a funduscopic exam. Depending on the impression based on the history and exam of the eyes, it may be necessary to extend the assessment to the skin, ears, nose, throat, and joints to assess for infections, allergy, or rheumatic disorders.

Diagnostic studies are generally not warranted for eye redness. However, it may prove necessary to obtain a culture from the conjunctiva or to determine the intraocular pressure through tonometry. If foreign body or corneal abrasion is suspected, the examination should include fluorescein staining and examination of the eye with Wood's lamplight. If a foreign body is suspected, a slit lamp exam is necessary and a referral to an ophthalmologist.

CONJUNCTIVITIS

The most common cause of eye redness is conjunctivitis, which causes an inflammation of one or more areas of the conjunctiva. It is important to discriminate between allergic, viral, bacterial, and other causes of conjunctivitis, in order to provide definitive treatment. Infectious conjunctivitis is usually caused by viral organisms, although bacterial infections are also common and can be secondary to viral infections. Allergies are the most frequent cause of noninfectious conjunctivitis. Other causes include chemical reactions.

Signs and Symptoms.

The primary symptom of conjunctivitis, eye redness, is fairly consistent between the various causes. However, the accompanying symptoms of eye discomfort, itching, and discharge, as well as the extraorbital symptoms, help to define the problem. Similarly, examination of the eyes provides important information to discriminate among the causes. Table 4-5 differentiates between the signs and symptoms of viral, bacterial, and allergic conjunctivitis.

Diagnostic Studies.

On occasion, it will be helpful to perform diagnostic tests to assess conjunctivitis. Studies can include viral and bacterial cultures of the conjunctiva or tests for atopy.

CORNEAL ABRASION

The cornea can become scratched or abraded by a variety of situations, including trauma and foreign bodies. A common foreign body involved in corneal abrasions is a contact lens. It is important to identify the situation that led up to the abrasion, in order to determine the risk of complications, including infection and ulceration. For instance, the abrasion is more likely to be contaminated and at risk for infection if caused by contact lenses or an animal scratch.

Signs and Symptoms.

The patient is likely to complain of either "scratchiness" or pain in the affected eye and the symptoms generally have a sudden onset after some exposure. There may be simply a complaint of the sense that there is a foreign body in the eye. Photophobia and significant tearing are common with abrasions. There will probably be decreased vision in the affected eye. The redness may be either diffuse or in a ciliary flush pattern. With fluorescein staining, there should be an obvious break in the corneal surface with uptake of the stain. Examination of the fundus will be normal. Unless the patient has delayed assessment, there should be no discharge or enlargement of the preauricular nodes, indicating infection.

Diagnostic Studies.

Unless there are signs of infection, diagnostic study is not indicated. With appropriate treatment, abrasions generally resolve in 24 hours. Patients should be rechecked, and if the abrasion has not resolved, the patient should be referred because ulceration is common.

Table 4-5. ■ Differentiating Conjunctivitis

Finding	Allergic Conjunctivitis	Bacterial Conjunctivitis	Viral Conjunctivitis
Pain/Discomfort	Itchy sensation	Burning or gritty sensation	Foreign body or gritty sensation
Discharge	Watery, thin, clear	Mucopurulent, viscous	Mucoid
Preauricular nodes	Nonpalpable/normal	Usually nonpalpable; Palpable in hyperacute cases	Palpable
Accompanying symptoms	History of allergies, recurrent	May have URI symptoms	May have URI symptoms

SUBCONJUNCTIVAL HEMORRHAGE

Subconjunctival hemorrhage, although an impressive sight, is usually a benign and self-limiting condition. Subconjunctival hemorrhage is caused by rupture of small capillaries and may follow trauma and can also be triggered by episodes of coughing, sneezing, or rubbing of the eye. Also, scuba diving and childbirth are often associated with the development of a subconjunctival hemorrhage. Often, the cause is not determined. It is important to exclude other eye symptoms and signs, however, to make sure that abrasion, perforation, or other conditions are not overlooked by the distraction associated with the very reddened eye.

Signs and Symptoms.

There is no visual disturbance associated with a subconjunctival hemorrhage and no photophobia or pain. The onset of the redness is sudden and typically limited to one eye; it may be localized to one region of that eye. With the exception of the deep redness, the findings are otherwise within normal limits.

UVEITIS

Uveitis involves inflammation of the uveal tract, including the iris, and thus includes iritis, as well. The inflammation may be caused either by infection or as part of a systemic reaction associated with a systemic disorder. For instance, there is an increased incidence of uveitis in patients with autoimmune disorders, such as Crohn's disease, ankylosing spondylitis, and HIV infection. It is important to identify any systemic source for the problem, as well as to refer the patient for a thorough ophthalmic examination.

Signs and Symptoms.

Uveitis affects the vision because with it there is limited responsiveness of the pupil and lens. Patients commonly experience both photophobia and eye pain. There is a ciliary flush and usually a constricted pupil. Precipitates may be visible on the posterior surface of the cornea. The patient may complain of other systemic symptoms, including joint pain, altered bowel habits/abdominal pain, and so on, if an autoimmune disorder is involved.

Diagnostic Studies.

The ophthalmologist will perform diagnostics related to the eye disorder, but if the uveitis is recurrent and/or has a suspected systemic cause, further diagnostic studies should be considered, including sedimentation rate, autoimmune panel, and HIV.

KERATITIS

Disorders in this category result in inflammation of the cornea and can lead to blindness in the affected eye. Keratitis can be caused by herpetic and other infections, ischemia, chemical exposures, and foreign bodies or corneal abrasions; it can be triggered by eye dryness or denervation; and it may also be secondary to conjunctivitis. A major difference that makes keratitis noteworthy is that it can lead to ulcerations, opacities, and blindness of the affected eye; thus, patients suspected of this disorder should be immediately referred to an ophthalmologist.

Signs and Symptoms.

Patients with keratitis may complain only of a foreign body sensation or may complain of severe pain. Ask about trauma associated with contact lens wear. Although vision may not be initially affected, it can be altered as the condition advances. Gray infiltrate may be visible on examination, and there may be a ciliary flush. If ulcerative keratitis is involved, perforations may be evident on staining. A hypopyon ulcer may develop, with pus collecting in the anterior chamber.

Diagnostic Studies.

On referral, the ophthalmologist will perform a variety of studies to identify the causative agent of the situation, including bacterial, fungal, and viral cultures and slit lamp exam.

SCLERITIS AND EPISCLERITIS

Scleritis and episcleritis are inflammatory problems involving the sclera and episclera, respectively. Most cases of scleritis are associated with chronic autoimmune disorders, such as rheumatoid arthritis, systemic lupus erythematosus, and sarcoidosis, in contrast to episcleritis, which is self-limiting and not associated with chronic disorders. They are best differentiated by the degree of involvement. Although they do not typically affect the vision, both conditions are often chronic and warrant referral to an ophthalmologist. With time, scleritis can evolve to cause cataracts and/or glaucoma.

Signs and Symptoms.

As noted above, the vision generally remains normal with both scleritis and episcleritis. Whereas episcleritis is generally painless, patients with scleritis may complain of extreme pain. And although photophobia is not common with either disorder, it is more likely to occur with scleritis. Neither disorder is associated with altered pupils, and the redness may be localized or diffuse. However, the redness associated with scleritis may be very deep in intensity—almost purple—and is darker than is typically seen with episcleritis. The discoloration lies immediately below the conjunctiva, and the sclera may develop inflammatory nodules and engorged vessels. Episcleritis, in contrast, is more localized, and can also be associated with localized engorged vessels and nodular changes. The visual acuity may be affected when scleritis has progressed.

Diagnostic Studies.

Episcleritis requires no specific diagnostic studies. However, if scleritis is suspected or the diagnosis is uncertain, the patient should be referred to an ophthalmologist for definitive diagnosis and treatment. Laboratory studies should include complete blood count, sedimentation rate, and antinuclear antibody; in addition, rheumatoid factor should be considered.

Eye Pain

Eye pain can be caused by urgent problems that threaten vision, such as acute angle-closure glaucoma, various traumatic injuries, and infectious agents. There is a lot of overlap among the disorders that cause eye pain and those causing eye redness; thus, the history and physical exam are similar for both complaints.

History

When the chief complaint includes eye pain, first establish whether there is a history of chemical exposure or burn, trauma, or vision loss. In the case of chemical burn, further assessment must be delayed until the eye has been thoroughly irrigated. Once chemical exposure and/or trauma has been excluded, explore the onset and characteristics of the pain. For instance, determine whether the pain had sudden onset or developed gradually. Have the patient describe the type of pain experienced, for instance, whether it is sharp, dull, throbbing, or aching, as well as whether it is superficial, deep, or diffuse. Identify any associated symptoms, including malaise, vision change, discharge, photophobia, and redness.

Physical Examination

Test visual acuity, if tolerated, before proceeding with further examination. Carefully inspect the accessory and external eye structures. Note any lacerations, lesions, discolorations, swelling, redness, and discharge. Assess the size, shape, and responsiveness of the pupils. If there is a history of trauma to the eye, the corneal surface should be carefully assessed. Grossly inspect for signs of perforation, such as bleeding or "leakage" from the globe, altered shape, and obvious entry points. If perforation can be excluded by history and exam, fluorescein stain should be applied so that the corneal surface can be inspected using Wood's lamplight. Assess the cornea for clarity, and note the anterior chamber depth. If tolerated, a funduscopic exam should be performed.

CHEMICAL BURNS

Chemical burns can occur from topical contact from many agents. Chemical burns make up the majority of ocular burns. Whereas acid burns do not penetrate the eye structures, alkali burns do cause penetrating injuries.

Signs and Symptoms.

Observe the face and periorbital region for blisters, redness, and other signs of a burn. The patient may not be able to hold the eye open. There may be significant redness, tearing, pain, and swelling of the eye and accessory structures. It is essential that the offending chemical be identified whenever, and as soon as, possible and that the appropriate decontamination measures be instituted immediately. It may be impossible to clearly assess visual acuity, owing to photophobia, pain, and tearing, which can blur vision.

HERPES ZOSTER

Herpes zoster, caused by the varicella-zoster virus, can affect the ophthalmic branch of the fifth cranial nerve. Ophthalmic involvement is often heralded by lesions on the tip of the nose.

Signs and Symptoms.

There is usually a period of several days during which the patient experiences malaise and neuralgia along the affected nerve root, preceding the development of skin lesions. The pain is severe and is often accompanied by systemic symptoms, including fever and fatigue. The patient may exhibit photophobia, and the accessory structures may be inflamed and/or swollen. Vision may be altered in the affected eye.

Diagnostic Studies.

Whenever eye involvement of herpes zoster is suspected, the patient should be referred to an ophthalmologist. Although the actual diagnosis may be evident, referral will allow specialized examination—including slit lamp, to assess the degree of involvement—and the timely initiation of appropriate and individualized treatment to minimize complications.

Acute Angle-Closure Glaucoma

Acute angle-closure glaucoma is described under Eye Redness, pp. 64–66.

Corneal Abrasion and Erosion

Corneal abrasions are discussed under Eye Redness, p. 67.

Conjunctivitis
Conjunctivitis is discussed under Eye Redness, pp. 66–67.

Uveitis, Iritis, and Scleritis
Each of these inflammatory disorders affecting the eye is covered in the section on Eye Redness, pp. 68–69.

Trauma
Trauma should always be considered with presentation of eye pain.

Eye Discharge

Eye discharge is most commonly associated with infectious disorders but can also be associated with other inflammatory conditions or systemic diseases affecting the eye. By far the most common causes of eye discharge are the various forms of conjunctivitis.

History
Ask about the onset of the discharge. It is important to know whether the discharge is persistent or, instead, occurs in certain settings. Determine whether there are any associated eye symptoms, such as pain, altered vision, photophobia, or swelling. Ask about extraocular symptoms, such as sneezing, itching, fever, malaise. Determine past history of atopic disorders and exposure to infectious diseases.

Physical Examination
Test visual acuity, and then perform a general inspection, observing for the quality and location of any discharge and noting the consistency and color. Although not generally necessary, a culture of the discharge may be warranted. To obtain a culture, retract the lower lid and place a conjunctival swab in the palpebral space.

DACRYOCYSTITIS

Dacryocystitis is an infection of the lacrimal sac and is most common in infants, secondary to congenital stenosis of the lacrimal duct. In adults, it can be caused by hypertrophic rhinitis, polyps, or trauma. Older adults lose the elasticity of the drainage system, so that the duct is not flushed by tears, and dacryocystitis may result.
Signs and Symptoms.
If the duct is occluded, constant tearing may occur. The lacrimal sac may be edematous, red, and tender. Pressure over the sac produces purulent discharge. The surrounding area can also become inflamed, tender, and swollen. Associated conjunctivitis or blepharitis may be present.
Diagnostic Studies.
Diagnostic studies are generally not warranted.

ERYTHEMA MULTIFORME—STEVENS-JOHNSON SYNDROME

Erythema multiforme involves inflammation of the mucous membranes and skin. It is often related to an infection or can be due to almost any medication. Often, no specific cause is identified. The most severe form is called Stevens-Johnson syndrome. Because the condition can be fatal, it is important to immediately recognize and treat.
Signs and Symptoms.
In Stevens-Johnson syndrome, conjunctivitis with copious amounts of purulent discharge may occur. The eyes become painful. Conjunctival bullae and ulcerations may

develop. Patients develop erythematous lesions and bullae over the skin and hemorrhagic lesions of the mucous membranes. The patient appears acutely ill and has systemic symptoms, including malaise, fever, and arthralgias.

Diagnostic Studies.

The diagnosis is often made by identifying the classic skin lesions, which consist of red-centered bullae, surrounded by white areas. In addition to the eye tissue, the palms, soles, anus, vagina, nose, and mouth are commonly affected.

Conjunctivitis

See the section on Eye Redness, pp. 66–67, for differentiation of allergic, bacterial, and viral conjunctivitis.

Ptosis

Ptosis, or drooping of an eyelid, can be related to simple aging, with natural loss of elasticity and lid drooping or it can result from a variety of other causes. The causes of ptosis that are neither congenital nor acquired include trauma, conditions that add mass to the eyelid, and conditions that affect the nerves or muscles controlling the lid's position. In 75% of the cases, in fact, the first manifestation of myasthenia gravis is ptosis.

History

It is important to determine how and when the ptosis developed. Determine whether the onset was sudden or gradual. Identify any associated altered vision and whether the patient believes the vision has been altered by the drooping eyelid. Ask about all other medical disorders and medications. Determine whether the patient has a history of hypertension, peripheral vascular disease, or any other risk factors for stroke, or a history of myasthenia gravis. Ask about the history of any recent trauma to the head or eye region.

Physical Examination

Assess visual acuity. Closely inspect the lids, noting the degree of ptosis and location of the lid margin to other eye structures, such as the iris or pupil. Measure the palpebral fissure, comparing one eye with the other. While inspecting the lids and determining the degree of asymmetry, ensure that there is not merely an illusion of ptosis, caused by a contralateral retraction of the opposite lid as seen in conditions causing exophthalmos. Palpate the lids for masses or swelling; observe for redness and discoloration. Assess cranial nerve III and muscle function by testing extraocular movements. Perform a general assessment of the face and cranial nerves. Assess the pupils for symmetry, shape, and reaction to light.

HORNER'S SYNDROME

Horner's syndrome is caused by decreased sympathetic innervation to the structures of the eye. Horner's syndrome can be caused by a variety of lesions, including trauma, tumors, and ischemia.

Signs and Symptoms.

The symptoms vary, but usually include unilateral ptosis, reduced sweating of the face, and miosis. The ptosis is typically incomplete and, although there is no true enophthalmos, the eye appears to have receded. The pupil reaction to light and accommodation remain intact.

Diagnostic Studies.
   A complete history and physical exam should be performed to identify likely etiologies. Based on findings, referral and/or imaging studies should be ordered.

MECHANICAL PTOSIS
   Lacrimal gland tumor is an example of a mechanical cause of ptosis, adding bulk to the upper lid. The degree of ptosis will depend on the size of the tumor. Other causes include a chalazion or hordeolum.
Signs and Symptoms.
   There is often pain associated with a lacrimal gland tumor, as well as with many of the inflammatory causes, such as from a chalazion or hordeolum. When inflammation is involved, the abnormal lid may be reddened and tender. If lacrimal gland tumor is involved, there may be some degree of exophthalmos and deviation of the eye, depending on tumor size.

Aging
Senile involutional ptosis is a very common cause of ptosis, particularly in patients with advanced age.
Signs and Symptoms.
   The lids and other accessory structures will have a thin, inelastic appearance. No masses, inflammation, or systemic signs will be evident.

MYASTHENIA GRAVIS
   Myasthenia gravis causes skeletal muscle weakness owing to a dysfunction of the acetylcholine receptors; this dysfunction results in reduced muscle innervation. It is a common cause of ptosis. Ptosis is the most common initial sign of myasthenia gravis, which often occurs at an earlier age in women than in men.
Signs and Symptoms.
   In myasthenia gravis, patients often have intermittent diplopia, in addition to the ptosis. The ptosis is often intermittent. The patient may attempt to compensate by raising the opposite lid. The ptosis of myasthenia gravis can be accentuated by having the patient maintain an upward gaze or forcibly blink for an extended time. The pupils are within normal limits, and not affected by the disorder.
Diagnostic Studies.
   Myasthenia gravis is definitively diagnosed by the Tensilon test, which involves administration of edrophonium chloride, which counteracts acetylcholine. If myasthenia gravis is present, any mild weakness will rapidly become exaggerated for a brief period of time.

OCULOMOTOR NERVE DEFICIT
   The third cranial nerve, the oculomotor nerve, stimulates the majority of the extraocular muscles, so this disorder was chosen as an exemplar of cranial nerve disorders. Deficits can be caused by a wide range of problems, including diabetes and tumors.
Signs and Symptoms.
   The affected eye may have a "down and out" deviation, and the pupil will be dilated. The ptosis is significant, so that the lid occludes the pupil and the patient will be unable to see from the affected eye. Facial muscle movement and strength are affected, as is sensa-

tion. The exact findings depend on which cranial nerve(s) are affected, as nerves III, V, and/or VII may be involved.

BOTULISM

Botulism is caused by toxins from the bacillus *Clostridium botulinum*, which can be either food borne or a wound contaminant. Following ingestion of the botulism toxin, the incubation period ranges from hours to several days. The incubation period following wound contamination may be as long as 2 weeks.

Signs and Symptoms.

The earliest symptoms involve the cranial nerves, and neurologic involvement then follows a descending pattern. Symptoms are generally symmetrical. Ptosis is an early symptom and may be preceded by diplopia. When wound contamination is the source of the condition, symptoms are limited to the neurologic system. However, when ingested, such systemic symptoms as nausea, vomiting, and diarrhea occur. Immediate referral should be made because botulism can be life threatening.

Double Vision

Double vision, or diplopia, is the condition in which the extraocular muscles do not work in a coordinated manner and the patient sees one object as two. There are a variety of causes for diplopia, including both neurological and muscular disorders.

History

For the complaint of double vision, it is important to fully analyze the symptom, determining how severe the visual disturbance is, when it occurs, and so on. Determine any associated symptoms, such as other weaknesses, headache, or pain. Explore whether the diplopia most commonly occurs in certain circumstances, including particular times of day. Ask about substance use/abuse, including alcohol intake. Identify any history of systemic disorders, including neuromuscular, endocrine, and neurological diseases.

Physical Examination

The physical examination should start with visual acuity testing. Determine whether the diplopia occurs only when the patient uses both eyes or whether it is limited to only one eye. Carefully assess the placement and symmetry of the eyes, performing a cover/uncover test and observing for the corneal light reflex. Note any lack of conjugate movement as the patient follows an object through the six cardinal fields of gaze.

PROPTOSIS AND EXOPHTHALMOS

Proptosis is the general term used to describe anterior displacement of the eye, whereas exophthalmos is used specifically to describe proptosis related to endocrinopathy, usually thyroid disease. In thyroid disorders, the eye muscles thicken and thereby move the eyes forward so that their ability to move conjugately is affected, and the lids may fail to close completely. Movement in all directions may be affected, although most commonly the patient finds it difficult to look upward. In addition to diplopia, patients may experience dry eyes, ulcerations, and diminished vision. Less common causes of proptosis include infections and tumors.

Signs and Symptoms.

The patient may complain of signs of thyroid disease, primarily those of hyperthyroidism, such as nervousness, anxiety, weight loss, and so on. The thyroid may be nodular or enlarged, the heart rate elevated, and a fine tremor may be present. A fever may accompany the proptosis, regardless of whether the cause is from thyroid disease or infection. There may also be complaints of visual disturbances in addition to the diplopia, a dry/gritty sensation, and eye tenderness.

Diagnostic Studies.

The initial tests would be to assess thyroid function, with complete blood count and other studies obtained subsequently, as needed. A Hertel exophthalmometer can be used to measure the degree of anterior displacement.

OCULOMOTOR NERVE DISORDERS

Lesions of the third, fourth, or sixth cranial nerves may result in diplopia, either vertical or horizontal. The third, fourth, or sixth cranial nerve palsies are usually benign, self-limited, and resolve in weeks to months. They commonly occur in patients who have hypertension and/or diabetes. However, a mass-occupying lesion should be excluded.

Signs and Symptoms.

If the third cranial nerve is affected, there is usually accompanying ptosis, so that the lid obscures the vision in the affected eye and the patient's main complaint may not be double vision. If the fourth nerve is involved, the diplopia will be vertical, whereas sixth cranial nerve palsy results in horizontal diplopia. Depending on the cause, the patient may exhibit signs or complaints consistent with herpes zoster, other infections, or neurological involvement.

Diagnostic Studies.

The patient who experiences new onset of diplopia related to nerve disorder should be promptly referred to an ophthalmologist for further evaluation and determination of subsequent assessment needs.

Myasthenia Gravis
See p. 73.

Botulism
See p. 74.

 SUGGESTED READINGS

Bickley, L.S., & Szilagyi, P.G. (2003). *Bates' Guide to Physical Examination and History Taking.* Philadelphia: Lippincott, Williams, and Wilkins.

Crouch, E., & Berger, A. (2001). Ophthalmology. In Rakel, R.E. (Ed.), *Textbook of Family Practice.* Philadelphia: Saunders.

Dillon, P.M. (2003). *Nursing Health Assessment. A Critical Thinking, Case Studies Approach.* Philadelphia: F.A. Davis.

Horton, J.C. (2001). Disorders of the eyes. In Baunwald, E., Fauci, A.S., Kasper, D.L., Hauser, S.L., Lange, D.L., & Jameson, J.L. (Eds.). *Harrison's Principles of Internal Medicine*. New York: McGraw Hill.

Roy, F.H. (2002). *Ocular Differential Diagnosis*. Philadelphia: Lippincott, Williams and Wilkins.

Swartz, M. H. (2002). *Textbook Of Physical Diagnosis: History And Examination*. Philadelphia: Saunders.

Yanoff, M., & Duker, J. (2004). *Ophthalmology*. Philadelphia: Mosby.

Chapter 5

Ear, Nose, Mouth, and Throat

Karen Koozer Olson, Randolph F.R. Rasch, & Mary Jo Goolsby

Upper respiratory complaints make up a significant component of the primary care provider's daily patient encounters. Figures 5-1, 5-2, and 5-3 identify the major landmarks of the upper respiratory system. The most common complaints of childhood include: earache, sore throat, and symptoms of allergy and "common cold." Elderly clients frequently present with complaints of hardened cerumen and decreased hearing resulting from cerumen impaction aggravated by hearing aid wear. All ages have significant sensory compromise associated with complaints of the ear, nose, mouth, and throat. The ability to maintain homeostasis related to breathing and nourishment may also be affected. Other issues are frequency of lost days of work or school related to allergies and upper respiratory infections.

HISTORY
General History
A general history of the ear, nose, mouth, and throat should include current or recent exposure to respiratory infections, such as the flu or colds; complaints of ear, sinus, or throat pain; nasal or ear discharge, including color changes; changes in hearing, taste, or smell; and tinnitus. A history of nausea and vomiting, cough, or elevated temperature is relevant. A history of flu, upper respiratory infection, frequent sinus infections, allergies, and dental care is also important. A history of exposure to mononucleosis or strep and a history of smoking are also important.

History of the Present Illness
When a patient presents with a complaint related to the ears, nose, mouth, or throat, a symptom analysis is indicated. The framework suggested is the "P, Q, R, S, T." Ask the patient to describe what, if anything, has been noticed to make the symptoms worse or better.

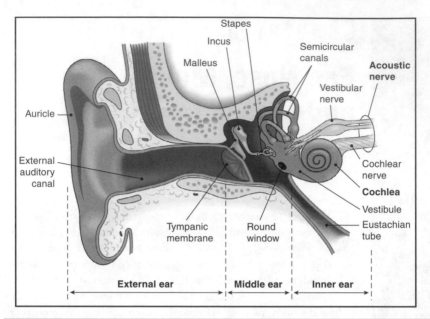

Figure 5-1. ■ Anatomy of the ear. (From Dillon, P.M. Nursing health assessment: A critical thinking, case studies approach. Philadelphia: F.A. Davis, 2003. Reprinted with permission)

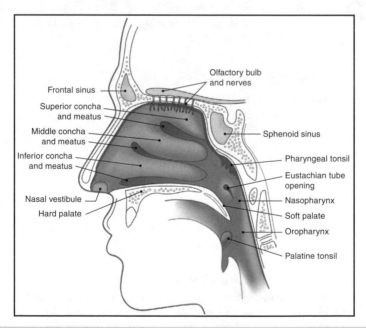

Figure 5-2. ■ Anatomy of the nose. (From Dillon, P.M. Nursing health assessment: A critical thinking, case studies approach. Philadelphia: F.A. Davis, 2003. Reprinted with permission)

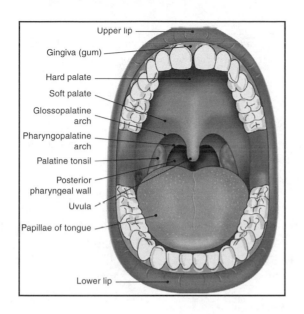

Figure 5-3. ■ Anatomy of the mouth and oropharynx. (From Dillon, P.M. Nursing health assessment: A critical thinking, case studies approach. Philadelphia: F.A. Davis, 2003. Reprinted with permission)

Ask about any self-treatment the patient may have attempted and the response. Determine whether the symptoms tend to happen only on exposure to certain allergy triggers, such as dust or pets. Have the patient quantify the symptoms, for instance, by rating the severity of ear or throat pain, congestion, or fullness/pressure. When pain is present, determine where, exactly, it is located, as well as any areas of radiation. With ear, nose, and throat complaints, patients commonly experience multiple complaints. Ask about any associated symptoms. Include systemic symptoms such as fatigue, fever, myalgia, malaise, and headache, as well as symptoms related to the ears, nose, mouth, and throat. Ask about pain or discomfort (mouth, nose, sinus, ear, throat, etc.); nasal congestion or discharge; sinus pressure; postnasal drainage; ear fullness, drainage, or tinnitus; ulcerations of the lips, mouth, or throat; swollen or tender nodes; hoarseness; cough; and/or sneezing. Finally, determine when the complaint(s) were first noticed and how they have progressed since first noticed.

Past Medical History

Ask about recent exposure to others with similar symptoms or potentially contagious conditions. Ask about frequency of upper respiratory infections, such as strep throat, sinusitis, and otitis media. Determine whether the patient has ever had surgery or other procedures performed on the ears, nose, mouth, or throat. Include cosmetic/aesthetic procedures, as well as therapeutic ones. Identify any other major medical conditions. Ask about history of rhinitis or other atopic conditions, such as asthma, allergic conjunctivitis, and atopic dermatitis. Determine whether the patient has a prior history of skin or other malignancies. Ask about any disorders that would affect the immune system, including HIV/AIDS. Obtain a history of all current and recent medications. An immunization/vaccination history should also be obtained. Prior audiology and other hearing tests should be determined, along with the results. The use of hearing aids should be noted.

Family History

A family history of hearing disorders and conditions, such as tinnitus, Ménière's disorder, allergies, malignancies, and asthma. Determine whether others in the family are ill with similar symptoms.

Habits

Patient exposure to recreational and occupational noise is important to discern. Assess whether the patient works in an area that requires hearing protection and the type of protection used. Ask about activities that involve barometric pressure changes, such as scuba diving and flying, which may affect ear equilibrium. Determine whether the patient's activities involve exposure to toxins, trauma, or chemicals and any protection used. Ask about the use of smoked and smokeless tobacco, alcohol, and recreational drugs. Determine the patient's living conditions, including the method of cooling and heating the home and any exposure to pets or dust. Determine whether the patient has pets. Determine how often the patient sees a dentist, and identify any dental conditions.

Review of Systems

Based on the initial history, complete a review of other systems.

PHYSICAL EXAMINATION

Order of the Examination

Note the patient's vital signs, and complete a general survey. Develop a systematic approach to examining the ear, nose, mouth, and throat. These components are often incorporated into the exam of the head, face, and neck. Those exams are described in Chapter 3.

Examination of the Ears

The ear examination begins with inspection of the external ear. Note the placement of the ears and compare the ears for symmetry. Inspect the external ears, noting the condition of the skin and the integrity of the structures. Assess any skin changes as described in Chapter 2. Identify any deformities, lesions, areas of enlargement, or other abnormalities. Observe for inflammation, signs of a foreign body, and drainage. If piercings are present, they should be assessed for healing and signs of tearing. Palpate the external ear, noting any areas of tenderness or deformities. Palpate the pre- and postauricular lymph nodes for size, tenderness, and mobility.

The otoscope is then used to examine the canal and middle ear. If symptoms are unilateral, assess the asymptomatic ear first and then proceed to the area of complaint. Use the largest ear speculum that is comfortable. The canal and associated structures are assessed for patency, erythema, tenderness, exudate, deformity, and drainage. Note the quality of the tympanic membrane (TM) light reflex and the integrity of its structure. Note the visibility and placement of the bony landmarks posterior to the TM. The TM is evaluated for inflammation, retraction, or bulging. In children, observe for the presence of pressure-equalizing tubes. Look for any bubbles behind the eardrum, air-fluid level, and/or discoloration. The use of a pneumonic otoscope may be used to evaluate TM motility. Table 5-1 depicts some abnormalities detected on the ear exam.

Table 5-1. ■ Abnormalities of Inspection: Ear

Finding	Significance
External swelling and redness	Malignant otitis externa or mastoiditis
Light yellow to dark brown matter that occludes the eardrum	Cerumen impaction
Bloody discharge	External ear canal wound, skull fracture, traumatic perforation of the TM
Purulent discharge	Infection or a foreign body
Whitish plaques on the eardrum	Scars from earlier infection
Dark area on the eardrum with drainage	Old or current perforation
Diffuse light reflex	Bulging eardrum
Bubbles on the eardrum	Serous fluid in the middle ear
Erythema of the TM	Otitis, crying, or fever

Red Flags: Warnings for the Ear

- *Red, warm, and very painful auricle.* Such a condition can be associated with malignant otitis externa and/or mastoiditis and warrants immediate referral.

- *Auricular lesions.* Cancerous lesions are most often found in the helix of the auricle. They are associated with sun exposure and should be assessed using the ABCD cancer-screening criteria. Tophi are auricular lesions associated with gout.

- *Clear fluid.* Clear fluid emitting from the ear may be associated with cerebral injury.

Hearing can be grossly assessed using the whisper test, watch ticking, and tuning forks (see next subsection). If screening indicates deficit or if the patient complains of hearing loss, an accurate assessment of hearing requires audiogram with proper equipment.

Special Maneuvers

WEBER TEST

The Weber test is performed with a tuning fork (500–1000 Hz). The test measures the patient's ability to hear sound bilaterally. The tuning fork is tapped gently and the base of the tuning fork is placed on the midline of the patient's head. The patient should hear the vibration equally.

RINNE'S TEST

This test uses the tuning fork to assess and compare the patient's ability to hear both through bone and air conduction. The vibrating tuning fork is placed on the patient's mastoid bone. The patient indicates when the tuning fork is no longer heard. The examiner then positions the tines of the fork in front of the ear until the patient signals that the sound is no longer heard and notes the amount of time the patient hears the vibration in both positions. This maneuver is repeated on the opposite side. Air conduction should be twice as long as bone, and the results should be similar for both ears.

HEARING TESTS

A skilled examiner using a soundproof booth should conduct audiometry. Before the audiogram is performed, ears should be examined for any cerumen buildup. Patients should be free from upper respiratory infection and the exacerbations of allergies. Patients should not have been exposed to loud noise activities for several days before the examination.

TYMPANOCENTESIS

Tympanocentesis should be considered in patients with recurrent otitis media to identify the causative organisms.

PNEUMATIC OTOSCOPY

Pneumatic otoscopy should be used to determine whether the TM is mobile.

Examination of the Nose and Sinuses

The exam of the sinuses begins with inspection, noting any swelling or edema. Palpate over the frontal and maxillary sinuses, noting any tenderness. Unless tenderness is elicited by palpation over the sinuses, proceed with percussion of the sinuses. Ask the patient to notify you of tenderness and observe the facial expression for signs of discomfort. A sinus that is thickened or full may percuss dull, compared with the resonant tones usually associated with percussion of the sinuses. If sinus thickening or fullness is suspected, the sinuses can be transilluminated using a penlight, otoscope, or transilluminator.

Observe the external nose for placement and any obvious deformity or discharge. Observe the patient's respiratory pattern, noting whether the patient is mouth breathing or is able to breath through the nose. Identify any flaring of the nostrils. If drainage is identified, note the color, and consistency. Palpate the external nose, noting any deformities, masses, or tenderness.

If the patient is experiencing significant nasal symptoms, the internal examination of the nose is best accomplished after asking the patient to blow his or her nose. Examine any discharge for color, consistency, and odor. To observe the internal structures, the patient's head should be tilted backward. The examiners nondominant hand and thumb can be used to stabilize the nose and forehead, respectively, with slight pressure of the thumb upward on the nose tip to facilitate inspection. A nasal speculum can be gently inserted to observe the nasal mucosa and turbinates.

The mucosa should be assessed for integrity, color, moistness, and edema/lesions. The nasal septum is assessed for patency and the turbinates should be assessed for color and size. Pale boggy turbinates are suggestive of allergies. Erythematous, swollen turbinates are often seen with infection. Any discharge should be noted. Clear, profuse discharge is often associated with allergies. Table 5-2 identifies several abnormalities that can be identified during examination of the nose.

Red Flags: *Warnings for the Nose and Sinuses*

- *Epistaxis*—persistent, recurrent, or profuse.
- *Severe maxillary pain.*
- *Thin, honey-colored sinus drainage following head trauma* may indicate skull fracture.

Table 5-2. ■ Abnormalities of Inspection: Nose

Finding	Significance
Transverse nasal crease	Allergic salute
Skin lesions	Skin cancer
Redness, papules, hyperplasia	Rosacea
Telangiectasia	EtOH abuse, Rendu-Osler-Weber
Crooked or asymmetric nose	Past or recent trauma
Erythematous turbinates	Infection
Pale boggy turbinates	Allergies
Clear copious discharge	Allergies

Olfactory sensation is typically a component of the cranial nerve exam. However, depending on the patient's complaints, it may be part of the limited ear, nose, and throat (ENT) exam.

Special Maneuvers Transillumination of the sinuses is accomplished in a slightly darkened room. A bright, focused light—an otoscope can be used—is placed directly on the cheek over the maxillary sinuses. The patient's mouth is opened and the examiner looks for a light glow on the roof of the mouth. Diminished light may indicate full sinus cavities. Unequal light may indicate unilateral sinus fullness.

Examination of the Mouth and Throat

The examination of the mouth and throat should begin with an inspection of all the structures that can be observed without touching, followed by an examination that requires touching and moving of the structures in order to facilitate the examination. The examination should end with palpation of the structures, paying particular attention to observed abnormalities. Gloves should always be worn during palpation. Ask the patient to remove any dental appliances, and proceed to systematically examine the mouth and the pharynx. The use of a tongue depressor facilitates complete examination of the inner cheeks/buccal mucosa, the floor and roof of the mouth, the gums, posterior mouth, and tongue.

The examination should include an inspection of the size, shape, and symmetry of the lips. Obvious lesions should be noted and their characteristics recorded. To inspect the oral cavity and the pharynx, use a good light source.

First, note the general condition of the internal structures of the mouth including the tongue, the buccal mucosa, hard and soft palates, gums, and teeth. Note any abnormalities, such as lesions, ulcers, masses, exudate, inflammation, and missing or decayed teeth. Identify any tongue or lip piercings, which may cause microscopic enamel cracks to teeth as a result of constant abrasion. Using a tongue depressor to displace the lips and cheeks, inspect areas of the buccal mucosa that are not otherwise visible, including the sites of the Stensen's and Wharton's ducts. Also observe as the patient lifts the tongue to touch palate, sticks it out, and moves it side-to-side. Also observe the lateral and ventral surfaces of the tongue during these motions, as well as the sublingual mucosa and the frenulum. As the oral cavity is inspected in this manner, the general integrity of the mucosal coverings and structures should be continually noted.

Inspect the oropharynx, tonsils, and uvula, taking care not to trigger an unwanted gag reflex. Observing the mucosa, identify any inflammation, petechia, ulcerations, discolorations, edema, swelling, asymmetry, lesions, and exudate or postnasal drainage. Observe the movement of the uvula as the patient says "ah." Identify whether the tonsils are present and, if present, their size, symmetry, color, and presence of exudate. Smell the breath for acetone, ammonia, or foul breath (fetor oris).

Finally, accessible structures should be palpated, including the tissue between the cheeks and buccal mucosa, the floor of the mouth, and the tongue. To palpate the floor of the mouth, use both hands, with one hand placed externally below the area being palpated and applying upward pressure, so that any masses will be displaced upward and toward the palpating hand. Use a similar technique to apply external, lateral pressure when palpating the buccal mucosa, so that masses are not pushed away by the examining hand. Note any areas of tenderness and masses. Masses should be assessed for consistency, dimensions, mobility, tenderness, and shape.

Red Flags: *Warnings for the Mouth and Throat*

- *Persistent, painless mouth lesions or lesions* consistent with malignancy require referral.
- *Sore throat associated with drooling or stridor* indicates potential epiglottitis or peritonsillar abscess.
- *Sore throat lasting more than 1 week* suggests untreated streptococcal pharyngitis and/ortonsillitis.

DIFFERENTIAL DIAGNOSIS OF CHIEF COMPLAINTS: EAR

Ear Pain (Otalgia)

Ear pain is one of the most common complaints seen in primary care practice. It is most often seen in children and is usually associated with bacterial or viral upper respiratory infection. Complaints of ear pain in the summer are often associated with otitis externa owing to swimmer's ear. Although common in children, complaints of primary ear pain decline with age and, in adults, are more likely associated with secondary conditions, such as sinus infection; dental disease; malignancy; other disorders of the head, face, and neck; and nervous and vascular symptoms.

History

The history should include information related to the pain: location, quality, quantity and/or severity, onset, timing, and duration. The presence of sinus and nasal congestion is relevant because otitis media is typically secondary to a cold or sinus infection. Other historical information includes air travel and deep sea diving. In adults, consideration should be given to possible underlying conditions, such as a diabetes mellitus, and chronic inflammatory conditions, such as psoriasis. A child's history should include exposure to second-hand smoke, day care, and swimming. A compromised immune status should be considered in those patients with atypical otitis media or who do not respond to therapy.

Physical Examination

The physical examination should include inspection of the external auditory structures, palpation and manipulation of the tragus and auricle, and otoscopic inspection of the canal and TM. Attention should be paid to detecting inflammation and/or exudate in the canal, and the condition of the TM, noting color, light reflex, translucency, and perforation. The exam should also include screening for hearing acuity.

Diagnostic Studies
Diagnosis is based on findings from the physical examination. A culture and sensitivity should be considered if there is a purulent discharge. If a complete blood count (CBC) is done, there may be an associated leukocytosis and elevated erythrocyte sedimentation rate.

ACUTE OTITIS MEDIA

Acute otitis media (AOM) involves infection of the fluid in the middle ear space. The three bacterial organisms most often associated with AOM include streptococcal pneumonia, *Haemophilus influenzae*, and *Moraxella catarrhalis*. Frequently, viral organisms coexist with one of the preceding bacterial causes.

Signs and Symptoms.
The patient often complains of unilateral ear pain, which may radiate to the neck or jaw. There is commonly a current condition or recent history of associated symptoms of an upper respiratory infection, including nasal congestion, sinus pressure/fullness, or sore throat. General hearing acuity may be diminished on the affected side, with bone conduction enhanced on that side. The external ear will have a normal appearance, unless there is drainage from perforated TM. The TM is typically dull, may be inflamed, and bulges so that the posterior landmarks are obscured. The light reflex will be distorted or obscured. If myringitis (inflammation of the TM) is present, the TM will be reddened. Purulent or yellow fluid may be evident posterior to the TM, with diminished TM mobility. The exam is often associated with increased pain. There are often other findings of upper respiratory infection. With eustachian tube dysfunction, otitis media with effusion (OME) may result, and this condition is discussed subsequently, with ear fullness/hearing loss. See Figure 5-4.

Diagnostic Studies.
Usually no diagnostic studies are indicated. However, tympanocentesis can be performed to alleviate discomfort and/or obtain culture in recurrent disease or when anticipated response to therapy is not achieved.

OTITIS EXTERNA

Otitis externa (OE) is inflammation of the external ear, more specifically, the canal. Frequent causes include pseudomonas and fungal organisms. It is frequently associated with swimming, as well as trauma, which may occur through attempts to clean the ear with

Figure 5-4. ■ Acute otitis media. (From Dillon, P.M. Nursing health assessment: A critical thinking, case studies approach. Philadelphia: F.A. Davis, 2003. Reprinted with permission)

cotton-tipped swabs or objects such as paper clips. In immunocompromised patients, necrotizing otitis can occur and extend to the temporal bone, so it is important to monitor response to therapy.

Signs and Symptoms.

Common findings include pain, particularly when the auricle or tragus is touched or moved, as well as itching. The pain can be very severe. Depending on the amount of edema and exudate, there may be a significant sensation of stuffiness and/or decreased hearing. Drainage may be present. On exam, there is increased pain as the tragus is manipulated and the examination may be quite uncomfortable. The canal is inflamed and often edematous. If exudate is present, it may range from purulent, to cheesy, to serous. Depending on the amount of swelling and exudate, the distal portion of the canal may not be visible. An odor may be present. See Figure 5-5.

Diagnostic Studies.

There is usually no indication for diagnostic studies, although exudate can be cultured, along with sensitivity. With failure to respond to treatment, referral to a specialist should be considered.

BAROTRAUMA

Barotrauma refers to injury to the structures of the ear resulting from exposure to differing atmospheric pressures, such as those associated with flying or deep sea diving. Onset typically occurs within 24 hours of the exposure to an extreme of atmospheric pressure.

Signs and Symptoms.

Complaints include ear pressure, pain, altered acuity of hearing, tinnitus, sinus pain/pressure, and headache. Vertigo may be present. The TM is often inflamed and may be perforated. A hemorrhagic collection may be present posterior to the TM. Benign positional vertigo may be evident and/or sinus tenderness.

Diagnostic Studies.

No specific diagnostics are warranted, providing the patient does not also have symptoms consistent with decompression sickness.

TRAUMA

Direct trauma as a cause of ear pain is most commonly seen in children, who frequently insert foreign objects into their ears. However, it may occur in adults as the result of overzealous ear cleaning with hairpins and sometimes from cotton-tipped applicators. Indirect trauma can be associated with blunt blows to the head, jaw, or ear.

Figure 5-5. ■ External otitis. (From Dillon, P.M. Nursing health assessment: A critical thinking, case studies approach. Philadelphia: F.A. Davis, 2003. Reprinted with permission)

Signs and Symptoms.

The signs and symptoms are dependent on the structures injured by the trauma. In cases of direct trauma, the pain is consistent with OE or perforated TM. In blunt trauma, the signs and symptoms are consistent with the history of the injury. The actual findings may be from a source of referred pain (a fractured jaw, for instance) or from resultant perforation of the TM. The history of the traumatic event is important.

Diagnostic Studies.

Often no diagnostic studies are warranted. However, in the case of trauma to the head, diagnostics should be accomplished as recommended in Chapter 3.

MASTOIDITIS

Mastoiditis refers to infection of the mastoid bone, which is almost always a complication of AOM.

Signs and Symptoms.

The patient complains of ear pain, with radiation, that has persisted for days to weeks. The pain is persistent, severe, deep, and often worst at night. Fever is associated with mastoiditis. The hearing on the affected site is usually significantly diminished. As the condition progresses, it is accompanied by swelling, erythema, and tenderness over the mastoid bone. The swelling can be so advanced as to displace the auricle; complications include paralysis resulting from facial nerve involvement and infection of the labyrinth or cerebrospinal fluid, causing meningitis or brain abscess.

Diagnostic Studies.

The patient should be referred to a specialist for definitive diagnosis and treatment. On referral, diagnostics will likely include CBC, culture of fluid, and computed tomographic (CT) scan to determine the degree of involvement.

FOREIGN BODY

Any foreign body in the ear canal, such as beads, cotton, insects, or toys, can cause pain. The presence of a foreign body is most common in young children.

Signs and Symptoms.

Pain is often the presenting complaint and may be associated with unilateral, purulent discharge from the canal. Other symptoms include altered hearing acuity. Physical findings often include tenderness on manipulation of the ear and with the examination, as well as the foreign body. Depending on the amount of trauma that has been caused by the offending object, the canal may be inflamed, edematous, and have exudate consistent with a resultant OE.

Diagnostic Studies.

Diagnostic studies are typically not warranted.

Referred Pain

A variety of conditions can result in pain that is referred to the ear. Theses include temporomandibular joint pain, dental pain, neck mass/pain, carotodynia, tonsillitis, temporal arteritis, and trigeminal neuralgia. The variety of conditions are beyond the scope of the discussion for ear pain but can be found in other chapters, particularly Chapter 3.

Ear Discharge (Otorrhea)

Discharge emanating from the ear can come from several sources and often indicates a condition warranting urgent diagnosis and treatment. In addition to stemming from conditions affecting the external and middle ear, otorrhea may indicate leakage of cerebrospinal fluid. Purulent discharge is most often related to an infectious process or a foreign body. Bloody discharge that is associated with recent head trauma may be indicative of a skull fracture.

History

Immediate proximal causes for ear discharge should be investigated, such as OM with perforation, OE, mastoiditis, and a foreign body. One should consider more serious conditions such as head trauma if an immediate proximal cause is ruled out. Ask about how and when the discharge was first noticed, as well as the patient's perceived health preceding that event. Explore the possibility of direct or indirect trauma, as well as secondary or complicated infections. Obtain a history of previous episodes of ear discharge, as well as of previous ear infections or conditions. A thorough review of systems is warranted, particularly as related to other components of the upper respiratory and neurological systems.

Physical Examination

Physical examination usually involves the head, ears, nose, and throat. Begin by assessing the patient's general health and mental status. If there is no history of head trauma and the patient's general neurological status is intact, proceed to the examination of the ears. Observe both external ears, comparing for symmetry of appearance. Identify areas of inflammation, swelling, deformity, or distortion of landmarks, signs of trauma. Identify the color, odor, and consistency of any discharge that is visible. Palpate the structures of the external ear, noting any tenderness or palpable abnormalities. Observe the distal portion of the canal for swelling, erythema, and discharge, as well as any obvious foreign body. Complete the otoscopic examination, noticing the condition of the canal walls, TM, and visible portion of the middle ear structures.

Diagnostic Studies

Diagnosis is usually made based on history and physical examination. Some specific diagnoses are discussed in preceding subsections along with other conditions that can be associated with discharge.

Aom With Perforation

Particularly in children, spontaneous rupture of the TM may occur owing to the pressure in the middle ear, resulting in a white or purulent discharge from the ear. In addition to the typical findings of AOM, there may be a visible perforation (Figure 5-6). See preceding subsection on AOM.

Cerebrospinal Fluid Leakage

Cerebrospinal fluid (CSF) leaks are associated with head trauma or surgery. If the history and/or physical examination suggest the potential for leakage of CSF, the drainage can be tested for glucose. Providing the patient is stable, a referral is warranted for definitive diagnosis, as CSF leakage indicates a heightened potential for the development of meningitis, in addition to the condition responsible for the leakage. Further diagnostic studies, including imaging, will be completed following referral.

Figure 5-6. ■ Perforated tympanic membrane. (From Dillon, P.M. Nursing health assessment: A critical thinking, case studies approach. Philadelphia: F.A. Davis, 2003. Reprinted with permission)

CHOLESTEATOMA

A cholesteatoma is an abnormal growth of epithelial tissue in the middle ear. The tissue can grow to invade surrounding bone and/or extend into the inner ear. Surgical excision is usually indicated, so the patient should be referred when this is suspected.

Signs and Symptoms.

The patient often presents with a history of drainage from the ear. There may be associated sense of aural fullness and/or decreased hearing in the affected ear. Over time, pain can develop, as well as dizziness. The examination will reveal drainage and/or granulatory tissue in the canal. The drainage is often mucopurulent. If there is an associated infection, inflammatory changes may be evident, as seen with AOM. The cholesteatoma may be visible behind the TM. Because of the risk of permanent hearing loss and invasiveness, the patient should be referred for definitive diagnosis and surgical intervention. See Figure 5-7.

Diagnostic Studies.

None indicated in primary care setting.

Otitis Externa
See pp. 85–86.

Mastoiditis
See p. 87.

Foreign Body
See p. 87.

Figure 5-7. ■ Cholesteatoma. (From Dillon, P.M. Nursing health assessment: A critical thinking, case studies approach. Philadelphia: F.A. Davis, 2003. Reprinted with permission)

Decreased Hearing or Hearing Loss

A decreased ability to hear is most often associated with aging, with onset noticed in the sixth decade. In children, hearing deficits are often associated with middle ear effusions. Other reasons for decreased hearing include repetitive exposure to loud noise, which may occur with recreational activities such as concert attendance, firearms use, all terrain vehicle riding, and the operation of woodworking equipment, as well as other outside equipment and occupational exposure. Mechanical obstruction of the ear canal by cerumen or a foreign body may also cause hearing impairment. Indeed, the list of conditions and factors that can result in an altered sense of hearing is extensive. It includes a variety of infectious diseases, autoimmune disorders, chronic systemic diseases (diabetes, thyroid disease, and vascular and neurological conditions), and many more. Types of deafness can be categorized as conductive, nerve, and central (see Figure 5-8). Examples of conductive deafness include perforated TM, serous otitis, and cerumen impaction. Examples of nerve deafness include presbycusis, acoustic neuroma, and medication-related changes. Examples of central deafness include losses stemming from infections, such as meningitis, and stroke.

History

It is essential to explore the onset and progression of the hearing loss, determining whether the onset was progressive over a period of time or was acute and, regardless of the onset, how it has progressed since first noticed. Determine what the patient means by "hearing loss" and whether the symptom involves one ear or both. To rate the severity, include questions to determine the impact of the hearing loss on the patient's ability to communicate. The presence of associated symptoms is important to determine, including ringing in the

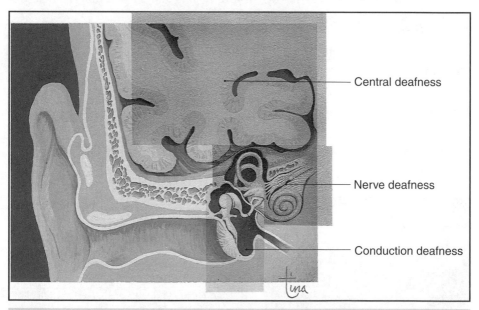

Figure 5-8. ■ Types of deafness. (From Scanlon, V.C. & Sanders, T. Essentials of anatomy and physiology, 4th ed. Philadelphia: F.A. Davis, 2003. Reprinted with permission)

ear(s), pain, fullness, or drainage. In addition to the typical symptom analysis, have the patient identify all prescribed, over-the-counter, and recreational substances used before and since onset as possible causative agents. Medications with ototoxic effects include aminoglycoside antibiotics; platinum-based antineoplastics and methotrexate; loop diuretics; salicylates and antiinflammatories; and quinine-based medications such as quinine, chloroquine, hydroxychloroquine, and mefloquine.

Explore the patient's general state of health from the period just before and since the altered sense of hearing was noticed, asking about other conditions and infections, including upper respiratory infections, Ménière's disease, OE, and OA. Identify the history of systemic disorders, such as diabetes, malignancies, hypertension, and vascular disorders. Ask about recent barotrauma, as well as other trauma to the head or ear.

Physical Examination

An audiogram is required to quantitatively assess the hearing acuity. However, it is reasonable to first grossly test hearing with the whisper test, ticking watch, or fingers being rubbed together. The type of loss (sensorineural or conductive) may be grossly evaluated using tuning fork examination techniques. Based on the results to these gross screenings, an audiogram can be obtained and/or the patient referred for more comprehensive hearing tests, if a self-limited condition is not identified.

A complete examination of the ears should be performed, along with assessment of the other upper respiratory structures, particularly in younger patients. As indicated by the patient's age and/or presenting history, general appearance, and ear findings, consider expanding the examination to include neurological, cardiovascular, and other systems.

Diagnostic Studies

As noted earlier, audiometric examination is essential to objectively measure the acuity of hearing and to determine affected frequencies. Other diagnostic procedures will depend on the suspected cause of hearing loss and can include vascular studies or neurological imaging, as well as laboratory studies, including serum glucose, thyroid studies, tests for autoimmune diseases, CBC, and others.

CERUMEN IMPACTION

Cerumen impaction is a common cause of altered hearing, particularly in older patients.

Signs and Symptoms.

The patient typically complains of progressive decreased hearing acuity, although the deficit may be suddenly noticed. The cerumen may cause discomfort and/or itching in the canal. In older patients, there is often a history of previous impactions. Hearing loss is conductive. The exam reveals the mass of cerumen within the canal. On occasion, the cerumen causes excoriation of the canal walls.

Diagnostic Studies.

No studies are indicated.

PRESBYCUSIS

Presbycusis is an age-related cause of decreased hearing acuity. Although the changes associated with presbycusis often start in early adulthood, the decreased acuity of hearing is usually not noticed until the individual is older than 65. In addition to changes associated with aging, onset can be associated with exposure to environmental noise and influenced by genetic predisposition. The condition involves sensorineural loss owing to diminished hairy cell function within the cochlea, as well as decreased elasticity of the TM. When presbycusis is suspected, the patient should be referred to a specialist for definitive diagnosis and assessment for use of hearing aid(s).

Signs and Symptoms.

Onset is usually gradual. The patient may have a family history of hearing loss, and/or a personal history of atherosclerosis and/or diabetes. The physical examination is normal, with exception of audiometric studies, which quantify the hearing loss and affected ranges. Presbycusis is a condition diagnosed by exclusion.

Diagnostic Studies.

Audiometric studies identify the degree of hearing loss, usually affecting the higher frequencies.

OTOSCLEROSIS

Otosclerosis involves the bony structures and results in gradual onset of hearing deficit. It occurs most frequently in women and Caucasians. It seems to be related to estrogen and can be accelerated by pregnancy. Risk factors include family history. Onset is earlier than presbycusis and lower frequencies are affected first. Otosclerosis involves degenerative changes to the middle ear bones such that they lose their vibratory ability.

Sign and Symptoms.

The patient typically complains of painless, progressive changes in hearing. Symptoms are usually bilateral, and tinnitus may be present. The physical examination is usually normal, with the exception of the hearing acuity test. The ear has a normal appearance and the TM mobility is normal.

Diagnostic Studies.

Audiometry quantifies the deficit, which usually involves the lower frequencies. A referral to a specialist is warranted, as surgical intervention is often successful. The specialist may order images to determine the degree of change.

OTITIS MEDIA WITH EFFUSION (OME)

Otitis media with effusion, or serous otitis media, results from one or both dysfunctional eustachian tubes and may follow or contribute to the development of AOM. The presence of residual middle ear fluid can cause significant conductive hearing loss. This condition is most common in children.

Signs and Symptoms.

Parents and/or teachers often relate that the patient does not listen well. There is an associated sense of ear fullness and a need to "pop" the ear(s). Physical examination reveals decreased acuity of hearing on the affected side. The external ear and canal are normal in appearance. The TM may be bulging and has a yellowish hue from the fluid collected posteriorly in the middle ear chamber. The TM mobility is diminished or absent on pneumatic otoscopy. Figure 5-9 depicts otitis with effusion.

Diagnostic Studies.

A tympanogram reveals decreased compliance.

INFECTIOUS DISEASES

A variety of infectious conditions can affect hearing acuity. These include the conditions that are usually responsible for AOM and OE (as described earlier in this chapter) as well

Figure 5-9. ■ Serous otitis with effusion. (From Dillon, P.M. Nursing health assessment: A critical thinking, case studies approach. Philadelphia: F.A. Davis, 2003. Reprinted with permission)

as the following: herpes simples, herpes zoster, syphilis, meningitis, mononucleosis, mumps, rubella, and rubeola. Infections are responsible for both conductive and sensorineural hearing loss.

Signs and Symptoms.

Complaints will be consistent with the specific infection, and may include malaise, fever, myalgia, headache, and pain. Similarly, findings will depend on the cause. Physical examination should reveal findings consistent with AOM or OE, if either of these conditions are present. In addition to physical ear findings, particularly when the infection is not limited to the ear(s), there may be generalized signs of upper respiratory infection, skin rash or lesions, lymphadenopathy, and other changes. Tuning fork tests may reveal either conductive hearing loss (associated with bacterial or viral AOM) or sensorineural loss (syphilis, meningitis, herpes zoster). It is possible that the signs of a causative infection may have resolved by the time the patient presents with hearing loss; thus, the history will be important in identifying this as a possible etiology.

Diagnostic Studies.

The selection of diagnostic studies will be guided by the history of exposure, symptomatology, and risk factors, as well as the physical findings.

ACOUSTIC NEUROMA

Acoustic neuromas are nonmalignant tumors affecting the acoustic nerve (cranial nerve [CN] VIII). The onset of symptoms usually occurs after age 30. Therapeutic interventions include surgery and radiation.

Signs and Symptoms.

Symptoms depend on the size of the tumor. Early complaints include unilateral hearing loss, tinnitus, and vertigo. As the tumor advances, symptoms may include headache, facial pain, ataxia, nausea/vomiting, and lethargy. The inspection of the ear structures yield normal findings. Audiogram will reveal diminished hearing acuity.

Diagnostic Studies.

The patient should be referred for definitive diagnosis and treatment. Magnetic resonance imaging (MRI) is useful in identifying the tumor.

MÉNIÈRE'S DISEASE

The exact cause of Ménière's disease is unknown. However, the symptoms are associated with increased fluid and pressure in the labyrinth.

Signs and Symptoms.

The triad of symptoms most commonly associated with Ménière's disease consists of severe vertigo, tinnitus, and hearing loss. The vertigo is transient but recurrent. The tinnitus and hearing loss may also be intermittent and/or recurrent but often become worse over time. Preceding an "episode," the patient may notice a sensation of ear fullness. During the episode, vertigo is often debilitating and is associated with nausea and vomiting. Although the tinnitus and hearing loss are usually unilateral, some patients experience bilateral symptoms. Vestibular maneuvers, including Nylen-Barany, are often positive, reproducing the patient's complaint.

Diagnostic Studies.

Because the symptoms and findings of Ménière's disease and acoustic neuroma are so similar, MRI is helpful to exclude tumor. A number of other studies are typically performed by specialists, including auditory evoked potentials.

Medications

A variety of medications can potentially affect hearing acuity. However, the most common are as follows: antibiotics (aminoglycosides); quinine derivatives; antineoplastics (platinum-based and methotrexate); loop diuretics; and nonsteroidal antiinflammatories, both salicylate-based and others. When hearing loss is identified, obtain a list of all agents taken by the patient and determine whether any have a potential ototoxicity. Medication-related ototoxicity can be permanent or reversible, depending on the agent.

Cholesteatoma

See p. 89.

Ringing (Tinnitus)

Ringing in the ears (tinnitus) is most often related to the use of ototoxic drugs. It is also associated with continued exposure to loud noise and environmental chemical exposure. Tinnitus refers to a wide range of sounds mimicking whistles, crickets, ringing, buzzing, and the like. It is typically persistent and bilateral. Tinnitus is associated with many of the causes of hearing loss.

History

Specific history should include current medications, the amount and frequency of dosing, and recent exposure to loud noise or chemical agents through activities including work, hobbies, or recreation. A history of other ear disorders and symptoms should be obtained, including labyrinthitis, Ménière's disease, or progressive hearing loss. Ask about ear pain, pressure, and drainage.

Physical Examination

A thorough ENT and neurological examination should be performed. Unless some abnormality of structure or infection is expected, the physical examination should be normal. There may be a decrease in gross hearing acuity and in performance during a tuning fork exam, as tinnitus is associated with the causes of hearing loss.

Box 5-1

Common Causes of Tinnitus

Ménière's disease
Acoustic trauma
Neoplasms
Cerumen or foreign body
Infections
Ototoxic medications

Diagnostic Studies

Diagnostic studies are related to the specific suspected etiology associated with the tinnitus but should include audiometry.

The major causes of tinnitus are listed in Box 5-1.

Ear Fullness

The etiology of ear fullness is multidimensional. Fullness can be related to fluid in the middle ear as a result of otitis media or changes in barometric pressure. The most common causes vary by age; children are more likely to experience ear fullness associated with OME, whereas older adults are more likely to have cerumen impaction.

History

Check for seven dimensions of the symptoms, and especially note the timing of the symptom. Ask whether the onset was gradual or sudden. Determine whether the fullness is affected by the patient's position. Identify any concurrent or recent other ENT symptoms or respiratory conditions.

Physical Examination

Examine the external ear structures. Manipulate the external ear to identify any tenderness before inserting the otoscope speculum. Examine the canal for masses or swelling. Observe the TM to detect any dullness, decreased light reflex, bulging, retraction, or inflammation, which may indicate fluid or infection.

Diagnostic Studies

Pneumatic otoscopy will assist in determining the presence of fluid in the middle ear.

The common causes of complaints of ear fullness are listed in Box 5-2.

Box 5-2

Common Causes of Ear Fullness

Ménière's disease
Infections (AOM, OE)
Otitis media with effusion
Allergies
Cerumen impaction or foreign body

DIFFERENTIAL DIAGNOSIS OF CHIEF COMPLAINTS: NOSE

Bleeding (Epistaxis)

Nosebleeds are a common complaint, with a variety of possible causes, and can occur at any age. Bleeding from the nose is bright red and often profuse, but can usually be controlled within a few minutes after applying pressure and cold. Bleeding deep in the inferior meatus may be more difficult to manage. Rarely do nasal polyps cause profuse bleeding, it is more likely to be vascular or tumor related. Nasal packing, and occasionally artery ligation, may be necessary to control the bleeding. Any unexplained, recurrent epistaxis warrants investigation and possible referral to an ENT specialist.

History

The past medical history should include medications the patient is taking that could be contributing, such as anticoagulants, aspirin, or NSAIDs, and the presence of other medical problems, such as hematologic disorders, or liver or vascular disease. Cocaine abuse is more common than might be expected and frequently causes epistaxis. There may be a need to explore this possibility with a patient. A complaint of recent trauma is a straightforward cause of epistaxis, and an x-ray should be taken to rule out fracture. Ask about frequent sinus infections and the use of nasal sprays, obtained by prescription or over the counter (OTC). Steroid or antihistamine nasal sprays can cause dryness, irritation, and bleeding. Ask whether this is the first episode of bleeding, and, if not, ask about the frequency at which it has occurred. Chronic epistaxis warrants referral to an ENT specialist to determine a structural or vascular cause. The history alone will often explain the bleeding.

Physical Examination

The physical examination should start with an inspection of the external nose for alignment and the presence of any skin lesions. If possible, the practitioner should try to visualize the nasal mucosa for redness, purulent discharge, or lesions, although visualization is difficult to accomplish with active bleeding.

Diagnostic Studies

X-rays or CT scanning of the nose and/or sinuses would assist in the diagnosis of fracture, infection, tumor, and polyps. Culture and sensitivity of nasal discharge could be taken for resistant infections. Complete blood count with differential, platelet count, and coagulation studies might be needed to rule out hematologic or vascular causes. A liver profile might be needed to identify a hepatic cause of the epistaxis.

Trauma

Bleeding accompanied by edema and asymmetry of the nose indicates a possible fracture, and x-rays of the nose are warranted. Ice and pressure on the sides of the nose usually will control the bleeding, at least temporarily. If not, packing or cautery may be necessary.

HISTORY

A history of a blow to the nose is given by the patient. If the cause of the trauma is not obviously reported by the patient, be alert for and inquire about any signs of abuse, particularly in women and children.

PHYSICAL EXAMINATION

Edema occurs rapidly after a blow to the nose and is obvious on visual inspection. There may be abrasions or lacerations present, and asymmetry is seen with fracture.

Diagnostic Studies.

An x-ray should be done to look for fracture. If the x-ray is positive for a fracture, the patient should be referred to the ENT and/or plastic surgeon.

Medication

Anticoagulant medications such as warfarin (Coumadin), heparin, or enoxaparin (Lovenox) are the most common medications to cause epistaxis. Other drugs that might cause bleeding include aspirin, NSAIDs, nasal sprays, and *Ginkgo biloba.*

HISTORY

A thorough medication history, including prescription and OTC/herbal preparations, will alert the practitioner to the cause of the epistaxis.

PHYSICAL EXAMINATION

Other than the nasal bleeding, the patient who is over-anticoagulated may have bruising over the body from everyday minor contusions, particularly on the limbs. Bleeding from the gums also is commonly seen with over-anticoagulation.

Diagnostic Studies.

If the patient is taking anticoagulants, a prothrombin time with international normalization ratio should be done.

Hematologic Disorders

The hematologic disorders that are likely to cause increased bleeding include thrombocytopenia, leukemia, aplastic anemia, and hereditary coagulopathies. Multiple hematologic disorders can be seen with liver disease, including anemia, thrombocytopenia, leukopenia, leukocytosis, and impaired synthesis of clotting factors causing increased prothrombin time.

HISTORY

A history of hematologic disorders will quickly point the practitioner toward the cause of the bleeding. Ask the patient about easy bruisability, fatigue, shortness of breath, fever, or frequent infections. Inquire as to a personal or family history of liver disease and about EtOH use and/or abuse. Determine whether there are any risk factors for hepatitis.

PHYSICAL EXAMINATION

Except for the epistaxis, the physical exam may be unremarkable. The patient could have fever, bruising, or petechiae that might indicate leukemia, thrombocytopenia, or coagulopathies. A rapid heart rate and/or heart murmur may be present with longstanding anemia. Check for any signs of cyanosis around the lips or nails. Check for brisk capillary refill. Examine the abdomen for hepatomegaly or ascites, which would indicate liver disease.

Diagnostic Studies.

If hematologic disorders are suspected, a CBC, platelet count, liver profile, and coagulation studies should be done. A bone marrow aspiration may need to be performed by the hematologist/oncologist to confirm the diagnosis.

Intranasal Drug Use

The clinician should be mindful of not stereotyping individuals whom he or she believes may or may not be at risk for cocaine abuse. Such abuse can run the gamut of socioeconomic class, age, and gender.

HISTORY

A history of any kind of illegal drug use or alcohol abuse should alert the practitioner to the possibility of cocaine use. Patients often are not forthcoming with information about drug use, so an astute practitioner should be alert for personality changes and other signs and symptoms that might raise a suspicion for cocaine use.

PHYSICAL EXAMINATION

Typical symptoms associated with cocaine use are tachycardia, tachypnea, elevated blood pressure, arrhythmias, dilated pupils, nervousness, euphoria, hallucinations, and friability of the nasal mucosa leading to epistaxis. An overdose may lead to tremors, seizures, delirium, respiratory failure, and cardiovascular collapse.

Diagnostic Studies.

A drug screening should be performed for those suspected of cocaine abuse. Electrocardiogram, blood pressure monitoring, and pulse oximetry may be necessary until the heart and respiratory rates and blood pressure return to a normal range.

Mucosal Dryness, Irritation, and Infection

Dry climates, especially during the winter months, may cause nasal mucosal irritation and bleeding. The bleeding is usually scanty rather than profuse, as might be seen with other causes of epistaxis. Over-the-counter nasal sprays and corticosteroid or antihistamine nasal sprays can lead to a drying of the mucosal lining of the nose and may cause bleeding. Infection, particularly if it has been recurrent or chronic, can lead to sinus and mucosal inflammation and irritation resulting in bleeding. Again, the bleeding tends to be scanty rather than profuse unless the infection is severe enough to erode the mucosal surface.

HISTORY

For those living in a dry climate, a history of outdoor work or hobbies or a work or home environment without a humidifier may lead to mucosal dryness. Ask about a history of sinus infections, fever, sinus pressure or pain, and purulent nasal discharge. With irritation and infection, the patient will usually report that the bleeding is caused or aggravated by blowing of the nose.

PHYSICAL EXAMINATION

Dry crusting found in the nares, along with areas of irritation, may indicate the etiology of the bleeding. Infections cause the nasal mucosa to look beefy red, and there may be areas that are raw and bleeding. With infection, there are usually objective findings of fever, sinus tenderness on palpation and/or percussion, decreased or absence of light with transillumination, and purulent discharge.

Diagnostic Studies.

The diagnosis can be made by the history and physical. Sinus x-rays or CT scanning may be necessary with treatment failure but are not always necessary for initial diagnosis and treatment.

Vascular Disorders

The most serious vascular etiology of epistaxis is Rendu-Osler-Weber disease, also known as hereditary hemorrhagic telangiectasia, an autosomal-dominant, hereditary disease caused by vascular malformation. It affects both men and women. It can cause severe recurrent epistaxis resulting from arteriovenous aneurysms in the mucous membranes. A less-common vascular cause is hypertension, particularly uncontrolled or episodic hypertension.

HISTORY

A thorough family history is essential to uncover the hereditary disease Rendu-Osler-Weber. The patient may give a history of recurrent, profuse nosebleeds. In hypertension, the patient may give a family or personal history of elevated blood pressure. Often these patients will admit to noncompliance with the recommended medical regimen, or they may be unaware of their hypertension. Occasionally, there may be complaints of headache, lightheadedness, and pounding or swishing sounds in the ears.

PHYSICAL EXAMINATION

Hypertension is easily uncovered with blood pressure measurement. In Rendu-Osler-Weber, small telangiectatic lesions on the face, lips, oral, nasal mucosa, fingertips, and toes are characteristic. The nosebleeds are profuse. Similar lesions occur internally in the mucosa of the GI tract, which can cause major GI bleeding.

Diagnostic Studies.

Diagnosis is usually made by history and physical exam. In Rendu-Osler-Weber, lab studies are normal except an iron deficiency anemia, which may be severe. For hypertension, blood chemistries and renal studies, including 24-hour urine for catecholamines, should be done to rule out kidney or adrenal disease.

Malignant Nasal and Sinus Tumors

The most common cancers seen in this area are squamous cell carcinomas. Less-common types in this area include adenocarcinoma, melanoma, sarcoma, and lymphoma. Neoplasias are most commonly seen in the nasopharynx, causing nasal obstruction and otitis media, but are also seen in the paranasal sinuses. Patients are often asymptomatic until late in the course.

HISTORY

Patients will often complain of persistent unilateral nasal, sinus, or ear congestion and/or pain that have failed symptomatic and antibiotic treatment. This is a red flag and warrants further investigation.

PHYSICAL EXAMINATION

The patient will commonly complain of nasal discharge, which may be unilateral. Sinus pain, and bleeding from the nose, particularly if it is unilateral, should alert the practitioner to the need for diagnostic studies. In advanced disease, there may be obvious swelling of the cheek or around the eye.

Diagnostic Studies.

Magnetic resonance imaging or CT scanning is needed to define the extent of the tumor. Biopsy is necessary to confirm the diagnosis and the type of neoplasm.

Congestion and/or Drainage

Nasal congestion with associated drainage is one of the common complaints seen in the family practice setting. It is common in the winter months with the concomitant increase in upper respiratory infections. Complaints of congestion and drainage in the fall and spring may be due to allergies, and a thorough history and physical exam will assist the practitioner in differentiating infection from allergy.

History

As with any history, start with the beginning of the symptoms, their frequency, persistence, and progression. Ask about the presence of fever and about the color and consistency of the mucous drainage. Persistent fever and thick, yellow-green mucus are indicative of bacterial infection. Inquire about allergies to plants and animals and about environmental exposures to chemicals or noxious fumes. Explore related symptoms, such as sore throat, ear pain, headache, or cough. Ask about the presence of facial and/or sinus pain, which might indicate impacted sinuses. Occasionally, patients will complain that their upper teeth hurt, which may indicate dental disease or sinus infection because the maxillary sinuses are located just above the upper teeth. Include questions regarding exposure to family members or coworkers with similar symptoms, and whether they are being treated.

Physical Examination

Vital signs are a good place to start looking for fever, which would indicate infection. Inspect the nasal mucosa with the nasal speculum as you look for septal deviation or lesions, redness, irritation, friability, and discharge. Nasal discharge should be assessed for its amount and color and any associated symptoms. Clear profuse discharge is allergic in nature; yellow-to-green purulent discharge indicates infection. Percuss the sinuses for tenderness. Impacted sinuses may require referral to the ENT. Examine the pharynx, ears, lungs, and lymph system in the head and neck.

Common Cold

Differentiating a cold, which is viral, from a true bacterial infection of the sinuses is one of the more challenging diagnostic exercises for any practitioner. The similarity of symptoms between viral and bacterial illnesses, accompanied by the patient expectation that antibiotics will cure all things, can make management difficult.

HISTORY

Aside from the history previously described, the practitioner should pay close attention to the duration and severity of the symptoms, along with the degree of malaise. If the patient experienced malaise and fever initially but feels well aside from the congestion, then it is likely viral in nature and generally can be successfully managed with antihistamines, decongestants, and cough suppressants.

A history of honey-colored sinus drainage following head trauma is a red flag warning because it may indicate a skull fracture.

PHYSICAL EXAMINATION

As previously detailed, the exam should include inspection of the nose, pharynx, ears, and transillumination of the sinuses. The sinuses should be percussed for tenderness, and the lymph nodes palpated for tenderness or enlargement. Auscultation of the chest is always necessary to rule out an accompanying respiratory infection. A physical exam that reveals no fever, TM dullness or redness, sinus pain, sinus tenderness, or chest congestion is likely viral.

Diagnostic Studies.

Sinus x-rays may be helpful to rule out sinusitis, but otherwise the diagnosis can usually be made with history and physical.

Sinusitis

Bacterial sinusitis is more common in persons with a long-term history of sinusitis, allergies, and asthma, with or without a history of smoking.

HISTORY

The patient will give a history of fever, frontal headache, severe sinus congestion, often sinus and ear pain and/or pressure, difficulty breathing, sore throat, purulent nasal discharge, and malaise. Inquire about the duration and severity of the symptoms. Viral illnesses generally run their course in 5–7 days; bacterial will worsen with time. A complaint of maxillary sinus pain without discharge is likely to be dental in origin. Examine the mouth and teeth for any obvious gum infection, or decayed or abscessed teeth. Significant periodontal infection puts the patient at risk for bacterial endocarditis, and antibiotics should be prescribed along with a prompt dental referral.

PHYSICAL EXAMINATION

The exam coincides with the preceding subjective information and may reveal fever; inflamed nasal mucosa; thick, colored discharge; sinus tenderness; an accompanying dull or inflamed tympanic membrane; and perhaps cervical lymphadenopathy.

Diagnostic Studies.

Simple sinusitis can be diagnosed by history and physical. Recurrent sinusitis or persistent sinusitis after a course of antibiotics should be further investigated with sinus x-rays or CT scanning of the sinuses. Complete blood count may confirm a bacterial cause, and a culture and sensitivity test of the nasal discharge may identify the organism responsible for chronic infections. Often, polyps are present, causing recurrent or prolonged symptoms. Tumor may be present, requiring prompt referral to the ENT. In extreme cases, chronic sinus infection can cause bone erosion and sinus or brain abscess.

Allergies

Allergies are more common in the fall and spring especially in damp, warm climates where foliage is thick and present year around. In tropical climates, mold may be present in homes and buildings, thereby causing allergy symptoms. Pets, especially cats, are commonly responsible for a patient's allergy symptoms, especially if they are new pets. People often become desensitized to pets that are in the house for long periods, but introducing a new pet may cause or exacerbate allergy symptoms.

HISTORY

A thorough history is necessary to determine the cause of the allergy, if possible. Plants, foods, and animals are the most common.

PHYSICAL EXAMINATION

With an allergic etiology, the patient may complain of fatigue, but will not have fever. The nasal mucosa will be boggy and pale, rather than inflamed. The nasal discharge will be clear and watery rather than purulent and yellowish green. The patient may complain of sore throat resulting from postnasal drip, and there may be a cobblestone look to the posterior pharynx. Ear congestion may be present. Sinus tenderness should not be present.

Diagnostic Studies.

RAST (radioallergosorbent test) studies performed on the blood will indicate the increased eosinophilia that is associated with allergies, and the use of skin testing will identify specific allergens.

Loss of Smell

A change in olfaction can accompany any of the conditions related to nasal congestion, or it can be a more serious problem related to injury to CN I from trauma or tumor.

Signs and Symptoms.

A closed head injury along with a complaint of the loss of smell may indicate an injury in the area of CN I. Other neurological complaints will likely be present because, in a closed head injury, it would be rare to have injury only to this small portion of the brain. In a patient without a history of trauma, an isolated complaint of olfactory changes without any accompanying symptoms of cold, allergies, or sinus congestion is a red flag finding suggesting a brain tumor. Brain tumors can cause either a decrease in olfaction or, in some cases, olfactory hallucinations. A complaint of a headache along with olfactory changes increases the index of suspicion for a tumor etiology.

Diagnostic Studies.

A CT or MRI of the head is necessary to determine the presence of a tumor. A thorough neurological exam should be performed to detect other neurological abnormalities.

See Chapter 14, on the neurological system, for a more in-depth discussion.

DIFFERENTIAL DIAGNOSIS OF CHIEF COMPLAINTS: MOUTH

Mouth Sores (Painful and Painless)

Many conditions manifest themselves with lesions on the lips and/or oral mucosa. Most of these are self-limiting conditions, such as aphthous ulcers, whereas others, such as Behçet's syndrome and oral cancers, can result in significant morbidity if not recognized and treated promptly. Oral lesions associated with pain can be very distressing to patients. Labial lesions (those on the lips) cause distress because they are obvious and difficult to conceal. Painful lesions, both on the lips and in the mouth, can significantly impair a patient's ability to take food and fluids by mouth. A diagnosis of herpes simplex can be very upsetting to a patient because of the association with herpes simplex and genital findings, as well as the chronicity of the condition.

History

When a patient presents with mouth sore(s), it is helpful to determine whether pain is associated with the lesion(s) early in the history, as certain conditions are more likely than others to cause painful lesions. It is important to obtain a thorough analysis of the symptom, including when the lesion was first noticed, whether the lesion's appearance was preceded by other symptoms, and whether there is a history of similar symptoms in the past. It is important to identify any associated symptoms, including fever, malaise, joint pain, shortness of breath, nausea, vomiting, diarrhea, photosensitivity, and so on. Identify any chronic or coexisting conditions, as well as any prescribed or OTC medications taken.

Physical Examination

The physical examination should include measurement of vitals signs, particularly noting the presence of fever. A thorough assessment of the specific lesion(s) should be performed, noting the type of lesion involved (ulcer, vesicle, papule, and so on), as well as the dimensions, coloring, shape, distribution, and other details. The surrounding tissue should be closely inspected, noting any edema, erythema, or pallor. A thorough examination of the entire oral mucosa is necessary, with careful palpation of all accessible areas to note indurations, thickenings, nodules, or other palpable changes. Cervical lymph nodes should be palpated. Depending on the patient's presenting history and findings, examination may include other systems.

Diagnostic Studies

For most mouth sores, diagnostic studies are not indicated. However, lesions can be cultured to provide definitive diagnosis of candida, herpes simplex, or other infectious causes. Biopsies may be indicated to diagnose or rule out malignancy.

Painful Mouth Sores

APHTHOUS ULCERS

The cause of aphthous ulcers is unclear. A number of theories exist, including infection, stress, and food sensitivities. They occur recurrently in some individuals. Episodes are self-limited. Onset is often in childhood.

Signs and Symptoms.

The ulcers are painful and usually small (less than 1 cm). The patient often has history of previous ulcers, which healed in approximately 1 week. The ulcer is shallow, surrounded by erythema and mild edema. The base of the ulcer is pale yellow or gray. Often only one ulcer is present, although patients may have multiple ulcers. On occasion, patients experience larger ulcers, which take longer to heal and are associated with increased pain. See Figure 5-10.

Figure 5-10. ■ Aphthous ulcer. (From Dillon, P.M. Nursing health assessment: A critical thinking, case studies approach. Philadelphia: F.A. Davis, 2003. Reprinted with permission)

Diagnostic Studies.
None are warranted. Occasionally, the ulcers can be cultured to rule out herpes simplex.

HERPES SIMPLEX
Orolabial ulcers are often caused by herpes simplex type 1 virus.
Signs and Symptoms.
The patient often complains of a history of intermittent mouth sores, with onset as a youth. The ulcers are typically preceded by a prodromal phase of tenderness, followed by edema at the site where an individual or cluster of vesicles forms and progresses to ulceration. The prodromal phase may also include malaise and fever. The vesicles have an erythematous base, and the ulcerated lesion often becomes crusted.
Diagnostic Studies.
None are usually warranted. The vesicles can be cultured for definitive diagnosis; a Tzanck smear can be performed in the office for rapid diagnosis.
Herpes Zoster Herpes zoster has been previously described in Chapter 2. Compared with other painful mouth lesions, herpes zoster typically occurs in older individuals. Because the virus affects a dermatome, there are usually extraoral findings and complaints.
Chemical and Thermal Burns As with any of the integument, the oral mucosa is at risk for chemical and thermal burns. The history is extremely important to identify whether the patient has been exposed to chemical agents or to a thermal source that would have resulted in the painful lesion. The distribution of the lesion(s) should be consistent with the history of exposure.

HAND-FOOT-AND-MOUTH DISEASE
Hand-foot-and-mouth disease is caused by a coxsackievirus. Outbreaks are most common in the summer and fall months. On occasion, the condition is associated with meningitis.
Signs and Symptoms.
Skin and oral lesions are often preceded by a period of malaise and fever. The patient often presents once the oral lesions appear on the lips and/or oral mucosa. The lesions erupt as vesicles, which later ulcerate. Multiple lesions are located on the lips and oral mucosa. As the condition's name implies, the lesions often appear on the hands and feet, as well as in the mouth. Lesions may also be evident on the genitalia and buttocks.
Diagnostic Studies.
Diagnostic studies are not usually warranted. The patient's hydration status should be monitored, if the lesions impair ability to take food and/or fluids by mouth.

CANDIDIASIS
Candidiasis is caused by a species of the fungal genus *Candida*. Risk factors for candidiasis include an impaired immune system, antibiotic therapy, malignancy, and recent surgery or trauma. Candidiasis affects a variety of systems and tissues, including the oral mucosa.
Signs and Symptoms.
Candidal infections of the oral mucosa take several forms. Thrush, or pseudomembranous candida, results in white patches or plaques overlying a very red base. Erythematous candida results in erythematous lesions and, on occasion, ulcerative lesions. Angular stomatitis results in lesions at the corners or angles of the mouth. The amount of associated pain is variable.

Diagnostic Studies.

Studies are not usually necessary, as the diagnosis is based on the findings. Fungal cultures can be used to isolate the specific organism.

BEHÇET'S SYNDROME

Behçet's disease is referred to as a syndrome because it involves a variety of problems, including oral lesions. Other findings that are characteristic of the condition include uveitis, arthralgia, genital lesions, and nongenital skin lesions. The condition affects males more often than females and is more common in young adults. Although rare, Behçet's can lead to significant morbidity and the patient should be referred to a specialist for definitive diagnosis and treatment if the condition is suspected.

Signs and Symptoms.

The patient complains of recurrent episodes of oral lesions that are consistent with aphthous ulcers. The size of the ulcers varies from less than to greater than 1 cm. Like aphthous ulcers, the lesions are well defined, with a pale yellow or gray base surrounded by erythema. The number of lesions ranges from one to several. The majority of patients also develop lesions on the genitals or other skin. Eye findings are varied, and include conjunctivitis, keratitis, uveitis, and others. The condition can, over time, lead to decreased visual acuity and blindness. A number of other miscellaneous findings and/or complaints are possible and include the gastrointestinal, musculoskeletal, neurological, and cardiovascular systems.

Diagnostic Studies.

There is no definitive laboratory test specific to Behçet's. Patients may have anemia, leukocytosis, elevated sedimentation rate, or elevated C-reactive protein. Rheumatoid factor and/or antinuclear antibody tests are negative.

ORAL LICHEN PLANUS

The exact cause of lichen planus is not known. The condition causes inflammatory changes in the mouth, with the development of mucosal changes that are primarily white in color. The condition is most common in adults older than 40 years of age. Although the relationship between lichen planus and oral cancers is not clear, there is a slight increased risk of malignancy in patients with lichen planus.

Signs and Symptoms.

The oral mucosa develops a variety of white lesions, ranging from papules, plaques, and patches. Erythemic and/or erosive lesions develop, often affecting the buccal mucosa. Although pain is not always an early symptom, many patients do complain of discomfort at the affected sites when, for instance, spicy foods are eaten. The more inflammatory and erosive lesions are usually painful. Episodes of lichen planus are often recurrent. Some patients develop extraoral pruritic skin lesions of the extremities, genitalia, and/or scalp, as well as nail changes. See Figure 5-11.

Diagnostic Studies.

Diagnostic studies are often not required. However, biopsies can be performed to rule out malignancy and to provide definitive diagnosis.

Erythema Multiforme Erythema multiforme is described in detail in Chapter 2. Oral lesions are common manifestations of erythema multiforme, ranging from shallow, crusted lesions of the lips, to deeper ulcerations of the lips and oral mucosa. Depending on the severity, lesions may have a necrotic appearance.

Figure 5-11. ■ Oral lichen planus. (From Dillon, P.M. Nursing health assessment: A critical thinking, case studies approach. Philadelphia: F.A. Davis, 2003. Reprinted with permission)

Infectious Causes of Oral Lesions In addition to the infections noted above, many others have painful oral mucosal manifestations. These include gonorrhea and chicken pox.

Noninfectious Systemic Conditions A wide range of systemic conditions are associated with oral lesions. Included are Crohn's disease, ulcerative colitis, anemia, and sarcoidosis. It is important to explore the potential other symptoms when the patient presents with unexplained oral lesions.

Painless Oral Lesions

LEUKOPLAKIA

The cause of most episodes of leukoplakia is not determined. However, this condition, which results in the development of white patches on the oral mucosa, is associated with an increased risk of oral squamous cell cancer. Risk factors for the development of leukoplakia include chronic/recurrent trauma to the affected site, as well as the use of smokeless and smoked tobacco and alcohol.

Signs and Symptoms.

The lesions are painless, so the patient will usually have noticed the lesion after looking in the mouth. Some lesions become rather "warty" and raised, and thus a patient can feel the lesion's presence. However, most are flat and smooth. Unlike thrush, these lesions cannot be rubbed or scraped away. See Figure 5-12.

Diagnostic Studies.

The diagnosis is usually made based on the history and physical. However, biopsy should be considered to rule out dysplasia.

Figure 5-12. ■ Leukoplakia. (From Dillon, P.M. Nursing health assessment: A critical thinking, case studies approach. Philadelphia: F.A. Davis, 2003. Reprinted with permission)

ERYTHROPLAKIA

Because erythroplakia is so frequently associated with malignancy, its causes are believed to be the same as those of oral squamous cell cancer. These lesions often coexist with leukoplakia, either in the form of "speckled leukoplakia," where leukoplakia lesions are superimposed on larger erythemic lesions, or the two lesions coexist.

Signs and Symptoms.

These lesions are painless, so the patient may not notice the lesion unless she or he has inspected the oral mucosa for some reason. The lesions are usually nonraised/flat and often have a velvety texture. Some erythroplakia lesions are "pebbly," with raised areas. The red lesions vary in size and are often very well demarcated.

Diagnostic Studies.

Biopsies are obtained on referral to a specialist, for definitive diagnosis and removal or destruction of the lesion.

MALIGNANCY

The most common form of oral cancer is squamous cell cancer. Most lesions occur on the lips or along the lateral aspects of the tongue. However, other forms of malignancy, including malignant melanoma, do affect the oral mucosa, and any of the tissue in the oral cavity can be involved. Because many oral cancers are not diagnosed until they are quite advanced, the prognosis can be poor.

Signs and Symptoms.

Most oral malignancies are painless until quite advanced, so patients are often unaware of the lesion unless the lip or anterior portion of the tongue is involved. The patient may become aware of the lesion if it bleeds. Squamous cell cancer lesions vary in appearance, from the reddened patches of erythroplakia to areas of induration/thickening, ulceration, or necrotic lesions. Lesions of malignant melanoma have varied pigmentation, including brown, blue, and black. Even lesions that appear flat and smooth may be nodular, indurated, or fixed to adjacent tissue on palpation. Even though patients with squamous cell malignancies often have a history of heavy alcohol use, tobacco use, or poor dentition, these are not risk factors for malignant melanoma. The regional lymph nodes may be enlarged and/or nodular. See Figure 5-13.

Diagnostic Studies.

Oral malignancy is diagnosed by biopsy.

KAPOSI'S SARCOMA

Kaposi's sarcoma is a vascular tumor that is often associated with HIV. It is believed that herpes virus is implicated in the development of this condition.

Figure 5-13. ■ Cancer of the tongue. (From Dillon, P.M. Nursing health assessment: A critical thinking, case studies approach. Philadelphia: F.A. Davis, 2003. Reprinted with permission)

Signs and Symptoms.

Like the other oral malignancies described in the preceding subsections, the lesions of Kaposi's sarcoma are usually painless. The lesions most commonly occur on the palate, which is not easily seen by the patient, although it can occur on any of the oral mucosa. Initially flat, the lesions often become nodular with time. The coloring of the lesions is consistent with a vascular tumor and range from deep reddish brown to purple. The patient may provide history of HIV.

Diagnostic Studies.

Diagnosis is made by biopsy.

DENTURE OR ORTHODONTIC DERMATITIS

Individuals wearing dentures and orthodontic devices are at risk for developing oral lesions, which may be related to an allergic reaction to a component of the device, or from chronic rubbing and irritation from the device.

Signs and Symptoms.

These lesions may result in mild discomfort or be painless. The history and physical findings should be consistent with use of the appliance that has caused the irritation.

Diagnostic Studies.

No diagnostic studies are indicated.

Mouth Pain Without Obvious Lesions

On occasion, patients present with mouth pain yet have no visible lesions. In this case, the history should be directed to a careful analysis of the pain from the time it was first noticed. A thorough review of systems is necessary, as well as a history of present illness and medications taken. Ask the patient about recent trauma or previous episodes of similar pain.

A careful examination of the mouth should be conducted. Most patients experiencing mouth pain without the clinical signs to guide diagnosis should be referred to a dentist for dental imaging and assessment.

TOOTHACHE

Toothache can result from tooth decay, infection, fracture, and/or related abscess. The pain is related to nerve irritation, pressure, and inflammation or to periodontal injury.

Signs and Symptoms.

The patient typically complains of unilateral mouth pain and/or toothache. The pain may be worsened by hot or cold food or by chewing. The source of the discomfort may be evident on exam, such as from tooth decay, fracture, periodontal inflammation, or loss of a filling. The affected tooth may be loose. If abscess is involved, there will usually be marked edema and inflammation of the surrounding gum. Cervical lymphadenopathy may be present.

Diagnostic Studies.

No diagnostic studies are indicated. Dental images will usually be obtained by dentist on referral.

HERPES

Both herpes simplex and herpes zoster affect the oral mucosa. The appearance of skin lesions is often preceded by a prodromal phase that may include significant pain.

Signs and Symptoms.

Preceding an eruption of herpetic lesions, the patient with herpes simplex may report a history of recurrent painful mouth sores that are often preceded by discomfort. A patient who is developing herpes zoster may describe pain distributed along a specific dermatome. There may be some palpable induration and lymphadenopathy, particularly with herpes simplex infections. Mouth pain may be the presenting complaint in a patient who is experiencing postherpetic neuralgia after the visible signs of herpes zoster have resolved.

Diagnostic Studies.

There are no diagnostic studies warranted if either early herpes simplex or early herpes zoster is suspected. Follow-up should be arranged to confirm diagnosis.

PAROTITIS

Parotitis involves inflammation of the parotid salivary glands. The condition most commonly affects children, who often have recurrent episodes. The etiology is often uncertain, although some cases, particularly in adults, are caused with the development of salivary stones, which obstruct the outflow of saliva from the affected duct.

Signs and Symptoms.

The patient complains of painful swelling that is worsened by chewing. Fever may be present. There is an area of fullness or edema and often obvious redness and/or warmth. The parotid gland is extremely sensitive and any manipulation triggers pain. The patient's ability to fully open the mouth is often limited by swelling and pain. Pressure over the parotid gland may result in purulent matter expressed from duct.

Diagnostic Studies.

Diagnostic studies are usually not necessary. If the condition fails to respond to initial treatment, imaging should be performed for definitive diagnosis.

BURNING MOUTH SYNDROME

Burning mouth syndrome is characterized by burning pain of the oral structures. The onset is typically sudden and is sometimes variable through the day. The cause is uncertain, although there are several theories under consideration, including nutritional deficit, dry mouth, and emotional disorders.

Signs and Symptoms.

The patient complains of significant burning pain that may affect the ability to sleep or to focus on normal daily activities. Many patients also complain of altered taste. There are no visible clinical signs or abnormalities.

Diagnostic Studies.

The condition is a diagnosis of exclusion. The patient should be referred for specialist assessment.

DIFFERENTIAL DIAGNOSIS
OF CHIEF COMPLAINTS: THROAT
Sore Throat or Throat Pain

Sore throat is a very frequent complaint in primary care settings. Most episodes of sore throat are associated with self-limited viral upper respiratory infections, although there are a number of more serious causes.

History

The history should begin with a thorough analysis of the throat pain, including determining what is meant by "sore throat," which may be used to describe sensations ranging from a mild, scratchy sore throat to excruciating throat pain. In addition to determining the characteristics of the pain, identifying all associated symptoms is helpful in narrowing the differential diagnosis. It is important to identify any other recent illnesses, as well as recent exposures to others who are ill. Determine whether the patient is experiencing any dysphagia or respiratory difficulty.

Physical Examination

The physical examination for sore throat should include comprehensive assessment of the upper and lower respiratory systems, including ears, nose, mouth, throat, and lungs. The neck assessment should include, at a minimum, assessment of the cervical lymph nodes. A more-thorough neck assessment is indicated if carotidynia or thyroiditis is suspected.

Diagnostic Studies

Strep screens, throat cultures, and mononucleosis screens are common diagnostic studies used to narrow the differential diagnosis of sore throat. Complete blood counts with differential counts are helpful in determining the cause of sore throat.

INFECTIOUS PHARYNGITIS

Most cases of pharyngitis are viral in origin, and any number of the respiratory viruses can cause inflammation of the throat. The majority of viral pharyngitis cases are self-limited. Herpes infections can also affect the pharynx. Group A beta-hemolytic streptococcal (GABHS) pharyngitis is a bacterial infection of the pharynx, commonly referred to as strep throat. Complications of GABHS pharyngitis, although rare, include rheumatic heart disease and glomerulonephritis and the condition requires prompt diagnosis and definitive treatment. Most patients with GABHS pharyngitis are children and youths. Other bacterial causes of pharyngitis include mycoplasmal pneumonia, gonorrhea, and diphtheria.

Signs and Symptoms.

Because pharyngitis is most commonly caused by respiratory viruses, the complaints typically include malaise, headache, rhinitis, and/or cough in addition to the throat pain, which can range from mild scratchy discomfort to severe pain. The onset can be sudden, as with influenza, but symptoms may develop over many hours. Fever and chills may be present. In all cases of pharyngitis, the pharynx is reddened and tender lymphadenopathy is often present. Depending on the cause, other findings may be present. The findings associated with varied causes of non-GABHS pharyngitis are summarized in Table 5-3.

The classic symptom of GABHS is a severe sore throat, with sudden onset. The patient often also complains of nausea, vomiting, fever, headache, and malaise. Unlike other forms of pharyngitis, the patient does not usually experience rhinitis or cough. The patient often appears quite ill and lethargic. The findings of GABHS include very inflamed pharynx, uvula, and tonsils. The tonsils are enlarged, usually with a white or gray-white exudate. There is tender cervical lymphadenopathy. Although some patients with viral pharyngitis may have an exanthem, GABHS can present with a fine scarlatinal rash, often described as "sand paper" rash owing to the tiny, punctate pink-red lesions.

Diagnostic Studies.

With GABHS pharyngitis, a throat culture and/or rapid strep assay is positive. If monospot is performed to rule out mononucleosis, it is negative.

Table 5-3. ■ Differential Diagnosis of Infectious Pharyngitis

Cause	Onset	Associated Symptoms	Pharyngeal Signs	Anterior Lymphadenopathy
Respiratory Viruses	Variable	Headache, fever, chills, malaise, rhinitis, conjunctivitis, cough, nausea, diarrhea	Inflamed pharynx	Present
Herpes pharyngitis	Evolves with prodromal phase	Malaise, fever	Inflamed with ulcerative lesions	Present
Herpangitis or hand-foot-and-mouth disease	Evolves over few days	Malaise, lesions in mouth, on hands, feet, buttocks, and/or genitalia	Inflamed with ulcerative lesions	Present
Diphtheria	Evolves over 1–2 days	Headache, rhinitis, fever/chills, dysphagia, difficulty breathing	Inflamed pharynx with thick gray membrane	Present
GABHS	Sudden onset	Malaise, nausea/vomiting, headache, sand-paper rash. No rhinitis, cough, conjunctivitis, diarrhea	Inflamed uvula, pharynx, tonsils. White-gray tonsillar exudate	Present

MONONUCLEOSIS

Mononucleosis is usually caused by the Epstein-Barr virus (EBV), although it can result from other viruses. Even though complications are rare, they can lead to significant morbidity, as well as death. The potential list of complications is broad and includes hepatitis, splenic rupture, myocarditis, meningitis/encephalitis, and hemolytic anemia.

Signs and Symptoms.

The patient often complains of an onset over several days or more than a week. The sore throat may be preceded by prodromal symptoms that include malaise, generalized aches, and headache. Throat pain is usually severe and is associated with lymphadenopathy of the posterior cervical nodes, in addition to generalized lymphadenopathy. The pharynx is inflamed and the tonsils are usually involved, with inflammation and exudate that ranges from white to yellow or green. The pharynx is often very similar in appearance to that of GABHS. Petechiae over the palate are often identified. There frequently is a maculopapular generalized rash. Other skin changes may include jaundice. Whereas splenomegaly is common, hepatomegaly may also be present.

Diagnostic Studies.

The white blood cell count is increased, with an increased ratio of lymphocytes. A rapid monospot is often positive in the clinical setting. Liver function tests are often elevated. Depending on the degree of findings suggesting the development of one of the potential complications listed above, consultation of or referral to the appropriate specialist should be completed.

TONSILLITIS

Tonsillitis involves infection of the tonsils, usually by GABHS, although viral tonsillitis (often associated with EBV) is more common in very young children. Most cases of tonsillitis are diagnosed in school-aged children and adolescents. Patients can develop chronic tonsillitis and/or have frequent recurrences of the condition.

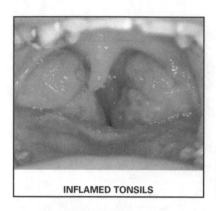

INFLAMED TONSILS

Figure 5-14. ■ Enlarged tonsils. (From Venes, D. Taber's cyclopedic medical dictionary. Philadelphia: F.A. Davis. Reprinted with permission)

Signs and Symptoms.

The patient presents with complaint of severe sore throat and difficulty swallowing. A fever is present and the patient appears ill. The patient is usually mouth breathing and has a deepened voice and may have difficulty articulating and moving the mouth because of the swelling and pain. The tonsils are edematous and have exudate that varies in color. If EBV is present, palatal petechiae may be visible. If herpes virus is present, tonsillar ulcerations are visible. Lymphadenopathy is present and the patient limits neck motion owing to pain. The history may reveal previous episodes.

Diagnostic Studies.

Definitive diagnosis is made by throat culture, rapid strep, and/or monospot test. See Figures 5-14 (enlarged tonsils) and 5-15 (exudative tonsillitis).

PERITONSILLAR ABSCESS

Peritonsillar abscesses may occur at any age, although most cases involve adults. Many cases evolve as a complication of tonsillitis, yet others develop as peritonsillar abscess without a history of tonsillitis. The condition involves infection of the peritonsillar space. A number of pathogens cause peritonsillar abscesses, although the most common cause is GABHS.

Signs and Symptoms.

The patient describes onset over several days of sore throat, fever, and malaise. Over time, the sore throat becomes very severe and localized to one side. It becomes increasingly difficult to move the neck, speak, and to swallow. The patient's breath is fetid and the patient is often drooling, unable to swallow saliva. Fever is present and respiratory distress

Figure 5-15. ■ Exudative tonsillitis. (From Dillon, P.M. Nursing health assessment: A critical thinking, case studies approach. Philadelphia: F.A. Davis, 2003. Reprinted with permission)

is possible. Pharyngeal examination can be very difficult, as the patient may have trismus, an inability to move the jaw due to the swelling. On examination of the pharynx, the area adjacent to the tonsil is swollen and the tonsil is often displaced and the uvula is deviated away from the site. The patient's voice is muffled. The tonsil may be enlarged, with exudate. There may be signs consistent with dehydration, including dry skin and tachycardia.

Diagnostic Studies.

The patient should be referred to a specialist, who may aspirate the abscess to obtain a culture or obtain a culture at the time of therapeutic incision and drainage. White blood count is elevated. An ultrasound or CT scan are used to confirm diagnosis.

EPIGLOTTITIS

Epiglottitis is rare, but it carries the potential for causing significant respiratory obstruction and death. The condition can occur at any age.

Signs and Symptoms.

The patient presents with the complaint of rapidly developing sore throat, fever, cough, and difficulty swallowing. The patient's voice is muffled and there is drooling. Stridor and/or varying signs of respiratory distress may be evident. The patient often assumes a posture of sitting while leaning forward, to maximize airway opening. The patient has a very ill appearance and gentle palpation over the larynx causes significant pain.

Diagnostic Studies.

The patient should be closely monitored for complete airway obstruction, but urgent referral for emergency care via an ambulance is indicated prior to performing any diagnostic evaluation, as the potential exists for sudden loss of airway. An ENT specialist should be informed to meet the patient at the emergency department.

THYROIDITIS

Painful subacute thyroiditis involves inflammation of the thyroid gland. It is a self-limiting condition. The condition includes a hyperthyroid phase, followed by a period of hypothyroidism, before the patient regains a euthyroid state. More women than men are affected. A variant, called postpartum thyroiditis occurs within six months of giving birth, is generally not associated with pain. Although the etiology of the painful subacute thyroiditis is not clear, it may have viral trigger.

Signs and Symptoms.

Patients commonly complain of pain in the throat and/or neck, with radiation to an ear. Onset is described as relatively sudden and associated symptoms include fever, malaise, and achiness. The throat pain may be associated with dysphagia. The patient may not complain of symptoms of hyper- or hypothyroidism during those phases; however, the severity of metabolic symptoms is quite variable. On physical examination, the thyroid region is very tender and enlarged.

Diagnostic Studies.

Depending on the phase during which diagnosis is made, thyroid studies may indicate an increase or decrease. Sedimentation rate is usually elevated. If radioactive iodine uptake is performed, uptake will be low. Thyroid antibodies may be elevated in painful thyroiditis.

CAROTIDYNIA

Carotidynia is a self-limiting condition with unknown origin.

Signs and Symptoms.

The patient presents with sudden onset of sore throat and/or unilateral neck pain. The pain may radiate to the jaw or ear on the affected side. The pain may be worsened or triggered by exposure to cold temperature or by chewing or neck movement. The patient is afebrile, and physical findings include a normal oropharynx. The thyroid is nonpalpable, and there is no lymphadenopathy. However, palpation along the course of the carotid is quite painful.

Diagnostic Studies.

No studies are indicated.

Hoarseness

While the causes of hoarseness are typically self-limiting, it is important to consider a range of potential causes: laryngeal growths; gastroesophageal reflux; vocal cord paralysis; and tumors of the larynx, lung, or mediastinum.

History

When a patient presents with complaint of hoarseness or voice alteration, it is important to obtain an explanation of how the voice has changed—whether in tone, volume, and so on. Determine whether the onset was sudden or gradual, as well as whether the change has been constant or intermittent. It is also essential to determine the patient's typical pattern of voice use, including whether any unusual use occurred before the onset of hoarseness. Examples of voice use would include singing, lecturing, shouting, and similar. The presence of associated symptoms, such as sore throat, neck pain, postnasal drainage, heartburn, and/or cough, is important. Identify use of alcohol and tobacco. Identify past medical history of such conditions as thyroid disorders, pulmonary disease, gastroesophageal reflux, and malignancy. Ask about previous surgical history, as well as any trauma to the neck or chest.

Physical Examination

The physical examination specific to a complaint of hoarseness should include the ears, nose, throat, neck, and lungs, as well as cranial nerves (particularly CNs IX and X). When hoarseness is persistent or laryngeal structural disorders are considered, laryngoscopy should be performed to view any redness, edema, motion, and masses or polyps.

Diagnostic Studies

Diagnostic studies are not warranted for most cases of hoarseness, but chest radiographs are recommended to rule out pulmonary or mediastinal masses when the symptom persists or in individuals with history of smoking.

OVERUSE

Voice overuse/stress is a common cause of hoarseness. It can occur at any age and may be a recurrent problem for patients who use their voice extensively in lecturing, singing, or speaking in loud environments.

Signs and Symptoms.

The patient provides history consistent with voice overuse or abuse. The hoarseness may tend to occur toward the end of the day and be better the next morning after some period of rest. The hoarseness may be associated with a sensation of muscle tension and/or discomfort in the neck. The physical findings are benign.

Diagnostic Studies.
   None are warranted.

POSTNASAL DISCHARGE

Postnasal discharge (PND) associated with allergies or upper respiratory infections can cause hoarseness. Hoarseness associated with PND is usually relieved by clearing the throat.
Signs and Symptoms.
   The patient complains of intermittent hoarseness with associated sensation of mucus or matter in the back of the throat. There may be mild to moderate throat discomfort associated with the drainage. The physical examination is usually benign, although there may be mild erythema and/or cobblestoning of the posterior pharynx and the PND may be present.
Diagnostic Studies.
   None are warranted.

Gerd

Gastroesophageal reflux can result in reflux laryngitis. GERD is described in Chapter 9.

Infectious Laryngitis

A number of pharyngeal and upper respiratory infections can also involve the larynx, resulting in hoarseness. The findings will be consistent with the descriptions in the foregoing sections.

VOCAL CORD PARALYSIS

Vocal cord paralysis can be caused by malignancies, trauma, surgery, infections, and neurological conditions.
Signs and Symptoms.
   The patient may complain of either a change in the character of the voice or in the intensity or volume. In addition to hoarseness, the patient may experience associated painless difficulty swallowing and respiratory stridor or dyspnea. The pharynx will appear within normal limits.
Diagnostic Studies.
   The patient should be referred to a specialist for diagnostic studies and definitive diagnosis. In addition to laryngoscopy, other diagnostic studies may include imaging, bronchoscopy, and/or esophagoscopy.

TUMOR AND MALIGNANCY

Hoarseness may result from squamous cell cancer of the larynx, as well as malignancies within the pulmonary tree, neck, and throat. The risk of malignancy as a cause for hoarseness is greatest in patients with a history of cigarette smoking and/or alcohol abuse.
Signs and Symptoms.
   The history usually reveals a progressive onset of hoarseness that has persisted for weeks. There is usually no associated pain. Other associated symptoms and physical findings will depend on the type of malignancy, although no abnormal findings may be evident on routine examination.
Diagnostic Studies.
   The patient with persistent hoarseness should be referred to a specialist for laryngoscopy, other diagnostic studies, and definitive diagnosis.

SUGGESTED READINGS

Bickley, L.S., & Szilagyi, P.G. (2003). *Bates' Guide to Physical Examination and History Taking*. Philadelphia: Lippincott, Williams, and Wilkins.

Dillon, P.M. (2003) *Nursing health assessment: A critical thinking, case studies approach*. Philadelphia: F.A. Davis.

Rubin, M.A., Gonzales, R., & Sande, M.A. (2005). Infections of the Upper Respiratory Tract. In Kasper, S.L., Braunwald, E., Fauci, A.S., Hauser, D.L., Longo, D.L., & Jameson, J.L. (Eds.). *Harrison's Principles of Internal Medicine*. New York: McGraw-Hill.

Isaacson, J.E., & Vora, N.M. (2003). Differential diagnosis and treatment of hearing loss. *American Family Physician*, 68, 1125–1132.

Lalwani, A.K., & Snow, J.B. (2005.) Disorders of smell, taste, and hearing. In Kasper, S.L., Braunwald, E., Fauci, A.S., Hauser, D.L., Longo, D.L., & Jameson, J.L. (Eds.). *Harrison's Principles of Internal Medicine*. New York: McGraw-Hill.

O'Handley, J.F., Tobin, E., & Tagge, B. (2001). Otolaryngology. In Rakel, R.E. (Ed.). *Textbook of Family Practice*. Philadelphia: Saunders.

Shohet, J.A., & Scherger, J.E. (1998). Which culprit is causing your patient's otorrhea? *Postgraduate Medicine*, 104 (3), 50–55.

Steyer, T.E., & Hueston, W.J. (2003). Otitis media and otitis externa. In Hueston, W.J. (Ed.). *20 Common Problems: Respiratory Disorders*. New York: McGraw-Hill.

Swartz, M.H. (2002). *Textbook of Physical Diagnosis: History and Examination*. Philadelphia: Saunders.

Temte, J.L. (2003). Pharyngitis. In Hueston, W.J. (Ed.). *20 Common Problems: Respiratory Disorders*. New York: McGraw-Hill.

Vincent, M.T., Celestin, N., & Hussain, A.N. (2004). Pharyngitis: Problem oriented diagnosis. *American Family Physician* 69 (6), 1465–1470.

Chapter 6

Cardiac and Peripheral Vascular Systems

Laurie Grubbs

CARDIAC SYSTEM

Cardiovascular disease (CVD) is the leader in all-cause morbidity and mortality across ages and genders. It accounts for approximately 5 million hospital admissions and over 800,000 deaths annually, not to mention lost work and reduced quality of life. Men are affected more than women especially before age 50 years. Cardiovascular disease often goes undetected, especially among females. Early detection and intervention can save many lives. Heart disease is one of the areas where advanced practice nursing can have a significant impact in terms of prevention, early detection, and treatment.

The New York Heart Association classifies heart disease into four functional categories according to the limitation on activity (Hurst, Morris & Alexander, 1999):

Class I: No limitation. Ordinary physical activity does not cause undue fatigue, dyspnea, or anginal pain.

Class II: Slight limitation. Ordinary physical activity results in symptoms.

Class III: Marked limitation. Comfortable at rest, but less than ordinary activity causes symptoms.

Class IV: Unable to engage in any physical activity without discomfort and symptoms are present at rest.

ANATOMY AND PHYSIOLOGY

Figure 6-1 illustrates the anatomy of the heart.

Heart Sounds

S_1, the closing of the mitral valve (in the following diagram, M_1) and the tricuspid (T_1) valve, together known as the atrioventricular valves.

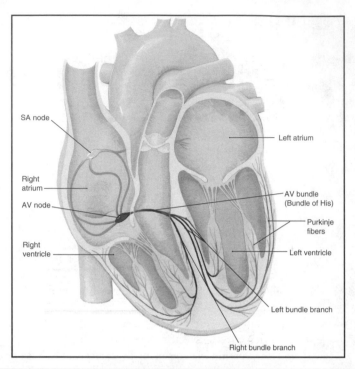

Figure 6-1. ■ Anatomy of the heart. (From Scanlon, V.C. & Sanders, T. Essentials of anatomy and physiology, 4th ed. Philadelphia: F.A. Davis, 2003. Reprinted with permission.)

S_2, the closing of the aortic (A_2) and pulmonic (P_2) valves, together known as the semilunar valves.

S_1 represents the beginning of systole; S_2 represents the beginning of diastole.

$$\underline{\quad}\frac{S_1}{M_1T_1}\underline{\quad}\text{systole}\underline{\quad}\frac{S_2}{A_2P_2}\underline{\quad}\text{diastole}\underline{\quad}\frac{S_1}{M_1T_1}\underline{\quad}\text{systole}\underline{\quad}\frac{S_2}{A_2P_2}\underline{\quad}\text{diastole}$$

Normally, the S_1 and S_2 occur as single sounds. There are conditions in which these sounds may be split and occur as two sounds. There are also conditions in which there are third and fourth heart sounds that occur under both normal and pathologic conditions. In healthy young adults, a physiologic split of S_2 may be detected in the second and third left interspaces during inspiration as a result of changes in the amount of blood returned to the right and left sides of the heart. During inspiration, there is an increased filling time and, therefore, increased stroke volume of the right ventricle, which can delay closure of the pulmonic valve, thus causing the second heart sound to be split. This physiologic split differs from other splits that are pathologic in origin because it occurs with inspiration and disappears with expiration.

Pathologic split heart sounds include the following.

- **Split S_1** may occur in right bundle branch block (RBBB), and with premature ventricular contractions (PVCs).

- **Fixed splitting of S$_2$** occurs with atrial septal defect and right ventricular failure.
- **Wide splitting of S$_2$** is associated with delayed closure of the pulmonic valve and can be caused by pulmonic stenosis and right bundle branch block, or by early closure of the aortic valve in mitral regurgitation.
- **Paradoxical splitting of S$_2$** occurs only on expiration and is associated with delayed closure of the aortic valve usually as a result of left bundle branch block (LBBB).

In addition to the first and second heart sounds, there are two additional heart sounds, S$_3$ and S$_4$, heard both in normal and pathologic conditions. Both S$_3$ and S$_4$ occur during diastole: an S$_3$ is heard early in diastole right after S$_2$, and an S$_4$ is heard in late diastole just before S$_1$. An S$_3$ can occur physiologically or pathologically depending on the age and disease status of the patient; an S$_4$ usually occurs under pathological conditions.

- **Physiologic S$_3$** is generally confined to children, young adults, and pregnant women as a result of rapid early ventricular filling. It is low pitched and is heard best at the apex or left sternal border with the bell of the stethoscope.
- **Pathologic S$_3$**, also referred to as a ventricular gallop, is heard in adults and is associated with decreased myocardial contractility, heart failure, and volume overload conditions as can occur with mitral or tricuspid regurgitation. The sound is the same as a physiologic S$_3$ and is heard with the patient supine or in the left lateral recumbent position.
- **S$_4$**, also referred to as an atrial gallop, occasionally occurs in a normal adult or well-trained athlete, but is usually due to increased resistance to filling of the ventricle. Possible causes of a left-sided S$_4$ include hypertension, coronary artery disease, cardiomyopathy, or aortic stenosis. Possible causes of a right-sided S$_4$ include pulmonic stenosis and pulmonary hypertension. Heard with the patient supine or in the left lateral recumbent position.

Other heart sounds may occur in pathological conditions and include opening snaps and pericardial friction rubs.

- **Opening snap** is caused by the opening of a stenotic mitral or tricuspid valve and is heard early in diastole along the lower left sternal border. It is high pitched and heard best with the diaphragm of the stethoscope.
- **Friction rubs** occur frequently after a myocardial infarction (MI) or with pericarditis. The sound is a high-pitched grating, scratching sound—resulting from inflammation of the pericardial sac—that issues from the parietal and visceral surfaces of the inflamed pericardium as they rub together.

The Cardiac Cycle

The cardiac cycle is diagramed in Figure 6-2. Blood is returned to the right atrium via the superior and inferior vena cava, and to the left atrium via the pulmonary veins. As the blood fills the atria during early diastole, the pressure rises until it exceeds the relaxed pressure in the ventricles, at which time the mitral and tricuspid valves open and blood flows from the atria to the ventricles. At the end of diastole, atrial contraction produces a slight rise in pressure termed the "atrial kick." As ventricular contraction begins, the rise in pressure in the ventricles exceeds that of the atria, causing the mitral and tricuspid valves to close. This closure produces the first heart sound (S$_1$). As ventricular pressure rises, it exceeds the pressure in the aorta and pulmonary artery, thus forcing the aortic and pulmonic valves to open. As the blood is ejected from the ventricles, the pressure declines until it is below that of the aorta and pulmonary artery, causing the aortic and pulmonic valves to close and thus

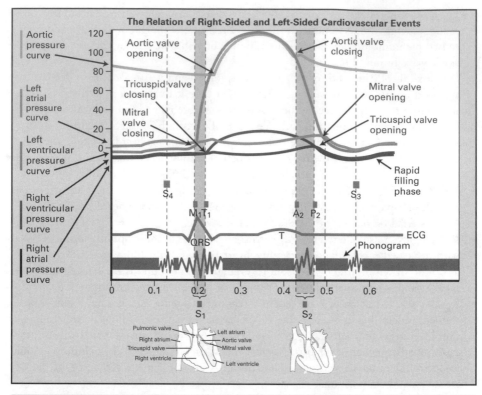

Figure 6-2. ■ The cardiac cycle and mechanisms of heart sounds. (From Dillon, P.M. Nursing health assessment: A critical thinking, case studies approach. Philadelphia: F.A. Davis, 2003. Reprinted with permission.)

producing the second heart sound (S_2). As the ventricles relax, the pressure falls below the atrial pressure, the mitral and tricuspid valves open, and the cycle begins again.

HISTORY
General History
In many instances, the history may be more telling than the physical exam. It is important to take a thorough history for signs and symptoms of heart disease, but also to alert the clinician to the need for lifestyle education or further evaluation in regards to smoking, a history of hypertension, exercise habits, diet, and professional and personal life behavior. Investigate any complaints of chest pain, pressure, or heaviness; left arm or jaw pain or numbness; dyspnea on exertion; cough; paroxysmal dyspnea; hemoptysis; syncope; palpitations; fatigue; or edema. Complaints indicating peripheral vascular disease also should be investigated, such as claudication, skin changes especially in the lower extremities, dependent edema, or pain. Determine the date of the last chest x-ray and electrocardiogram (EKG). Inquire about any comorbid conditions or other factors that may increase the patient's risk for heart disease and peripheral vascular disease (see Box 6-1).

> ### Box 6-1
> #### Risk Factors for Heart and Peripheral Vascular Disease
>
> Hypertension
> Smoking
> Diabetes
> Obesity
> Dyslipidemia
> Sedentary lifestyle
> Hostility
> Age >45 years for males and >55 years for females
> Gender: males and postmenopausal females
> Positive family history
> Increased C-reactive protein

Past Medical History

Past history of heart disease includes any previous diagnoses of congenital heart disease, murmurs, palpitations, arrhythmias, abnormal EKGs, unstable angina, MI, angiography, angioplasty, or coronary artery bypass graft.

Family History

Family history is particularly important for cardiac assessment because cardiovascular disease, hypertension (HTN), hyperlipidemia, and other vascular diseases often have a familial association that is not easily ameliorated by lifestyle changes. If there are deaths in the family related to CVD, determine the age and exact cause of death because CVD at a young age in the immediate family carries an increased risk compared with CVD in an elderly family member. Ask about sudden death, which might indicate a congenital disease, such as Marfan's. This is especially important to ask for pre-sports physicals because sudden death in athletes is often related to congenital or familial heart disease. Familial hyperlipidemia is autosomal dominant, and often leads to coronary artery disease (CAD) and MI at a young age. Family history of obesity and Type 2 diabetes are also secondary risk factors for heart disease because the familial tendency for these is strong. Ask about smoking in the house because second-hand smoke has been shown to be a risk factor for respiratory and cardiac disease.

Habits

The social history should include habits or behaviors that increase the risk for heart disease, include smoking, sedentary lifestyle, high-fat diet, drug or EtOH abuse, and stress.

PHYSICAL EXAMINATION
General Assessment

General signs of heart or circulatory disease include pallor, cyanosis, diaphoresis, edema, restlessness, and confusion. Vital signs should be thoroughly assessed. Blood pressure readings in the prehypertensive stage of 120–139/80–89 (Chobanian et al., 2003) should be further evaluated, and patients should be educated on lifestyle modifications. Heart rates above 90 may be seen in noncardiac conditions, such as fever, anxiety, pain, medication, thyroid disease, dehydration, anemia, or pulmonary disease, but if other clinical signs or symptoms are present, an EKG is warranted. Heart rates below 50 can be seen in young trained athletes, but otherwise, there should be a high index of suspicion for other causes, such as heart block, and an EKG is recommended. Any diminished or accentuated peripheral pulses, pulsus paradoxus (decreased pulse amplitude at the end of inspiration, associated with pericarditis), pulsus alternans (alternating weak and strong pulsation, associated with left ventricular failure), and a bisferious pulse (having two systolic peaks, associated with aortic regurgitation or hypertrophic cardiomyopathy) are indicative of valvular heart disease or tamponade. Jugular venous distention and hepatojugular reflux suggest an increase in right ventricular pressure. Wheezes, rhonchi, crackles, or any significant increase in respiratory rate should alert the examiner to the possibility of pulmonary disease or heart failure.

Inspection

A general inspection of the patient is necessary as one looks for any particularly short or tall stature, which may be associated with Turner's or Marfan's syndrome—both linked to congenital heart defects. Inspect the skin for changes in temperature, color, and ulcerations or sores that will not heal. Pallor, coolness, ulcerations, or hyperpigmentation of the extremities suggests arterial or venous insufficiency. Cyanosis of the nail beds or, in more severe cases, circumoral cyanosis suggests hypoxia. A red, ruddy complexion can be seen in HTN and in EtOH abuse. Inspect the skin around the eyes for xanthelasma seen in hyperlipidemia. Inspect the configuration of the chest, noting any thoracic scoliosis or pectus excavatum that may be associated with restrictive lung or cardiac disease. Inspect the respiratory rate and effort, looking for dyspnea. Inspect the point of maximal impulse (PMI) and the precordium for any visible heaves or lifts, seen in ventricular hypertrophy. The apical impulse is easily observed in the pediatric client but not always visible in the adult. An accentuated or displaced apical impulse may be indicative of ventricular hypertrophy. Inspect the neck for the jugular venous distention seen in right-sided heart failure.

Auscultation

Auscultation is generally the most useful part of the cardiac exam. First, identify the rate and rhythm of the heart. Identify S_1 (heard louder at the apex), and S_2 (heard louder at the base). Determine if these are heard as single sounds or if there are any splits. A physiologic split of the second heart sound is common and varies with respiration in that S_2 splits on inspiration and is heard as a single sound on expiration. This is due to changes in intrathoracic pressure during inspiration that cause increased filling time of the right ventricle and therefore increased stroke volume, and thus a slightly later closing of the pulmonary valve (P_2). Note any fixed splitting of the first and second heart sounds, which can occur in a variety of pathologic conditions, including right and left bundle branch block, premature ventricular contraction, right ventricular failure, atrial septal defect, pulmonic stenosis, and mitral regurgitation. Next, identify any extra sounds, such as an opening snap heard early in diastole in mitral or tricuspid stenosis, an early systolic ejection click heard in aortic or pulmonic stenosis, the mid-systolic ejection click of mitral valve prolapse, a ventricular gallop (S_3), or an atrial gallop (S_4), or a systolic or diastolic murmur. Auscultating the carotid arteries for bruits and amplitude is an important part of the cardiovascular exam. Audible bruits should be further evaluated with a carotid duplex scan to assess the amount, if any, of carotid artery stenosis or occlusion. Occlusion of the carotid artery should alert the examiner to the increased risk of stroke in these patients, and prompt referral should be made to the surgeon.

Palpation

It is important to palpate the precordium because palpation of a sustained apical or ventricular impulse can give information about heart size. A lift or heave caused by right ventricular hypertrophy can be palpated along the left sternal border, and a left ventricular lift or heave at the apex. Thrills associated with Grade IV, V, and VI murmurs are palpated over the precordium and are vibratory in nature. Palpate the carotid, femoral and dorsalis pedis arterial pulses for amplitude and regularity.

Percussion

Percussion of the heart borders is not often performed owing to its low sensitivity. However, in some conditions it may be useful—such as in pericardial effusion with or without cardiac tamponade—and especially in emergency situations when x-ray is not readily available. In addition, when the heart is either located or displaced to the right of the sternum, as in dextrocardia or tension pneumothorax of the left chest, percussion can be helpful.

CARDIOVASCULAR LABORATORY TESTS

Table 6-1 presents normal values for common laboratory tests used in assessment of the cardiovascular system, along with the significance of each test.

Table 6-1. ■ Cardiovascular Laboratory Tests

Lab	Normal	Significance
Test	Value	
LDH	45–90 U/L	An enzyme released when organ or tissue is destroyed, particularly myocardial tissue. Can also be elevated in hemolytic states, hyperthyroidism, renal disease, gastric malignancy, and megaloblastic anemia.
CPK	5–75 mU/mL	Elevated in MI, but not specific to myocardial damage. Also seen with skeletal muscle damage owing to excessive exercise or rhabdomyolysis.
CK-MB	0–3 µg/mL	A cardiac isoenzyme called myocardial band creatine kinase. It is most sensitive in detecting myocardial injury within the first 4 hours after onset of chest pain.
Troponin I (cTnI)	<0.35 ng/mL	This index is useful in the diagnosis of acute myocardial injury. After 4 hours, it is equally as sensitive as CK-MB up to 48 hours. Troponin I remains elevated longer than CK-MB and is more cardiac specific.

(Continued on following page)

Table 6-1. ■ Cardiovascular Laboratory Tests *(Continued)*

Lab Test	Normal Value	Significance
Troponin T (cTnT)	<0.2 µg/L	The sensitivity of Troponin T for detecting AMI is 100% from 10 hours to 7 days after onset. The sensitivity begins to decrease after 7 days.
Potassium (K⁺)	3.5–5.0 mEq/L	Most importantly, elevated K⁺ levels can cause ventricular fibrillation. Other changes in the EKG include: widened P waves, peaked T waves, widened QRS complex, depressed ST segment, and heart block. Decreased K+ can cause inverted T waves, U waves, and depressed ST segment.
Sodium (Na⁺)	135–145 mEq/L	Important for fluid balance particularly when dehydration may be an issue or in heart failure.
Calcium (Ca⁺)	8.5–10.6 mg/dL	The hypercalcemic effects on the heart include shortening of the QT interval, and AV block. The effect of hypocalcemia is prolongation of the ST segment.
Glucose	70–100 mg/dL	Changes in blood glucose can have indirect effects on the heart. Diabetes significantly increases the risk for MI and hyperlipidemia.
Creatinine	0.6–12 mg/dL	Renal disease may elevate BP, which, over time, will increase the risk for CVD. Also important when prescribing certain meds for HTN and CHF, particularly ACE inhibitors and diuretics.
Cholesterol	Total, <200 mg/dL LDL, <130 mg/dL HDL, >40 mg/dL	Increased total and LDL cholesterol and decreased HDL increase the risk for CAD. Cause may be inherited or acquired, secondary to obesity, thyroid disease, or high-fat diet.
Triglycerides	<200 mg/dL	Elevated levels increase the risk for heart disease.
TSH	0.4–4.2 mIU/L	In the elderly, hypothyroidism may contribute to the development of CHF. Hyperthyroidism may present as atrial fibrillation or other arrhythmias in patients over 50 years.
Hgb	11.5–15.0 g/dL	Anemia may be a cause or a result of many forms of heart disease.
Hct	34.0%–44.0%	Anemia may be a cause or a result of many forms of heart disease.
O₂ saturation	95%–97%	Pulse oximetry can be helpful in patients with severe myocardial damage and CHF to evaluate clinical status.

DIFFERENTIAL DIAGNOSIS OF CHIEF COMPLAINTS
Palpitations or Arrhythmia

The Conduction System

The conduction pathway of the heart begins in the sinoatrial (SA) node, travels through the atria to the atrioventricular (AV) node, the bundle of His, the bundle branches, the Purkinje fibers, and finally, to the ventricular muscle. When the electrical impulse travels normally through this pathway, it is considered a normal sinus rhythm (NSR), with a rate of 60–100 beats per minute, but perhaps lower in patients taking beta-blockers or in athletes.

Figure 6-3. ■ The electrocardiogram. (From Scanlon, V.C. & Sanders, T. Essentials of anatomy and physiology, 4th ed. Philadelphia: F.A. Davis, 2003. Reprinted with permission.)

The EKG

Following are the elements of the EKG (also see Figure 6-3).

- **P wave:** represents depolarization of the atria. The absence of P waves may indicate atrial fibrillation or an idioventricular rhythm.
- **P-R interval:** 0.12–0.20 second, measured from the beginning of the P wave to the beginning of the QRS. Prolongation of the P-R interval indicates a conduction delay producing first-, second-, or third-degree heart block. A shortened P-R interval is seen in Wolff-Parkinson-White and Lown-Ganong-Levine syndromes.
- **QRS duration:** 0.08–0.12 second. The QRS represents depolarization of the ventricles. A wide QRS is seen in conduction delays in the ventricles, such as with bundle branch blocks and complete heart block, and in ventricular ectopic beats, such as with PVCs.
- **T wave:** represents repolarization of the ventricles. Repolarization of the atria is not represented on the EKG tracing because it takes place within the QRS complex. Configuration should be upright. Myocardial ischemia, injury, and necrosis cause inversion of the T wave as a result of altered repolarization. Hyperventilation may also cause flipped T waves.
- **QT interval:** <0.05 seconds. Prolongation may result in syncope and sudden death.
- **QRS complex:** the amplitude of the R wave is decreased in MI owing to altered depolarization, decreased myocardial contractility, or in pericardial effusion.
- **S-T segment:** should be isoelectric. Myocardial injury causes elevations in the S-T

segment in the leads that reflect the area of injury and reciprocal S-T depression in the leads opposite the area of infarct.
- **Q wave:** represents death (infarction) of the muscle and is due to the absence of depolarization in dead tissue. A pathological Q wave measures >0.04 second and is $>^1/_3$ the height of the QRS.

Each small block on the EKG represents 0.04 second, and each large block represents 0.20 second.

History

Occasional palpitations occur physiologically in the majority of the population or as a result of other noncardiac conditions, such as anxiety, exercise, hyperthyroidism, and anemia. They can also occur with valvular heart disease, increased or decreased stroke volume, and arrhythmias. The patient may complain of palpitations or skipped beats, or an arrhythmia may be seen on EKG. Patients are often aware if their heart rate is slower or faster than normal, or if it is irregular. With some arrhythmias, patients may complain only of fatigue, shortness of breath, weakness, or syncopal episodes. These are common symptoms in patients who have atrial fibrillation, and, if the ventricular response is slow, the patient may be unaware of the arrhythmia. Ask the patient about the frequency and duration of the palpitations and the presence of any associated symptoms, such as loss of consciousness, lightheadedness, chest pain, shortness of breath, nausea, or vomiting.

Inquire as to any history of MI or valvular heart disease. In young women, mitral valve prolapse is a common cause of palpitations, which are benign in nature but are unsettling to the patient. Ask patients how long they have had the symptoms and whether they are constant or intermittent. Paroxysmal supraventricular tachycardia (PSVT) occurs intermittently and lasts anywhere from several seconds to several hours. Determine whether there is any chest pain because myocardial ischemia predisposes the patient to ventricular arrhythmias. Age and other risk factors are important to the history. Occasionally, young, healthy patients will have fairly frequent PVCs that are benign in nature, but warrant investigation to rule out serious causes.

Physical Examination

Although the EKG remains the major diagnostic tool, a thorough cardiac exam is necessary, including vital signs, carotid and jugular venous pulsation (JVP), as well as an examination of the extremities and peripheral vascular system.

Irregular Pulse

BRADYARRHYTHMIAS

A pulse rate of <60 bpm is considered bradycardia although many trained athletes normally have a sinus bradycardia. In an elderly or untrained individual, it is more concerning. The underlying cardiac history is of utmost importance. Sinus node pathology and heart blocks should be suspected in the elderly or in patients with underlying heart disease. A thorough medication history is also imperative because many medications, including many heart medications, can cause arrhythmias. Electrolyte imbalance, particularly potassium (K^+), should be excluded. A temporary or permanent pacemaker is often necessary for treatment of bradyarrhythmias. See Table 6-2 for common causes of bradyarrhythmias.

Table 6-2. ■ Common Causes of Bradyarrhythmias

Cause	Description
Sick sinus syndrome	This term is used to describe sinus arrest, sinoatrial block, and persistent sinus bradycardia of unknown origin. Often caused or exacerbated by drugs, particularly digitalis, calcium-channel blockers, beta-blockers, and antiarrhythmics.
First-degree heart block	This rhythm is characterized by a lengthening of the P-R interval >0.20 second.
Second-degree heart block • Mobitz Type I or Wenckebach • Mobitz Type II	In Mobitz Type I, the P-R interval progressively lengthens until a QRS complex is completely dropped, and the pattern is repeated. In Mobitz Type II, there is a regular P-R interval, and a QRS is absent on a regular interval.
Third-degree (complete) heart block	There is a complete dissociation between the atrial and ventricular rhythms. None of the electrical activity originating in the SA or AV node is being conducted through the ventricles. The atria continue beating at the normal rate while the ventricles are beating at rate of 30–40.
Interventricular conduction defect/bundle branch block	A condition in which the electrical impulse is slowed or blocked in one of the branches of the bundle of His. The right and left ventricles will not beat in complete synchronization, causing a widened and slightly delayed QRS.

Signs and Symptoms.

Fatigue and shortness of breath are common symptoms of bradyarrhythmias. In the elderly, weakness, confusion, and syncope may occur as cerebral perfusion is decreased due to decreased cardiac output. Congestive heart failure may ensue in elderly patients or patients who already have some degree of cardiac compromise.

TACHYARRHYTHMIAS

A pulse rate over 100 is considered tachycardia. Pulse rates increase with age, but a rate over 100 should be investigated. Tachycardia can be a result of many noncardiac conditions, including hyperthyroidism, respiratory disease, anemia and blood loss, illegal drugs, prescription medications, heat exhaustion, emotions, and exercise. The underlying cardiac history is also important to rule out a cardiac origin. See Table 6-3 for common causes of tachyarrhythmias.

Signs and Symptoms.

The symptoms vary greatly depending on the cause of the arrhythmia, the ventricular rate, and the cardiac output. Those with mild-to-moderate increases in ventricular rate may be asymptomatic. With higher rates, patients will complain of weakness, dizziness, syncope, and shortness of breath, and they may lose consciousness.

Diagnostic Studies for Bradyarrhythmias and Tachyarrhythmias

- EKG: An EKG is the first step in diagnosing arrhythmias. If the problem is intermittent, however, it may not show on a single EKG.
- Holter monitor: This device gives a continuous EKG reading for 24 hours or more and is useful in those arrhythmias that are paroxysmal.

Table 6-3. ■ Common Causes of Tachyarrhythmias

Cause	Description
Sinus tachycardia	When the heart rate is >100 bpm, but the impulse is via the normal sinus pathway, it is a sinus tachycardia. This is due to outside influences, such as fever, pain, anemia, volume depletion as in shock, or volume overload as in CHF, thyrotoxicosis, drugs, fear or other emotions, and exercise.
Supraventricular tachycardia	The heart rate ranges from 140 to 240 bpm and may last a few seconds to several hours. The usual mechanism is reentry, which is initiated by a premature atrial or ventricular beat involving dual pathways within the AV node. Most do not involve structural heart disease. SVT may be a result of digitalis toxicity. Patients may complain of dizziness, shortness of breath, or mild chest pain, or they may be asymptomatic except for the sense of a racing heart rate.
Ventricular tachycardia	The usual ventricular rate is 160–240 bpm and results in syncope owing to decreased stroke volume. The usual mechanism is reentry, which is initiated by a premature atrial or ventricular beat. Causes include MI, cardiomyopathy, myocarditis, and, occasionally, mitral valve prolapse.
Atrial fibrillation	Atrial fibrillation may or may not result in tachycardia. Although the atria are not beating regularly, there may be a controlled ventricular response. In some cases, there is a rapid ventricular response resulting in tachycardia.
Atrial flutter	In atrial flutter, the atrial rate is often over 250, but there is a variable ventricular response. In 2:1 or 3:1 flutter, the ventricular response may be close to normal and the patient may have few or no symptoms

- Electrolytes: An electrolyte panel, particularly to obtain the K^+ level, is necessary because problems with potassium balance can cause arrhythmias. Medications such as diuretics can lead to hypokalemia.
- Thyroid functions: TSH, T_3, and T_4 will alert you to thyroid disease as a cause for the arrhythmia.
- Medication levels: It may be necessary to draw blood levels of certain medications that can cause arrhythmias, for example, digoxin and theophylline. There are many other medications that may affect cardiac rhythms and patients' medication lists should be carefully reviewed.

Chest Pain

The coronary arteries supply blood to the heart muscle. A blockage in one of the coronary arteries results in decreased blood supply and, when the lesion becomes significant, myocardial ischemia and chest pain occur. Blockage in the right coronary artery (RCA) results in damage to the posterior/inferior area of the heart. Blockage in the left main coronary artery (LCA) results in damage to the atrial, apical, lateral, and septal areas and is usually fatal. Blockage in the left anterior descending artery (LAD) results in damage to the anterior portion of the heart. Blockage in the circumflex branch (CFX) results in damage to the posterior and lateral areas.

History

Any complaint of chest pain should be thoroughly investigated in all patients. Initially, determine whether the patient is having an acute episode of cardiac chest pain, and the need for emergent referral. Although it may be a low likelihood in certain seemingly young, healthy patients, a cardiac origin for the chest pain should always be kept on the list of differential diagnoses. Start by asking the patient about current medicines and comorbidities. Ask whether this is the first episode of chest pain that the patient has had or whether this is a recurrent attack. Ask how long the pain has been going on, whether it is constant or intermittent, and whether it radiates to either arm, back, neck, or jaw. Ask how long the pain lasts, what the pain is like, and where the level of pain lies on a scale of 0 to 10. Inquire about any associated symptoms, such as shortness of breath, sweating, dizziness, syncope, nausea, vomiting, palpitations, or cough. Is there anything that seems to bring the pain on or is it associated with certain activities, such as exercise, sexual intercourse, eating, sleeping, stress, or strong emotions. Be sure to inquire about sports or exercise activities that could have resulted in injury to the intercostal muscles, ribs, or chest wall. Ask about alleviating or aggravating factors and whether the patient is taking any kind of medicine for the pain, either prescription or over the counter, or any other alternative treatment.

Strong suspicion of a cardiac origin of the pain warrants prompt evaluation by a cardiologist or a referral to the emergency room. Characteristics that indicate angina include: crushing, substernal pain with radiation to the neck or left arm, a score of >7 on the pain scale, an association with exertion or stress with relief on rest, a duration of minutes and associated symptoms of nausea, diaphoresis, weakness, or shortness of breath (SOB).

Physical Examination

The physical exam is not definitive for ruling out myocardial infarction as the cause of the chest pain. Assess the patient's level of pain and any associated signs, such as changes in color, looking for any paleness or cyanosis, and the presence of dyspnea, diaphoresis, nausea, or vomiting. Listen to the heart and note any murmurs, arrhythmias, bradycardia, or tachycardia. Auscultate the lungs for rales/crackles or decreased breath sounds that might alert you to a pulmonary origin for the chest pain. If a pulmonary origin is suspected, percuss the lungs for any areas of dullness and assess for voice sounds. For any patients with obvious dyspnea, a pulse oximetry reading would give useful information. Palpate the chest wall for any tenderness. The EKG, chest x-ray, and cardiac enzymes are most helpful in determining whether there is a cardiac origin for the chest pain.

With angina and myocardial infarction, changes can be seen on the EKG. Each lead reflects an area of the heart, and EKG can determine the location of the ischemia. The lateral wall of the heart is reflected in Leads I, aVL, V_5, and V_6. The inferior wall is reflected in Leads II, III, and aVF. The anterior wall is reflected in Leads V_1, V_2, V_3, and V_4. The posterior wall is reflected in Leads V_1, V_2, and V_3. Reciprocal EKG changes can be seen in the area of the heart opposite the injured area.

ANGINA AND MYOCARDIAL INFARCTION

With a complaint of chest pain, the most life-threatening diagnosis should be ruled out first. A thorough history identifying the quality and quantity of the pain, alleviating and aggravating factors, and associated symptoms will assist in raising or lowering your index of suspicion for a myocardial origin of the pain. Also, the age, gender, weight, vital signs, family history, and past medical history will assist you in diagnosis.

Signs and Symptoms.

Signs and symptoms that are suspicious for myocardial ischemia include crushing substernal chest pain that may radiate into the neck or left arm, diaphoresis, nausea, shortness of breath, and, perhaps, weakness. Pain that increases with physical activity and disappears at rest can be indicative of myocardial ischemia. Pain that occurs in the early morning or wakes a patient at night can also be cardiac in origin. Pain at rest is worrisome as it may signify unstable angina.

GASTROESOPHAGEAL REFLUX (GERD) AND PEPTIC ULCER DISEASE (PUD)

It is often difficult to differentiate the pain of GERD or PUD from cardiac pain. A good history and diagnostic tests are necessary. Patients with a history of GERD or PUD should still be worked up for a cardiac origin, particularly if the characteristics of the pain or the history have changed to raise the index of suspicion for cardiac disease.

Signs and Symptoms.

The pain of GERD and PUD can be quite severe and anxiety provoking. It is substernal and may be accompanied by nausea and diaphoresis, if severe enough. Unlike cardiac pain, GERD tends to be worse at night when the patient is lying down, which will help in differentiating it from cardiac pain. Pain relieved with nitro or a "GI cocktail" cannot rule in or rule out a cardiac origin because both GERD/PUD and angina often will respond to either or both treatments.

CHOLECYSTITIS

The history and location of the pain are good indicators for differentiating the symptoms of cholecystitis from angina. It is more common in young to middle aged women, and is seen more in those with a positive family history.

Signs and Symptoms.

The pain of cholecystitis is generally colicky in nature and localized to the right upper quadrant. It is often accompanied by nausea and vomiting, and Murphy's sign is positive. Often there is fever and an elevated white count. Attacks are intermittent and are usually related to large or fatty meals. See Chapter 9 for further detail.

PANCREATITIS

Alcohol abuse accounts for more than 80% of pancreatitis, making the history most helpful. Other causes include hyperlipidemia, drugs, toxins, infection, structural abnormalities, surgery, vascular disease, trauma, hyperparathyroidism and hypercalcemia, renal transplantation, and hereditary pancreatitis.

Signs and Symptoms.

The pain of pancreatitis is severe, steady, and "boring"—radiating from the epigastric region through to the back. It is usually accompanied by nausea and vomiting. In addition to the nausea and vomiting, some of the other symptoms mimic those of MI, such as tachycardia, hypotension, and diaphoresis. However, exquisite abdominal tenderness is present, which assists in differentiating it from cardiac pain. See Chapter 9 for details.

CHEST WALL PAIN AND COSTOCHONDRITIS

Chest wall pain can often be differentiated from cardiac pain through history. A history of injury; heavy lifting; contact sports; excessive coughing; or even late-stage pregnancy, which stretches the intercostal muscles, leads the examiner to consider chest wall pain versus cardiac pain. This often occurs in a younger population with no cardiac risk factors.

Signs and Symptoms.

One of the most helpful differentiating symptoms is the fact that the pain is increased with movement, cough, or in some cases, respiration. The pain tends to be less severe than with other causes and, generally, there are no accompanying symptoms.

THORACIC AORTIC ANEURYSM

Thoracic aneurysms account for less than 10% of aortic aneurysms, are rarely symptomatic, and are usually found in routine exams for other reasons. The history should include any chest trauma; hereditary connective tissue disorder, especially Marfan's or Ehlers-Danlos syndrome; congenital cardiac anomalies, such as coarctation, patent ductus arteriosus, or bicuspid aortic valve; or severe, long-standing hypertension.

Signs and Symptoms.

Symptoms that could occur include substernal or back pain, as well as symptoms related to pressure on the trachea or esophagus, such as dyspnea, cough, hoarseness, and dysphagia. Superior vena cava syndrome may accompany thoracic aneurysm. The systolic murmur of aortic regurgitation may be heard in aneurysms of the ascending aorta. The risk of rupture depends on the diameter of the aneurysm. The long-term prognosis is generally poor. Surgical intervention is also risky, with a high rate of morbidity and mortality. Control of hypertension is imperative to prevent progression of the aneurysm.

PULMONARY DISEASE

There are several pulmonary conditions that can cause chest pain, most commonly, pulmonary embolism, pneumonia, pleurisy, or tumor. The symptoms vary widely depending on the underlying disease. See Chapter 7 for details.

Signs and Symptoms.

Except in the case of pulmonary embolism, in which the pain can be quite sudden and severe, the pain accompanying pulmonary disease is often more insidious in onset, localized to the area of disease, less acute in nature, and less severe than is the pain of myocardial ischemia. Shortness of breath is almost always an accompanying symptom, and, in some cases, cough is present. For details, see Chapter 7.

Diagnostic Studies for Chest Pain

- MB CK—the serum level of myocardial band creatine kinase is elevated 10–25 times above the normal level in the first few hours after myocardial infarction and returns to normal within 2–4 days. The levels can also be elevated following trauma or with progressive muscular dystrophy.
- Troponin—an inhibitory protein found in muscle fibers. It is elevated in within 4 hours of a myocardial infarction and stays elevated for several days. It is more specific for cardiac muscle than is CK.
- EKG—can aid in diagnosis, and the practitioner should look for signs indicative of MI, such as ST-segment elevation or depression, arrhythmias, and conduction delays.
- ABGs—arterial blood gases evaluate oxygenation and acid–base balance, and can assist in ruling out pulmonary disease.
- Chest x-ray—this test can identify the presence of pneumonia, pulmonary masses or other pulmonary disease, heart size, and aortic aneurysms.
- CT or MRI—these diagnostic tests are helpful in detecting aortic aneurysms or other structural abnormalities in the chest.
- Cardiac catheterization—if the chest pain is due to myocardial infarction, the cardiac catheterization can assess the need for revascularization or coronary artery bypass graft. Revascularization must be performed promptly, within a few hours of onset of the MI, in order to minimize the amount of cardiac muscle damage.

- Endoscopy—once a cardiac origin has been ruled out, endoscopy will rule out a gastric cause for the pain.

Patient History of Heart Murmur

Heart murmurs fall into two general categories, systolic and diastolic. Systolic murmurs are further categorized into pathologic, functional, and innocent murmurs. Diastolic murmurs are generally not considered to be functional or innocent. The following are the broad categories of the causes of murmurs with parenthetical examples:

- Flow across a partial obstruction (valvular stenosis)
- Flow across a valvular irregularity (bicuspid aortic valve)
- Increased flow through normal structures (anemia, pregnancy)
- Flow into a dilated chamber (aneurysm)
- Backward or regurgitant flow across an incompetent valve (valvular incompetence)
- Shunting of blood out of a high pressure chamber through an abnormal passage (atrial or ventricular septal defect)

Grading of murmurs is based on a scale of I through VI. Grading murmurs is an experiential process, but the following characteristics can be used as a guide:

- Grade I   very faint, not heard in all positions
- Grade II   soft, but easily heard
- Grade III   moderately loud
- Grade IV   loud and may be associated with a thrill
- Grade V   very loud, may be heard with the stethoscope barely on the chest, associated with a thrill
- Grade VI   may be heard with the stethoscope off the chest, associated with a thrill

Murmurs should be described as to grade (intensity), location, radiation, pitch (high, medium, low), quality (blowing, rumbling, harsh, musical), and where they occur in the cardiac cycle.

History

One of the first questions to ask when a murmur is heard on examination is whether or not the patient has ever been told that he/she has a murmur and if any diagnostic testing has been done, particularly an echocardiogram. Inquire about palpitations, weakness or syncope, cough, exercise intolerance, endocarditis, or respiratory problems. A past medical history is important for congenital anomalies or rheumatic fever.

Physical Examination

A thorough cardiac exam is performed with the patient sitting, leaning forward, lying, and in the left lateral recumbent position. Some murmurs are heard better in different positions. Listen over the carotids for radiation of an aortic or pulmonic murmur, in the left midaxillary line for radiation of a mitral murmur, and in the aortic area for a bruit indicating an aneurysm. Assess the peripheral vascular system for bruits, pulses, and edema. Auscultate the lungs for crackles, which might indicate respiratory involvement.

Systolic Murmurs

Systolic murmurs occur between S_1 and S_2, and are broken down into ejection murmurs and regurgitant murmurs. Because systolic ejection murmurs are often physiologic, especially in children and pregnant women, they are further classified as to whether they are pathologic, functional, or physiologic/innocent.

Systolic Ejection Murmurs Ejection murmurs are the most common type of systolic murmurs and are associated with forward flow through the semilunar valves. They have a crescendo–decrescendo pattern.

PATHOLOGIC EJECTION MURMURS.

Murmurs result from obstruction to forward flow through the semilunar valves. The causes of this obstruction are aortic stenosis, pulmonic stenosis, and idiopathic hypertrophic subaortic stenosis (IHSS), also called asymmetrical septal hypertrophy.

Aortic Stenosis.

Aortic stenosis (AS) is heard best in the second right intercostal space with the client leaning forward. The murmur is harsh, loud, and often associated with a thrill. It may radiate to the neck, left sternal border, and, in some cases, to the apex. Associated physical findings include the following: an early ejection click, a diminished S_2, a heave or sustained apical impulse with left ventricular hypertrophy (LVH), crackles at the lung bases with left ventricular failure; jugular venous distention, hepatomegaly, and peripheral edema with right ventricular failure.

Diagnostic Studies.

- Chest x-ray—is helpful for outlining the heart border in LVH. Calcification of the aortic valve may be visible on x-ray.
- EKG—may show evidence of left ventricular hypertrophy. On exam, look for other signs of left ventricular hypertrophy, such as a left ventricular heave and an S_4.
- Echo—echocardiography is a simple, noninvasive, diagnostic test to determine the presence or absence of aortic stenosis, but has little value in determining the severity.
- GXT—a graded exercise test is helpful in determining the severity of aortic stenosis.
- Cardiac catheterization—this is the definitive study for the severity of aortic stenosis by measuring systolic blood flow across the aortic valve along with pressure differences between the left ventricle and the aorta.

Pulmonic Stenosis.

Pulmonic stenosis (PS) is less common than AS, is heard best at the third left intercostal space. The quality of the murmur is harsh, of medium pitch, and if loud, may be associated with a thrill. It is the second most common form of congenital heart disease, it is more common in women, and about two-thirds of adults are hemodynamically insignificant. In patients with severe pulmonic stenosis, dyspnea, cyanosis, syncope on exertion, palpitations, and right heart failure can occur.

Diagnostic Studies.

- Chest x-ray—unless right ventricular failure occurs, the heart may not appear enlarged on x-ray. Pulmonary artery dilatation is commonly seen but does not reflect the severity of the disease.
- EKG—the electrocardiographic changes in mild PS are minimal, but in severe obstruction to right ventricular flow, peaked P waves can be seen and, sometimes right bundle branch block.
- Echo—electrocardiography can be helpful in determining the degree of right ventricular hypertrophy and to distinguish PS from other lesions.
- Cardiac catheterization—as in AS, cardiac catheterization is the definitive diagnostic test for the presence and severity of PS.

Ideopathic Hypertrophic Subaortic Stenosis (IHSS).

Sometimes called asymmetrical septal hypertrophy, there has been controversy surrounding the exact nomenclature that would best describe obstructive cardiomyopathy. Clinical findings include a Grade 4/6 systolic murmur heard at the left sternal border that increases when upright and decreases with squatting, and an S_4. For this text, the term hypertrophic obstructive cardiomyopathy will be used. The cause is unknown, but is thought to be genetic, and familial. Manifestations may not be apparent until adulthood, and it is generally seen in conjunction with essential hypertension. The most common presenting symptoms are dyspnea on exertion and chest pain. Although the chest pain mimics that of angina, it is not relieved by nitroglycerin. Syncope is also a common complaint and may be more severe after exertion. Both atrial and ventricular arrhythmias can occur and are problematic. Atrial fibrillation may occur as a result of a chronic elevation of left atrial pressure. Ventricular arrhythmias can cause sudden death especially after extreme exertion. This illuminates the importance of a good history and physical for athletic screening. Questions regarding a family history of sudden death, dyspnea on exertion, syncopal episodes during or after exercise, and chest pain warrant diagnostic testing.

Diagnostic Studies.

- Echo—in the case of IHSS, electrocardiography is diagnostic and, generally, more invasive studies are not necessary. Echo findings include asymmetric left ventricular hypertrophy, a hypercontractile left ventricle and delayed diastolic filling of the left ventricle.
- Cardiac catheterization—cardiac catheterization may be helpful but generally is not necessary for diagnosis.

PHYSIOLOGIC OR FUNCTIONAL MURMURS.

This term refers to systolic murmurs that are due to a temporary increase in blood flow rather than to any structural change abnormality and include such conditions as anemia, hyperthyroidism, pregnancy, and fever.

INNOCENT MURMURS.

This type of systolic murmur results from turbulent blood flow and is not associated with heart disease. They occur commonly in children and young adults and reflect the contractile force of the heart resulting in greater velocity of flow during early systole. They are heard best in the second and third left interspaces along the left sternal border or at the apex. They are short, heard in early systole and are less than Grade III. Innocent murmurs disappear with patient in the sitting position.

SYSTOLIC REGURGITANT MURMURS

When the valves fail to close completely in systole, the blood is forced backward into the atrium, resulting in a murmur, volume overload, and ventricular hypertrophy. The following regurgitant murmurs occur in systole.

Mitral Regurgitation.

The murmur of mitral regurgitation is heard best in the apex often with radiation to the left axilla. It is pansystolic, high pitched, and blowing and may be associated with a thrill. There may be a decreased S_1, an S_3, and a sustained apical impulse owing to left ventricular hypertrophy. There is secondary left atrial enlargement resulting from systolic backflow into the left atrium. Dyspnea is the most common presenting symptom. Palpitations are common, and atrial fibrillation may develop. Complications include embolism, usually secondary to the atrial fibrillation. Bacterial endocarditis occurs most frequently (20%) in patients with mitral incompetence.

Diagnostic Studies.

- Chest x-ray—the left atrium and left ventricle are enlarged proportionate to the severity of the disease.
- EKG—atrial arrhythmias are common, particularly atrial fibrillation. Right and left bundle branches are uncommon. The main change seen is higher voltage.
- Echo—in addition to visualizing the diseased valve itself, echocardiography can assist in determining the size of the left atrium and left ventricle.
- Cardiac catheterization—in patients with hemodynamically significant mitral regurgitation, cardiac catheterization is the definitive choice for determining the need for surgical intervention.

MITRAL VALVE PROLAPSE.

Mitral valve prolapse, also termed "click-murmur syndrome" is a variant of mitral regurgitation that is generally hemodynamically insignificant and characterized by normal heart size and dynamics, although the process can progress to hemodynamically significant mitral regurgitation. Characteristically, a portion of the mitral valve balloons into the left atrium giving rise to a midsystolic click followed by a soft Grade I murmur that crescendos up to S_2. It is high-pitched and is heard best at the apex or left sternal border. Some patients with mitral valve prolapse have only a murmur and no click, and others have only a click and no murmur. Patients are usually asymptomatic but may complain of palpitations. It is of concern only in that antibiotic prophylaxis is needed in some cases for surgical and dental procedures to avoid the rare chance of subacute bacterial endocarditis.

TRICUSPID REGURGITATION.

The murmur of tricuspid regurgitation is heard best at the left sternal border, and may radiate to the right of the sternum. It is pansystolic, high-pitched, and blowing, and it increases with respiration. Tricuspid regurgitation may be associated with right ventricular hypertrophy resulting in a right parasternal lift. When right ventricular failure occurs, jugular venous distention occurs with a prominent *v* wave, and liver enlargement may be present. There may be secondary right atrial enlargement owing to backflow into the right atrium. The most common initiator is pulmonary hypertension; it may also be a secondary result of left ventricular failure. Symptoms are consistent with the underlying cause.

Diagnostic Studies.

- Chest x-ray—the right atrium and right ventricle are enlarged proportionate to the severity of the disease.
- EKG—atrial arrhythmias are common, particularly atrial fibrillation. Right and left bundle branches are uncommon. The main change seen is higher voltage.
- Echo—in addition to visualizing the diseased valve itself, echocardiography can assist in determining the size of the right atrium and right ventricle.
- Swan-Ganz pressure readings—the *v* peak and the *y* trough are exaggerated during inspiration.

Diastolic Murmurs

Unlike some physiologic causes of functional or innocent systolic murmurs, diastolic murmurs almost always indicate pathology.

Diastolic Stenotic Murmurs

MITRAL STENOSIS.

Mitral stenosis results from thickening and stiffening of the mitral valve, usually secondary to rheumatic fever. The murmur is generally Grade I to IV, low pitched and, therefore, is heard better with the bell at the apex in the left lateral recumbent position. The first heart sound (S_1) is loud, followed by S_2 and a loud opening snap that precedes the murmur. The most common presenting symptoms are dyspnea on exertion and hemoptysis due to pulmonary congestion. The pulmonary congestion is caused by increased left atrial pressure related to the decrease in left atrial emptying. Crackles may be heard at the lung bases but are not present in all patients with pulmonary congestion. Orthopnea may be present because the lungs become more congested in the recumbent position. In instances where the heart rate is increased as a result of fever, exertion, anxiety, or infection, congestion worsens and pulmonary edema may result. In addition, atrial fibrillation often develops in patients with mitral stenosis, which, in turn, worsens the pulmonary congestion. Over time, increased pulmonary vascular resistance may lead to right ventricular hypertrophy.

Diagnostic Studies.
- EKG—broad, notched P waves will provide evidence that mitral stenosis exists, but the EKG is not helpful in determining the severity. If right ventricular hypertrophy is present, it is manifested by right axis deviation.
- Chest x-ray—the heart size may be normal or there may be enlargement of the left atrium, but enlargement of the pulmonary artery is usually not seen until the pressures in the pulmonary artery are high. Radiographic changes in the chest that signify chronic pulmonary congestion are Kerley B lines, which are seen as thickened, interlobular septa, particularly at the outer edges of the lungs.
- Cardiac catheterization—heart catheterization is the definitive diagnostic study to determine the severity of the mitral stenosis.

TRICUSPID STENOSIS.

Tricuspid stenosis is most often caused by rheumatic fever and almost always accompanies the dominant mitral stenosis. The right atrium becomes hypertrophied with a small right ventricle. Signs and symptoms include a mid-diastolic murmur that is low-pitched and rumbling, heard at the left sternal border in the fourth interspace that increases with inspiration. The duration of the murmur is related to the severity of the stenosis and the stroke volume. Patients complain of fatigue and possible right upper quadrant discomfort related to an enlarged liver. There will be an accentuated *a* wave in the jugular venous pulse.

Diagnostic Studies.
- EKG—the EKG will show peaked P waves in the inferior leads because of an overload of the right atrium.
- Chest x-ray—reveals an enlarged superior vena cava and enlarged right atrium.
- Cardiac catheterization—is helpful in determining the pressure gradients across the tricuspid valve, and assists in determining the severity of the valvular stenosis.

Diastolic Regurgitant Murmurs

AORTIC REGURGITATION AND INSUFFICIENCY.

Aortic regurgitation results from failure of the leaflets of the aortic valve to close completely during diastole. This causes a backflow of blood from the aorta into the left ventricle. The murmur of aortic regurgitation is heard best in the second fourth interspaces, just to the left of the sternum. The quality is blowing, high-pitched, usually Grade III or less. It may radiate to the apex, and having the patient sitting and leaning forward will aid in hearing the murmur. Volume overload of the left ventricle occurs owing to the backflow of blood, which can lead to left ventricular hypertrophy. In this case, the apical impulse will be accentuated, and a left ventricular heave will be seen. An accompanying S_3 or S_4 indicate significant regurgitation. There may be an associated midsystolic murmur caused by the increased volume of blood flowing through the aortic valve. The most common cause of aortic insufficiency is infective endocarditis associated with rheumatic fever. In acute infectious destruction of the aortic valve, dyspnea, orthopnea, and cough are the most common presenting cardiac symptoms, resulting from pulmonary edema. This is often life threatening, and prompt treatment is necessary. In chronic aortic regurgitation, patients often complain of palpitations. If these are caused by ventricular arrhythmias, a thorough investigation is necessary to avoid a lethal ventricular arrhythmia. If left ventricular hypertrophy and failure develop, the symptoms typically are dyspnea and chest pain. An unexplained symptom of patients with aortic incompetence is increased sweating, which is thought to involve the cholinergic sympathetic vasodilator fibers. The greater volume of blood being pumped out of the ventricle increases the systolic pressure causing a widened pulse pressure.

Diagnostic Studies.

- EKG—in patients with hemodynamically significant aortic regurgitation, left ventricular hypertrophy is reflected on the EKG by increased height of the R waves in the left-sided chest leads, increased depth of the S waves in the right-sided chest leads, and associated S-T changes.
- Chest x-ray—in chronic, severe aortic regurgitation, the chest x-ray shows an enlarged left ventricle and aortic dilatation. Confirmation with EKG is prudent.
- Cardiac catheterization—is preferred over echocardiography for definitive diagnosis that the aortic valve is diseased and is the cause of rapid aortic runoff. It is also useful in determining heart pressures and pulmonary vascular resistance.

PULMONIC REGURGITATION AND INSUFFICIENCY.

Pulmonary insufficiency rarely occurs in patients without pulmonary hypertension and is usually seen in conjunction with right ventricular hypertrophy. This diastolic murmur is high pitched, heard best at the base, and difficult to distinguish from aortic incompetence.

Ventricular Septal Defect.

Ventricular septal defect (VSD) is a congenital heart defect in which oxygenated blood is shunted from a higher-pressured left ventricle to a lower-pressured right ventricle through an abnormal opening in the ventricular septum. This left-to-right shunt causes an increased blood flow across the pulmonic valve. The signs and symptoms depend on the size of the defect and the age of the patient. Characteristic of a VSD is a loud, harsh, pansystolic murmur at the lower left sternal border usually accompanied by a thrill. If the shunt is large, there is a mid-diastolic murmur of mitral flow heard at the apex, elevated pulmonary artery pressure, and possible heart failure. Adult patients with large defects will usually complain of dyspnea on exertion. In children, VSDs are often accompanied by other congenital anomalies and can be life threatening if not surgically repaired. Small defects can be clinically insignificant and may become smaller or even close as the child grows.

DIAGNOSTIC STUDIES.

- EKG—initially, the EKG shows signs of left ventricular hypertrophy (tall R waves and inverted T waves in Leads II, III, aVF, and V_6), but as right ventricular and pulmonary artery pressures increase, changes consistent with right ventricular hypertrophy are seen (tall R wave in V_1, small R wave in V_6, prominent S wave in V_6, and right axis deviation).
- Chest x-ray—on x-ray, left and right ventricular enlargement is seen, cardiomegaly, and an enlarged pulmonary artery.
- Cardiac catheterization—a heart catheterization is necessary prior to corrective surgery to determine the size and location of the VSD, the severity of pulmonary vascular resistance, and the presence of other congenital anomalies, such as patent ductus arteriosus or coarctation of the aorta.

Atrial Septal Defect.

Atrial septal defect (ASD) is a congenital abnormality in which oxygenated blood is shunted from a higher-pressured left atrium to a lower-pressured right atrium through an abnormal opening in the atrial septum. This causes an increased blood flow across the tricuspid valve and to the lungs. Atrial septal defects are often accompanied by other congenital heart defects, but, in an uncomplicated lesion, patients are often asymptomatic until early adulthood, when they present with dyspnea on exertion or palpitations resulting from atrial arrhythmia. Because patients may be asymptomatic for many years, right heart failure can be the first sign and patients may present with edema and ascites. A visible pulsation over the second–third left intercostal space may be seen because of an increased right ventricular stroke volume. A pulmonic systolic ejection murmur is present owing to the increased blood flow through the pulmonary valve. Tricuspid stenosis likewise develops as a result of the increased diastolic flow across the tricuspid valve, producing a diastolic murmur. There is fixed splitting of the second heart sound. Atrial arrhythmias, especially atrial fibrillation, are common in the adult population with atrial septal defect.

DIAGNOSTIC STUDIES.

- EKG—a majority of patients with ASD will have a right ventricular conduction defect, and, in older patients, a prolonged P-R interval is also common. Evidence of right ventricular hypertrophy may be present.
- Chest x-ray—the heart is usually enlarged and the pulmonary artery and branches are dilated. The right atrium and ventricle are enlarged, although right atrial enlargement can be difficult to determine.
- Echo—is helpful to visualize right ventricular enlargement and movement of the mitral and tricuspid valves.
- Cardiac catheterization—although the above procedures are helpful in diagnosis, cardiac catheterization is essential for confirmation of ASD.

Elevated Blood Pressure

From the Seventh Report of the Joint National Committee (JNC 7, 2003) on detection, education, and treatment of high blood pressure, the classification and follow-up of blood pressure measurements are as follows.

Category	Systolic Blood Pressure, mm Hg*	Diastolic Blood Pressure, mm Hg*	Follow-Up
Normal	<120	<80	Recheck in 2 years.
Prehypertension	120–139	80–90	Recheck within 2 months. Lifestyle modifications.
Hypertension Stage 1	140–159	90–99	Confirm within 2 weeks. Single drug treatment necessary.
Stage 2	≥160	≥100	Two-drug combination for most patients. Recheck 1–2 weeks.

*Classification is based on the average of two or more readings on two or more occasions after initial screening.

History

It is important to determine whether there is a past history or family history of hypertension. Identify the medications the patient is taking. Ask about lifestyle behaviors including smoking, alcohol, drugs, and exercise. Inquire about the presence of any chronic disease in the patient or family that may cause or contribute to hypertension. The subjective complaints depend on the type of hypertension.

Physical Examination

The blood pressure should be measured in both arms and lying, sitting, and standing. Measure temperature, pulse, and respirations, and note fever, tachycardia, or tachypnea. Upper and lower extremity pulses should be compared to look for coarctation. The abdomen should be auscultated for aortic and renal artery bruits. The heart should be examined for an S_3 or S_4 indicating decreased compliance of the left ventricle and ventricular hypertrophy, a systolic ejection murmur that might indicate aortic stenosis, or the diastolic murmur of aortic insufficiency. The eyes should be examined for exophthalmos, and the retinas inspected for such hypertensive changes as hemorrhages, exudates, A-V nicking, copper or silver wire appearance, or papilledema, which might point to a more serious neurologic cause.

PRIMARY (ESSENTIAL) HYPERTENSION

Approximately 10%–15% of Caucasians and 20%–30% of African Americans in the United States have primary HTN. The pathophysiology of primary HTN is varied. Genetic factors are significant contributors especially if both parents are hypertensive. Other factors include sympathetic nervous system hypersensitivity, decreased ability to balance sodium and calcium, and a renin-angiotensin-aldosterone imbalance. Factors that may exacerbate the predisposition to develop HTN include a sedentary lifestyle, obesity, smoking, alcohol, sodium intake in some individuals, low potassium intake, polycythemia, and long-term use of NSAIDs.

Signs and Symptoms.

In primary hypertension, symptoms may be absent. Some patients complain of a throbbing headache that is usually worse in the morning. Occasionally a patient will complain that they can hear their heart beating in their ears when it is quiet or when they go to bed at night.

SECONDARY HYPERTENSION

A small percentage of patients have specific, identifiable causes of hypertension, particularly those who develop hypertension at an early age with no family history, those whose previously controlled hypertension suddenly becomes uncontrolled, and those who first develop hypertension after age 50. There are several causes of secondary hypertension, including renal parenchymal disease, such as glomerulonephritis, pyelonephritis, tuberculosis of the kidney, or scarring from trauma; renal arterial disease, such as renal artery stenosis, aneurysm, embolism, or infarction; renal tumors; coarctation of the aorta; endocrine disorders, such as pheochromocytoma, primary aldosteronism, Cushing's syndrome, thyroid disease or acromegaly; hypercalcemia; pregnancy; neurologic disorders, such as tumor or trauma causing increased intracranial pressure; and medications, such as hormone replacement therapy, oral contraceptives, prolonged use of corticosteroids, NSAIDs, theophylline, or cold preparations containing ephedrine.

Signs and Symptoms.

In secondary hypertension, the symptoms are consistent with the underlying etiology. Listen for complaints such as nervousness, diaphoresis, palpitations, dyspnea, tremor, muscle weakness, polyuria, nocturia, nausea, or vomiting.

Diagnostic Studies for Elevated Blood Pressure
- TSH, T_7—to identify thyroid disease
- Electrolytes—K^+ is decreased and Na^+ increased in hyperaldosteronism
- Fasting blood glucose—hyperglycemia is seen in pheochromocytoma
- Renal chemistries—to identify renal parenchymal disease
- Urinalysis—to identify low specific gravity, proteinuria, hematuria, or casts that might indicate renal parenchymal disease
- 24-Hour urine for catecholamines—to identify pheochromocytoma
- Echo—to identify heart defects
- Renal Doppler ultrasound—to identify renal vascular disease
- Renal arteriography—to identify renal vascular disease
- CT or MRI—to identify renal vascular disease, adrenal adenoma, adrenal hyperplasia, or pheochromocytoma
- Chest x-ray—to visualize coarctation of the aorta
- EKG or Echo—to identify ventricular hypertrophy or valvular disease in patients with known cardiac disease

History of Elevated Lipids

Dyslipidemia can be defined as a disproportionate amount of deleterious lipids in the blood leading to an increase in atherosclerotic heart disease. The amount of HDL and LDL seem to be most important for both primary and secondary prevention of heart disease. The aim for primary prevention is to keep LDL levels below 130 mg/dL (<100 = optimal) and HDL levels above 40 mg/dL. Although primary prevention lowers a person's risk of heart disease and MI, it has shown only small, if any, effect on all-cause mortality. In patients with known coronary disease or diabetes, the target cholesterol levels are more stringent, and aim for a LDL level below 100 mg/dL and an HDL level above 60 mg/dL. Raising HDL seems to be more important to protect against heart disease than lowering LDL, and this is particularly true for women. The complete guidelines for management of hyperlipidemia can be found in the National Heart, Lung, and Blood Institute ATP III Guidelines (2003).

Patients over the age of 40 years should be screened every 1–2 years and elevated lipids treated aggressively with diet and exercise, weight loss, and lipid-lowering drugs when necessary. The relationship of hyperlipidemia to heart disease lessens with age and, therefore, patients over 75 years of age without heart disease or other risk factors are treated less aggressively.

History

The history includes screening for the following risk factors in addition to any past history in the patient of elevated lipids. See Box 6-2 for risk factors for dyslipidemia.

Physical Examination

The physical exam includes measurement of height and weight to calculate body mass index (BMI). The formula for calculating BMI is $wt(kg)/ht(m^2)$. A waist/hip ratio is also an indicator for risk of heart disease. A ratio of >0.85 for women and >0.95 for men is considered to place individuals at increased risk, especially if accompanied by hyperinsulinemia or diabetes. These are part of a constellation of symptoms, termed Syndrome X, or metabolic syndrome, that indicate the greatest risk for the development of heart disease.

SYNDROME X, OR METABOLIC SYNDROME

A cluster of risk factors known as Syndrome X, or metabolic syndrome, when occurring together, seem to dramatically increase the risk for coronary artery disease, diabetes, and stroke. Lack of physical activity and poor dietary habits lead to a positive energy balance, increased body fat, and insulin resistance. Therefore, obesity may be the underlying factor causing the regulation defect in the insulin receptor, thus promoting insulin resistance. The more calories that are consumed, the more insulin is needed to store the glucose and break down protein and fat. As fat cells become full, they become less sensitive to insulin, leading to an increased need for more insulin in order to perform the same work. Eventually, the body loses its ability to increase insulin secretion. Decreased secretion and insulin resistance impair sugar storage leading to increased circulating glucose and a tendency for the

---

Box 6-2
Risk Factors for Dyslipidemia

Obesity
Sedentary lifestyle
Diabetes
Positive family history
High-fat diet
Tobacco
Hypothyroidism
Chronic renal disease
Medications, particularly progestins,
    androgenic steroids, β-blockers

Characteristics of Syndrome X

Hypertension
Dyslipidemia
Central obesity
Glucose intolerance with hyperinsulinemia

increased sugar to be converted to fat, thus increasing the risk for Type 2 diabetes and dyslipidemia, which leads to atherosclerosis.

Treating only one of these risk factors does not lower morbidity, and in some cases, makes other risk factors worse. Weight loss through diet and exercise has been found to be the most important factor in the prevention of the progression of this syndrome. Insulin sensitivity increases with weight loss and is thought to be due to the loss of visceral fat. The target BMI is less than 22 kg/m^2 for women and less than 27 kg/m^2 for men. Weight loss will also reduce hypertension and improve the lipid profile. Aerobic and resistance exercise assists in weight loss and improves carbohydrate and lipid metabolism. Medication for hypertension and dyslipidemia may be necessary in patients who do not make necessary lifestyle changes or who are slow to make significant improvement.

Signs and Symptoms.

Generally, patients are made aware of their hyperlipidemia only from laboratory blood tests. Occasionally, there are lipid plaques around the eyes, called xanthelasma, but these are not apparent until hyperlipidemia has been present for some time.

Diagnostic Studies for Dyslipidemia

- Lipid panel—measures triglycerides, total cholesterol, HDL, LDL, and a TC/HDL ratio as a risk for heart disease. More sophisticated lipid profiles measure particle size, which gives a more accurate picture of cardiac risk.
- Glucose—fasting glucose should be measured because Type 2 diabetes is often responsible for hyperlipidemia.
- Insulin—insulin levels are not part of a routine workup, although they are helpful in detecting hyperinsulinemia and early Type 2 diabetes.
- Thyroid panel—hypothyroidism affects lipid levels and should be ruled out before placing a patient on lipid-lowering drugs.

Difficulty Breathing and Shortness of Breath

Dyspnea, or shortness of breath, has many causes, including cardiac or pulmonary disease, anxiety, obesity, and anemia. Patients with a cardiac cause may also complain of increased symptoms with exertion and dyspnea that wake them up at night and that are relieved by sitting up. This paroxysmal nocturnal dyspnea (PND) is one of the early signs of heart failure and, therefore, is more specific for cardiac disease. Dyspnea that is due to cardiac disease results most commonly from left ventricular dysfunction and/or valvular disease.

History

The history should include any past history of respiratory disease, heart failure, MI, heart murmur, arrhythmias, rheumatic fever, angioplasty, or cardiac surgeries. Inquire about other serious illnesses or hospitalizations and about current medicines, both prescription and over the counter. The review of systems should include chest pain, HTN, palpitations, dyspnea on exertion (DOE), PND, cough, fatigue, weight gain or loss, and last EKG. A thorough respiratory review of systems should also be done, which includes history of productive cough, asthma, wheezing, pleurisy, bronchitis, pneumonia, hemoptysis, tuberculosis, last chest x-ray, and PPD. A smoking history is also essential.

Physical Examination
The general survey includes any acute respiratory distress at rest, cyanosis, anxiety, restlessness, or confusion. Monitor vital signs for tachycardia, tachypnea, hypotension, or narrow pulse pressure, which could indicate ventricular dysfunction. A thorough examination of the lungs, heart, neck, abdomen, and extremities should be done. Auscultate the lungs for adventitious sounds, particularly crackles at the bases, which might indicate heart failure. Other adventitious sounds could indicate a respiratory rather than cardiac cause. Keep in mind that obstructive lung disease is often complicated by cardiac disease, so there may be more than one disease process occurring. Percuss the lungs for areas of dullness, indicating fluid or solid mass, such as pneumonia, pleural effusion, cancer, or pulmonary fibrosis. If possible, pulse oximetry would give valuable information about oxygenation. Inspect the precordium for a parasternal lift or accentuated apical impulse indicating ventricular hypertrophy. Palpate the precordium for a thrill that would indicate at least a Grade IV murmur. Auscultate all cardiac areas for murmurs that would indicate valvular heart disease, an S_3 related to volume overload and heart failure, an S_4 usually heard in diastolic failure, and any arrhythmias that could be either a cause or a result of heart failure. The neck should be examined for jugular venous distention with the patient's head elevated to 30 degrees. This is a sign of right-sided heart failure. Auscultate the carotids for bruits or murmurs that may radiate into the neck, usually aortic in origin. Palpate the thyroid for enlargement or nodules because hyper- and hypothyroidism can both cause heart failure. The abdomen should be examined particularly for right upper quadrant (RUQ) discomfort related to hepatic congestion and enlargement, secondary to right heart failure. Check for hepatic jugular reflux by placing sustained pressure on the liver while observing for JVD. In right heart failure, ascites may also be present. Examine the extremities for pitting edema seen in heart failure.

CONGESTIVE HEART FAILURE

Congestive heart failure (CHF) can occur at any age depending on underlying diseases, but as a primary diagnosis, it is more common in the elderly. There are four main determinants of systolic function:

1. Myocardial contractility—a decrease in contractility can result from a loss of functional muscle resulting from MI or other diseases affecting the myocardium. A decrease in contractility results in decreased stroke volume.
2. Heart rate—when the stroke volume decreases, the heart attempts to compensate by increasing heart rate. When this does not occur, cardiac output decreases, leading to heart failure. Bradycardia can occur in a number of cardiac conditions, which are outlined in this chapter in the subsection on arrhythmia. Also, bradycardia in a nonathlete can lead to decreased cardiac output and ensuing heart failure.
3. Preload—is determined by the end-diastolic stretch of the ventricular muscle fibers. This is equal to the end-diastolic volume or pressure. If preload is excessively elevated,

pump failure can result. This occurs with valvular regurgitation. Starling's law states that the force of the heartbeat is determined by the length of the fibers constituting the muscular wall; that is, an increase in diastolic filling increases the force of the heartbeat.

4. Afterload—the ventricular wall tension during systole, which determines the impedance to ejection of blood from the left ventricle. If afterload is excessive, the heart fails to be able to pump adequately against increased resistance. This can be seen in severe hypertension or aortic stenosis.

Heart failure also can occur when supply cannot meet demand as a result of high output states, such as severe anemia and thyrotoxicosis. Other, less-common causes of high output states are AV shunting and Paget's disease of the bone.

Signs and Symptoms.

One of the early signs of CHF is paroxysmal nocturnal dyspnea. Patients also may complain of DOE, nonproductive cough, and fatigue. Signs include ankle or pretibial edema, rapid weight gain that is due to fluid retention, bibasilar crackles, tachycardia with a gallop rhythm, and hypoxia. By symptom, left ventricular failure is most commonly characterized by DOE, cough, fatigue, orthopnea, paroxysmal nocturnal dyspnea, cardiac enlargement, crackles, gallop rhythm, and pulmonary congestion. Right ventricular failure is more commonly characterized by dependent edema, elevated venous pressure, hepatomegaly, and possibly ascites. Although left and right failure can occur independently, they often occur together, and left ventricular failure is the most common cause of right ventricular failure.

Respiratory Disease

Dyspnea is a symptom in many respiratory diseases, which are covered in Chapter 7. A holistic look at the patient—including age, past history, such habits as smoking and EtOH, and comorbid conditions—can assist the practitioner in differentiating a cardiac versus a respiratory origin for dyspnea.

Liver Disease

Severe liver diseases, resulting in ascites, can cause venous congestion, and dyspnea. This generally occurs in end-stage liver disease and is a secondary symptom to the more serious symptoms of liver disease, such as jaundice, bleeding, RUQ pain, and encephalopathy. Liver disease is easily diagnosed by laboratory tests, ultrasound, and biopsy, if necessary.

Renal Disease

As in liver disease, dyspnea is a secondary symptom in renal failure as a result of fluid retention. Renal failure can be a cause of heart failure, and dyspnea is one of the early symptoms. Laboratory testing for renal function, as well as urinalysis, will assist in diagnosis.

Diagnostic Studies for Dyspnea

- Complete blood count (CBC) should be done to check for anemia, which could cause or worsen dyspnea and heart failure.
- Chemistry panel should be ordered to check renal function, liver function, and electrolyte balance—particularly hypokalemia, which can cause arrhythmias.
- Thyroid profile is wise to rule out hyper- or hypothyroidism.
- Pro-brain natriuretic peptide (pro-BNP)—for patients with comorbid respiratory disease,

this blood test can assist in the differentiation of a cardiac versus respiratory etiology of dyspnea.
- Chest x-ray—most importantly, the x-ray will show the presence of cardiomegaly that can assist in the diagnosis of heart failure as a cause of the dyspnea. Look for fluid at the bases, flattening of diaphragms in COPD, tumors in cancer, increased markings, interstitial edema, atelectasis, or pneumonia. Pulmonary vasculature may be normal especially in chronic heart failure. Pleural effusions indicate heart failure or metastatic cancer, and thoracentesis is indicated to examine the fluid for malignant cells.
- Echo—shows the size and function of the ventricles if heart failure is thought to be the cause of the dyspnea. Echo can also be helpful in detecting shunts and pericardial effusion, and for visualizing the heart valves for abnormalities.
- Cardiac catheterization—may be necessary only when valvular disease is thought to be the cause of the dyspnea or if left ventricular dysfunction is caused by myocardial ischemia and revascularization is a treatment consideration.

Acute and Subacute Bacterial Endocarditis

Bacterial endocarditis is a microbial infection of the endocardium. The most common causative organisms are *Staphylococcus aureus*, Group A streptococcus, pneumococcus, and gonococcus. Although the incidence of subacute bacterial endocarditis has been fairly stable over the last few decades, the incidence has increased in the elderly owing to stiff, sclerotic valves. Other risk factors include IV drug use, dental disease, and in those requiring invasive diagnostic procedures. Nosocomial infections have increased in open-heart surgery patients. Initially, the signs and symptoms are similar to those of other systemic illnesses, including fever, chills, arthralgias, malaise, and fatigue. Petechiae, anemia, weight loss, new or worsening heart murmur, and emboli alert the examiner to a more serious disease process. Emboli may cause life-threatening events, such as stroke or myocardial infarction. Hematuria or proteinuria may result from a renal embolism or acute glomerulonephritis. Endocardial vegetation may occur, causing valvular incompetence or obstruction. The disease may be acute or subacute, and recurrences are not uncommon. If untreated, bacterial endocarditis is fatal because of a variety of complications. Prompt referral and hospitalization are necessary for antibiotic therapy and other supportive measures. As prevention against bacterial endocarditis, patients with valvular disorders or septal defects should have antibiotic prophylaxis prior to dental or surgical procedures.

PERIPHERAL VASCULAR SYSTEM

The assessment of the peripheral vascular system includes the following.
- Inspection and palpation of the peripheral pulses for strength and quality
- Inspection and palpation of the skin for color, texture and temperature changes
- Inspection of the extremities for edema, open sores, ulcers, pressure areas
- Auscultation of the arteries for bruits
- Questioning the patient for subjective complaints of discomfort or pain at rest and with exercise

Note that arterial and venous insufficiency present with different signs and symptoms. See Table 6-4.

Table 6-4. ■ Differentiation of Arterial and Venous Insufficiency

Sign	Arterial Insufficiency	Venous Insufficiency
Pulse	Decreased/absent	Normal
Edema	Absent or mild	Significant
Pain	Severe	Absent/mild
Temperature	Cool	Normal
Color	Pallor with elevation; Dusky red on dependency	Hyperpigmented; Cyanotic on dependency
Skin	Thin, atrophic; risk of gangrene	Thick; risk of stasis ulcers

DIFFERENTIAL DIAGNOSIS OF CHIEF COMPLAINTS
Peripheral Edema
In ambulatory patients, fluid collects dependently in the lower extremities or in the sacral area in nonambulatory patients. Nonpathologic causes of edema include poor venous return in prolonged standing or sitting. Pathologic causes of edema result from right and left heart failure, kidney disease, liver disease, or tumors that obstruct venous return. One of the early signs of congestive heart failure is pretibial and ankle edema. Renal failure causes fluid retention and hepatic disease may cause ascites, which contribute to peripheral edema.

History
The age and general health of the patient can lead to either a high or low index of suspicion for cardiac causes of edema. Older patients and those with comorbid conditions have a greater risk of a cardiac cause for the edema. Ask the patient about past history of respiratory, cardiac, renal, liver, or vascular disease. Certainly, a history of heart failure makes a recurrence likely. Ask about any history of cancer, particularly abdominal or genitourinary. Ascites can occur with these cancers, thus causing lower extremity edema. Determine how many pillows the patient sleeps on at night and ask about the presence of paroxysmal nocturnal dyspnea, another early sign of CHF. Inquire about daily activities, exercise, and occupation to determine a simple, mechanical cause of the edema. Psychosocial data is important, such as EtOH intake and sexual practices, which might lead to a suspicion of a possible hepatic cause. A positive smoking history is a significant contributing factor in peripheral vascular disease. Note any symptoms of intermittent claudication, such as complaints of cramping, aching, or pain in the ankle, calf, or thigh that occur with exercise and are promptly relieved with rest.

Physical Examination
Assess the extent and magnitude of the edema. Is it confined to the ankles, or does it extend up the leg to include pretibial edema or higher? Grade the edema on a scale of 1+ to 4+, or mild to pitting. Assess the peripheral pulses and major arteries for bruits, that is, the abdominal aortic, renal, iliac, and femoral arteries. Stenosis or occlusion of any of these arteries can have an effect on distal pulses. Assess capillary refill time and pallor or rubor of the skin on elevation and dependence.

Assess the skin integrity as you look for thinning, ulcers, or necrosis, which often occur in peripheral vascular disease. Hyperpigmentation and atrophic skin changes are common in venous insufficiency. Note any change in temperature of the skin. Cellulitis can sometimes mimic peripheral vascular disease (PVD) and would cause increased temperature. Coolness of the skin suggests circulatory impairment. Ulceration or necrosis are serious signs of circulatory impairment and must be promptly treated to avoid amputation.

Many people have dependent edema in the absence of heart disease that is due to prolonged sitting and standing or poor venous return, but a thorough exam of the heart, lungs, and abdomen is warranted. If the edema is accompanied by congestive heart failure, crackles may be heard at the lung bases. Listen for other adventitious sounds, such as wheezes or decreased breath sounds that might indicate obstructive lung disease, often complicated by right heart failure. Auscultate all cardiac areas for murmurs that would indicate valvular heart disease, an S_3 related to volume overload and heart failure, an S_4 usually heard in diastolic failure, and any arrhythmias that could be either a cause or a result of heart failure. Palpate the precordium for a thrill that would indicate at least a Grade IV murmur. Inspect the precordium for a parasternal lift or accentuated apical impulse indicating ventricular hypertrophy. The neck should be examined for jugular venous distention with the patient's head elevated to 30 degrees. This is a sign of right-sided heart failure. Auscultate the carotids for bruits or murmurs that may radiate into the neck, usually aortic in origin. Palpate the thyroid for enlargement or nodules because hyper- and hypothyroidism can both cause heart failure. The abdomen should be examined particularly for RUQ discomfort related to hepatic congestion and enlargement secondary to right heart failure. Check for hepatic jugular reflux by placing sustained pressure on the liver while observing for JVD. In right heart failure, ascites may also be present.

Congestive Heart Failure
See the section on dyspnea in this chapter, pp. 142–145.

Renal Disease
See the section on dyspnea in this chapter, pp. 142–145.

Liver Disease
See the section on dyspnea in this chapter, pp. 142–145.

Peripheral Vascular Disease (PVD)
See pp. 148–150. for a discussion of PVD.

Diagnostic Studies For Peripheral Edema
- A CBC should be done to check for anemia, which could cause or worsen heart failure of which edema is a symptom.
- A chemistry panel should be ordered to check renal function, liver function, and electrolyte balance.
- A thyroid profile is wise to rule out hyper- or hypothyroidism.
- A chest x-ray—most importantly, the x-ray will show the presence of cardiomegaly, which that can assist in the diagnosis of heart failure as a cause of the edema. Look for fluid at the bases, flattening of diaphragms in COPD, pleural effusion, tumors in cancer, increased vascular markings, interstitial edema, atelectasis, or pneumonia.

Pulmonary vasculature may be normal especially in chronic heart failure. Pleural effusions indicate heart failure or metastatic cancer, and thoracentesis is indicated to examine the fluid for cancer cells.
- Echo—shows the size and function of the ventricles if heart failure is thought to be the cause of the edema. Echocardiography can also be helpful in detecting shunts, pericardial effusion, and for visualizing the heart valves for abnormalities.

Leg Pain

Consider a vascular origin for leg pain that is not musculoskeletal in nature. Pain or weakness that occurs in the calves, and sometimes thighs or buttocks, with exercise and dissipates at rest is most likely related to peripheral vascular disease. If it is related to arterial insufficiency, the pain comes on rapidly during exercise, is quickly relieved by rest, and usually increases as the intensity and duration of the exercise increases. This is termed intermittent claudication. If the leg pain is due to venous insufficiency, the picture is quite different. The onset of the pain is gradual, and may not even occur until some time after exercise. There is greater variability of the pain in response to duration and intensity of exercise. The pain tends to be a constant ache that may last hours to days. A potentially life-threatening complication of venous insufficiency is thrombophlebitis.

THROMBOPHLEBITIS

In addition to arteriovenous insufficiency, other risk factors for thrombophlebitis include immobility, orthopedic surgery, malignancy, congestive heart failure, smoking, pregnancy, oral contraceptive use, advanced age, and clotting disorders. The majority of cases occur in the deep veins of the calf, and the remainder from the iliac or femoral veins. The prognosis of thrombophlebitis is good unless the patient develops pulmonary embolism. Recurrent pulmonary embolism may occur. Deep vein thrombosis (DVT) can be a result of or a cause of chronic venous insufficiency. Thrombolytic therapy should be instituted to avoid the complication of chronic venous insufficiency.

Signs and Symptoms.

The signs and symptoms of DVT include swelling, tenderness, and inflammation of the calf, and often pain with ambulation. In about 50% of the cases, symptoms are absent and pulmonary embolism may be the first sign. Pulmonary embolism should be suspected with a complaint of acute onset of shortness of breath, chest pain, or hemoptysis in a person with any of the above risk factors. Preventive measures include early mobilization of postsurgical patients, raising the foot of the bed, and antiembolism hosiery, especially for patients who have a history of venous insufficiency, and for people traveling long distances by plane.

Diagnostic Studies.
- Calf measurement—a simple measurement with a measuring tape of both calves for comparison should always be performed in the clinical setting. Deep vein thrombosis will cause swelling and redness of the affected leg.
- Duplex Doppler ultrasound—Because of its sensitivity, specificity, and noninvasive method, duplex ultrasound is the recommended diagnostic test for venous thrombosis. It gives segmental readings on blood flow both distal and proximal to the thrombus. It is most accurate for clots in the veins proximal to the popliteal; however, it is not a reliable indicator of small thrombi in the calf veins.

- Venography—contrast venography remains the most accurate diagnostic procedure for DVT. It gives information regarding location, extent, and degree of attachment of the thrombus. Venography is particularly useful when there is a strong clinical suspicion of a calf thrombosis and when Doppler ultrasound has not given adequate information.

ARTERIAL INSUFFICIENCY

Patients with peripheral arterial disease will often have underlying atherosclerosis. Other diseases such as diabetes, HTN, and obesity should also raise the index of suspicion for arterial insufficiency. Smoking is a risk factor for all vascular disease. A history of significant trauma or surgeries may be a risk factor.

Signs and Symptoms.

See Table 6-4 for the signs and symptoms of arterial insufficiency.

Diagnostic Studies.

- Ankle-brachial index (ABI) - the ankle-brachial index is currently the easiest, least expensive, noninvasive method for diagnosing peripheral vascular disease and is particularly helpful in the office and home settings. The ABI is obtained by the following steps:
  1. Obtain brachial systolic pressure in both arms. Select the higher of these two values.
  2. Use Doppler stethoscope to obtain systolic pressure in the dorsalis pedis or posterior tibialis vessel.
  3. Divide ankle pressure by the higher brachial pressure.
  4. The index should be 1.00 or higher. If it is less than 0.5, impairment to blood flow is significant. An abnormal ABI indicates the need for a vascular consult.

The ABI may be falsely elevated in diabetic patients because calcification of the vessels raises the pressure, especially in the ankle. Doppler ultrasound is also helpful, but requires specialized equipment.

- Duplex Doppler ultrasound—a relatively inexpensive, accurate method for the diagnosis of arterial insufficiency, often making arteriography unnecessary. Flow velocity can be measured, and arterial stenosis and occlusion can be detected.

CHRONIC VENOUS INSUFFICIENCY

Chronic venous insufficiency can be a long-term complication of venous thrombosis owing to the destruction of valves in the deep veins. The calf muscle pump that returns blood from the lower legs is damaged, thus increasing ambulatory pressure in the calf veins. A constellation of symptoms is set up: aching or pain in the lower legs, edema, thinning and hyperpigmentation of the skin, superficial varicosities, venous stasis, and ulceration. Ankle edema is often the earliest sign. Other causes of chronic venous insufficiency include trauma, pelvic neoplasm, and occasionally secondary to superficial venous disease. Prompt treatment of DVT with thrombolytics decreases the risk for chronic venous insufficiency. General measures for symptom management include the following: elevation of the legs intermittently during the day and at night, avoidance of prolonged sitting or standing, and support or compression stockings. Wearing a unaboot is valuable and successful in the treatment of stasis ulcers.

Signs and Symptoms.

Stasis dermatitis and stasis ulcers are common in chronic venous insufficiency. See Table 6-4 for signs and symptoms of venous insufficiency.

Diagnostic Studies.
- Duplex Doppler ultrasound—owing to its sensitivity, specificity, and noninvasive method, duplex ultrasound is recommended for the diagnosis of venous disease. It gives segmental readings on blood flow and is accurate for the diagnosis of occlusion. It is most accurate for clots in the veins proximal to the popliteal; however, it is not a reliable indicator of small thrombi in the calf veins.
- Venography—contrast venography remains the most accurate diagnostic procedure for venous disease. Venography is particularly useful when there is a strong clinical suspicion of a calf thrombosis and when Doppler ultrasound has not given adequate information. It gives information regarding location, extent, and degree of attachment of the thrombus.

VARICOSE VEINS

Often a precursor to chronic venous insufficiency, varicose veins are usually caused by occupations that involve prolonged standing or sitting in one place, overweight, pregnancy, or a familial tendency. They may increase the patient's risk for DVT, or they may occur secondary to a DVT. Blockage to lymphatic flow can cause varicosities as seen with pelvic neoplasm. They appear as long, dilated tortuous veins in the lower extremities.

Signs and Symptoms.

Although cosmetically unsightly, varicose veins may be completely asymptomatic or the patient may complain of aching or fatigue in the legs particularly with standing. The same general measures should be applied that are used with chronic venous insufficiency.

Diagnostic Studies.

Usually the physical exam is enough for the diagnosis, but ultrasound or venography may be warranted if thrombosis is suspected. Excision of the varicosity and ligation of the vein are possible for symptom relief or for cosmetic reasons, and rarely to prevent complications. For small varicosities, compression sclerotherapy is helpful.

References

Chobanian, A.V., et al. (2003). The Seventh Report of the Joint National Committee on Prevention, Detection, Evaluation, and Treatment of High Blood Pressure (JNC 7). *JAMA*, 289, 2560–2572.

Hurst, J.W., Morris, D.C., & Alexander, R.W. (1999). The Use of the New York Heart Association's Classification of Cardiovascular Disease as Part of the Patient's Complete Problem List. *Clinical Cardiology*, 22, 385–390. www.clinicalcardiology.org/briefs/9906briefs/22–385.html.

National Heart, Lung and Blood Institute Third Report of the Expert Panel on Detection, Evaluation, and Treatment of High Blood Cholesterol in Adults (ATP III). http://www.nhlbi.nih.gov/guidelines/cholesterol/attp_iii.htm

 SUGGESTED READINGS

Bates, B. (2002). *A Guide to Physical Examination and History Taking* (8th ed.). Philadelphia: J.B. Lippincott Co.

Beers, M., Berkow, R. & Burs, M. (Eds.). (1999). *Merck Manual of Medical Therapeutics* (17th ed). Rahway, NJ: Merck & Co., Inc

Sokolow, M., & McIlroy, M.B. (1979). *Clinical Cardiology* (2nd ed.). Los Altos, CA: Lange Medical Publications.

Tierney, L.M., McPhee, S.J., & Papadakis, M.A. (Eds.). (2002). *CURRENT Medical Diagnosis & Treatment.* New York: Lange Medical Books/McGraw Hill.

Chapter 7

Respiratory System

Mary Jo Goolsby

Respiratory complaints are commonly encountered in most health care settings. Chronic obstructive pulmonary disease (COPD) affects over 12 million adults in the United States and is now the fourth leading cause of death (NHLBI, 2003). Pneumonia is currently the sixth leading cause of death in the United States and the greatest cause of infection-related deaths (CDC, 2004). The prevalence of asthma is also increasing, and the number of individuals diagnosed with the condition has doubled, from 7 million in 1980 to over 14 million in 1996 (NHLBI, 2002).

Respiratory complaints, such as dyspnea and cough, can be vague and quite nonspecific. In addition to potentially stemming from many extrapulmonary systems, including cardiac, neurologic, and upper respiratory, they may be psychogenic in origin. A careful and detailed history and physical examination, with attention first to the respiratory system, enable accurate diagnosis. For instance, the history of uncontrolled hypertension and previous myocardial infarction (MI) in a nonsmoker, paired with the complaint of cough or sudden onset of dyspnea direct the examiner to consider the potential for congestive heart failure, whereas a similar complaint in an otherwise healthy appearing teen would be more likely to suggest asthma or bronchitis.

HISTORY

Symptom Analysis

Regardless of the chief complaint, a thorough symptom analysis is warranted. It is important to get an understanding of when the complaint started, and how the onset occurred. Determine how it has evolved, starting with the initial episode or awareness of the problem. Ask whether the problem is constant or intermittent. Determine whether a similar problem has been experienced in the past. It is important to learn whether anything in particular, such as emotions, exposure to outdoor allergens, or fatigue, tends to precipitate or accelerate the complaint. Also determine whether the symptoms tend to be tied to any particular time of day, such as the night, early morning, or immediately following a meal. Another timing-related issue involves whether the complaint has continued essentially unchanged, worsened, or improved since first noticed.

The quality of the symptom is important. For chest discomfort, it is important to determine whether the pain or discomfort is sharp, dull, or aching. If the complaint is a cough, the potential qualities include whether the cough is mild and tickling versus sharp and paroxysmal. For some complaints, such as wheezing and tightness or pain, it is also necessary to determine the exact location of the symptom, as well as whether the patient has noticed any radiation to other sites and how it relates to respirations. The severity is always important to establish.

As with other symptoms, it is always important to ask about any self-treatment the patient may have tried and the response. For instance, determine what the patient has done to minimize the symptoms, including whether he has altered normal activity or taken any medications (prescribed or over the counter). Include questions to identify any herbal agents, illicit drugs, and/or complementary therapies tried.

When asking about the existence of any associated symptoms, the pulmonary review of symptoms should be performed. There is a long list of symptoms that should be explored during this part of the history. Determine whether the patient has experienced any shortness of breath and, if so, record the amount of work/effort that causes this symptom. Ask about nocturnal orthopnea or related difficulty sleeping. Specifically, ask about the number of pillows the patient uses to sleep as well as (and/or) the sleeping position. A patient may use no pillows, but rest comfortably only in a recliner. Determine whether the patient has had a cough and whether any cough has been associated with the production of sputum or with hemoptysis. Also ask about wheezing, chest tightness, and sense of congestion. Ask whether the patient has had a fever, as well as any chills or night sweats. In addition to asking about symptoms related to the lower respiratory tract, other systems should be explored, based on the presenting symptom and symptom analysis.

Past Medical and Family History

The past medical history should identify any history of allergies, emphysema, bronchitis, asthma, pneumonia, recent or recurrent upper respiratory infections, and tuberculosis. Ask about the history of malignancy. Conditions stemming from other systems are often important to specifically address, including heart failure, gastroesophageal reflux disease (GERD), and allergies. During this part of the history, determine the approximate date of the patient's last chest x-ray and skin test for TB and the results of the tests. The family history should be explored. Ask about whether there is a family history of the conditions just mentioned.

Habits

The patient's habits are important in the assessment of respiratory complaints. Always establish the patient's smoking history, calculating pack years. Also determine any occupational or recreational exposures to toxins. The travel history is often significant, particularly for exposure to various infectious disorders affecting the lungs. Knowledge of the patient's exposure to pets is important, as it can suggest exposure to infectious diseases or allergens. Identify all medications/drugs taken, including prescribed, over-the-counter, and recreational drugs, as well as any herbal or alternative therapies.

PHYSICAL EXAMINATION

The historical findings should guide attention within the physical exam. However, regardless of the complaint, a thorough and orderly approach is recommended. In addition to the respiratory examination, a more comprehensive approach is usually necessary, regardless of whether the symptoms are mild or severe, acute or chronic. Other systems that should often be included are: cardiac, musculoskeletal, neurological, and ear/nose/throat (upper respiratory).

The examination actually starts during the history, as the examiner observes the patient's general condition. For instance, note whether the patient is able to provide a history without shortness of breath. Notice the patient's demeanor and apparent energy level. Assess the patient's breathing pattern and general coloring as he talks.

In assessing the lungs and chest, it is important that the patient be disrobed from the waist up and examined in an area with good lighting. The assessment of the chest involves all four components of physical assessment: inspection, palpation, percussion, and auscultation.

Inspection

Start by observing the patient's quiet respirations. Notice the rate, rhythm, depth, and amount of effort required. Determine whether there is any obvious use of accessory muscles, as might be seen in a number of pulmonary conditions, including asthma, COPD, and pneumonia. Notice the movement of the chest and whether it is symmetrical. Identify any intercostal inspiratory retractions or expiratory bulges, which may indicate asthma, a tumor, tracheal/bronchial occlusion, or COPD. The chest configuration should be determined, including whether the chest is symmetrical and noting the ratio of the anterior-to-posterior (AP) diameter compared with the transverse chest diameter. An asymmetric configuration is often seen in scoliosis or kyphosis, both of which may restrict respiratory effort. Increased AP diameter is indicative of COPD, as well as pectus carinatum.

Palpation

Following inspection, gently palpate any area of discomfort or pain. Examples would include intercostal tenderness, which could indicate inflamed pleurae, or costal-sternal border pain, indicating costochondritis. Next palpate any area of visible deformity. The respiratory excursion, or expansion, is determined by placing hands around the patient's posterior rib cage with the thumbs at the level of the 10th rib and sliding them together so that a "pinch" of skin is raised between the thumbs, and then asking the patient to take a deep breath and observing the movement of the hands. The motion should be symmetrical. Less than anticipated movement occurs with COPD and pleural effusions. Asymmetry of movement occurs with atelectasis, pneumothorax, and fibrosis.

The quality of tactile fremitus is determined by palpating symmetrical areas with the palmar surface of the hands and fingers, as the patient is directed to speak, usually repeatedly saying "99" or "one, two, three" in a loud and a low voice. This maneuver provides only a rough estimate of lung condition, but is useful in guiding further assessment. Areas of increased fremitus should raise the suspicion of conditions resulting in increased solidity or consolidation in the underlying lung tissue, such as in pneumonia, tumor, or pulmonary fibrosis. Conversely, areas of decreased fremitus raise the suspicion of abnormal fluid- or air-filled spaces, such as occurs with pleural effusion, pneumothorax, or emphysema. In the instance of an extensive bronchial obstruction, there will be no palpable vibration in the related field.

Percussion

Percussion provides an estimate of the relative amounts of air, fluid, and solid matter in a space and is helpful in identifying the margins of organs, including the lungs. The lung fields should be percussed starting from the superior-most areas at Kronig's isthmus, the area superior to the clavicles that connects the anterior and posterior aspects of the chest. Percussion should then proceed downward to the level of the diaphragm. Areas of hyper-resonance suggest air trapping, which occurs with COPD, as well superior to an area of atelectasis or pleural effusion. Dullness is detected over the actual site of atelectasis and pleural effusion, as well as tumors or the consolidation/pneumonia.

Auscultation

Finally, the most helpful assessment maneuver involves auscultation of the lung fields. The general lung fields should be auscultated, with special attention paid to any areas where previous abnormalities were detected. With the patient breathing fully through an open mouth, a full inspiratory and expiratory cycle should be assessed at each site. During auscultation, the examiner should first notice the qualities associated with the breath sound itself, then assess for the presence of any adventitious lung sounds.

Breath sounds vary in intensity, volume, and duration, depending on the site along the tracheobronchoalveolar system. In the upper part of the respiratory tree, over the trachea, breath sounds should be "bronchial," meaning they are loud and that the inspiratory component is shorter than the expiratory component. Over the bronchi, the bronchovesicular sounds are of a medium intensity and are of equal duration in the inspiratory and expiratory components. Finally, the vesicular sounds over the peripheral lung tissue are, by comparison, softer in volume and have a shorter expiratory phase. Increased breath sounds over peripheral lung regions indicate consolidation, which may occur with tumor, pneumonia, or atelectasis. Decreased, or softer, peripheral breath sounds indicate bronchial obstruction or shallow breathing.

Adventitious breath sounds are those extra and abnormal sounds that are detected in addition to the expected breath sounds. The terminology used to describe these adventitious sounds varies and includes the terms rales, rhonchi, wheezes, and crackles. The terms rales and rhonchi are confused by some and are more or less synonymous with crackles and wheezes, respectively. Regardless of the terminology used, it is important to provide as many descriptors relative to the adventitious sound, as possible. Descriptors can include details of the detected pitch, amplitude, and quality of the sound. For instance, crackles can be described as loud or soft, coarse or fine. Wheezes, or rhonchi, can be described as loud or soft, high- or low-pitched, coarse/sonorous, squeaking, or hissing/sibilant. Another important characteristic to note is whether adventitious lung sounds occur early or late in the respiratory cycle. All of these characteristics are helpful in determining the cause. Table 7-1 describes potential adventitious sounds tied with some respiratory disorders.

Table 7-1. ■ Adventitious Sounds

Description	Significance
Crackles (Rales)	
Low pitched, coarse, early inspiratory	Bronchial; bronchitis
Medium pitched, mid-inspiration	Smaller bronchial branches; bronchiectasis
High pitched, fine, late inspiration	Bronchioles/alveoli; emphysema, atelectasis, pneumonia, CHF, pulmonary fibrosis
Wheezes (Rhonchi)	
Low pitched, early, deep	Bronchi; bronchitis
High pitched, hissing	Smaller airways; asthma
Friction Rub	
Loud, grating; late inspiratory–early expiratory	Inflamed pleura; pneumonia, pleuritis, malignancy

Because mobile bronchial secretions can cause both crackles and wheezes, ask the patient to take a deep breath and cough if these are detected. This often clears the airway and eliminates or changes the adventitious sounds. The effect of cough (or lack of) on the adventitious sounds is important to record. Failure to have the patient clear the airway of mobile secretions could result in a misdiagnosis.

A final adventitious sound is the pleural friction rub, which is typically a loud, grating sound that is produced when the two inflamed and roughened surfaces of the visceral and parietal pleurae rub together. A friction rub is usually noted in the late inspiratory and early expiratory phases and in the lower anterolateral lung fields. Examples of conditions that result in a pleural rub include pneumonia and malignancy.

Depending on the findings associated with the exam up to this point, the examiner can decide whether to proceed with auscultated spoken sounds: bronchophony, egophony, and/or whispered pectoriloquy. If the exam has been normal up to this point, there is no need to proceed with spoken sounds. However, if an abnormality has been detected, this maneuver may provide valuable data that will help to further narrow the assessment. As with tactile fremitus, the patient is again directed to repeatedly say "99" or "1-2-3", as the examiner auscultates the lung fields. The expected norm is that the volume and clarity of the transmitted speech sounds are uniform throughout the lung fields. If there is an increased volume in one area, this is called bronchophony, suggesting an area of consolidation or effusion. Whispered sounds are also auscultated, as the patient whispers "99" or "1-2-3". Any area of increased clarity is positive for whispered pectoriloquy, another indication of consolidation. Finally, the lung fields can be auscultated as the patient repeats "E - E - E." If the detected sound is heard as "A - A - A" with a nasal quality over a particular area, indicating egophony, this is a final indication of consolidation.

Diagnostic Studies.

Diagnostic studies are often helpful in making definitive diagnosis for pulmonary conditions. Spirometry provides a range of information about the lung function and is important in differentiating among causes of respiratory complaints. An increasing number of portable and accurate devices are available. Arterial blood gases provide data on a patient's acid–base balance and whether or not disturbances stem from respiratory or metabolic derangements. Pulse oximetry provides a portable, simple method to determine the percentage of hemoglobin saturated with oxygen.

Imaging Studies

A wide range of imaging studies are useful in assessing respiratory complaints. In addition to plain films, CT, MRI, and PET scans provide noninvasive ways to assess pulmonary tissue and space.

DIFFERENTIAL DIAGNOSIS OF CHIEF COMPLAINTS
Cough

Cough is an extremely common and potentially nonspecific complaint. Whereas the cough serves as an important defense mechanism, it is often the major reason a patient seeks diagnosis and treatment of many self-limiting and minor complaints, as well as many life-threatening ones. Cough is classified as acute (less than 3 weeks in duration) and chronic (3 or more weeks in duration), and this distinction helps to narrow the potential differential diagnoses. However, patients with chronic cough may present acutely, as some component of their problem is exacerbated.

The history and physical are essential in eliminating potential causes and identifying the most likely causes of cough. For instance, when a person presents with a cough after being prescribed an angiotensin-converting enzyme inhibitor (ACEI), a thorough history and physical help the provider ensure that there is no other likely coexisting problem triggering and/or causing the cough.

The history should include a thorough analysis of the cough, including a determination of how long it has persisted. It is essential to determine any associated symptoms, including shortness of breath, wheezing, orthopnea, fever, chills, chest pain or discomfort, sputum production, and hemoptysis. The past medical history should be comprehensive, with a particular focus on the potential for asthma, emphysema, chronic or acute bronchitis, heart failure, GERD, recent upper respiratory infections, or atopy. The medication history will not only exclude the potential for ACEI-induced cough, but also identify other problems for which medications are taken. The patient's prior self-treatment or prescribed treatment of cough should be explored, including the response and tolerance of the treatment.

POSTNASAL DISCHARGE SYNDROME

Postnasal discharge is the most common cause of chronic cough.
Signs and Symptoms.
The patient complains of a chronic cough that is often associated with sensation of the drainage in back of the throat and/or the need to clear the throat frequently. There may be accompanying hoarseness. Depending on the cause of the postnasal discharge syndrome (PNDS), the patient will have complaints of symptoms consistent with allergic rhinitis, chronic sinusitis, or other condition, such as cold or viral upper respiratory infection (URI). Although no sputum is produced, there is a potential that secretions will be cleared

from the posterior pharynx by the coughing effort. Common signs include throat clearing, drainage on the posterior pharynx, and hyperemia and/or cobblestoning of the posterior pharynx, with a negative chest exam.

Diagnostic Studies.

None are usually warranted initially. Response to treatment for PNDS provides presumptive diagnosis. Depending on the patient's risk factors, specific diagnostic studies can be considered to rule out other causes, which could coexist with PNDS, and/or contributing factors. These include allergy testing and radiographs of the sinuses or chest.

ASTHMA

Asthma is a chronic condition that involves inflammation of the airways, with varying degrees of airway obstruction and hyperresponsiveness. The incidence of asthma is increasing in the United States, and it affects people of all ages. Although typically associated with wheezing, a cough may be the primary complaint associated with asthma.

Signs and Symptoms.

The patient complains of intermittent sensation of chest tightness, cough, shortness of breath, and/or wheezing. The cough is nonproductive. The symptoms may become relatively persistent and affect quality of life. Symptoms often worsen with activity, viral infections, exposure to allergens, or other triggers. Exam may reveal wheezes. Deep respiratory effort may trigger paroxysmal coughing. The "rule of twos" is helpful in discriminating between intermittent and persistent asthma. (See Box 7-1). There are often other signs of atopy, including allergic rhinitis or atopic dermatitis.

Diagnostic Studies.

Pulmonary functions provide diagnosis, with the FEV_1 diminished, indicating restricted outflow. There is some degree of reversibility occurring with administration of bronchodilators. Chest films are generally within normal limits, unless there is significant air-trapping. Peak flow meters are not typically used in the initial diagnosis, but are important in monitoring ongoing symptoms and determining the response to therapy, particularly once a patient's "personal best" is determined.

CHRONIC OBSTRUCTIVE PULMONARY DISEASE

Chronic obstructive pulmonary disease is most commonly caused by smoking, with the onset of symptoms typically beginning in middle age. When younger patients or nonsmokers develop findings consistent with COPD, alpha-1-antitrypsin deficiency should be suspected. Chronic obstructive pulmonary disease is actually made up of two related and

---

Box 7-1

Rule of Twos

Rule of Twos: Patients Meeting Any of the Following Criteria Have Persistent Asthma

Use 2 or more canisters of beta-2-agonist per year
Use 2 or more doses of beta-2-agonist per week
Experience 2 or more nocturnal awakenings per month because of asthma symptoms
Require 2 or more unscheduled asthma-related visits per year
Require 2 or more bursts of prednisone per year

often coexisting problems: chronic bronchitis and emphysema. The condition is progressive and, overall, irreversible.

Signs and Symptoms.

The symptoms of COPD include chronic cough usually following years of smoking and with sputum production. The symptoms are worse on exertion and are usually progressive over time. There is often a history of exacerbations, during episodes of acute bronchitis. On physical exam, lung sounds are diminished. Crackles are more common than wheezes. The patient develops a "barrel chest," in which the AP chest diameter is greater than the lateral diameter. Progressive disease results in right heart failure, with abdominal distention, liver tenderness, and edema.

Diagnostic Studies.

Spirometry should be performed to confirm diagnosis. The ratio of forced expiratory volume in 1 second (FEV_1) to forced vital capacity is decreased from the norm of 80% to 60% or lower. Unless there is some degree of asthma, postbronchodilator spirometry does not improve more than 12%. Chest radiographs reveal hyperinflation of lungs, with flattened diaphragm. If alpha-1-antitrypsin deficit is suspected, a qualitative serum should be performed as a screen, followed by quantitative study, as indicated.

PNEUMONIA

Pneumonia involves inflammation and consolidation of lung tissue. Pneumonia is broadly categorized by whether it occurs outside of the hospital (community-acquired pneumonia) or within the hospital (nosocomial, or hospital-acquired, pneumonia). The cause is most often *Streptococcus pneumoniae*, *Haemophilus influenzae*, or *Staphylococcus aureus*. Atypical pneumonia involves infection of mycoplasma, legionella, or chlamydia. However, pneumonia can be caused by a wide range of microorganisms, including other bacteria, viruses, and fungi.

Signs and Symptoms.

The symptoms of pneumonia are quite varied. Commonly, the patient complains of cough associated with fever, malaise, shaking chills, rigors, and/or chest discomfort. The patient often appears ill. Abnormal vital signs include tachycardia and tachypnea, and fever. There is uneven fremitus and the area over the consolidation percusses dull. On auscultation, there are bronchial breath sounds, often with crackles. Bronchophony, egophony, and whispered pectoriloquy are often present.

Diagnostic Studies.

Chest film typically reveals an area of infiltrate. Cultures and Gram stains of sputum are usually not ordered for outpatients. The white blood cell count is often elevated.

ACUTE BRONCHITIS

Acute bronchitis is commonly encountered in ambulatory care and affects persons of all ages. It involves inflammatory processes of the bronchial smooth muscles and is associated with a wide range of microorganisms.

Signs and Symptoms.

Cough is the most common symptom of bronchitis and may persist for several weeks after the initial infection is resolved. During the acute phase, the cough may be productive. There may be associated symptoms including fever, malaise, chest discomfort, chills, and headache. The chills and chest discomfort are mild in comparison to the symptoms of pneumonia. There may be wheezes and/or crackles on auscultation, which disappear or alter with cough effort. Fremitus is equal and there is no egophony.

Diagnostic Studies.

None are necessary, unless chest radiology is needed to rule out pneumonia. Spirometry can be performed to rule out asthma and/or monitor response to therapy.

Congestive Heart Failure

Congestive heart failure (CHF) often results in cough, associated with the other symptoms and findings common to CHF. See Chapter 6, pp. 143–145.

Gastroesophageal Reflux Disease (GERD)

GERD is a common cause of chronic cough. The mechanism by which GERD causes cough usually involves vagal stimulation rather than aspiration. Although cough may be the only symptom of GERD, patients usually also complain of heartburn or other GI symptoms. See Chapter 9, pp. 198–199.

BRONCHIECTASIS

Bronchiectasis involves dilation of one or more bronchi. Congenital bronchiectasis affects infants and children. Acquired bronchiectasis involves older children and adults and stems from infections, bronchial obstruction, and cystic fibrosis.

Signs and Symptoms.

There is usually a history of chronic, productive cough. Sputum is typically mucopurulent. Other common findings include hemoptysis, shortness of breath, wheezing, fatigue, pleuritic pain, and weight loss. Physical exam reveals crackles and/or wheezing. In advanced disease, clubbing and cyanosis may be present.

Diagnostic Studies.

Chest films reveal linear markings, atelectasis, and/or pulmonary cysts. To confirm diagnosis, CT scan is used. Sputum studies may include positive cultures. Complete blood count may identify either anemia or polycythemia and increased white blood cell count. Pulmonary functions vary. Diagnostic studies are further needed to identify the cause of the condition.

TUBERCULOSIS

Tuberculosis is caused by a mycobacterium and frequently affects the lungs, although other organs may be involved. Risk factors include low socioeconomic status, impaired immune system, and crowded conditions. Tuberculosis presents a significant public health threat, and early diagnosis and treatment is important.

Signs and Symptoms.

Many times, patients with active tuberculosis are essentially symptom free. Some complain of malaise and/or fevers, but have no significantly disruptive complaints. When respiratory symptoms occur with tuberculosis, cough is common; the cough is nonproductive at first and is later associated with sputum production. Additionally, patients with tuberculosis may experience progressive dyspnea, night sweats, and weight loss, as well as hemoptysis.

Diagnostic Studies.

Plain chest films reveal multilobular granulomas, particularly of the upper lungs. For this reason, it is important to include a lordotic view with the usual AP and lateral views. Tuberculin skin testing is positive. Sputum reveals acid-fast bacilli. Sputum culture requires up to 3 weeks for definitive diagnosis, but should identify *M. tuberculosis*.

MALIGNANCY

Pulmonary malignancies may arise anywhere from the tracheobronchial tree to peripheral lung tissue.

Signs and Symptoms.

There may be few symptoms until the condition is advanced. Common complaints include dyspnea, cough, hemoptysis, fatigue, wheezing, and chest discomfort. Suspicion of potential malignancy should be heightened in patients who present with cough and hemoptysis, paired with history of recurrent respiratory infections. Physical signs depend on the area of involvement, and the exam may be entirely normal. However, patients with pulmonary malignancy may appear ill, have unexplained weight loss, and a variety of abnormal pulmonary findings, including asymmetrical breath sounds, adventitious sounds and/or stridor.

Diagnostic Studies.

Pulmonary functions vary depending on the location and size of mass. Chest films are often nondiagnostic, although they may reveal a nodule, mass, or other abnormality. A CT scan of the chest is typically used diagnostically and can be followed by MRI if the CT does not identify a mass. Diagnosis is made on biopsy and histopathy, with samples obtained by fine needle aspiration, bronchoscopy, mediastinoscopy, or thoracentesis.

PHARMACOLOGIC AND ACE INHIBITOR–INDUCED COUGH

Although cough can be associated with a variety of other medications, including aspirin, ACE inhibitors are a common cause of chronic cough. ACE inhibitors allow kinins to accumulate in the respiratory tract, causing a cough in 10%–20% of patients who are prescribed these agents.

Signs and Symptoms.

The cough associated with ACE inhibitors is dry and intractable and often worst at night. Aspirin is a common trigger of asthma, and a cough due to aspirin or NSAIDs is often tight and dry, accompanied by wheezing. The history is of cough onset soon after newly prescribed agent.

Diagnostic Studies.

None warranted, other than to rule out other causes. Diagnosis is typically made by discontinuing the offending agent. Aspirin-associated cough may persist for a considerable time following elimination of the agent.

PSYCHOGENIC COUGH

The term psychogenic cough is used to describe the situation in which there is no apparent organic cause for a cough. This may be associated with psychological disorders. Sometimes, patients develop a nervous habit cough. These causes must be considered after other organic causes have been ruled out.

Sign and Symptoms.

Patients may complain of chronic cough or family members may complain that the patient has persistent cough. There are usually no other related symptoms, and the physical exam is negative.

Diagnostic Studies.

Based on the patient's risk factors and exposures, diagnostic studies may be necessary to exclude other causes. The results of diagnostic studies should be within normal limits.

Shortness of Breath and Dyspnea

Dyspnea is the subjective sense of discomfort or difficulty breathing. Commonly, patients with dyspnea may present with complaint of shortness of breath, chest tightness, or simply difficulty breathing or catching the breath. With this presentation, it is essential that the symptom be thoroughly explored, in order to help the patient definitively define the complaint. The setting in which the dyspnea occurs is important, including whether it occurs in specific situations or activities, is persistent or intermittent, and has any associated symptoms. In addition to the history and physical specific to the respiratory system, a comprehensive assessment must be included, because the causes of dyspnea may stem from many extrapulmonary conditions. In assessing the dyspnea, there are a variety of measures that can be used. For instance, the patient can be asked to identify the point along a 10-cm visual analog scale that best depicts the dyspnea experienced, with one pole representing absence of shortness of breath or dyspnea and the other pole representing the worst dyspnea imaginable. Other scales depend on numerical rating and/or are specific to dyspnea related to a particular condition, such as asthma or cancer. A thorough medication history must be obtained.

Pneumonia

Pneumonia often causes acute dyspnea. See previous discussion on pneumonia, p. 159.

Congestive Heart Failure

Dyspnea is associated with congestive heart failure. See pp. 143–145.

PLEURAL EFFUSION

Pleural effusions involve an abnormal collection of fluid in the pleural space. Effusions are usually secondary to another condition, such as malignancy, heart failure, cirrhosis, trauma, and infections.

Signs and Symptoms.

Dyspnea is the most common symptom associated with pleural effusion, but effusion may be accompanied by cough, pain, and systemic symptoms, such as malaise and fever. Abnormal physical findings become evident as the effusion increases in volume. These include decreased lung sounds, dullness over the effusion, decreased fremitus, egophony, and whispered pectoriloquy. With extremely large effusions, the mediastinum and trachea may shift to the opposite side. The exception involves effusion related to malignancy, in which case the mediastinum and trachea may be pulled toward the malignancy.

Diagnostic Studies.

Chest films reveal the fluid collection as an increased area of density, blunting of costophrenic angle, and/or elevation of the hemidiaphragm. Plain films may also reveal a potential cause, including a mass or malignancy, infiltrates of pneumonia, or cardiomegaly of heart failure. A consultant may perform a thoracentesis to remove the effusion for observation and therapy. Observations include determining whether the fluid is purulent, bloody, milky, and/or malodorous. Testing could involve Gram stain, cultures, pH, cytology, and chemical studies.

PULMONARY EMBOLISM

Pulmonary emboli (PE) are life-threatening events, stemming from venous thrombi. The symptoms associated with pulmonary emboli range from very dramatic to nonspecific, making them sometimes difficult to diagnose.

Signs and Symptoms.

There may be a history of immobility, surgery, pregnancy, hypercoagulability, deep venous thrombosis, or other condition(s) associated with the development of emboli. Dyspnea is common to PE, as is pain. Patients may have no symptoms at all or only non-specific dyspnea. However, in severe cases, the patient presents with a sudden onset of severe dyspnea, associated with cough, chest pain, and, potentially, hemoptysis. Physical findings also vary. The patient is often tachycardic and tachypneic. Crackles and chest tenderness are common. There may be findings consistent with pleural effusion on the affected side (see preceding subsection).

Diagnostic Studies.

Plain chest films are usually normal, but may reveal atelectasis, pleural effusion, or infiltrates. Ventilation/perfusion (V/Q) scanning reveals a perfusion defect. Arterial blood gases are nonspecific, but reveal respiratory alkalosis, with hypoxemia and hypocapnia. Spiral CT with contrast has high sensitivity and specificity for PE.

RESTRICTIVE LUNG DISEASE

Both pulmonary and extrapulmonary disorders can result in diminished lung capacity and restrictive lung disease. Pulmonary disorders that affect the compliance of the lung tissue result in decreased ventilation, as do extrinsic conditions, such as kyphosis. Onset may be gradual for lung problems such as pneumonitis, pulmonary fibrosis, and sarcoidosis, as well as extrinsic problems causes, such as kyphosis or obesity.

Signs and Symptoms.

There may be a family history of intrinsic restrictive lung disease or personal history of occupational exposure to toxins. Patients with neuromuscular disorders often have symptoms of generalized fatigue and weakness. With extrinsic conditions, such as kyphosis or obesity, physical findings are usually evident. Examination reveals restricted respiratory excursion and, often, crackles.

Diagnostic Studies.

Appropriate studies vary depending on the suspected cause of restricted airway disease. Spirometry reveals decreased FEV_1, total lung capacity, and/or forced vital capacity.

PNEUMOTHORAX

Pneumothorax involves air in the pleural cavity. A pneumothorax can occur spontaneously in otherwise healthy individuals or be secondary to trauma or intrinsic lung disease.

Signs and Symptoms.

There is history of sudden onset of shortness of breath, associated with chest pain. The patient usually presents in great distress, with tachycardia and tachypnea, and is often splinting the chest. There is decreased fremitus and increased hyperresonance on the affected side. Lung sounds are diminished or absent. The trachea may shift away from the affected side if a large pneumothorax is present.

Diagnostic Studies.

Plain chest films usually reveal the pneumothorax, with an absence of lung markings in the affected area and shift of the mediastinum.

FOREIGN BODY ASPIRATION

Aspiration of a solid or semisolid object can be life threatening. Foreign body aspiration can occur at any age. However, young children, who have a tendency to put objects in their mouths, have the highest incidence of foreign body aspiration and associated mortality. Onset of symptoms may be sudden, if the object obstructs airway. However, if the airway is not significantly obstructed, symptoms may develop more slowly, as the aspiration results in pneumonia.

Signs and Symptoms.

There may be a witnessed episode of sudden difficulty breathing and/or choking, accompanied by inability to speak; cyanosis; coughing; and/or loss of consciousness. If the airway obstruction is complete, respiratory arrest occurs. If obstruction is partial, there will be varying degrees of coughing, wheezing, stridor. If obstruction is not significant, the patient may present with complaints of cough, increasing dyspnea, fever, and symptoms consistent with pneumonia. Physical findings depend on the degree of obstruction and can include stridor, wheezing, diminished lung sounds, cyanosis, and/or findings consistent with pneumonia.

Diagnostic Studies.

Plain chest films may reveal air trapping or atelectasis, as well as the radiolucent object. A CT scan may be necessary to identify radiopaque objects. A bronchoscopy may be necessary to identify and/or remove a foreign object.

Malignancy

Pulmonary and nonpulmonary malignancies may result in difficulty breathing. See previous discussion, p. 161.

Asthma

Shortness of breath or dyspnea is extremely common in asthma. See previous discussion of asthma, p. 158.

COPD

Progressive dyspnea is a common finding of COPD. See previous discussion, pp. 158–159.

Anemia

Anemia can result in dyspnea or a sense of "air hunger." See the discussion of anemia in Chapter 15, p. 382.

Wheezing and Chest Tightness

Wheezing is an audible respiratory sound, often associated with a sense of chest tightness and/or dyspnea. Many of the conditions included in the preceding discussions of cough and dyspnea also cause wheezing and chest tightness. For this reason, the history and physical assessment for this complaint are the same as for the other respiratory complaints and should be thorough.

LARYNGEAL OR TRACHEAL OBSTRUCTION

Obstruction of the large airways can occur with many conditions, including inflammation, malignancy, laryngospasm, and foreign body aspiration.

Signs and Symptoms.

The symptoms and signs will vary dependent on the condition responsible for the obstruction. The wheezing will be evident over the major airways, and the sound is often more harsh and stridorous than typical wheezing.

Diagnostic Studies.
   Appropriate diagnostic studies will depend on suspected cause.

Asthma
Wheezing is commonly associated with asthma. See previous discussion, page XX.

Acute Bronchitis
See previous discussion, page XX.

COPD
Wheezing often occurs with COPD, particularly chronic bronchitis. See page XX.

Malignancy
Bronchial and pulmonary tumors can present with wheezing. See page XX.

Hemoptysis

Hemoptysis can be associated with a wide range of pulmonary disorders, which have been described in this chapter. With presentation of a hemoptysis complaint, it is essential that the history identify associated symptoms, in addition to the analysis of hemoptysis. Investigate recent exposures to other persons with infectious diseases. Patients living in close proximity to others are at increased risk for contracting infectious respiratory disorders. A history of smoking is important; history of tuberculosis or positive skin tests must be identified. A thorough examination of the respiratory system provides data important to narrowing the differential diagnosis. Diagnostic studies often include plain radiographs of the chest.

Tuberculosis
Hemoptysis is a late symptom of tuberculosis, which is described on page XX.

Pneumonia
Pneumonia may result in hemoptysis and is described on page XX.

Malignancy
Malignancy should be considered for patients with hemoptysis. See page XX.

Bronchitis
Bronchitis can result in hemoptysis. See page XX.

Pulmonary Emboli
See page XX.

Pleuritic Pain

Pleuritic pain is associated with respiratory movements and breathing. Although the cause is often respiratory in nature, pleuritic pain is also associated with chest trauma and inflammation, as well as gastrointestinal and cardiac disorders. Pleuritic pain can be very distressful and can also cause great anxiety. A thorough symptom analysis is necessary. Through the history, determine whether there have been recent symptoms of respiratory infection, trauma to the chest, or extrapulmonary symptoms consistent with musculoskeletal, gastrointestinal, or cardiac problems. A comprehensive physical assessment is necessary.

COSTOCHONDRITIS

Costochondritis is pain at a costosternal cartilage site. It can follow trauma to the chest wall, but the cause is often not identifiable. The symptoms may follow a period of strenuous exercise or coughing.

Signs and Symptoms.

The patient reports pleuritic pain that is affected by breathing or chest motion. The site of tenderness is limited and the pain is reproducible with firm pressure to the site. On occasion there are signs of inflammation at the tender area, but generally the physical exam is otherwise negative.

Diagnostic Studies.

Generally no diagnostic studies are warranted.

PLEURISY

Pleurisy involves inflammation of the pleura and is often related to underlying infectious process.

Signs and Symptoms.

The patient complains of severe and sharp pleuritic pain, with acute onset. The pain may be noted only with cough, respiration, or maneuvers causing chest motion. However, there may be a sense of vague consistent pain that becomes pronounced with respiratory motions. The patient often splints the chest, attempts shallow respirations to limit the discomfort. A pleural friction rub can be auscultated. Pleural effusion may develop, with physical findings of percussive dullness, decreased fremitus, egophony, and decreased breath sounds at the site.

Diagnostic Studies.

The diagnosis is usually based on the history of definitive pleuritic pain and physical findings. However, chest films can be obtained and will vary from being within normal limits to revealing pleural effusion.

CHEST TRAUMA

Direct trauma to the chest can result in pain that is worsened with respirations owing either to rib fracture or injury to the intercostal muscles

Signs and Symptoms.

The history should reveal the offending trauma, with physical findings consistent with the injury.

Diagnostic Studies.

Diagnostic studies should be determined by the history of trauma.

Pericarditis

Pericarditis involves inflammation of the pericardium. Pericarditis can be associated with infectious disorder, as well as a variety of other conditions. See the discussion in Chapter 6.

Pulmonary Emboli

See previous discussion, pp. 162–163.

Malignancy

See previous discussion, p. 161.

References

CDC. (2004). Centers for Disease Control and Prevention. *National Vital Statistics Report*, 53 (5).

NHLBI. (2003). *Fact Sheet: Chronic Obstructive Pulmonary Disease Data*. Bethesda, MD: National Heart, Lung, and Blood Institute.

NHLBI. (2002). *Asthma Data and Prevalence*. Accessed online at URL www.nhlbi.nih.gov/health/prof/lung/asthma/surveil/htm on November 1, 2004.

 # SUGGESTED READINGS

Bickley, L.S., & Szilagyi, P.G. (2003). *Bates' Guide to Physical Examination and History Taking*. Philadelphia: Lippincott, Williams, and Wilkins.

Dillon, P.M. (2003). *Nursing Health Assessment: A Critical Thinking, Case Studies Approach*. Philadelphia: F.A. Davis.

Hah, D.L. (2003). Evaluation and management of acute bronchitis. In W.J. Hueston (Ed). *20 Common Problems: Respiratory Disorders*. New York: McGraw-Hill.

Hebbar, K. (2003). Pulmonary embolism. In W.J. Hueston (Ed). *20 Common Problems: Respiratory Disorders*. New York: McGraw-Hill.

Holmes, R.L., & Fadden, C.T. (2004) Evaluation of the patient with chronic cough. *American Family Physician* 69 (9), 2159–2166.

Hueston, W.J. (2003). Dyspnea and shortness of breath. In W.J. Hueston (Ed). *20 Common Problems: Respiratory Disorders*. New York: McGraw-Hill.

Morgan, W.C., & Hodge, H.L. (1998). Diagnostic evaluation of dyspnea. *American Family Physician*, 57 (4), 711–718.

National Asthma Education and Prevention Program. (2002). *Expert Panel Report: Guidelines for the Diagnosis and Management of Asthma: Update on Selected Topics 2002*. Bethesda, MD: National Heart, Lung, and Blood Institute.

NHLBI/WHO. (2004). Global Strategies for the Diagnosis, Management and Prevention of Chronic Obstructive Pulmonary Disease: Updated 2004. Bethesda, MD: National Heart, Lung, and Blood Institute.

Swartz, M.H. (2002). Textbook of Physical Diagnosis: History and Examination. Philadelphia: Saunders.

Turino, G.M. (2004). Approach to the patient with respiratory disease. In L. Goldman & D. Ausiello (Eds.). *Cecil Textbook of Medicine*. Philadelphia: Saunders.

Chapter 8
Breasts

Mary Jo Goolsby

Women in the United States have a one-in-eight chance of being diagnosed with breast cancer during their lifetime. In 2003, the American Cancer Society (ACS, 2003) estimated the diagnosis of over 211,000 cases of invasive breast cancer in addition to almost 56,000 cases of in situ cancer. Breast cancer is responsible for over 40,000 deaths each year. Whereas most breast cancer occurs in women, 1% of all breast cancer is diagnosed in men.

The role of mutations in the breast cancer susceptibility genes (including *BRCA1* and *BRCA2*) is being explored. Although fewer than 1% of women have mutations in these genes, between 5% and 10% of the women diagnosed with breast cancer are found to have a mutation. And although genetic testing for mutations in *BRCA1* became available in the mid-1990s, the application of genetic testing as it relates to the risk for developing breast cancer remains controversial. Women with a mutation have an increased risk for developing breast cancer, but other variables are involved and a positive finding is not clearly predictive of breast cancer. Similarly, testing negative for the mutated genes does not ensure that one will not develop breast cancer.

Another controversial technique that is currently being tested to determine its ability to predict breast cancer is ductal lavage. The premise is that 95% of breast cancers begin in the ducts and that identification of atypical cells should warrant further diagnostic investigation. The test involves a catheter being threaded into the breast duct through the nipple, allowing the duct to be lavaged and cells collected for cytology.

It is important to remember that the majority of breast complaints and findings are related to benign conditions. Whereas it is crucial to recognize and respond appropriately to potential signs of malignancy, it is also vital that providers recognize the range of other common breast conditions and their indications.

HISTORY

In addition to intrinsic breast disease, the function and structure of the breasts are influenced by changes in many other body systems.

For example, disorders of the musculoskeletal, respiratory, cardiovascular, or nerological systems can result in chest discomfort that is perceived as mastalgia, having breast origin. Endocrine problems, both reproductive and nonreproductive, may result in changes to breast tissue, comfort, and/or secretions. When assessing problems related to the breasts, it is important to consider the range of disorders that may influence breast health.

General History: Symptoms Analysis and Review of Systems

When obtaining a history related to a breast complaint, always complete a symptom analysis, using the PQRST sequence. The analysis of individual symptoms will be addressed in detail later in this chapter. When a patient complains of one breast symptom, it is important to obtain a complete review of other possible symptoms, including pain, mass, nipple discharge, skin changes, and recent nipple inversion. It is also important to ask about the presence of general and nonspecific symptoms, such as fatigue, fevers, appetite change, and weight loss. These will often be helpful in identifying potential endocrine problems or malignancy, which may present with nonspecific complaints.

Past Medical History

Ask about reproductive and menstrual history, including, as appropriate, age at menarche and at menopause. Ask about pregnancies, including the age at each pregnancy and whether the pregnancy resulted in a live birth. Assess the history of breastfeeding. Have the patient identify all previous breast surgeries or procedures. Include questions about breast augmentation, biopsies, and diagnostic studies. Determine the history of trauma to the chest/breasts. Obtain a history of chronic or current acute illnesses, particularly those of the reproductive/endocrine system. If the patient complains of breast pain, ask about musculoskeletal, cardiac, and neurologic disorders. During the medical history, obtain a history of all medications prescribed and/or taken by the patient. Many pharmacological agents have the potential to affect breast function, including hormone replacements, contraceptives, antidepressants and psychoactives, and antihypertensives. Moreover, the medication history may also help to identify a previously undisclosed health problem.

Family History

The family history should identify any breast problems, as well as disorders that might influence the breasts. Ask about the history of breast cancer and fibrocystic breasts, as well as any reproductive and endocrine disorders.

Habits

Obtain a history of caffeine and alcohol intake, as well as all over-the-counter and recreational drugs. Identify the level of physical activity, as well as any occupational or recreational activities that might place the patient at risk for trauma to the chest area.

PHYSICAL EXAMINATION

Although the examination of the female breasts is described, the same assessment should be performed for both men and women, particularly when the male patient presents with any of the symptoms described in the complaint section of this chapter.

Gail Model for Breast Cancer Risk Assessment

The Gail model is a clinical prediction rule used to estimate a patient's risk of breast cancer. The model identifies the relative risk associated with three factors obtained through history: age at menarche, number of previous breast biopsies, and the age at first live birth. The model combines the three risks to determine the woman's overall relative risk for her current age. Although applying the model is somewhat cumbersome, electronic calculators based on the model, some with slight adaptations, are readily available. One source is the calculator available at the National Cancer Institute's Web site, where individuals and providers can enter the information pertaining to each identified risk factor and receive the patient's risk for developing breast cancer within the next 5 years and by age 90.

Order of the Examination

Examination of the breasts typically includes only inspection and palpation. You will want to inspect the breasts with the patient in sitting and supine positions, and to palpate once the supine position is assumed.

Inspection

Observe the breasts as the patient is at rest, comparing for symmetry of size and contour. While the breasts are often slightly different in size, the difference is typically not excessive and is long-standing, as opposed to a recent development. Continue to inspect the breasts as the patient moves her arms through various motions: raising arms overhead, lowering the arms so that she presses palms together in front of her, and then pressing the hands downward against hips. Finally, ask the patient to lean forward at the waist. Through each motion, inspect the breast contours individually, observing for retractions, dimples, and irregularities of contour while also comparing the breasts with each other for symmetry. The motions cause constriction/motion of the breasts' underlying musculature, which may result in a "pulling" from any abnormal mass so that a retraction or dimple becomes evident. If normal, the breasts should move freely and the contours should remain smooth throughout the movement.

Following this surface inspection, assist the patient in assuming a supine position. Inspect the breasts again for general symmetry, comparing one with the other. Then inspect each breast individually, noting the skin's color and apparent texture, the general contour and smoothness, vascular pattern, areola, and nipple. Carefully note any irregularities or suspicious areas for detailed palpation. Identify any areas of retraction, dimpling, swelling, lesions, or discharge. Recent nipple inversion, retraction, or excoriation should be identified. Observe for other skin changes, including the peau d'orange condition, in which the skin of the breast is swollen so that the hair follicles look like "dimples" and the skin develops the texture of an orange peel.

Palpation

Before palpating either breast, ask the patient to raise her arm on the side to be examined, placing her hand behind her head. This maneuver extends the shoulder to approximately a 90-degree angle, providing better access to the breast region because it flattens the breast tissue across the chest wall. Examination of the breast should include the region from the midsternal line to the midaxillary line, from the subclavicular to approximately the 6–7th rib, or the "bra line." Several systems provide good coverage of the breast region. The specific sequence of palpation is unimportant, although each practitioner should become comfortable with a sequence that seems logical for him or her and that ensures palpation of the full breast region. Each individual examiner should be consistent with one approach. Palpation of the breast should also include attention to the axillary and subclavicular lymph nodes.

Regardless of the approach used, light, medium, and deep pressure should be applied at each palpation point. By varying the palpation pressure, you are more likely to detect masses—whether they are superficial or deep. Compress the area immediately beneath each areola, and gently squeeze each nipple. Breast tissue may be normally somewhat nodular or irregular, but the texture should be generally consistent between the breasts. Ask the patient to inform you of any areas of tenderness or pain elicited with the examination. Note any masses, areas of firmness, or nodules. Any mass should be assessed for size, consistency, mobility, margins/borders, shape, and delineation. It is sometimes helpful to palpate symmetrical areas of breast tissue simultaneously to assess areas of thickening or fullness.

As you palpate each breast, identify any discharge, which is most likely to be produced with pressure over the areola and/or when the nipple is gently squeezed. If any discharge is detected, assess its color, consistency, and odor, as well as the number of ducts from which the discharge appears. To collect the discharge, press a clean glass slide lightly against the nipple. In addition to facilitating the ability to judge the color and consistency of the discharge, the slide can also be used for cytology testing, if warranted. When there is discharge from multiple ducts, there is a higher likelihood of a cause such as fibrocystic change or galactorrhea. Malignancy should always be considered in the differential diagnosis for nipple discharge, although the likelihood of malignancy increases when the discharge is from only one duct.

Special Considerations

Women for whom special consideration is warranted include those who have had a mastectomy or breast-sparing surgery; those who have had breast augmentation, both cosmetic and postmastectomy; and women who have had breast reduction surgery. In these cases, careful history and examination relevant to the breasts are indicated.

For women who have previously been diagnosed and treated for breast cancer, the frequency at which they should have a clinical breast exam may often be greater than the usual. The unaffected breast should be examined using standard technique. Any remaining tissue on the affected side, including the axilla, should also be carefully examined.

Following breast augmentation, the ability to examine the breast tissue is somewhat dependent on the type and placement of the implant or augmentation. The history should include questions to detect any difficulty the woman may have experienced at the time of the procedure or implant, as well as current symptoms. The examination should be performed with the recognition that access to certain tissues may be occluded by the implant.

Following breast reduction, there is the potential for deep scarring and adhesions, which may confound the ability to palpate a mass. There may also be voids in the breast tissue, particularly in the tissue underlying the area of scarring, such that the normal and regular distribution of tissue is altered. When mammograms or other imaging studies are ordered on women following mastectomy, breast-sparing procedures, and breast augmentation or reduction surgeries, these details of the woman's history should be clearly noted.

DIFFERENTIAL DIAGNOSIS OF CHIEF COMPLAINTS
Breast Mass

Breast tissue is normally glandular and may have a rather nodular consistency. The degree of nodularity tends to fluctuate through the menstrual cycle in premenopausal women. Masses are most often significant when their characteristics are different from the surrounding area, are discrete, and tend to persist throughout the hormonal cycle. The term dominant breast mass describes a mass that persists throughout a woman's hormonal cycles, is larger and firmer than other irregularities, and differs from rest of the breast tissue. Dominant masses typically fall into the following categories: fibroadenomas, cysts, fibrocystic changes, fat necrosis, and malignancy. Whenever a breast mass is identified, it should be followed to diagnostic resolution. Breast cancer is always included in the differential diagnosis, and diagnostic efforts should definitely include either ruling out the existence of a malignancy or identifying it in a timely manner. Missed or delayed diagnoses can have catastrophic results and are, in fact, consistently among the most frequent causes of malpractice suits.

History

As with other breast symptoms, it is essential to obtain a complete reproductive and menstrual history, as well as to ascertain the symptoms associated with the discovery of the mass. Determine how long the mass has been present and whether it has changed since first noticed. If present for a while, ask whether any of its characteristics fluctuate in relation to the menstrual cycle. Identify any accompanying symptoms, such as pain, nipple discharge, or skin changes. Ask about recent trauma to the breast. The presence of systemic symptoms is important, as these may be signs of advanced breast cancer. These include loss of energy, altered appetite, weight loss, and fever.

Physical Examination

It is important to perform a complete breast exam for any complaint of breast mass. Throughout the examination, be attentive for changes in the skin; the contours of the breasts, including dimpling or retractions; nipple discharge; eczematous or similar rash or erosions around the nipple; and palpable axillary or subclavicular lymph nodes. It is crucial that the examiner confirm the presence of a palpable mass, carefully noting its location, and other characteristics.

The dimensions, mobility, consistency/texture of each palpable breast mass must be identified and are important in determining further diagnostic work-up. For any mass, determine whether it is soft, rubbery, firm, or hard; whether it is fixed and immobile or moves freely; whether it has smooth or irregular margins; and whether it is tender, painful, or painless. Determine whether the skin overlying an identified mass moves independently of the mass or, instead, is connected to the mass so that they move together. As the mass is palpated, try to determine whether it is cystic or solid. Any patient with a dominant breast mass should be referred for definitive diagnosis.

Diagnostic Studies

All patients with a palpable dominant breast mass should be referred. Imaging and other studies, such as biopsies, are necessary to discriminate among potential causes when a breast mass is detected either by the patient or provider. Unfortunately, both palpation and mammography, alone or together, are inadequate to definitely identify the cause of a breast mass and to rule out malignancy. Indicated for the assessment of a breast mass are mammography, ultrasound, aspiration, and biopsy. The "triple test" for evaluation of a breast mass involves clinical examination, either ultrasound or mammogram, and aspiration. The determination of whether an ultrasound or mammography is recommended is based on age and other situations. Women under 30 years of age have more dense breasts, and ultrasound is therefore more often useful than a mammogram. Ultrasounds are often helpful in determining whether or not a mass that feels potentially "cystic" is fluid filled or solid. The patient should be referred to a surgeon for definitive diagnosis, through fine needle aspiration (FNA) or core biopsy. If an FNA reveals only nonbloody aspirate and the mass appears to be resolved following aspiration, the surgeon may decide to recheck the patient in approximately 1 month. If the mass is still resolved at the follow-up visit, a decision may be made to do no further follow-up at that time, but instead to perform serial examinations over time. If an FNA reveals bloody aspirate or reveals a solid mass (suggested by inability to aspirate the mass), or if the cyst returns following aspiration, a biopsy is indicated. It is crucial that the term "diagnostic mammogram" not be interpreted to suggest that the procedure can diagnose whether or not a malignancy exists. A mammogram is a screening tool and is never diagnostic regarding the existence or absence of a malignancy.

MALIGNANCY

In the United States, breast cancer is responsible for over 40,000 deaths annually. It is the most common form of cancer among women and the second leading cause of cancer deaths. The differential diagnosis should include malignancy when a woman complains of or the practitioner identifies a breast mass. A thorough history and careful physical exam are essential if breast cancer is suspected.

Signs and Symptoms.

A breast lump is the most common presenting complaint in breast cancer and is usually the only presenting complaint. More rarely, the presentation may include complaint of discomfort, skin change, or discharge. If the cancer is advanced, the patient may have extra-breast symptoms, such as fatigue, weight loss, and bone pain. The typical malignant mass is solitary, non-tender, hard, immobile or fixed, and poorly defined. It may be accompanied by nipple erosion or other inflammatory skin changes, as seen in Paget's disease (an advanced example is illustrated in Plate 20, in Chapter 2), nipple discharge, skin thickening or dimpling, retraction, and palpable axillary nodes. Although most malignant masses are painless, associated discomfort does not exclude the potential for breast cancer.

Diagnostic Studies.

Any breast mass, particularly those that are solitary, noncyclic, and non-tender, should trigger a mammogram or ultrasound. The patient should be referred to a surgeon who will determine the need for FNA, biopsy, or other diagnostic studies.

FIBROADENOMA

Fibroadenomas are common, benign neoplasms that usually occur in premenopausal women. Women with fibroadenomas have a slightly higher than average lifetime risk of developing breast cancer. These changes usually appear in the second or third decade of life.

Signs and Symptoms.

There are usually no complaints other than the mass. Although fibroadenomas are usually solitary, they can be multiple. The lump is generally mobile, rubbery, and non-tender; has discrete and smooth borders; and is less than 5 cm in diameter. However, fibroadenomas may also have irregular borders.

Diagnostic Studies.

A mammogram or ultrasound is usually ordered to confirm the diagnosis and rule out malignancy. Even when a newly identified mass is consistent with a fibroadenoma and imaging supports the diagnosis, a surgical consult should be considered for definitive diagnosis.

FIBROCYSTIC CHANGE

Fibrocystic breast changes include a variety of histoplastic variations, with fibrotic thickening often paired with the development of cysts. This condition, however, is considered benign and/or physiologic rather than pathologic.

Signs and Symptoms.

The nodularity is usually associated with tenderness. The nodularity and tenderness are both cyclic in nature, fluctuating with the menstrual cycle. The symptoms are usually most severe just before menses. The lumps or nodules may fluctuate in size and or in number during the cycle. The changes are usually bilateral. Breast discharge may also occur cyclically before menses and is usually serous.

Diagnostic Studies.

In young women who have lumpy breasts with multiple areas of thickening and a cyclic component, with or without tenderness, immediate diagnostic studies are not generally necessary. The patient should be instructed to complete a breast symptom calendar for at least 2 months; the calendar can then be studied to confirm the cyclic nature of the symptoms. If there is a dominant mass identified or some other diagnostic uncertainty exists, a surgical consult should be obtained.

TRAUMA

Trauma to the anterior chest area may result in a palpable breast mass. An automobile accident in which the female sustains injury from contact with her seat belt, air bag, steering wheel, or dashboard is a common source of breast trauma. The trauma may result in a variety of injuries, and deeper damage should be considered, with assessment for musculoskeletal and lung injury. When a palpable mass results from chest trauma, it typically represents either a hematoma or area of secondary fat necrosis. Even when a mass is identified subsequent to direct trauma, the provider must remain suspicious for the possibility of malignancy that preexisted but was undetected before the accident.

Signs and Symptoms.

When a palpable mass is due to trauma, there will typically be associated chest wall and breast discomfort. There may be an area of ecchymosis or discoloration in the distribution of trauma. Patients with large breasts are more likely to develop fat necrosis than are those with small breasts. A palpable mass associated with trauma is often poorly defined and immobile. An area of fat necrosis is typically superficial and may develop calcified margins. It can be difficult to differentiate between isolated trauma and a potential for malignancy. Serial examinations should demonstrate a solution of the hematoma and/or no increase in mass size.

Diagnostic Studies.

Because the potential for malignancy is not easily excluded, an ultrasound or mammogram should be considered. Additional imaging may include plain films to assess the condition of ribs and other bones, as well as to exclude pneumothorax or hemothorax resulting from trauma.

Breast Pain

Breast pain—mastalgia or mastodynia—is the most common breast complaint. The most common type of breast pain is cyclic mastalgia, which occurs in premenopausal women and is associated with hormonal fluctuations. In contrast, noncyclic breast pain is often unilateral and may be described in many ways, including sharp, burning, aching. Many benign breast changes are associated with noncyclic mastalgia, including cysts, mastitis, trauma, abscess, duct ectasia, and fibroadenoma. Breast pain tends most often to be mild in severity but can be quite severe. Both noncyclic and cyclic breast pain may be associated with certain variables, such as the intake of methylxanthine/caffeine-containing products. Although pain is not commonly associated with the diagnosis of breast cancer, it may accompany malignancy and is sometimes the presenting complaint. A complaint of breast pain may also represent pain referred from another origin, usually related to some musculoskeletal or neuropathic disorder.

History

It is important to have the patient describe the pain in detail, through a symptom analysis, identifying any palliative/provocative factors, actual quality and type of pain, the primary region of pain and any radiation, the severity of the pain and any associated breast or systemic symptoms, and the timing. Any history of prior breast complaints, disorders, surgeries, and procedures should be determined. It may be appropriate to explore symptoms associated with other systems, including cardiac, neurological, and musculoskeletal. The menstrual history is important. If the patient has an infant, determine the history of lactation. The family history should include questions about breast cancer and fibrocystic breasts. It is important to identify any current medications, particularly hormonal contraceptives.

Physical Examination

A general survey should be completed to determine the patient's overall appearance. The exam should focus on the breasts and should be expanded, as indicated. Observe for masses, skin texture changes, redness/inflammation, and discharge. Notice whether any of the motions involved in the inspection phase of the examination seem to elicit discomfort.

Ask the patient to point to the area of discomfort. If the patient has complained of discomfort limited to a specific region, palpate the opposite breast first, before proceeding to the non-tender portion of the affected breast. Gently palpate the area of tenderness or pain, noting the boundaries of the discomfort, and assess the underlying tissue for any change in texture, or for masses.

Diagnostic Studies
A variety of diagnostic studies may be appropriate for the assessment of breast pain. If the pain is cyclic in nature and related to menses, there is generally no indication to order diagnostic studies. A diary of the breast discomfort may prove helpful, however. If the patient is over 30 and has not had a recent mammogram, it would be appropriate to order a routine mammogram, just as a part of normal care. If a solid mass or cyst is suspected, the pain is noncyclic, or the patient is postmenopausal, a surgical consult should be obtained. If the patient is under 30, an ultrasound would be appropriate in lieu of the mammogram. If mastitis is suspected, a white blood count is indicated.

HORMONAL, CYCLIC MASTALGIA

Although it is broadly assumed that cyclic mastalgia is related to fluctuating hormones, the mechanisms resulting in the discomfort are unknown. There does not seem to be a direct correlation between fluid retention, for instance, and breast tenderness or pain. Women who experience cyclic mastalgia usually have onset as a teen or young adult. It is important to determine menstrual and reproductive history and to identify all phamacologic agents taken. A complete breast examination should be performed.

Signs and Symptoms.
The pain associated with hormonal fluctuation most commonly occurs during the second half of the woman's cycle. The variability of the signs and symptoms is identified with a symptom calendar. Cyclic mastalgia pain is typically poorly localized, bilateral, and nonspecific. It may be accompanied by a sense of breast fullness. The exam may identify the multiple, bilateral nodularities associated with fibroadenomas or fibrocystic changes.

Diagnostic Studies.
The breast pain diary identifies the cyclic nature of the pain and its association with the menstrual cycle. If a mammogram or ultrasound is obtained, there is no indication of malignancy or mass other than fibroadenomas or cysts.

Fibroadenomas and Fibrocysts
As noted in the preceding, two benign causes of breast pain include fibroadenomas and fibrocystic breasts. Although fibroadenomas are not typically painful, they can be accompanied by discomfort. Both conditions are described in the previous section on breast masses.

MASTITIS

Mastitis is an inflammatory breast disorder, typically occurring in lactating women (puerperal mastitis) and caused by either a streptococcal or staphylococcal infection. The cause likely stems from altered nipple/areola skin integrity, with retrograde infection. Although rare, mastitis can occur in nonlactating females, and, in this situation, it often stems from duct ectasia (see later discussion on breast discharge), with an anaerobic microbe. It is important to recognize mastitis so that it can be promptly treated. Because mastitis does occur only rarely in nonlactating women, providers should remain suspicious of the potential for inflammatory breast cancer in women who are not nursing, particularly if there are no systemic symptoms of infection.

Signs and Symptoms.

The patient typically complains of unilateral pain, redness, and swelling of one breast. Systemic symptoms include fever, chills, and myalgia. The examination reveals a wedge-shaped area of redness that is swollen and very tender. Because the patient is typically nursing, there is often visible discharge of milk, which may be spontaneous as the breast becomes engorged.

Diagnostic Studies.

A white blood count should be obtained and is usually elevated. Even though the breast milk can be cultured, this is not generally recommended. If the presentation is atypical—that is, the patient is not lactating—and there are no associated systemic signs or symptoms, a consultation should be obtained and mammography ordered to determine the definitive diagnosis and rule out malignancy.

CHEST WALL PAIN AND COSTOCHONDRITIS

Costochondritis is a condition in which there is usually localized discomfort, often quite sharp in nature, along the costochondral and/or costosternal cartilages. The cause of the pain is unknown. Costochondritis is one form of chest discomfort that can mimic breast pain. Others include posttrauma pain, as described earlier.

Signs and Symptoms.

The patient usually has well-localized pain, often with point tenderness. The pain often worsens with straining and/or motion of the chest wall, for instance, during coughing or deep breathing. There are typically no physical signs, other than pain on palpation of the affected site. Exceptions might occur if, rather than costochondritis, the chest wall pain were due to recent trauma, in which case signs of trauma might be present.

Diagnostic Studies.

The diagnosis is generally made by the history and physical, with no diagnostic studies warranted.

RADICULAR NERVE PAIN

Nerve root inflammation or impingement can result in pain that radiates or is experienced in the region of breasts. Thoracic lesions may radiate to the chest.

Signs and Symptoms.

Pain is typically sharp or burning in nature. The discomfort is often worsened by movements that narrow the intervertebral space. If inflammation is involved, for instance, with herpes zoster, nerve root discomfort or neuralgia often precedes the onset of skin changes, which follow with the development of erythematous skin and progress to vesicles along the dermatome. The patient may also complain of malaise and fever, common to viral disorders.

Diagnostic Studies.

If nerve root compression is suspected, thoracic images should be obtained to confirm or rule out the cause. Herpes zoster is diagnosed based on the presentation and skin changes, with no diagnostic studies indicated.

Cardiac Pain

Ischemic heart pain can be misinterpreted as breast pain. When the presentation involves atypical breast pain and/or occurs in a patient at high risk for cardiac disease, cardiac pain should be strongly considered in the differential diagnosis. Cardiac pain is described in Chapter 6.

Breast Discharge

Although breast discharge may occur without pathology, it may be indicative of serious disorders. Categories of breast or nipple discharge include galactorrhea, physiologic discharge, and pathologic discharge. Galactorrhea can be caused by a variety of endocrine disorders. Causes of pathologic discharge include ductal papilloma, duct ectasia, and fibrocystic changes. Discharge may be present at the diagnosis of breast cancer. However, the vast majority (95%) of breast discharge cases are from benign causes. In over 50% of females, a very small amount of discharge (one or a very few drops) can be produced by manipulating the breast and nipple, but this is not considered spontaneous.

History

Determine whether the discharge is bilateral or unilateral and whether it comes from single or multiple ducts. Ask whether or not it comes from the same site on the nipple each time. Determine whether the discharge is spontaneous or comes after breast manipulation. The color and consistency of the discharge are important characteristics and should be determined, as should the presence of any other breast symptoms, including pain, retraction, skin changes, or mass. The menstrual, reproductive, and lactating histories are important. A thorough medication and substance history is crucial, as breast discharge can be caused by several agents. Similarly, discharge is a sign of other conditions, including renal, endocrine, and idiopathic disorders. Ask about a history of headaches, visual changes, recent trauma, and thyroid symptoms or disorders. Determine whether the patient participates in high-intensity exercise and, if so, what type of bra is worn.

Physical Examination

The breast exam should be thorough and include manipulation intended to produce discharge. If no discharge is produced by the general breast examination, finally depress the areolar region and note any discharge. If milky discharge is produced, milk production can be confirmed by microscopic identification of fat globules. In addition to the breast exam, the assessment should include a general physical assessment, noting facial features, skin, and visual fields because acromegaly, hypothyroidism, and pituitary tumors are commonly associated with galactorrhea. The examiner should also be attentive for signs of other endocrine disorders, including Cushing's syndrome, and signs of renal failure, liver failure, and sarcoidosis.

Diagnostic Studies

Pregnancy should be excluded. If pregnancy is excluded, additional studies should include a prolactin level and thyroid studies. Pituitary imaging should be considered if the prolactin level is elevated. If thyroid and pituitary studies are negative, renal and liver function tests should be ordered. A mammogram should be obtained to exclude malignancy, even if a palpable mass is not identified.

GALACTORRHEA

Galactorrhea is characterized by bilateral and milky discharge from multiple ducts in a woman who is neither pregnant nor lactating. Causes of galactorrhea include a variety of drugs, as well as an elevated prolactin level, associated with pituitary tumor or hyperthyroidism. The drugs associated with galactorrhea include antidepressants (amitryptyline, imipramine), psychoactives (haloperidol, thioridazine), hormones (estrogens, progestogens), antiepileptics (valproic acid), and antihypertensives (verapamil). This list is not exhaustive.

Signs and Symptoms.

If associated with prolactin elevation, there may be symptoms of a pituitary tumor, including headaches, vision change, relative infertility, and amenorrhea. The signs of thyroid disease or acromegaly may be present. If acromegaly is involved, the woman may admit to recent changes in shoe or ring size, as well as other structural changes. The history may identify one or more of the medications that are commonly associated with galactorrhea. The breast examination is negative, with the exception of possibly stimulating the production of milky discharge.

Diagnostic Studies.

Laboratory studies should include a pregnancy test, prolactin level, and thyroid functions.

PHYSIOLOGIC DISCHARGE

As noted earlier, physiologic discharge is not rare. Physiologic discharge may be associated with fibrocystic breasts or gynecomastia, or it may exist with no other breast complaints. In addition to squeezing of the breast, physiologic discharge may be caused by trauma or exercise. It may occur in response to hormonal changes at puberty or menopause.

Signs and Symptoms.

Physiologic discharge is not spontaneous but is triggered by manipulation and/or excessive movement. It is bilateral, comes from multiple ducts, and is serous in appearance. The patient may complain of cyclic symptoms of mastalgia or lumpy breasts.

PATHOLOGIC DISCHARGE

Pathologic discharge is most often unilateral, spontaneous, and limited to one duct, although multiple ducts in a limited area may be involved. It can be intermittent and persistent. The color of pathologic discharge ranges widely and can be watery, cloudy, bloody, serosanguineous, green-gray, and multicolored. In spite of the term "pathologic," the cause is usually benign and frequently includes duct ectasia or an intraductal papilloma. Duct ectasia results in dilation of one major breast duct and causes approximately one-third of the cases of pathological discharge. Because the discharge associated with ductal ectasia is often stagnant, the discharge is cheesy in appearance. Papillomas are responsible for 44% of pathologic discharge. The discharge associated with papillomas ranges from serous to bloody.

Signs and Symptoms.

The discharge associated with duct ectasia comes from one duct and is "cheesy" in consistency. It is often associated with noncyclic breast discomfort and a subareolar lump, at the site of the dilated duct. Papillomas can occur singly or in multiples; the intraductal papilloma is generally located proximal to the nipple. Because one major duct is involved, the discharge comes also from one duct or nipple area. However, in contrast to the discharge associated with duct ectasia, papillomas cause discharge that ranges from serous, to serosanguineous, to bloody. A clean glass slide is used to collect discharge for inspection and any subsequent analysis.

Diagnostic Studies.

A mammogram should be ordered, and it will reveal the dilated duct or the papilloma. Surgical consultation is indicated to determine the need for excision.

Malignancy

Breast discharge is also a potential sign of malignancy (11%). Up to 5% of women diagnosed with breast cancer have nipple discharge as part of their presentation, although it is rarely a solitary symptom or sign. Cytology of the discharge is diagnostic in only approximately 50% of cases in which cancer is present and is, therefore, not reliable in diagnosis. Mammography should be performed to begin discrimination among benign causes, such as mammary duct ectasia, cancer, and other possibilities. However, a negative mammogram does not exclude malignancy. In fact, of those women who presented with nipple discharge and were diagnosed with cancer, only approximately 50% had an abnormal mammogram. Thus, if a benign explanation is not identified for the discharge, the woman should be referred to a surgeon for further evaluation.

Male Breast Enlargement or Mass

As noted previously, although the risk for developing breast cancer is much lower in men than in women, 1% of all breast cancer is diagnosed in men. In addition to the potential for a malignancy, complaints of breast changes in men may indicate hormonal disturbances, adverse effects of medications, and systemic symptoms of liver or renal disease. Complaints of breast enlargement or mass should trigger careful investigation.

The general term for male breast enlargement is gynecomastia, which can be present in one or both breasts. Even though hormone-related gynecomastia is relatively common, particularly in pubertal and older adult males, it must be differentiated from adipose tissue, lipoma, hematoma, malignancy, and systemic conditions.

History

Obtain a full history of the breast enlargement, including when it was first noted, any subsequent changes in the area, and any associated symptoms. When asking about associated symptoms, include skin changes, discharge and pain or tenderness, as well as systemic symptoms that would indicate extramammary conditions. Identify any history of previous breast changes or procedures and the family history of breast disease. The past medical history should be directed toward identifying all current and previous medical problems and a list of all medications/drugs currently taken.

Physical Examination

A complete examination of the breasts should be performed. The male breasts are best examined with the patient resting supine, with his arm raised over his head. The same examination techniques should be incorporated, including careful inspection for any skin changes, retractions, areas of thickening, bulges, or visible masses. The palpation should include comparison of breast tissue consistency between the breasts and identification of any palpable masses and their characteristics. The axillary nodes should be assessed. Obese men are more likely to have "fatty breasts" than true gynecomastia. It is often helpful to compare the consistency of the affected breast(s) with the consistency of the tissue in the anterior axillary fold region, to determine whether or not adipose tissue is involved.

Diagnostic Studies

If a palpable mass is discovered that is not consistent with gynecomastia (see the following section), imaging studies (an ultrasound or mammogram) should be obtained to determine the cause. A surgical consult should be obtained if a benign diagnosis is not certain.

GYNECOMASTIA

Gynecomastia most often occurs during infancy, puberty, and senescence. It is caused by an altered balance between estradiol and testosterone levels. Although it can be an indication of primary hypogonadism (see Chapter 11), hyperthyroidism, cirrhosis, or renal disease, the majority of the cases are specific to hormonal changes of puberty, are drug induced, or are idiopathic. With the presentation of breast enlargement in a male, malignancy must always be considered.

Signs and Symptoms.

The enlargement associated with gynecomastia presents as a disk-shaped rubbery area of tissue that is centered beneath the areola, extending out centrifugally. The thickened area of tissue may be tender, and there may be associated nipple discharge. Other times, there are no other findings or symptoms except for the area of enlargement. If the enlargement is due to some condition other than gynecomastia, the mass or enlargement will be found in an area remote from the areola and can be hard, irregularly shaped, or immobile. If drug induced, the patient may identify one of the many drugs known to cause gynecomastia, such as phenytoin, cimetidine, estrogens, calcium-channel blockers, ACE inhibitors, spironolactone, finasteride, methyldopa, or marijuana. If the drug is eliminated, the enlargement may resolve. If related to cirrhosis or renal failure, other physical signs of the etiologic condition should be evident.

Diagnostic Studies.

If the mass or enlargement is consistent with gynecomastia, there is no need to perform diagnostic studies. However, ultrasound or mammography should be considered, if necessary, for either definitive diagnosis or reassurance of the patient. The provider should be alert to the remote potential that the gynecomastia stems from cirrhosis or renal disease and determine whether renal or liver function studies should be ordered.

PSEUDOGYNECOMASTIA

Pseudogynecomastia refers to fatty deposits and enlargements of the breast that are related to obesity.

Signs and Symptoms.

The patient will have no tenderness, discharge, or other symptoms related to the breast enlargement. The area of enlargement will have a consistency similar to the patient's other fatty areas, for instance, the tissue in the immediate region of the anterior axillary fold. There will be no palpable rubbery disk of thickening beneath the areola and no signs of malignancy will be present, including retractions, dimpling, nipple discharge, or a discrete palpable mass.

Diagnostic Studies.

There are no diagnostic studies indicated for pseudogynecomastia.

MALIGNANCY

On average, 1500 new cases of male breast cancer are diagnosed each year in the United States, and there are over 400 related deaths (ACS, 2002). Men develop the same types of breast cancer as women. Therefore, it is important to include malignancy in the differential diagnosis when a man complains of breast enlargement. Factors that increase the risk of breast cancer in men include a previous history of breast or testicular disease and Klinefelter's syndrome. A history of gynecomastia is not associated with an increased risk for breast cancer.

Signs and Symptoms.

The man may complain of breast tenderness, skin changes, and/or nipple discharge. There may be associated systemic symptoms of fatigue, weight loss, and so on. The mass may be more evident in a male patient who has less breast tissue than a woman. The mass will usually lie in a location that is inconsistent with gynecomastia. However, regardless of the site, any firm or hard mass should trigger investigation for malignancy. Nipple discharge associated with malignancy is often bloody.

References

American Cancer Society. Cancer Facts & Figures, 2003. America Cancer Society, Atlanta, GA, 2003.

 SUGGESTED READINGS

Apantaku, L.M. (2000). Breast cancer diagnosis and screening. *American Family Physician*, 62, 596–602.

Bickley, L.S., & Szilagyi, P.G. (2003). *Bates' Guide to Physical Examination and History Taking*. Philadelphia: Lippincott, Williams, and Wilkins.

Bland, K.L., & Copeland, E.M. (2004). *The Breast: Comprehensive Management of Benign and Malignant Disorders*. Philadelphia: Saunders.

Dillon, P.M. (2003). *Nursing Health Assessment: A Critical Thinking, Case Studies Approach*. Philadelphia: F.A. Davis.

Donegan, W.L., & Spratt, J. S. (2002). *Cancer of the Breast* (5th ed). Philadelphia: Saunders.

Morrow, M. (2000). The evaluation of common breast problems. *American Family Physician*, 61, 6371–6378.

Poole, G.V. (1999). Benign breast disorders. In Rivlin, M.E., & Nartin, R.W. (Eds.). *Manual of Clinical Problems in Obstetrics and Gynecology*. Philadelphia: Lippincott, Williams, & Wilkins.

Swartz, M.H. (2002). *Textbook of Physical Diagnosis: History and Examination*. Philadelphia: Saunders.

Poole, G.V. (1999). Malignant breast disease. In Rivlin, M.E., & Nartin, R.W. (Eds.). *Manual of Clinical Problems in Obstetrics and Gynecology*. Philadelphia: Lippincott, Williams, & Wilkins.

Chapter 9

Abdomen

Mary Jo Goolsby & Laurie Grubbs

In 2001, digestive disease accounted for 31.6 million office visits, 3 million outpatient department visits, and 3.3 million emergency department visits (CDC, 2003). Diarrheal conditions are the most prevalent gastrointestinal problems in the United States, with over 200 million cases occurring annually, when causes both food-borne and otherwise are combined. These are followed in prevalence by gastroesophageal reflux (GERD), diseases of the gall bladder, and irritable bowel syndrome (IBS). The most costly digestive disease is GERD, with annual direct costs of over $9 billion. Other costly gastrointestinal conditions include gall bladder disease, colorectal cancer, and peptic ulcer disease (PUD), with direct costs of $5.8 billion, $4.9 billion, and $3.1 billion, respectively (AGA, 2001). Over 110,000 cases of digestive tract cancer are diagnosed each year, of which approximately 65,000 are cancers of the colon and rectum, combined (CDC, 2000).

The causes of abdominal complaints can range from very mild, self-limited problems to those that can be disabling or result in mortality. In addition to digestive diseases, abdominal complaints may be indicative of musculoskeletal, neurologic, genitourinary, reproductive, cardiovascular, or respiratory disorders.

HISTORY
General History
A general history for the abdominal exam should include any reports of nausea and/or vomiting; current bowel habits, including diarrhea, changes in bowel or bladder habits, or constipation; and pain, weight loss or gain, change in appetite, bloating, excessive gas or belching, dysphagia, heartburn or indigestion, rectal bleeding, or black stools. Ask about past history of jaundice, liver disease, hepatitis, gallbladder disease, fever, or malaise. As specific complaints are discussed subsequently in the chapter, further symptom analysis will be described.

Past Medical History

A general past medical history should include any history of jaundice, liver disease, hepatitis, gallbladder disease, infectious diseases, PUD, GERD, bleeding or platelet disorders, trauma, or previous surgeries with the emphasis on abdominal surgeries.

Family History

Identify any history in the family of liver or gallbladder disease, hepatitis, or cancer. There is a familial predisposition to certain diseases of the digestive tract, such as inflammatory bowel disease, polyposis, and cancer of the colon. There is an increased risk of hepatitis among family members in the same household, especially hepatitis C.

Habits

Habits may be particularly important for certain abdominal complaints, especially the use of tobacco, caffeine, and alcohol. Also important are a list of all medications/drugs, activity, exercise, and sleep patterns. Identify usual dietary intake. Explore sexual habits. Ask about travel patterns and recent exposures.

PHYSICAL EXAMINATION

The abdominal exam begins with inspection, followed by auscultation, percussion, and palpation. Auscultating before percussion or palpation allows the examiner to listen to the abdominal sounds undisturbed. Moreover, if pain is present, it is best to leave palpation until last and to gather other data before possibly causing the patient discomfort. When examining the abdomen, it often helps to break the abdomen down into quadrants, or regions, in order to consider which organs are involved (see Figure 9-1).

Order of the Examination

Inspection

Inspect for scars, striae, venous pattern, rashes, contour, symmetry, masses, peristalsis, pulsations, or discolorations. The use of tangential lighting is helpful when observing for peristalsis and pulsations. See Table 9-1 for abnormalities found on inspection.

Auscultation

Perform before palpation so as to hear unaltered bowel sounds. Listen for bruits over the aorta and the iliac, renal, and femoral arteries. See Table 9-2 for abnormalities found on auscultation.

Percussion

Percuss for areas of dullness, indicating fluid or solid, rather than air. See Table 9-3 for normal percussion tones.

Palpation

Both light and deep palpation are necessary to detect tenderness tumors, or changes in underlying structures. Note any areas of tenderness, any changes in contour, and the presence of masses—and if masses are present, their consistency, size, shape, location, and delineation. See Table 9-4 for abnormalities found on palpation.

- Light palpation—helpful in detecting tenderness and guarding
- Deep palpation—usually required in order to delineate masses

Rectal Examination

A digital rectal exam is included in the abdominal exam. Note any skin changes or lesions in the perianal region, or the presence of external hemorrhoids. Insert the gloved index

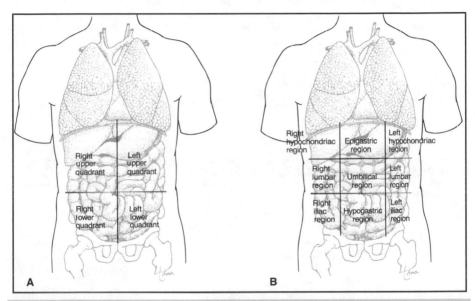

Figure 9-1. ■ Areas of the abdomen: (A) Four quadrants. (B) Nine regions. (From Scanlon, V.C., & Sanders, T. Essentials of anatomy and physiology, 4th ed. Philadelphia: F.A. Davis. 2003. Reprinted with permission)

Abdominal Regions

RUQ	_Epigastric_	_LUQ_
Liver	Stomach	Spleen
GB	Pancreas	Pancreas
Tip of Right Kidney		Tip of Left Kidney
Diaphragm		
Right Lumbar	_Umbilical_	_Left Lumbar_
	Uterus	
	Bowel	
	Aorta	
RLQ	_Suprapubic_	_LLQ_
Appendix	Bladder	Left Ovary
Right Ovary	Uterus	Bowel
Bowel		

Table 9-1. ■ Abnormalities on Inspection

Physical Finding	Cause
Scars	Indicating past surgery or trauma.
Striae	Includes obesity, ascites, pregnancy, tumor, Cushing's disease, and steroid use.
Venous Pattern	May be prominent in fair-skinned people or due to congested portal circulation.
Discoloration	Consider jaundice, Addison's disease, von Recklinghausen's disease, trauma, or other rashes or lesions.
Visible Peristalsis	In an older adult, consider bowel obstruction. In newborns, upper-abdominal peristalsis is diagnostic for pyloric stenosis.
Pulsations	Visible aortic pulsations may be normal in thin individuals but, in others, may indicate aortic aneurysm.
Distention	For changes in contour or symmetry, consider the Fs of abdominal distention: fat, fluid, feces, fetus, flatus, fibroid, full bladder, fatal tumor, false pregnancy.

Table 9-2. ■ Abnormalities on Auscultation

Physical Finding	Cause
Bruits	A swishing sound heard over the aortic, renal, iliac, and femoral arteries, indicating narrowing or aneurysm.
Pops/Tinkles	These high-pitched sounds suggest intestinal fluid and air under pressure as in early obstruction.
Rushes	Rushes of high-pitched sounds that coincide with cramping suggest intestinal obstruction.
Borborygmi	These increased, prolonged gurgles occur with gastroenteritis, early intestinal obstruction, and hunger.
Rubs	Grating sounds that vary with respiration. Indicate inflammation of the peritoneal surface of an organ from tumor, infection, or splenic infarct.
Venous Hum	A soft humming noise often heard in hepatic cirrhosis that is caused by increased collateral circulation between portal and systemic venous systems.
Succussion Splash	A splashing noise produced by shaking the body when there is both gas and fluid in a cavity, or free air in the peritoneum or thorax.
Decreased/Absent Sounds	Occurs with peritonitis or paralytic ileus.

Table 9-3. ■ Normal Tones Produced by Percussion

	Most Dense	←	→	Least Dense	
Tone	*Flat*	*Dull*	*Resonant*	*Hyperresonant*	*Tympanic*
Intensity	Soft	Medium	Loud	Very Loud	Loud
Pitch	High	Medium	Low	Very Low	High
Duration	Short	Medium	Long	Very Long	Medium
Area	Muscle, Bone	Liver, Spleen	Lung	Emphysematous lung	Gastric air bubble

Table 9-4. ■ Abnormalities on Palpation

Condition	Description	Characteristics
Hepatomegaly	Liver enlargement can be detected by percussion and/or palpation and can be caused by cirrhosis, hepatitis, right heart failure, cysts, and malignancy.	Cirrhosis produces an enlarged, firm, nontender liver. Hepatitis and right heart failure are characterized by a smooth, tender liver. Cysts may not be palpable but will produce RUQ pain and tenderness. A malignancy typically produces a firm, irregular liver surface.
Splenomegaly	The causes of an enlarged spleen include infectious or inflammatory diseases, such as mononucleosis, infectious hepatitis, SBE, psittacosis, TB, malaria, sarcoidosis, amyloidosis, SLE; lympho- and myeloproliferative diseases, such as lymphoma, leukemia, polycythemia, and myelofibrosis; hemolytic anemias and hemoglobinopathies; splenic cysts; and storage diseases, such as Gaucher's, Niemann-Pick, and Hand-Schuller-Christian diseases.	Other symptoms in addition to an enlarged and usually tender spleen are early feeding satiety, splenic friction rub, epigastric and splenic bruits, and cytopenias.
Aortic Aneurysm	Arteriosclerosis is the most common cause of aortic aneurysm. Aging, cigarette smoking, and HTN are contributing factors. Trauma, syphilis; congenital connective tissue disorders, such as Marfan's; and positive history of aneurysm also increase the incidence.	A prominent lateral pulsation suggests an aneurysm.
Tumor	Caused by any benign or malignant growth in any of the abdominal organs.	Variable according to the affected organ but include pain, bloating, obstruction, anorexia, and changes in bowel or GU functioning.

finger into the anus with the patient leaning over the exam table or side-lying on the exam table, and note any internal hemorrhoids or fissures. Check the stool for occult blood. For males, the rectal exam is necessary for direct examination of the prostate.

Special Maneuvers

Rebound tenderness Tested by slowly pressing over the abdomen with your fingertips, holding the position until pain subsides or the patient adjusts to the discomfort, and then quickly removing the pressure (Figure 9-2). Rebound pain, a sign of peritoneal inflammation, is present if the patient experiences a sharp discomfort over the inflamed site when pressure is released.

Rovsing's sign Appendicitis is suggested when there is referred rebound pain in the *right* lower quadrant when the examiner presses deeply in the *left* lower quadrant and then quickly releases the pressure (Figure 9-2).

Figure 9-2. ■ Testing for rebound tenderness, specifically for Rovsing's sign. (From Dillon, P.M. Nursing health assessment: A critical thinking, case studies approach. Philadelphia: F.A. Davis, 2003. Reprinted with permission.)

Heel strike	Ask the patient to stand with straight legs and to raise up on toes. Then ask the patient to relax, thus allowing the heel to strike the floor thus jarring the body. Positive in appendicitis and peritoneal irritation. Alternatively, strike the plantar surface of the heel with your fist while the patient rests supine on the exam table.
Obturator sign	Pain is elicited in appendicitis by inward rotation of the hip with the knee bent, so that the obturator internus muscle is stretched (Figure 9-3).
Psoas sign	Place your hand on the patient's thigh just above the knee and ask the patient to raise the thigh against your hand (Figure 9-4). This contracts the psoas muscle and produces pain in patients with an inflamed appendix.
Murphy's sign	Pain is present on deep inspiration when an inflamed gallbladder is palpated by pressing the fingers under the rib cage (Figure 9-5). Positive in cholecystitis.
Hepatojugular reflux	Elicited by applying firm, sustained hand pressure to the abdomen in the mid-epigastric region while the patient breathes regularly. Observe the neck for elevation of the jugular venous pressure (JVP) with pressure of the hand and a sudden drop of the JVP when the hand pressure is released. The hepatojugular reflux is exaggerated in right heart failure.
"Scratch" test	An alternative to palpation/percussion to determine hepatic size when necessary. The scratch test is performed by placing the stethoscope over the liver and then lightly scratching up the

Figure 9-3. ■ Testing for the obturator sign. (From Dillon, P.M. Nursing health assessment: A critical thinking, case studies approach. Philadelphia: F.A. Davis, 2003. Reprinted with permission.)

Figure 9-4. ■ Testing for the psoas sign. (From Dillon, P.M. Nursing health assessment: A critical thinking, case studies approach. Philadelphia: F.A. Davis, 2003. Reprinted with permission.)

Figure 9-5. ■ Testing for Murphy's sign. (From Dillon, P.M. Nursing health assessment: A critical thinking, case studies approach. Philadelphia: F.A. Davis, 2003. Reprinted with permission.)

Figure 9-6. ■ Performing the scratch test. (From Dillon, P.M. Nursing health assessment: A critical thinking, case studies approach. Philadelphia: F.A. Davis, 2003. Reprinted with permission.)

abdomen on the right side, using a fingertip or tongue depressor (Figure 9-6). The sound you hear through the stethoscope will be intensified over the liver.

Shifting dullness   Test to differentiate ascites: test for shifting of the peritoneal fluid to the dependent side by rolling the patient side to side and percussing for dullness on the dependent side of the abdomen. Note: This maneuver is nonspecific and has, for the most part, been replaced by ultrasonography of the abdomen.

DIFFERENTIAL DIAGNOSIS OF CHIEF COMPLAINTS
Abdominal Pain
Abdominal pain is one of the most common complaints in primary care and can be functional or organic in cause, and acute or chronic in nature. Even though the causes of

Table 9-5. ■ Normal Laboratory Values for Differential Diagnosis of the Abdomen

Test	Normal Value
AST (SGOT)	≤42 units/L
ALT (SGPT)	<48 units/L
Alkaline Phosphatase	25–150 units/L
Albumin	3.5–5.0 g/dL
Globulin	1.5–4.5 g/dL
A/G Ratio	1.1–2.5
Total Serum Protein	6.0–8.5 g/dL
Total Bilirubin	<1.3 mg/dL
Amylase	30–170 units/L
Lipase	7–60 units/L
BUN	7–30 mg/dL
Serum Creatinine	≤1.2 mg/dL
Uric Acid	Female: 2.5–7.5 mg/dL Male: 4.0–8.5 mg/dL
WBC	$3.8–10.8 \times 10^3/\mu L$
Hgb	Female: 12.0–15.6 g/dL Male: 13.8–17.2 g/dL
Hct	Female: 35%–46 % Male: 41%–50%
CA 125	<35 units/mL
CEA	Non-smoker: <2.5 ng/L Smoker: <5.0 ng/L

abdominal pain are often self-limiting, the pain can also indicate a life-threatening situation and must be carefully assessed. When a patient complains of abdominal pain, it is essential to rule out indications for an emergency referral by carefully reviewing the history of the complaint, including the general description of the pain, quantity, quality, location, timing, onset, and associated symptoms. Although the physical exam may suggest the cause, the exam may be normal even with underlying pathology. Laboratory studies and diagnostic testing may be necessary to pinpoint the actual cause and rule out the more serious causes. Table 9-5 presents normal values for some of the lab tests commonly used in differential diagnosis of the abdomen.

There are three major categories used to classify abdominal pain: visceral, somatoparietal, and referred. Referred pain is simply pain radiating or referring from a site external to the abdomen. See Table 9-6 for differentiating common characteristics of visceral and somatoparietal pain.

Right Upper Quadrant Pain or Discomfort
The conditions of the underlying organs are key to identifying the etiology of right upper quadrant (RUQ) pain. Consider diseases of the gallbladder, liver, pancreas, or lung as the most likely cause of pain. As is true of other complaints, a thorough history and physical are necessary. In the case of the RUQ, laboratory testing can be most helpful and often diagnostic.

History
Begin with the exact location of the pain, onset, timing, quality and quantity, and alleviating or aggravating factors—particularly if the pain is related to meals or movement. Ask if there has been any nausea, vomiting, anorexia, or change in urine or stool color, indicating liver or gallbladder disease. A pleuritic cause for the pain should be considered, and you should inquire as to the presence of cough, shortness of breath, or fever. Include a smok-

Table 9-6. ■ Differentiating Types of Abdominal Pain

Visceral	Somatoparietal
Poorly localized	Localized
Vague	Intense
Often midline	Guarding
Crampy	Patient often still
Burning	
Patient often restless	
Associated with:	Worsened by:
Diaphoresis	Movement
Pallor	Respirations
Nausea	Cough
Caused by:	Caused by:
Inflammation or injury to solid or hollow organs	Inflammation of the parietal peritoneum

ing history. Ask about the diet history, particularly in regards to a high-fat diet or fad diets that might exclude food groups, or be very low in calories. This might increase the likelihood of gallbladder disease. Inquire about sexual practices, EtOH, and drugs (prescription and illicit) that might alert you to an increased risk for liver disease, particularly hepatitis. Ask about travel because hepatitis is endemic in certain areas and often the standards for food preparation are not the same as in North America. Ask about patient and family history of breast or colon cancer, gallbladder or liver disease, and general disorders of the digestive tract.

Physical Examination

A thorough abdominal exam should be performed with particular attention to the RUQ, assessing for tenderness, rebound, masses, and organ enlargement or nodularity. A respira-

Red Flags for Abdominal Pain

Pain that awakens patient

Pain that persists more than 6 hours and progresses in intensity

Pain that changes location

Associated syncope

Pain followed by vomiting or intractable vomiting

Hematemesis

Black, tarry stools

Progressive abdominal distention

Pain worsened by movement, respirations

Radiation of the pain to shoulder (cholecystitis) or back (pancreatitis/aneurysm)

Decreased urine output

Fever, leukocytosis, granulocytosis

Pain associated with signs of hypovolemic shock

tory exam should include auscultation for adventitious breath sounds and the presence of friction rubs or voice sounds. Table 9-7 summarizes differential diagnosis for RUQ (and left upper quadrant) pain.

Laboratory Tests for RUQ Pain

- CBC—complete blood count, particularly to determine elevated white blood cells (WBCs) in infection.
- Liver function tests.
  - ALT—alanine aminotransferase, primarily for the diagnosis of liver disease, but will detect biliary obstruction.
  - AST—aspartate aminotransferase, primarily for the diagnosis of liver disease, but elevations are also associated with acute common bile duct obstruction. Levels of AST may be affected by statin drugs, acetaminophen, and EtOH.
  - Alkaline phosphatase—used as a tumor marker and an index of liver and bone disease or metastasis in correlation with other findings.

Table 9-7. ■ Differential Diagnosis for Right and Left Upper Quadrant Pain

Disease	History	Diagnostic Studies	Physical Findings
Cholecystitis	RUQ pain, anorexia, nausea, vomiting, fever.	CBC, LFTs, amylase, GB ultrasound, HIDA scan.	↑ neutrophilic leukocytes, ↑ AST/ ALT, ↑ amylase with common duct obstruction, ultrasound will show nonvisualization of the GB and wall thickening.
Liver disease	RUQ pain, sexual practices, travel, EtOH use, history of malignancy, nausea, vomiting, anorexia, drugs, raw shellfish ingestion, change in color of urine or stools, weight loss, abdominal distention.	LFTs, hepatitis profile, abdominal US or CT.	↑ LFTs, ↑ IgM and specific antigens will be present for A, B, and C; US or CT may show cysts or tumors, obstruction.
Pancreatitis	Epigastric pain, EtOH abuse, liver or GB disease, jaundice, hyperlipidemia.	Amylase, lipase, LFTs, plain abdominal films, abdominal US or CT, chest x-ray.	↑ Amylase and lipase, ↑ LFTs, ↑ WBC, epigastric tenderness, pancreatic or biliary obstruction on US/CT.
Pleurisy	Respiratory disease, such as URI or pneumonia, SOB, chest trauma, other systemic disease	Chest x-ray.	If there is air or fluid in the pleural space, investigate other more serious diagnoses.
Hypersplenism	LUQ pain, anorexia, fever, fatigue, weight loss, recent infection, bruising or bleeding, lymphadenopathy, jaundice.	CBC, platelet, SPE, amylase, B_{12}, uric acid, bone marrow aspiration, abdominal CT.	Picture is varied depending on underlying cause: Cytopenias or myelo- or lymphoproliferation, ↑ B_{12} in leukemias and polycythemia, ↑ uric acid in proliferative disorders, monoclonal gammopathy or ↓ immunoglobulins on SPE, abnormalities on CT and bone marrow aspirate.

- GGT—gamma-glutamyltransferase, used to determine liver cell dysfunction and to detect alcohol-induced liver disease. The GGT can be helpful as a confirmatory test.
- LDH—lactate dehydrogenase, a widely distributed enzyme that is elevated with cellular damage of the liver, kidney, skeletal muscle, and heart.
- Bilirubin—evaluates liver function, biliary obstruction, and hemolytic anemia.
- Albumin—influenced by nutritional state, and hepatic and renal function.
- Amylase—useful to distinguish pancreatitis from other causes of abdominal pain.
- Lipase—assists in diagnosis of pancreatitis. Lipase stays elevated longer than amylase, but is not specific and also may be elevated in biliary and hepatic disease, DM, and gastric malignancy.
- Hepatitis Profile—detects acute or chronic, active and previous disease, carrier state, and immunity to Hepatitis A, B, C.

Diagnostics Tests for RUQ Pain
- GB ultrasound—gallbladder ultrasonography, a simple, noninvasive test if cholecystitis is suspected. Demonstrates cholelithiasis (95% sensitive), GB wall thickening, and biliary dilatation. There are no contraindications or risks.
- HIDA scan—hepatobiliary iminodiacetic acid, assesses hepatobiliary function, but does not demonstrate the causes of obstruction. Advantages: no IV contrast used, rapid, and not dependent on intestinal absorption. Disadvantages: may give false-positive results in acute pancreatitis, contraindicated in pregnancy, more expensive than ultrasound.
- Abdominal ultrasound/CT scan—if the signs and symptoms do not typically point to cholecystitis, an abdominal ultrasound or computed tomographic (CT) scan will allow visualization of the entire abdomen. Ultrasound gives information on the condition of the liver, GB, pancreas, spleen, aorta, kidneys, and appendix. There are no contraindications, but bowel gas may obscure organs. A CT scan is more comprehensive and includes morphologic evaluation of all abdominal and pelvic organs, and can assist in the staging of renal and GI carcinomas. A CT scan is contraindicated in pregnancy and is more expensive than ultrasound.
- Chest x-ray—if there are any signs of respiratory involvement, a chest x-ray is recommended

GALLBLADDER DISEASE

A mnemonic used to describe a common presentation for cholecystitis is "female, fat, and forty," although it can occur in much younger and older individuals after surgery, trauma, burns, sepsis, or critical illness. Young people have shown an increased incidence of cholecystitis if they are adhering to any of the more drastic weight-loss diets that are extremely low in fat and calories.

Signs and Symptoms.
Initially, acute colicky pain is localized in the RUQ and is often accompanied by nausea and vomiting. Murphy's sign is frequently present. Fever is low grade, and the increase in neutrophilic leukocytes in the blood is slight. Acute cholecystitis improves in 2–3 days and resolves within a week; however, recurrences are common. If acute cholecystitis is accompanied by jaundice and cholestasis (arrest of bile excretion), suspect common duct obstruction.

Diagnostic Studies.
A diagnosis can usually be made with ultrasound or hepatobiliary scanning (HIDA scan).

Decision Rule for Gallbladder Disease

Ebell (2001) reports a decision rule for common bile duct lithiasis developed by Houdart, Perniceni, Dame, et al. The prediction rule was developed on a sample of 503 patients and validated on a group of 279 patients. They found that patients were at low risk (0.6%) for common bile duct lithiasis if they presented with no jaundice and normal transaminases, had a common bile duct diameter of less than 8 mm, and had no ultrasound-demonstrated intrahepatic duct enlargement. In contrast, patients who had jaundice, abnormal transaminases, a common bile duct diameter of greater than 8 mm, and intrahepatic duct enlargement were categorized as "at risk" (39%).

LIVER DISEASE

Liver diseases include viral hepatitis (hepatitis A, B, C, D, E), EtOH hepatitis, cirrhosis, hepatic cysts, and malignancy (primary or metastatic).

Signs and Symptoms.

The major clinical manifestations of liver disease include jaundice, hepatomegaly, cholestasis, portal hypertension, ascites, and encephalopathy. Symptoms vary with the cause but many are insidious, especially with hepatitis. Liver disease is often discovered on routine exam or laboratory testing.

Diagnostic Studies.

If liver disease is suspected, begin with liver function tests (LFTs) and a hepatitis profile. This will give you valuable information on most liver diseases, except hepatic cysts, which generally do not alter liver functions. If cirrhosis, malignancy, or a hepatic cyst is suspected or should be eliminated, include an abdominal ultrasound or CT scan.

Those found to have hepatitis B or C should be referred to a gastroenterologist or infectious disease specialist. Hepatitis A is usually self-limiting and can be managed by the nurse practitioner or family physician.

PANCREATITIS

Biliary tract disease and alcoholism account for ≥80% of the pancreatitis admissions. Other causes include hyperlipidemia, drugs, toxins, infection, structural abnormalities, surgery, vascular disease, trauma, hyperparathyroidism and hypercalcemia, renal transplantation, and hereditary pancreatitis. The most common cause of pancreatitis is alcohol abuse.

Signs and Symptoms.

Pancreatitis is characterized by severe abdominal pain often with radiation through to the back usually accompanied by nausea and vomiting. The pain is steady and boring (piercing, penetrating) often refractory to narcotic pain medicines, and persistent for many days. Fever is present within a few hours, tachycardia, rapid and shallow respirations, postural hypotension, diaphoresis, blunted sensorium, abdominal distention, tenderness, hypoactive bowel sounds, and possibly ascites.

Diagnostic Studies.

There is no single test to diagnose pancreatitis, but several tests support the clinical impression, including serum amylase and lipase, WBC count, supine and upright plain films of the abdomen, chest x-ray, and ultrasound. Lipase and amylase are usually quite elevated, as is the WBC. Ultrasound imaging will detect an enlarged pancreas, as well as the presence of gallstones and biliary obstruction. A CT scan can be used in lieu of ultrasound to image the pancreas, but it is less helpful in identifying gallstones as the potential cause.

PLEURISY

Pleurisy may result from a) an underlying lung process, b) an infection or irritation in the pleural space, c) the transport of an infectious or other disease agent, or neoplastic metastases to the pleura, and d) trauma, especially rib trauma. Basilar pleurisy may produce referred pain to the abdomen.

Signs and Symptoms.

Differentiated from abdominal disease by chest x-ray or evidence of a respiratory origin, such as increased pain with deep breathing and coughing, shallow or rapid breathing, the absence of nausea or vomiting, or a tendency toward relief of pain with pressure on the chest wall or abdomen. A pleural friction rub is pathognomonic.

Diagnostic Studies.

Pleurisy may not be evident on any thoracic imaging and may be a diagnosis made by history and physical exam. A chest x-ray or CT of the chest showing inflammation or pleural thickening will be helpful in some cases.

Left Upper Quadrant Pain or Discomfort

Diseases and disorders of the spleen, stomach, and pancreas are the most likely culprits in LUQ pain (see Table 9-7). Also consider colon and kidney disease, which are covered in this chapter under lower quadrant pain. For disorders of the spleen and pancreas, laboratory evaluation is helpful along with the history and physical. For the stomach, more-definitive diagnostic tests may need to be performed.

History

Left upper quadrant pain is often associated with causes that are outside the abdomen. Hematopoietic malignancies, such as lymphomas and leukemias, and other hematologic disorders, such as thrombocytopenia, polycythemia, myelofibrosis, and hemolytic anemia, often cause enlargement of the spleen leading to left upper quadrant pain. In addition to questions about the specific characteristics of the pain, it is important to ask the patient about fever, unusual bleeding or bruising, recent diagnosis of mononucleosis, fatigue, malaise, lymphadenopathy, cough, arthralgias, anorexia, weight loss, jaundice, high blood pressure, and headache.

Decision Rule for Pancreatitis

Ebell (2001) reports a prediction rule developed by Balthazar, Robinson, Megibow, and Ranson to determine the severity of acute pancreatitis. The rule is based on 88 patients and was not validated on a second group. The rule uses a score determined by CT scan results, with an index possible range of 0 to 10. A categorization of patients indicates the risk of both mortality and complication from the disease. Patients at the low end of the index (1–3) are predicted to have a low risk of mortality (3%) and complications (8%), whereas patients scoring at the high end (7–10) of the index are predicted to have a higher incidence of mortality (17%) and/or complications (92%).

Physical Examination

A thorough abdominal exam is necessary with special attention to the left upper quadrant. A respiratory exam should be included to rule out referred pain. A hematopoietic cause can be explored only through laboratory tests.

Laboratory Tests for LUQ Pain

- CBC—for diagnosis of cytopenic and myeloproliferative disorders.
- Platelets—for diagnosis of thrombocytopenia or thrombocytosis.
- LFTs—will be elevated in cirrhosis or hepatic infiltration from miliary tuberculosis (TB) and from myeloproliferative and lymphoproliferative disorders. Also, they may be elevated if pancreatitis is the cause of LUQ pain.
- Serum protein electrophoresis—will assist in the diagnosis of lymphoproliferative disorders, amyloidosis, chronic infection, cirrhosis, sarcoidosis, and collagen vascular diseases.
- Uric acid—will be elevated in myeloproliferative and lymphoproliferative disorders.
- Vitamin B_{12}—may be elevated in myeloproliferative disorders, such as chronic myelogenous leukemia and polycythemia vera.
- Amylase—elevated in pancreatitis.
- Lipase—elevated in pancreatitis.

Diagnostic Tests for LUQ Pain

- Abdominal ultrasound/CT—determines splenomegaly, intrasplenic pathology, or pancreatic obstruction.
- MRI—magnetic resonance imaging, shows blood flow patterns if portal or splenic vein thrombosis is suspected.
- Bone marrow biopsy—will show specific abnormal cellular changes for many of the causes of hypersplenism.
- Endoscopy—if gastric pathology is suspected.

HYPERSPLENISM

Abnormalities are almost always secondary to other primary disorders, most commonly cytopenic hematologic disorders, such as lymphoma, leukemia, thrombocytopenia, polycythemia, myelofibrosis, and hemolytic anemias. Other causes include portal or splenic vein thrombosis; infection, such as mononucleosis, infectious hepatitis, subacute bacterial endocarditis (SBE), psittacosis, miliary TB, malaria, brucellosis, and syphilis; sarcoidosis; amyloidosis; connective tissue diseases, such as systemic lupus erythematosus (SLE) and rheumatoid arthritis; lipoid and nonlipoid storage diseases; and splenic cysts. Splenomegaly results from an increase in splenic workload by the trapping and destroying of abnormal blood cells or diverse abnormal circulating organisms.

Signs and Symptoms.

The signs and symptoms are highly variable and relate to the underlying cause. The patient may complain of early satiety or abdominal fullness, and LUQ pain. If the cause is infectious, a complaint of fatigue and/or fever is common. On physical exam, splenomegaly is present. An epigastric or splenic bruit may be present. The CBC may identify anemia, leukopenia, thrombocytopenia, or any combination of the three.

Diagnostic Studies.

There are several laboratory studies that may be needed to diagnose the numerous underlying causes of hypersplenism. Begin with a CBC and platelet count, which will likely give you the most information on how to proceed. If abnormal, a bone marrow examination is indicated. Other tests to consider would be serum protein electrophoresis, LFTs, uric acid, B_{12}, amylase, and CT or MRI of the abdomen.

Pleurisy

See RUQ Pain, p. 190.

Pancreatitis

See p. 194.

Stomach Conditions

See Epigastric Pain, in the following subsection.

Epigastric Pain or Discomfort

Epigastric pain can represent the heartburn or dyspepsia often associated with GERD, as well as several other diseases, including malignancies.

The epigastric region is a very common site of discomfort stemming from many digestive structures. Heartburn, often from GERD, is a very common complaint; patients may use alternative terms to describe this sensation, including "indigestion" or "sour stomach." Dyspepsia, as a term, covers a variety of complaints that include heartburn, as well as fullness, bloating, and upper abdominal pain. Because pain in this region provides little specificity on its own, the history is crucial in narrowing the differential diagnosis.

The physical examination is most helpful in eliminating some of the more rare causes of epigastric pain, as the common causes are typically associated with benign physical findings. A change in vital signs can point to cardiac or respiratory disturbances, as well as to potential fevers and infections. A positive Hemoccult on rectal exam may indicate an upper GI bleed or malignancy. Malignancy should also be suspected if there is weight loss and or a palpable abdominal mass. Be attentive for adventitious abdominal sounds, such as succussion splash, indicating air or fluid in the thorax or peritoneum, or aortic bruit heard in abdominal aneurysm. Be alert for a positive Murphy's sign, which is seen in cholecystitis. Note any abnormalities in skin tone and/or color that could indicate liver disease, cholecystitis, or hypoxia owing to respiratory or cardiac disease.

History

To differentiate between the causes of epigastric pain, have the patient clearly describe his or her complaint, particularly in the characteristics (whether sharp, dull, nagging, burning, steady, cramping, boring, etc.) and point to the exact location of the pain. Discomfort

---

Common causes of epigastric pain

Gastroesophageal reflux disease (GERD)
Gastric or duodenal ulcer
Gastric or duodenal malignancy
Esophageal spasm
Cholecystitis
Pancreatitis
Hepatitis/liver disease
Medication intolerance
Ischemic heart disease
Pregnancy

stemming from a serious disorder is often constant and intense and may radiate to the back. Determine what factors worsen and/or improve the discomfort, particularly any relationship to meals or activity. When rating the severity of the pain, determine what, if any, behaviors the pain has limited, including intake or physical activities. Establish the type of onset and progression, including whether the discomfort is intermittent, gradually increasing in severity, and so on. Finally, determine what, if any, associated symptoms the patient has noticed. Important considerations include vomiting, regurgitation, diaphoresis, dysphagia, blood in the stool or emesis, shortness of breath, fatigue, weight loss, and radiation to other sites (intra- and extra-abdominal). Ask about any new or current medications.

Physical Examination

A thorough exam of the entire abdomen is necessary, with special attention to the epigastric area. Tenderness can be present with peptic ulcer disease and pancreatitis. Auscultating for bruits in this area is vital; abdominal aortic aneurysm may present with epigastric pain. It is a life-threatening and possibly emergent problem. Vital signs and weight need to be recorded looking for any signs of infection, blood loss, or weight loss in the case of malignancy. A rectal exam for occult blood can add important information. In addition, a thorough respiratory, and cardiac history and exam should be performed because the pain may be referred. Depending on history and cardiovascular risks, consider an electrocardiogram (EKG) to rule out a cardiac source for the pain.

Laboratory Tests for Epigastric Pain

- CBC—to assess for anemia, which may accompany a malignancy or ulcer.
- A series of occult blood studies following careful instruction to the patient.
- *Helicobacter pylori*—serum blood test for common bacteria causing PUD.

Diagnostic Tests for Epigastric Pain

Often, the history and physical are adequate to rule out the need for diagnostic studies.

- Endoscopy—provides the most valuable information on the structures and provides the ability to obtain biopsies. It provides direct visualization of the esophagus and evidence to rule out other disorders.
- Upper GI series—gives information about structures but does not allow for biopsies. Provides information on structures, but with high potential to miss esophageal damage. Does not require any type of anesthesia.
- Ambulatory esophageal pH monitoring—may help to identify association between symptoms and reflux.

GASTROESOPHAGEAL REFLUX DISEASE

Gastroesophageal reflux disease is the most common organic cause of heartburn. Lower esophageal sphincter (LES) control can be decreased by several medications (examples include theophylline, dopamine, diazepam, calcium-channel blockers), foods and/or beverages (caffeine, alcohol, chocolate, fatty foods) and tobacco use. When LES tone is lower than normal, secretions are allowed to reflux into the esophagus, causing discomfort. Reflux is also promoted by weight gain and other variables causing greater pressure against the LES.

Signs and Symptoms.

The most common symptom of GERD is heartburn, which typically occurs after meals and is often relieved by antacids. Other symptoms include belching, regurgitation, and/or water brash. Respiratory and ear/nose/throat symptoms may develop, including cough, wheeze, aspiration, hoarseness, and globus sensation (fullness in the throat). Symptoms may occur primarily at night, when patients recline following a meal. See Box 9-1 for common triggers of GERD.

Diagnostic Studies.

Diagnosis can often be made by the history, although the degree of symptoms may not be consistent with the degree of esophageal injury. When gastroesophageal reflux is the most likely cause of acute epigastric discomfort, empiric treatment may include avoiding any triggers, as well as prescribing antacids and/or antisecretory agents, particularly for a young, otherwise healthy patient without known risk factors for more serious disorders. However, the risk of delaying the definitive diagnosis and treatment must be weighed when considering this route. Endoscopy provides direct visualization of the esophagus and evidence to rule out other disorders. Ambulatory esophageal pH monitoring may help to identify association between symptoms and reflux. Barium swallows have a high potential of missing esophageal damage.

PEPTIC ULCER DISEASE

Peptic ulcer disease (PUD) includes both gastric and duodenal ulcers. *Helicobacter pylori* and NSAIDs are common causes of both disorders, along with some probable genetic predisposition. Zollinger-Ellison syndrome commonly results in gastric ulcer development. The incidence of gastric ulcer is higher in persons who smoke and those with certain chronic disease, including cirrhosis, hyperparathyroidism, chronic renal failure, and lung disease.

Signs and Symptoms.

Epigastric pain is common with both gastric and duodenal ulcers and is described as a gnawing or burning sensation. Whereas the pain of gastric ulcer is usually worsened by intake, a duodenal ulcer usually causes pain on an empty stomach. It is not uncommon for the pain of duodenal ulcer to awaken the patient from sleep at 1 to 2 a.m. Antacids typically offer relief for both types of ulcer. Pain may be episodic, with symptom-free intervals. Pain may radiate to the back. Associated symptoms include bloating, belching, nausea, and loss of appetite. The physical examination is not usually positive, other than potentially identifying some degree of abdominal tenderness. As the mucosa erodes, bleeding may occur. If rupture occurs, pain acutely changes character and is intractable.

Box 9-1

Common Triggers for GERD

Tomato products
Citrus
Spicy foods
Coffee
Fatty foods
Peppermint
Chocolate
Alcohol
Smoking

Diagnostic Tests.

   Stool guaiac should be performed on any patient with epigastric pain. Peptic ulcer disease should be suspected in any patient with dyspepsia/epigastric pain who does not fit the profile associated with GERD and is >50 years old, has associated weight loss, or loss of appetite; direct endoscopy should be ordered. Biopsies will be taken of any erosive site, to rule out gastric malignancy. If PUD is diagnosed, testing for *H. pylori* should be performed. When patients with gastric ulcers have neither *H. pylori* nor a history of NSAID use, serum gastrin level should be determined, assessing for Zollinger-Ellison syndrome.

GASTRIC MALIGNANCY

   Although the incidence of gastric cancer is lower than in the past, the incidence has remained relatively steady for several years. It was anticipated that 21,700 cases would have been diagnosed in the United States in 2001, with 12,800 deaths. Suspected contributing factors, including excess salt intake and chronic gastritis, as is seen with *H. pylori*, can lead to the development of gastric cancer. The early stage of the disease is asymptomatic, and diagnosis is made usually only after significant advancement; the 5-year survival rate is 20.6%.

Signs and Symptoms.

   Cancers of the stomach are rarely symptomatic until the disease has progressed. Symptoms may be mild and consistent with heartburn or include more definite abdominal pain. Other symptoms include nausea and vomiting, diarrhea, constipation, fullness, anorexia, fatigue, and weight loss. Although the abdominal exam may be negative, tenderness and/or a palpable mass may be present.

Diagnostic Studies.

   The patient should be referred for endoscopy. A CBC should be ordered, any anemia assessed, and stool guaiac performed.

Pancreatitis

See p. 194.

Cholecystitis

See p. 224.

Hepatitis

See p. 223.

Lower Abdominal Pain

Lower abdominal pain can have a multitude of causes, including diseases or disorders of the appendix, colon, kidney, bladder, ureter, ovary, uterus, and prostate. Pinpointing the specific location of the pain is crucial to beginning the differential diagnosis; however, caution is recommended owing to the fact that abdominal pain can be referred from areas of the abdomen other than the point of origin. Because of the complexity of the differential diagnosis for lower abdominal pain, diagnostic tests are often necessary to confirm the findings of the history and physical.

History

There are a multitude of etiologies for lower abdominal complaints. It is important to begin with a thorough history. Although abdominal pain can often radiate to other areas or can present a vague and confusing picture, pinpointing the location of the pain is a prudent place to start. Question the patient about the onset of the pain and whether it is accompanied by fever, anorexia, nausea, or vomiting, which might lead you to suspect appendicitis, gastroenteritis, or obstruction. It is imperative to ask about the last menstrual period (LMP) and about birth control methods in order to rule out ectopic pregnancy. A history of miscarriages and/or sexually transmitted diseases (STDs) can give more clues for the risk of ectopic pregnancy. Safe sex practices and the number of sexual partners can alert the practitioner to the risk for pelvic inflammatory disease (PID). Ovarian tumors can go undetected for months, and the examiner must be alert to vague symptoms that might indicate a need for further investigation, such as bloating, gas, dyspepsia, and pressure type pain. These complaints in a postmenopausal woman should not be trivialized. A positive family history of ovarian cancer in a patient presenting with these complaints is a red flag. Urinary symptoms such as dysuria, hematuria, and a history of kidney stones indicate a risk for kidney stones. If the patient complains of pain with movement or exercise and gives a history of heavy lifting, then hernia may be suspected. Sudden onset of severe lower abdominal pain, nausea, and vomiting in a young male should alert the examiner to the possibility of testicular torsion. A complaint of fatigue, weakness, weight loss, or change in bowel or bladder habits is worrisome and a malignancy should be on the top of the list of differential diagnoses. Occasionally, hip disorders can present as lower abdominal pain.

Physical Examination

An entire abdominal exam is necessary with the addition of the genitourinary (GU) system. It is warranted in both males and females, but is of particular importance in females. *No complaint of lower abdominal pain in a female should be evaluated without performing a pelvic exam.* A rectal exam should be performed for occult blood, for palpation of the uterus or prostate, and for the presence of masses or tenderness. Although an unusual cause of lower abdominal pain, a musculoskeletal history and exam should be included, particularly when the pain is in the groin or hip area.

For clarity, the lower abdominal complaints will be broken down into the following regions: right lower quadrant (RLQ), left lower quadrant (LLQ), periumbilical, and suprapubic. For an overview and summary of the differential diagnosis of lower abdominal pain, see Table 9-8.

Laboratory Tests for Lower Abdominal Pain

- Serum/urine pregnancy—in ectopic pregnancy, levels of human chorionic gonadotropin (hCG) may not be at the levels appropriate for the number of weeks as estimated by LMP.
- CBC—white blood cells will be elevated in appendicitis and diverticulitis, and the hemoglobin and hematocrit (H & H) may be decreased in colon cancer.
- U/A—urinalysis, check for blood and WBCs indicating infection or renal calculi; increased specific gravity with dehydration.
- Wet prep, GC/chlamydial culture—gonococcal/chlamydial culture, may be positive in salpingitis/PID. If positive for STD, other considerations include rapid plasma reagin (RPR), HIV, and hepatitis profile.
- CEA—carcinoembryonic antigen, will be elevated in colon cancer.

Diagnostic Tests for Lower Abdominal Pain

- Abdominal, pelvic, renal ultrasound or CT for appendicitis, ovarian mass, ureteral stone, obstruction.
- Pelvic ultrasound to rule out ectopic pregnancy.
- Flat and upright x-ray of the abdomen to look for stone and bowel obstruction.
- Barium enema (BE) and/or colonoscopy to detect colon cancer or obstruction.

Table 9-8. ■ Differential Diagnosis of Lower Abdominal Pain

Disease	History	Diagnosis	Findings
Appendicitis	Anorexia, nausea, vomiting, fever, midline or RLQ pain worsening with cough or walking.	CBC, abdominal CT or US.	+ rebound tenderness, fever, leukocytosis of 10-20,000/μL, US/CT may be positive for perforation/abscess.
Ectopic pregnancy	Amenorrhea, severe RLQ or LLQ pain.	Pelvic ultrasound, urine and serum hCG.	A pregnancy outside the uterus, usually the tube, + hCG, + US, + rebound
Colorectal cancer	Weight loss, fatigue, change in bowel habits, anemia, + Hemoccult.	Hemoccult, CBC, CEA, flex. sig., colonoscopy.	+ Hemoccult, ↑ CEA ↓ H & H, + flex. sig. or colonoscopy.
Urinary calculi	+ history of stones, severe colicky flank pain.	U/A, plain abdominal x-ray, renal US, IVP.	Hematuria, + stone visualization with x-ray or US.
Ovarian tumor	+ family history, abdominal bloating, pain, or heaviness.	Pelvic exam, pelvic US, CT, CA-125.	↑ CA-125, mass on exam, CT or US.
Hernia	History of straining or heavy lifting, previous abdominal surgery, lower abdominal or groin pain.	Physical exam or US.	Palpable mass in the inguinal ring or femoral area.
Intestinal obstruction	History of abdominal surgery or inflammatory bowel disease, radiation, or impaction; abdominal pain or distention, vomiting; obstipation.	Flat & upright abdominal x-ray, BE, CBC, electrolytes, BUN, creatinine, U/A.	+ mass on exam, BE, or x-ray; tinkles, rushes, borborygmi, or absent bowel sounds, ↑ SG, ↑ BUN and creatinine; electrolyte imbalance; leukocytosis.
Diverticulitis	+ history of diverticulosis.	CBC, flexible sigmoidoscopy, BE, abdominal CT.	Leukocytosis, abdominal mass, stricture, hypertrophy of colonic musculature, possible free air in the abdomen.
Gastroenteritis	Sudden onset diarrhea, abdominal cramping, nausea, vomiting, fever.	CBC, stool for O & P, C & S.	Abdominal tenderness, borborygmi, possibly positive stool culture.

RLQ Pain/Discomfort

APPENDICITIS

Other than hernia, appendicitis is the most common cause of acute abdominal pain. It occurs most commonly between the ages of 10 and 30 years. Because gangrene, perforation, and peritonitis can develop within 36 hours if untreated, approximately 15% of patients sent to surgery with a diagnosis of appendicitis are falsely positive. Ultrasound and CT have decreased the incidence of overdiagnosis, but, in some cases, laparotomy or laparoscopy are still required for a definitive diagnosis. Gynecologic disorders and gastroenteritis are the most common causes of misdiagnosis.

Signs and Symptoms.

The pain of appendicitis usually evolves over a few hours and, initially, is poorly localized, midline, and vague; associated with some degree of nausea and/or loss of appetite. In
a matter of hours, the pain migrates to the RLQ, becoming more intense and localized, and
may increase with coughing or walking. Low-grade fever typically develops. The various
tests for peritoneal irritation (rebound tenderness, Rovsing's, heel strike, psoas, and obturator) will be positive.

Diagnostic Studies.

An elevated WBC and the physical exam are the two most important diagnostic tools.
If the diagnosis is still uncertain, an abdominal CT may be helpful.

COLON DISORDERS

See next section.

GENITOURINARY DISORDERS

See next section and Chapter 10.

OVARIAN DISORDERS

See next section and Chapter 12.

RLQ or LLQ Pain and Discomfort

ECTOPIC PREGNANCY

A pregnancy is considered ectopic if implantation takes place outside the cavity of the
uterus, with 98% of those being tubal. Conditions that predispose a woman to an ectopic
pregnancy are those that prevent the migration of the fertilized ovum to the uterus, and
approximately 50% are due to a previous tubal infection. Other risk factors include a history of infertility, PID, previous abdominal or tubal surgery, previous tubal pregnancy, and
the use of an intrauterine device (IUD).

Signs and Symptoms.

The most obvious sign of ectopic pregnancy is amenorrhea followed by spotting and
sudden onset of severe lower quadrant pain. A stat pregnancy test should be performed.
Backache may be present. There is tenderness on pelvic exam, and a pelvic mass may be
palpated. Blood is present in the cul-de-sac. Shock and hemorrhage occur if the pregnancy
ruptures. Abdominal distention with peritoneal signs will ensue. Immediate laparoscopy or
laparotomy is indicated because this is life threatening.

Diagnostic Studies.

A urine hCG or stat serum hCG, pelvic ultrasound, culdocentesis to detect blood in the
cul-de-sac.

COLORECTAL CANCER

Colorectal cancer is the second leading cause of death from malignancies in the United
States. Over half are located in the rectosigmoid region and are typically adenocarcinomas.
Risk factors include a history of polyps, positive family history of colon cancer or familial
polyposis, ulcerative colitis, granulomatous colitis, and a diet low in fiber and high in animal protein, fat, and refined carbohydrates.

Signs and Symptoms.

The cancer may be present for several years before symptoms appear. Complaints include fatigue, weakness, weight loss, alternating constipation and diarrhea, a change in the caliber of stool, tenesmus, urgency, and hematochezia. Physical exam is usually normal except in advanced disease, when the tumor can be palpated or if hepatomegaly is present owing to metastatic disease.

Diagnostic Studies.

Stool for occult blood is recommended, and a colonoscopy is diagnostic. A barium enema may be helpful initially, but if positive, colonoscopy will be necessary. Recommended labs include a CBC and CEA.

URINARY CALCULI

Men are more frequently affected, with a ratio of 4:1, until the sixth or seventh decade, when the risk equalizes. There are many factors contributing to the formation of stones, including geographic, diet, genetic, and occupational factors. Stones occur more frequently in people living in hot, humid climates. Diets high in salt and protein and, in some cases, oxalate and purines, can increase the risk of calculi. Despite previous beliefs, a diet high in calcium is a contributing factor only in selected individuals. Some stones may be genetically linked, particularly cystine stones, and persons in sedentary occupations are more likely to develop stones compared with manual laborers. The most common types of stones are made of calcium (calcium oxalate and calcium phosphate), with the other three types being struvite, uric acid, and cystine.

Signs and Symptoms.

Urinary calculi can occur anywhere in the urinary tract and therefore pain can originate in the flank or kidney area and radiate into the right or left lower quadrant and then to the suprapubic area as the stone attempts to move down the tract. The pain is severe, acute, and colicky and may be accompanied by nausea and vomiting. If the stone becomes lodged at the ureterovesical junction, the patient will complain of urgency and frequency. Blood will be present in the urine.

Diagnostic Studies.

The urinalysis typically shows hematuria. Infection needs to be ruled out because a combination of infection and obstruction requires prompt intervention to prevent pyelonephritis and kidney damage. A plain, flat plate of the abdomen or a renal ultrasound is the most helpful in diagnosing stones. If diagnosis remains uncertain, a noncontrast CT is indicated. Alternatively, an intravenous pyelogram (IVP) should be ordered if a CT is not available. Pain medicine is imperative if patients are to undergo lengthy diagnostic testing.

OVARIAN CYST AND TUMOR

Although there are no hard-and-fast rules, ovarian cysts are more likely to occur in the younger female, whereas ovarian cancer has a greater incidence in the postmenopausal female. Women with a positive family history of ovarian cancer have a 5% lifetime risk versus a 1.6% risk in those with no family history. The long-term use of oral contraceptives may decrease the risk of ovarian cancer.

Signs and Symptoms.

Ovarian masses are often asymptomatic, but symptoms may include pressure type pain, heaviness, aching, bloating. Cysts tend to be more painful than malignant tumors and often spontaneously resolve with the onset of the menstrual cycle. Masses are typically detected on pelvic exam. In advanced malignancies, ascites is often present.

Diagnostic Studies.

An elevated cancer antigen-125 (CA-125) result indicates the likelihood that the mass is malignant. A transvaginal pelvic ultrasound has a higher diagnostic sensitivity in women at high risk rather than low risk. If diagnosis is unclear, exploratory laparotomy can be performed.

INGUINAL AND FEMORAL HERNIA

In the majority of hernia cases, a history of heavy physical labor or heavy lifting can be elicited. Young children and individuals with a history of abdominal surgery are also at increased risk.

Signs and Symptoms.

Right or left lower quadrant pain that may radiate into the groin or testicle is typical. The pain is usually dull or aching unless strangulated, in which case the pain is more severe. The pain increases with straining, lifting, or movement of the lower extremities. Physical exam includes palpating the femoral area and inguinal ring for bulging or tenderness. Ask the patient to bear down against your hand.

Diagnostic Studies.

The physical exam is often all that is necessary for diagnosis, but ultrasound may be helpful.

GASTROENTERITIS

See section on nausea and vomiting, p. 207.

INTESTINAL OBSTRUCTION

See periumbilical pain in the following.

Periumbilical Pain and Discomfort

INTESTINAL OBSTRUCTION

The most common causes of mechanical obstruction are adhesions, almost exclusively in patients with previous abdominal surgery, hernias, tumors, volvulus, inflammatory bowel disease (Crohn's disease, colitis), Hirschsprung's disease, fecal impaction, and radiation enteritis.

Signs and Symptoms.

Initially, the patient complains of a cramping periumbilical pain that eventually becomes constant. There is abdominal distention, vomiting that may lead to dehydration, diarrhea in partial obstruction, and obstipation when there is complete obstruction. On physical exam, there is mild diffuse tenderness without peritoneal signs, and possibly visible peristaltic waves. In early obstruction, tinkles, rushes, and borborygmi can be heard. In late obstruction, bowel sounds may be absent. There is minimal or no fever. Carefully inspect and palpate for hernias and masses.

Diagnostic Studies.

The diagnosis can be made with flat and upright abdominal films, and with barium enema if the diagnosis is unclear. Complete blood count and electrolytes are recommended to look for leukocytosis and electrolyte imbalance; BUN, creatinine, and U/A are performed to detect extracellular volume loss.

PID/SALPINGITIS
See Chapter 12.
LLQ Pain and Discomfort

DIVERTICULITIS
Diverticular disease is prevalent in patients over 60 years of age. It is seen more commonly in Western countries and is thought to be due to a diet deficient in fiber. It most often affects the sigmoid colon. Patients with connective tissue disease, such as scleroderma, Marfan's syndrome, and Ehlers-Danlos syndrome are at increased risk.

Signs and Symptoms.
Although the pain can be generalized, it is typically localized to the left lower abdomen and is accompanied by tenderness, fever, and leukocytosis. These symptoms in a person with a known history of diverticulosis make the diagnosis almost certain for diverticulitis. Other symptoms can include constipation or loose stools, nausea, vomiting, and positive stool occult blood. With diverticulitis, there is a risk of perforation that presents with a more dramatic clinical picture as a result of peritonitis. Look for signs of peritonitis, such as a positive heel strike test and/or rebound tenderness.

Diagnostic Studies.
A CBC will show mildly elevated WBCs. Plain abdominal films should be obtained to look for an ileus; a small or large bowel obstruction; and free air in the abdomen, indicating perforation. Acute medical management is indicated, and, after 7–10 days, a flexible sigmoidoscopy and/or BE is recommended. These should not be done in the acute stage owing to an increased risk of perforation during the procedure. A CT is obtained to look for an abscess.

Pelvic or Suprapubic Pain and Discomfort
The following will be covered in detail in Chapter 10:
1. Inguinal and femoral hernia
2. Testicular torsion
3. Prostatitis
4. Prostate Cancer
5. Epididymitis
6. Urinary tract infection
7. PID/Salpingitis
8. Renal calculi

HISTORY
Ask about urinary symptoms, such as dysuria and frequency; any heavy lifting; contact sports; sexual practices; the presence of vaginal or penile discharge; and a history of STDs, kidney stones, or prostate disease.

PHYSICAL EXAMINATION
The physical examination should include a thorough abdominal exam, a pelvic and genital exam, and a rectal exam including prostate for males.

LABORATORY TESTS FOR PELVIC OR SUPRAPUBIC PAIN
- U/A, urine culture—looking for leukocytes, indicating infection, or for hematuria, indicating infection, calculi, or malignancy.

- CBC—to evaluate for anemia or leukocytosis.
- PSA—prostate-specific antigen, to evaluate for prostate cancer.
- Wet prep, GC/chlamydia—for STDs; if positive for STD, other considerations include RPR, HIV, and a hepatitis profile.

DIAGNOSTIC TESTS FOR PELVIC OR SUPRAPUBIC PAIN

- Stat nuclear medicine scan if torsion is suspected, or stat referral to surgery.
- Transrectal prostate ultrasound if PSA is elevated or there is strong suspicion of prostate disease by history and physical.
- Prostate biopsy if nodules or asymmetry is seen on ultrasound.
- Pelvic ultrasound if abnormalities are found on pelvic exam.

Nausea and Vomiting

Nausea and vomiting usually stem from gastrointestinal infections, but may reflect many categories of problems, including other infections, actual or functional gastrointestinal obstruction, metabolic disorders, central nervous system disorders, drugs, pain, pregnancy, and psychiatric disorders. A detailed list of potential causes is provided in Table 9-9. This section describes the basic approach to nausea and vomiting to differentiate between major potential causes. Table 9-9 summarizes common findings for each condition listed and will help you narrow your diagnosis and limit your work-up appropriately. The approach to nausea and vomiting should be determined by the patient's age, overall health, and past medical history.

History

A thorough symptom analysis should identify any triggering events, such as meals, offensive odors, motion, position changes, and pain. Determine what, if anything, relieves the symptoms, including any attempted self-treatments. Determine what is meant by a complaint of "nausea": loss of appetite, queasiness, sense of imminent vomiting, or retching. When vomiting has occurred, determine the color, amount, the presence of bile or undigested food, and the frequency/number of episodes. The severity of the nausea can be rated; the presence of associated symptoms is a very important consideration: fever, diarrhea, diaphoresis, syncope, or pain. When determining the temporal sequence, establish the relationship to meals, activity, or travel; the time of day when symptoms are the worst; when the symptoms were first noticed; sudden or gradual onset; and whether the patient has been exposed to others who are ill. Whereas nausea is commonly intermittent in nature, medications can cause unrelenting symptoms. Because many substances can cause nausea, the complete drug history is essential and should include prescribed, over-the-counter drugs, and recreational drugs and alcohol. Table 9-9 lists specific causes of nausea and vomiting and the common descriptions. The current and past health history may identify comorbid disorders that might cause nausea (renal failure with metabolic disturbances, diabetes with gastroparesis), as well as treatment modalities that might contribute to the nausea and/or vomiting.

Physical Examination

The physical examination should start with a general survey and vital signs. Pulse and blood pressure provide important information about hydration status and a fever may suggest infection; weight helps to determine any changes associated with decreased intake and/or significant vomiting. Even though the physical will be guided by the history and

Table 9-9. ■ Causes of Nausea and Vomiting

Cause	Examples	Typical Signs and Symptoms
Infection	Gastroenteritis (viral or bacterial), hepatitis, PID, viral syndrome, URI.	Abrupt onset, spontaneous vomiting, often accompanied by fever, malaise, and diarrhea.
Food poisoning	Bacterial sources: *C. botulinum*, staphylococcal. Nonbacterial sources: mushrooms, poisonous plants, fish, chemicals.	Symptoms occur hours to days after exposure, severe nausea and vomiting often with diarrhea, neurological symptoms, liver involvement.
Gastrointestinal obstruction	Gastric outlet obstruction related to PUD, GERD, malignancy, esophageal stricture, pyloric stenosis, or intestinal obstruction related to malignancy, intussusception, adhesions, and motility disorders.	Emesis containing undigested food, upper or lower abdominal pain and tenderness, absent bowel sounds, x-ray or CT showing bowel loops, ileus, mass, or stricture.
Metabolic disorders	Renal disease with uremia, hyperglycemia, ketoacidosis, Addison's disease, hyperthyroidism.	Mild nausea rarely accompanied by vomiting; fatigue, weakness, muscle cramping, skin changes, hypo- or hypertension, neuropathic changes, abnormal renal or endocrine lab studies.
Medication	Cardiac medicines, especially digitalis and quinidine, antihypertensives, antibiotics, bronchodilators, especially aminophylline, antineoplastic drugs, NSAIDs, MAO inhibitors, antidepressants, antiretrovirals, oral hyperglycemics.	Symptoms may be from central trigger zone stimulation or irritation to the gastric mucosa. Reactions to medicine generally cause a persistent nausea. If from gastric irritation, the nausea will worsen soon after medication administration. With trigger zone stimulation, nausea will often be delayed. If related to cardiac medicines or bronchodilators, there may be changes in heart rate and EKG changes are possible.
Central nervous system disorders	Meningitis, increased intracranial pressure, migraines, space-occupying lesion or fluid, Ménière's disorder, cerebellar disorders.	CNS-related vomiting is often projectile and not preceded by nausea. Vomiting caused by a space-occupying lesion is often worse upon arising due to a recumbent increase in ICP. Depending on the cause, accompanying symptoms include headache, visual disturbances, nystagmus, ataxia and, in meningitis, nuchal rigidity.
Cardiac disease	Myocardial infarction, congestive heart failure.	Often nausea only, but vomiting may occur in MI with severe pain. In CHF, the nausea is vague and persistent, accompanied by pain, diaphoresis, SOB, edema.
Pregnancy	Due to either hormonal or emotional changes.	Typically nausea without emesis often in the morning but may present with persistent or intermittent vomiting, missed or irregular menses, + hCG.
Psychogenic	Anorexia, bulimia, anxiety.	Usually promptly follows eating, may remit on hospitalization, more common in young women.
Cholecystitis/ pancreatitis	Due to infection, inflammation, or obstruction of the pancreas or GB.	Nausea and vomiting is intermittent and usually accompanied by RUQ or epigastric pain.

initial observations, signs of obstruction should be determined, including altered bowel sounds or succussion splash; scars should be noted as signs of surgery; percussion and palpation should be adequate to identify any tenderness, masses, or organomegaly.

Diagnostic Studies
Diagnostic studies may be warranted to discover the definitive diagnosis or the effect of the vomiting and any complications.

Laboratory Tests for Nausea and Vomiting
- U/A—an increase in urine specific gravity will be seen in dehydration.
- Electrolytes—assesses sodium, potassium, glucose, calcium, etc. Electrolytes are particularly important if the patient has had significant vomiting.
- CBC—helpful in determining the level of hydration and presence of infection.
- hCG—for a female patient of reproductive age; as the basis for symptoms and a consideration in treatment decisions.
- Depending on the associated symptoms and other information, you may choose to obtain labs specific to disorders such as pancreatitis (amylase/lipase), hepatitis (liver functions), and renal disease (BUN/creatinine). If medication-related toxicity is suspected, blood levels should be ordered.

Diagnostic Tests for Nausea and Vomiting
- Endoscopy—if PUD or malignancy is suspected.
- Barium swallow—will show structural changes in the esophagus or stomach; strictures of the esophagus are common in the elderly population.
- Barium enema—if obstruction or malignancy is suspected in the lower GI tract.
- Abdominal ultrasound/CT—to detect obstructive masses, malignancies, and pregnancy (either intrauterine or ectopic).
- CT—scan the head if a neurological cause is suspected.
- Flat/upright plain abdominal films—may be helpful in detecting obstruction, free air, gas, and renal stones.

INFECTIONS (NON-FOOD POISONING)
Signs and Symptoms.
  Nausea and vomiting associated with acute infections (viral and bacterial) may be accompanied by fever and diarrhea, as well as by other commonly associated symptoms, including malaise and fatigue. Nausea and vomiting from infections generally have a very abrupt onset; spontaneous vomiting may occur when the patient is unable to reach the toilet. The patient may be able to identify exposure to other persons with similar symptoms or other persons who ate the same meal and then developed nausea and vomiting. If hepatitis is involved, the predominant symptom(s) are usually nausea and/or anorexia, although vomiting may occur. Fever might be present. With dehydration, the patient may complain of light-headedness or dizziness; the pulse may be elevated and the blood pressure positive for postural changes. Mucous membranes may be dry, and skin turgor is diminished. Bowel sounds are often exaggerated; even without diarrhea; borborygmi may be present. The abdomen may be tender and/or distended.

Diagnostic Studies.
  Typically, common viral causes of nausea and vomiting require no diagnostic studies, as they resolve within 72 hours.

FOOD POISONING

Food poisoning can have either an infectious or noninfectious cause. Noninfectious causes occur when one eats food contaminated with chemicals or food that contains naturally occurring toxins, such as mushrooms or fish. The range of infectious causes is broad and includes staphylococcal and botulism. Onset may be days after the offending meal was ingested. For instance, whereas vomiting related to staphylococcal food poisoning often occurs only hours after the contaminated meal, vomiting caused by botulism occurs hours to days after ingestion.

Signs and Symptoms.

The presentation of food poisoning varies depending on the offending agent. When the organism is staphylococcal, symptoms include headache and fever, abdominal pain, and diarrhea. Although the disturbance is usually self-limited, severe fluid and electrolyte disturbances may occur. In contrast, a botulism-related attack usually begins with severe nausea, vomiting, and/or diarrhea, but these symptoms are often followed by neurologic symptoms. Staphylococcal food poisoning may result in fever, whereas vitals signs usually remain normal with botulism. When noninfectious poisons are involved, the symptoms may progress to profound neurological findings, liver damage, and even death, depending on the offensive toxin.

Diagnostic Studies.

When food poisoning is suspected, serum or fecal test for *Clostridium botulinum* should be performed, if symptoms warrant. Similarly, the food may be tested for staphylococci, as might the vomitus.

GASTROINTESTINAL OBSTRUCTION (REAL AND FUNCTIONAL)

Gastrointestinal obstructions cause vomiting when contents are unable to pass distally. Gastric outlet obstructions may be related to PUD. Intestinal obstructions often occur from adhesions from old surgical procedures; other causes include malignancy and intussusception. Functional obstruction can develop from motility disorders, such as gastroparesis, when smooth muscle contraction is diminished.

Signs and Symptoms.

The contents of the vomitus commonly vary according to the level of obstruction. Gastric outlet obstruction is associated with emesis containing undigested food. Proximal small intestinal blockage is likely to be bile-stained. Distal intestinal blockage is more likely to contain fecal matter. Proximal blockage may result in a large volume of emesis, as the stomach produces up to 1.5 L of secretions/24 hours. When real obstruction is involved, pain often builds in a crescendo fashion and is then intermittently relieved or lessened following emesis. The degree of cramping and pain is often related to the proximity of the obstruction, so that obstructions of the lower intestines may have less-severe cramping, vomiting, and/or pain. Bowel sounds will often be high pitched and metallic sounding, but may later become absent. Tenderness may be localized or diffuse. Distention may be present, as well as a succussion splash.

Diagnostic Studies.

Flat and upright plain films of the abdomen may depict dilated loops of bowels and ileus. A CT scan would determine the presence of a mass. Endoscopy can identify strictures associated with PUD. A barium swallow can monitor motility.

PREGNANCY

Hormonal changes associated with pregnancy are believed to contribute to nausea and vomiting, although other theories suggest some degree of emotional etiology.

Signs and Symptoms.

Although pregnant women may well present with persistent or intermittent vomiting episodes, pregnancy more commonly causes nausea, without emesis. The nausea can occur at any time of the day but occurs most often in the morning and without regard to meals. Although this may be the presenting symptom of pregnancy, the patient will have recently missed or had an irregular period.

Diagnostic Studies.

Perform urine or serum hCG.

METABOLIC DISORDERS

A variety of metabolic disorders can present with nausea and/or vomiting. Common examples include renal disease associated with uremia and many endocrine problems, such as hyperglycemia, ketoacidosis, Addison's disease, and hyperthyroidism.

Signs and Symptoms.

Nausea is more common than vomiting with metabolic disorders. With uremia of renal failure, other common symptoms are muscle cramping, neuropathic changes, hypertension, and skin changes. With diabetes, the patient may present with the classic symptoms of hyperglycemia. With adrenal insufficiency, or Addison's disease, common early symptoms include fatigue, weakness, hypotension, and skin changes.

Diagnostic Studies.

The diagnosis would depend on the suspected metabolic disorder. Consider BUN/creatinine, which will be elevated in renal disease. Order blood glucose and urine ketones, if diabetes is suspected with or without ketoacidosis.

CENTRAL NERVOUS SYSTEM DISORDERS

The range of neurologic disorders that result in nausea and/or vomiting is broad. Included are meningitis, increased intracranial pressure (ICP), migraines, a space-occupying lesion, and Ménière's disorder.

Signs and Symptoms.

Central nervous system–related vomiting is often projectile and may not be preceded by nausea. Associated complaints/findings depend on the causative lesion. Papilledema may accompany increased ICP. Neurologic deficits may be evident with increased ICP, space-occupying lesions, and meningitis. Nuchal rigidity is a classic finding for meningitis. With Ménière's or other forms of labyrinthitis, nystagmus and/or ataxia may be present. Migraines may be preceded with the classic visual disturbance or other auras and are typically unilateral. See Chapters 14 and 15.

Diagnostic Studies.

A CT scan of the head is warranted in most cases and, if meningitis is suspected, a lumbar puncture may be necessary.

DRUGS

Drugs are very common causes of nausea and vomiting. The nausea associated with medications may stem from either central trigger zone stimulation or irritation to the gastric mucosa. Drugs that are commonly associated with nausea and vomiting are listed in Table 9-9.

Signs and Symptoms.

Drugs, like other toxins, generally cause a persistent nausea. There may be associated findings related to the toxic level. For instance, with excessive levels of digitalis, vision may be altered and bradycardia evident. With excessive aminophylline, tachycardia and tremors may be manifested.

Diagnostic Studies.

The primary diagnostic study would be a level of the suspected agent.

PSYCHOGENIC CAUSES

Emotional disturbances may result in either chronic or recurrent episodes of vomiting. Examples include bulimia and extreme anxiety responses.

Signs and Symptoms.

Usually, psychogenic vomiting promptly follows eating and may occur during the meal; it is more common in young women. This vomiting is not urgent and can usually be suppressed; it may remit on hospitalization. The patient may show little concern regarding the vomiting. The patient may be very thin, but often in the case of bulimia, the patient is of normal weight. In other patients, vomiting occurs when there is acute anxiety associated with certain stressful situations or events, for instance, public speaking, interviews, and tests.

Diagnostic Studies.

When no organic cause is found to explain recurrent or chronic vomiting, a psychiatric history should be performed.

Cardiac Causes

Depending on the patient's health history and/or risk factors, you may include cardiac-related disorders in your differential diagnosis for nausea and/or vomiting. These can be associated with both myocardial infarction and congestive heart failure (see Chapter 6). Another potential cardiac-related source, mentioned above, includes cardiac medications.

GERD

See p. 198.

PUD, Gastritis

See p. 228, 226.

Cholecystitis

See p. 224.

Diarrhea

The causes of diarrhea are numerous and include bacterial, viral, organic, and functional. The mechanisms are due to 1) abnormal transport mechanisms; 2) a change in the osmotic mechanism, thus resulting in variations in absorption; 3) increased motility; and 4) exudative blood or pus, thereby decreasing absorption.

Most cases are self-limiting and resolve within days without medical intervention. When there is high fever, intractable vomiting, or severe dehydration, prompt attention is necessary, and, frequently, hospitalization is required—especially in the child or the geriatric patient.

History

Symptoms vary according to the cause of the diarrhea. A thorough symptom analysis should identify the time of onset, whether onset was sudden or gradual, and the duration of the symptoms. Determine severity according to whether the diarrhea is intermittent or persistent and according to the number of stools per day. Inquire as to associated symptoms, such as abdominal pain, fever, nausea, or vomiting, as well as whether there is any relation to meals. Ask the patient to describe the color of the stool, looking for reports of dark or bloody stools; consistency, as to formed, watery, fatty, or greasy; and the presence of mucus or odor. It is important to ask about recent meals or travel and if accompanying others may have similar symptoms; recent antibiotics or other new medications, either prescription or over the counter; and whether there is a history of EtOH abuse or PUD disease that could indicate a GI bleed. Dehydration and electrolyte depletion are concerns, and the volume of fluid intake should be determined. If diarrhea has been chronic, changes in weight or appetite should be recorded. Stress or anxiety may be a causative factor; therefore, the presence of psychosocial issues should be investigated.

Physical Examination

The physical exam should begin with vital signs, particularly determining the presence of fever, which might indicate infection, and tachycardia or orthostatic hypotension, which might indicate dehydration. Other signs of dehydration may include dry mucous membranes, light-headedness, syncope, lethargy, and oliguria. If there is accompanying electrolyte imbalance, cardiac arrhythmias, muscle weakness, tetany, or vascular collapse may occur particularly in young children, the elderly, or patients who are already debilitated. Listen for hypoactive or hyperactive bowel sounds, which could indicate early obstruction; palpate for abdominal tenderness, indicating infection or inflammation; perform a digital rectal exam, checking for heme-positive stool. Significant unexplained weight loss should be investigated.

Diagnostic Studies
Laboratory Tests for Diarrhea
- Stool for ova and parasites (O & P) and culture and sensitivity (C & S); Hemoccult.
- CBC to check for anemia, which might indicate malignancy.
- Chemistry panel and amylase to check for inflammatory, hepatic, pancreatic, or renal causes.

Diagnostic Tests for Diarrhea
- Sigmoidoscopy or colonoscopy if symptoms persist.

INFECTIONS (NON-FOOD POISONING)
Signs and Symptoms.

Diarrhea associated with acute infections (viral and bacterial) may be accompanied by fever, nausea, and vomiting; other commonly associated symptoms include malaise, fatigue, weakness, and light-headedness. Diarrhea from infections generally has a very abrupt onset; spontaneous diarrhea may occur and the patient is unable to reach the toilet. The patient may be able to identify exposure to other persons with similar symptoms or other persons who ate the same meal or traveled to the same area and then developed the diarrhea. If the diarrhea is severe, dehydration may ensue, causing tachycardia and postural hypotension. Mucous membranes may be dry and skin turgor diminished. Bowel sounds are often exaggerated, even without diarrhea; borborygmi may be present. The abdomen may be tender and/or distended. Several viruses have been identified as causing diarrhea: Norwalk virus, rotavirus, adenovirus, and enterovirus, with the latter two sometimes associated with respiratory symptoms. Common bacterial causes of diarrhea either from toxins or from mucosal invasion and ulceration include *Vibrio cholerae*, salmonella, shigella, *Escherichia coli*, and campylobacter, the most common.

Diagnostic Studies.

Typically, common viral causes of nausea, vomiting, and diarrhea require no diagnostic studies and will resolve within 72 hours. Bacterial causes will require antibiotics.

PARASITIC INFECTION

Signs and Symptoms.

Certain parasites, most commonly *Giardia lamblia*, transmitted by fecally contaminated water or food, can cause diarrhea, bloating, flatulence, cramps, nausea, anorexia, weight loss, greasy stools because of its interference with fat absorption, and occasionally fever. Symptoms usually occur about 2 weeks after exposure and can last 2–3 months. Often the symptoms are vague and intermittent, which makes diagnosis more difficult. There is no chemoprophylaxis, but boiling water deactivates the *Giardia* cysts. Anti-infectives are available for treatment.

Diagnostic Studies.

Serial stool samples for O & P should be ordered because a single sample may not reveal the *Giardia*. Duodenal contents can be sampled by the Enterotest, which collects the sample by having the patient swallow a nylon string with a weight on the end and then removing the string after a certain amount of time. This is more reliable than stool cultures, but the procedure is not desirable to the patient.

AMEBIC DYSENTERY

This particular type of dysentery is common in tropical climates but fairly rare in temperate climates.

Signs and Symptoms.

It is characterized by semifluid stools containing mucus, blood, and active trophozoites. This form of dysentery may become chronic, and the symptoms are those of recurrent abdominal cramping and soft stools. In the chronic state, weight loss is significant and anemia is present.

Diagnostic Studies.

The diagnosis is made by stool cultures, and three to six specimens may be needed before an accurate diagnosis can be made.

FOOD POISONING

Food poisoning can have either infectious or noninfectious cause. Noninfectious causes occur when one eats food contaminated with chemicals or that contains naturally occurring toxins, such as mushrooms or fish. The range of infectious causes is broad and includes staphylococcal, *C. botulinum, C. perfringens*, and *E. coli*. Onset may be days after the offending meal was ingested. For instance, whereas diarrhea related to staphylococcal food poisoning often occurs several hours after the contaminated meal, botulism causes diarrhea 2–8 days after ingestion.

Signs and Symptoms.

The presentation of food poisoning varies depending on the offending agent. When the organism is staphylococcal, symptoms may include headache and fever, abdominal pain, nausea, vomiting, and diarrhea. Although the disturbance is usually self-limited, severe fluid and electrolyte disturbances can occur. A botulism-related attack usually begins with severe nausea, vomiting, and/or diarrhea, but these symptoms are often followed by neurologic symptoms, such as diplopia, loss of accommodation, diminished pupillary reflex, and dysphagia. Staphylococcal food poisoning may result in fever, whereas vitals signs usually remain normal with botulism. *Escherichia coli* infection is characterized by acute onset, severe abdominal cramps, and watery/bloody diarrhea. Fever may be present. *Escherichia coli* infection can be complicated by hemolytic-uremic syndrome, which is characterized by hemolytic anemia, thrombocytopenia, and acute renal failure. The prognosis in these cases is grave. *Escherichia coli* infection can result in death with or without these complications, especially in children and the elderly. *Clostridium perfringens* symptoms can range from a mild self-limiting disease to a severe, fatal gastroenteritis. In severe cases, diarrhea, abdominal pain, distention, and vascular collapse can occur rapidly, and prompt supportive measures are necessary. When noninfectious poisons are involved, the symptoms may progress to profound neurological findings, liver damage, and even death, depending on the toxin.

Diagnostic Studies.

When food poisoning is suspected, serum testing or fecal culture for the suspected organism should be performed, if symptoms warrant. Similarly, the food could be tested, as could the vomitus.

DRUG REACTION/SENSITIVITY

Drugs are a very common cause of diarrhea. The diarrhea associated with medications may stem from either a generalized allergic reaction or irritation of the intestinal mucosa. Many drugs have the potential to cause diarrhea, but among the drugs that are commonly associated are quinidine, digitalis, antibiotics, metformin, and many SSRIs. A late sequela of antibiotic treatment—particularly with clindamycin, ampicillin, cephalosporins, erythromycin, tetracycline, and sulfamethoxazole/trimethoprim—is pseudomembranous colitis resulting from *Clostridium difficile*. An antibiotic-induced change in the intestinal flora is the predisposing factor. *Clostridium difficile* has been implicated in much of the nosocomial cases of diarrhea, in hospitals and nursing homes. In some instances, necrotizing colitis may ensue.

Signs and Symptoms.

Drugs, like other toxins, generally cause persistent diarrhea. Drugs that affect the lower GI tract often affect the upper GI tract as well, and it is common to find associated nausea or vomiting.

Diagnostic Studies.

A history of a new medication gives a high likelihood of that being the causative agent. Stopping the drug or replacing it with another category of drug should result in resolution of the diarrhea.

Gastrointestinal Surgery

Any surgery that affects intestinal transit, such as large bowel resection, gastric resection, gastric or intestinal bypass, pyloroplasty or vagotomy, may cause diarrhea. A history of any of these surgeries suggests that as the causative factor. Because malabsorption and malnutrition may result, patients need education on vitamin and mineral supplementation.

MUCOSAL DISEASES

There are several diseases that can cause mucosal inflammation and ulceration, resulting in intermittent, and often severe, diarrhea. These diseases include ulcerative colitis, Crohn's disease, regional enteritis, gastrointestinal TB, and carcinomas.

Signs and Symptoms.

The symptoms and severity of the diarrhea vary according to the underlying cause. The symptoms of carcinomas are generally insidious. The diarrhea is mild and intermittent. Often malignancies are found on routine Hemoccults, sigmoidoscopy, or colonoscopy. There should be a high index of suspicion with unexplained weight loss or new-onset iron deficiency anemia in a patient over 40 years old. With colitis, enteritis, Crohn's disease, and TB, the onset of the diarrhea may be sudden and severe, with fever and significant abdominal tenderness, or it may be slow in onset, with mild cramps and the urge to defecate. The stool is frequently bloody with pus and/or mucus. Malaise, fever, and weight loss are common. Initially, a history and stool examination are helpful in making a diagnosis. The stool is heavy with RBCs and WBCs, and usually overt blood and pus are present. Because bouts are recurrent, a positive history of these diseases supports an exacerbation. There is a risk of bowel perforation and resultant peritonitis, and, in these cases, mortality may be as high as 40%.

Diagnostic Studies.

A CBC and erythrocyte sedimentation rate (ESR) should be performed. Colitis is often accompanied by leukocytosis, anemia, and an elevated sedimentation rate. In malignancies, anemia is often the first sign found on routine laboratory studies. A variety of diagnostic tests may be helpful in making a definitive diagnosis, including abdominal CT, BE, sigmoidoscopy, or colonoscopy.

IRRITABLE BOWEL SYNDROME

Signs and Symptoms.

Irritable bowel syndrome is a motility disorder involving the upper and lower GI tracts that causes intermittent nausea, abdominal pain and distention, flatulence, pain relieved by defecation, diarrhea, and/or constipation. Symptoms usually occur in the waking hours and may be worsened or triggered by meals. It is three times more prevalent in women, accounts for more than half of all GI referrals, and is highly correlated with emotional factors, particularly anxiety and stress. These patients have a heightened sensitivity to food and parasympathomimetic drugs, which causes abnormalities in transit—increased in the diarrhea-predominant group and decreased in the constipation-predominant group.

Diagnostic Studies.

Digital rectal exam and 3-day Hemoccults for occult blood; stool for O & P and for C & S; CBC to check for anemia, which might indicate a malignant cause of the symptoms; and ESR, chemistry panel, amylase, and U/A to rule out inflammatory, hepatic, pancreatic, or renal causes. Sigmoidoscopy or colonoscopy is recommended.

CARBOHYDRATE INTOLERANCE

More commonly referred to as lactose intolerance, this actually represents a symptom complex resulting from a lack of intestinal enzymes (usually lactase) necessary to break down disaccharides. Unsplit disaccharides in the intestine retain water and result in diarrhea.

Signs and Symptoms.

Symptoms include nausea, diarrhea, abdominal cramps, borborygmi, bloating, and flatulence, which generally occur within 1–2 hours after eating the offending food, usually dairy products. Diarrhea may be severe, but the duration is relatively short.

Diagnostic Studies.

Acid stools with a pH < 6 are suspicious. The hydrogen breath test, if available, is easy and reliable. A lactose or glucose challenge is diagnostic when diarrhea occurs in about 30 minutes. Jejunal biopsies are generally not performed because they are invasive and expensive.

LAXATIVE USE AND ABUSE

Laxative abuse is often seen in the elderly, as caused by chronic or overtreatment of constipation. It is also seen in eating disorders, particularly bulimia, as a water and weight loss aid.

Signs and Symptoms.

May cause muscle weakness, lethargy, weight loss, electrolyte depletion, cardiac arrhythmias, changes in the intestinal mucosa, and bleeding.

Diagnostic Studies.

The diagnosis of laxative abuse is made by history. Those treating constipation should be educated regarding dietary changes, adequate fluid intake, and the proper use of bulking agents so as to avoid the need for laxative use. Overdependence on laxatives for regular bowel movements serves only to compound the constipation problem. Rarely does this type of laxative use cause serious electrolyte imbalance. In the eating disorder client, however, the abuse is significant and can lead to serious complications. Complete blood count and electrolytes will identify anemia or electrolyte depletion. Psychological counseling is necessary for eating disorder patients.

Constipation

Constipation is a common complaint generally used to describe excessively dry, small, or infrequent stools. According to a more specific definition, constipation is the presence of more than one of the following conditions for at least three months:

* Straining with bowel movements more than 25% of the time.
* Hard stools more than 25% of the time.
* Incomplete evacuations more than 25% of the time.
* Fewer than three bowel movements per week.

What is important is that the term constipation covers more than infrequent stools and must be addressed from the patient's viewpoint. Constipation is often a chronic condition. Patients often self-treat both real and perceived constipation; its presence may be identified when the history identifies frequent or chronic use of laxatives or cathartics. Lifestyle factors (nutritional and fluid intake, activity) often contribute to chronic constipation. The altered colonic transit time may also be associated with medications, endocrine disorders, neurologic deficits, and various gastrointestinal disorders; constipation may be one sign of an eating or psychiatric disorder. Acute-onset constipation may stem from bowel obstruction or ileus.

HISTORY

Establish what the term constipation means to the patient. Ask how long it has existed and whether it is constant or intermittent. Determine how, if at all, the patient's previous bowel patterns differed. Explore the current bowel history: frequency of bowel movements; any changes in caliber, color, quantity, or consistency (are the movements hard?); the need to strain; and whether there is complete evacuation. Ask about associated symptoms: abdominal bloating/fullness, rectal pain or bleeding, blood or mucus in the stool, altered appetite, and abdominal pain. Inquire about any preceding events: a newly prescribed or over-the-counter medication, or changes in diet or activity. Establish whether the constipation alternates with normal bowel pattern or diarrhea, or whether it is progressive. Include a review of systems, focusing on the gastrointestinal, endocrine, and neurologic systems. Find out whether the patient has experienced a weight loss because the potential for a malignancy must be considered. Establish the presence of any associated complications: hemorrhoids, fissures, or fecal incontinence. Obtain a history of endocrine, neurological, or gastrointestinal problems; abdominal surgeries; and currently prescribed or over-the-counter medications. Obtain a history of dietary and fluid intake, activity, and recreational drug use.

Physical Examination

The physical examination should start with a general survey—note the patient's overall appearance and whether she or he appears healthy or ill, has any obvious deficits, or exhibits physical signs of systemic disorders. Obtain a weight. Observe the skin and mucous membranes for signs of dehydration. Depending on the history and your general survey, you should examine other systems. Otherwise, the examination can focus on the abdomen and rectum.

Inspect and auscultate the abdomen first, noting any scars, distention, visible masses, and discoloration. If bowel sounds are not immediately evident, continue listening for at least 15 seconds in each quadrant before you conclude that they are absent; if sounds are present, determine the pitch and frequency. Identify areas of dullness over organs, and estimate organ size. Note any areas of dullness over the bowel. Palpate superficially at first, noting any guarding, rigidity, or tenderness. Palpate more deeply to assess organs and any other areas of firmness or mass. For any palpable mass, determine the consistency, size, shape, mobility, and margins. Perform an anorectal examination, inspecting the anus for tone, fissures, external hemorrhoids, or other defects. Palpate the rectum for masses and stool, noting the consistency of anything palpated; perform guaiac on any palpated stool.

Diagnostic Studies

Laboratory Tests for Constipation

Laboratory studies can include thyroid functions, renal studies, electrolytes, and CBC.

Diagnostic Tests for Constipation

Diagnostics are not usually warranted for the initial workup of constipation, provided that a probable contributing factor or cause has been determined. Providers typically recommend changes in diet and/or fiber intake, fluid intake, or medications and then determine the response before ordering studies. When appropriate, however, commonly ordered

imaging and visualization studies include plain abdominal films, ultrasounds, barium ene
mas, or flexible sigmoidoscopy/colonoscopy.

COLONIC MOTILITY DISORDERS

Disorders of the smooth muscle of the colon can cause hypotonia and decreased motility; examples include congenital and acquired myopathies and enteric nerve disorders, such
as Hirschsprung's disease. The result can be slowed transit time with greater intervals
between evacuations, the development of bowel dilation, or pseudo-obstruction.

Signs and Symptoms.

The history may identify a familial tendency to constipation. The patient may have previously attempted increasing dietary fiber and fluids, as well as maintaining a reasonable
activity level, without improvement.

Diagnostic Studies.

A barium enema can identify areas of colon dilation. Measurements of whole-gut transit time are available; serial radiographs identify the position of ingested radiopaque
marker(s) over time. There are a variety of specialized tests that provide information regarding the bowel motility and tone that are performed by gastroenterologist, on consultation.

INTESTINAL OBSTRUCTION

Obstructions of the colon cause a progressive constipation, which may be associated
with pain, nausea, or other symptoms. In older patients, constipation may be the presenting symptom of obstruction. Malignancy must be considered.

Signs and Symptoms.

There may be a history of the stool having become smaller in diameter, the term "pen-
cil" stool, as well as a history of decreasing frequency of bowel movements and/or blood in
the stool. Obstipation—extreme obstruction—leads to the failure to pass even gas. If a
volvulus is the cause, the symptoms may or may not include pain and discomfort.
Abdominal distention is marked in colonic obstruction. As the problem progresses, the
patient may develop signs of shock. A palpable mass may be evident in volvulus or malignancy. The degree of tenderness is variable. There may be high-pitched bowel sounds or
borborygmi, until a late stage, at which time bowel sounds are absent.

Diagnostic Studies.

Plain films of the abdomen should be ordered, looking for dilated loops of bowel, air-
fluid levels, and the absence of colonic gas. The nature of an obstruction can be identified
with a barium enema or colonoscopy/flexible sigmoidoscopy. If the obstruction is due to
strangulation, the CBC may show a leukocyte shift to the left. Never order a barium upper-
GI series until colonic obstruction has been ruled out.

RECTOCELE AND PROLAPSE

Structural disorders of the anorectum and/or pelvic floor can cause constipation. A rectocele occurs when the rectovaginal septum bulges anteriorly. Weakness of the pelvic floor
results in a widened anorectal angle, and thereby a weakened perineal body. The pelvic
floor may be weakened during childbirth, trauma, or repeated straining during bowel
movements (thus, the cause and effect are blurred). Once weakened, the pelvic floor resistance is lessened and the stool is not directed/extruded through the anal canal. Both problems are more common among females.

Signs and Symptoms.

Patients may complain of general constipation, but may also note that the problem is more related to the act of defecation, which is difficult. Women who have developed a rectocele may perceive that there is weakness in the perineal area and that a mass is evident at the introitus when they strain; some learn to support the introitus to facilitate defecation. The physical signs of rectocele are determined during the vaginal exam; refer Chapter 12.

Diagnostic Studies.

A barium enema provides evidence of rectocele with lateral view but is usually not warranted, as the physical examination identifies the change. When bleeding from a fistula or hemorrhoid occurs, a proctoscopic examination should be performed to ensure there is not also a malignancy or other mass.

MEDICATIONS

Many medications can cause or contribute to constipation. The medications most commonly associated with constipation are listed in Box 9-2.

Signs and Symptoms.

The presentation of constipation related to medications can be acute or chronic, either following the initial introduction of a new drug or after some time period has elapsed. The appearance of the abdomen and presence of bowel sounds are usually not altered. Depending on the severity of the constipation, the abdominal examination may be within normal limits; however, feces may be palpable and there may be some tenderness with deep palpation. The anorectal examination will typically be normal, although you may palpate hard, dry feces.

Diagnostic Studies.

There are usually no studies necessary. A common diagnostic effort would be to discontinue the suspected offending drug; however, it is not always possible to discontinue a medication in order to confirm the relationship (thus, other treatments/recommendations must be made to minimize the constipating effects of necessary drugs). If obstruction is suspected, refer to earlier section.

PSYCHIATRIC DISORDERS AND EATING DISORDERS

Constipation has been associated with depression. Patients with eating disorders commonly develop constipation, unless they are also using laxatives. Patients with vari-

---

Box 9-2

Medications Causing Constipation

Analgesics/narcotics
Antacids containing aluminum
Anticonvulsants
Antidepressants
Antihypertensives (calcium-channel blockers, beta-blockers)
Antiparkinsonism agents
Antispasmodics
Calcium supplements
Diuretics
Iron supplements
Sedatives/tranquilizers

ous psychiatric disorders may deny having bowel movements and fictitiously report constipation.

Signs and Symptoms.

The history is very important, in order to determine the actual pattern of bowel movements. Patients may give a history of frequency and characteristics of bowel habits that are well within normal range, but indicate dissatisfaction, or concern over some specific characteristic, such as the color or caliber, in spite of no report of a recent change. When a psychogenic cause is suspected, a psychiatric history is warranted. Look for indications of depression or obsessive-compulsive disorder. Be sure to perform a thorough overall history and physical, however, to ensure that an organic cause is not missed. Recognize, also, that often patients who initially develop real or perceived constipation associated with psychogenic causes, begin to use laxatives and cathartics progressively so that they develop a dependence on these agents.

Diagnostic Studies.

It is possible that a patient might underestimate the frequency of bowel movements. Consider having the patient monitor their bowel movements over several days, using a diary card. They should document each bowel movement and the volume and form of the stool. Although no specific diagnostic studies are necessary, you should order those that will allow you to exclude major organic causes—selecting based on the presentation and patient's history. Possible studies include: thyroid studies, electrolytes, CBC, abdominal imaging, sigmoidoscopy, and colonoscopy.

Endocrine Disorders

Both hypothyroidism and diabetes can contribute to or cause constipation by decreasing motility. In hypothyroidism, myxedematous tissue may infiltrate the gut, resulting in megacolon. Diabetes should be considered as contributory to constipation when patients have other signs of autonomic neuropathy. The hypercalcemia associated with hyperparathyroidism may cause constipation.

Neurologic Disorders

Many neurologic disorders can alter bowel patterns, including Parkinson's disease, multiple sclerosis, and spinal cord injuries. It is unknown whether the neurologic changes caused in the brain of a patient with Parkinson's disease also affect the enteric nerves or whether constipation is the result of increased pelvic floor muscle tone. Multiple sclerosis is believed to contribute to slow transit time, as well as altered pelvic floor muscle tone. The degree to which a spinal cord lesion affects bowel function depends on the level of injury; injuries may alter distal transit time, as well as sphincter responsiveness. See Chapter 14 for further discussion.

Irritable Bowel Disorder

See previous discussion, p. 216.

Jaundice

Jaundice, a yellow discoloration of skin and mucous membranes, stems from an elevation of either the unconjugated or conjugated bilirubin. Causes of unconjugated hyperbilirubinemia include both bilirubin overproduction, as occurs in several hemolytic disorders, and impaired bilirubin uptake, associated with inherited disorders. Conjugated hyperbilirubinemia is more common and stems from either impaired hepatic excretion or extra-hepatic obstruction. Hepatitis is the most common cause of jaundice (75%) among persons younger than 30. Obstruction is the most common etiology of jaundice (60%) after age 60, and the causes include gallstones, tumors, or strictures from past surgeries. Other relatively common causes in older adults include congestive heart failure (CHF) (10%) and metastatic malignancy (13%). Clearly, jaundice may be the presenting sign of serious disease in all age groups. With appropriate history, physical, and early diagnostic studies, the cause of jaundice usually can be correctly identified as either obstructive or nonobstructive.

History

The patient's age is an important consideration in differentiating among potential causes of jaundice. Find out when the discoloration was first noticed and whether other symptoms have developed or been associated with this finding. Important associated symptoms include pruritus, malaise, fever/chills, nausea, anorexia, change in the color of urine or feces, and abdominal pain. The medical history must address previous hepatic or biliary diseases, malignancy, hemolytic disorders, and surgeries, as well as other potential contributing disorders, including CHF. Obtain a family history of hemolytic, biliary, and hepatic disorders. Obtain a thorough medication history, including over-the-counter and herbal agents; determine the use of alcohol and recreational drugs, particularly IV drug use; and social risk factors for hepatitis, including sexual practices.

Physical Examination

The physical examination should include a general survey of the skin and mucous membranes, observing for discoloration, dryness, spider angiomas, petechiae, and xanthomas as well as excoriations indicative of pruritus (see also Chapter 2). The general survey should also include consideration of the patient's mental status as an indicator of liver disease. The lungs and heart should be assessed briefly to identify overall health and indications of heart failure (see also Chapter 6). Unless otherwise indicated by the history, the remainder of the physical should focus on the abdomen. Carefully observe for scars from previous surgical procedures. Percuss to determine organ size and any unexpected areas of dullness indicative of a possible mass. As you percuss, note any areas of tenderness, particularly over the liver. Palpate to further assess abdominal organs. As you palpate for the liver, be attentive for a positive Murphy's sign. If the liver is palpable, note the consistency and margins, in addition to the size.

Diagnostic Studies

Laboratory Tests for Jaundice

- CBC, liver profile, hepatitis screening, bilirubin, and prothrombin times to evaluate for liver disease.
- Serum studies that are less common, but that are very appropriate for certain causes of jaundice include iron, transferrin, ferritin, antimitochondrial antibodies, antinuclear antibodies, and ceruloplasmin.

Diagnostic Tests for Jaundice

- Helpful imaging studies include ultrasounds and CT scans to evaluate organomegaly or palpable masses. Ultrasound is more helpful when nonobstructive causes of jaundice are suspected.

- When the index of suspicion is high for obstructive causes of jaundice, either endo-scopic retrograde cholangiopancreatography (ERCP) or percutaneous transhepatic cholangiography (PTC) are appropriate initial imaging studies.
- Referral for liver biopsy if warranted.

HEPATITIS

Jaundice causing injury to the liver can have many potential sources; viruses and hepatotoxins are the most common causes. The viral diseases that can cause hepatitis include the identified hepatitis viruses (A, B, C, D, and E), as well as Epstein-Barr and cytomegalovirus. Hepatotoxins include numerous prescribed and over-the-counter med-ications, such as acetaminophen, methyldopa, isoniazid, and phenytoin; herbal remedies; alcohol; and, more rarely, chemical exposures.

Signs and Symptoms.

Explore potential sources of viral illness, including exposures to blood and body secre-tions and toxins through occupational, sexual, and/or recreational activities. Obtain a com-plete listing of all drugs and herbal agents ingested, as well as the use of alcohol. Viral causes of hepatitis with jaundice often have other accompanying symptoms of the virus, includ-ing malaise and myalgia, as well as right upper quadrant discomfort and anorexia. Past medical history should include any episodes of viral hepatitis or other hepatic injury. Assess for nonhepatic signs of viral illness, including fever, splenomegaly, and lymphadenopathy. Identify the size and condition of the liver, and the presence of discomfort.

Diagnostic Studies.

Obtain liver functions, including ALT and AST; a hepatitis screen; and total and direct bilirubin levels. Order a CBC. Consider abdominal/liver ultrasound or CT. Further diag nostic studies are generally obtained in consultation with or after referral to a gastroen-terologist.

HEPATIC AND PANCREATIC CANCERS

Primary or metastatic cancers of the liver and/or pancreas can cause obstructive hyper-bilirubinemia and jaundice. Jaundice may be either the initial sign of a malignancy or may follow the development of other symptoms.

Signs and Symptoms.

Ask about associated symptoms such as RUQ discomfort, nausea, fever, back pain, weight loss, fatigue/weakness, and pruritus. None of these symptoms are specific to malig-nancy; however, other causes of jaundice are less likely to be associated with weight loss. Review past medical history of malignancies, as well as the family history of cancer. A his-tory of previous malignancy should cause this to be a major consideration in the differen-tial diagnosis for unexplained jaundice. If hepatic or pancreatic cancer is suspected, a prompt, thorough physical exam is warranted owing to the potential for metastatic disease and the need to identify the primary site. During the abdominal examination, carefully palpate the area of the liver, as well as the remainder of the abdomen, being attentive for any masses or unexpected findings.

Diagnostic Studies.

In addition to a CBC, liver functions, amylase, and bilirubin levels, abdominal CT and/or ultrasound should be promptly ordered.

CIRRHOSIS

Cirrhosis develops with the replacement of normal liver tissue by regenerative, fibrotic nodules and may occur in the late phase of a variety of disorders that damage the liver, such as chronic viral hepatitis, Wilson's disease, and drug and alcohol toxicity.

Signs and Symptoms.

Symptoms may be subtle at first or dramatic. A patient may present with jaundice and describe an associated, progressive pattern of pruritus, weakness, anorexia, nausea, and weight loss. Alternatively, a patient with undiagnosed cirrhosis may present with jaundice and also with acute onset of ascites, bleeding varices, and/or severe RUQ discomfort. Include a mental status exam as well as an examination of the lung and heart. Assess for the presence of ascites. Determine the size and consistency of the liver, as well as any tenderness.

Diagnostic Studies.

In addition to AST and ALT, other diagnostic studies should include a CBC, alkaline phosphatase, bilirubin, albumin, and prothrombin time. An ultrasound of the abdomen should be done to further evaluate the liver size and structure.

CHOLECYSTITIS, CHOLELITHIASIS, AND CHOLANGITIS

Occlusion of the common bile duct may occur with disorders of the gall bladder and/or bile duct.

Signs and Symptoms.

All three conditions are generally accompanied by RUQ discomfort, anorexia, and nausea. Charcot's triad, which includes jaundice, RUQ pain, and fever/chills is common to problems resulting in obstructions of the bile duct. Identify any prior history of biliary surgery. Assess the abdomen, noting the condition of the liver, as well as testing for Murphy's sign. Observe the skin for xanthomas.

Diagnostic Studies.

Obtain an ultrasound of the gall bladder and biliary structures.

HEMOLYTIC DISORDERS

A variety of conditions causing hemolysis of the red blood cells can result in jaundice. These include acquired hemolytic anemia, sickle cell anemia, and hemolytic drug reactions, among others.

Signs and Symptoms.

If hemolytic anemia is involved, the history may also include weakness, fatigue, dyspnea, palpitations, or other symptoms common to anemia. Other symptoms may include abdominal pain, fever, and chills if hemolysis has been rapid. Patients with sickle cell disorder are usually able to provide a history of recurrent episodes of symptoms, including severe pain, weakness, dyspnea, swollen joints, and/or skin lesions—often requiring serial hospitalizations. The medication survey may identify medications with hemolysis as a potential adverse effect, such as sulfonamides and methyldopa. Assess for splenomegaly and hepatomegaly. Observe skin and mucous membranes for lesions, purpura, and/or pallor. Assess joints for swelling, inflammation, or tenderness. Assess heart and lungs; determine the presence of any associated cardiomegaly.

Diagnostic Studies.

Order a CBC, noting the hematocrit, red blood count and indices, hemoglobin, as well as a reticulocyte count. Tests for hemoglobinopathies may be indicated, as might an indirect Coomb's test for levels of antibodies to the red blood cells.

Pancreatitis
See earlier discussion, p. 194.

Gastrointestinal Bleeding

Patients with gastrointestinal bleeding may complain of hematemesis, melena, or hematochezia. Alternatively, they may have occult bleeding and be unaware of the problem. When a patient does present with a complaint of GI bleeding, the first step must be to determine the patient's hemodynamic stability before proceeding with further investigation. Stability is assessed, to a large extent, by consideration of the patient's vital signs and general appearance. This discussion does not apply to patients who present with significant, acute blood loss or who otherwise require urgent stabilization and treatment. Rather, this section will describe the approach for patients who appear stable and who present with a history of blood in emesis or stool, as well as those in whom occult bleeding is suspected or confirmed. It is important to be able to narrow the differential diagnosis to allow for a focused approach.

History

It is important to obtain a thorough symptom analysis of any complaint of GI bleeding, including the timing, progression, and description of the blood. Whether the blood is noticed in emesis and/or in stool, determine the amount, color, odor, and any other characteristics of the emesis and/or stool. The ability to differentiate between melena and hematochezia is helpful. When melena is present, the blood is likely to have been present for over 14 hours; therefore, the site of bleeding is most likely distant from the rectum (upper GI). When hematochezia is present, the blood is less likely to have remained in the bowel long enough for the hemoglobin to have degraded it, and thus the source is more likely to be nearer the rectum, usually in the colon. However, rapid upper-GI bleeding can result in hematochezia. Establish the history of bowel movements and previous episodes of emesis and/or retching. Identify other indications of bleeding, including bleeding gums, bruising, or epistaxis. Associated symptoms such as pain, weakness, constipation, or diarrhea must be identified. Prior history of gastrointestinal conditions, malignancies, bleeding disorders, comorbidities, and current medications must be determined. A review of habits should include diet, alcohol intake, and tobacco use. A history of any prior gastrointestinal diagnostic studies should be determined, along with the results.

Physical Examination

The physical examination must start with a general survey and accurate vital signs. Observe the patient's general overall appearance, as well as for any signs of pallor, weakness, or dyspnea. Obtain pulse and blood pressure lying, sitting, and standing, and note any postural changes. The heart and lungs should be assessed to provide an assessment of general well-being, as well as any compensatory changes related to bleeding. Finally, unless otherwise indicated, the examination should focus on the abdomen. Note any areas of discomfort, organomegaly, palpable masses, and unexpected dullness to percussion. A rectal examination must be performed, noting the presence of hemorrhoids, masses, and testing for occult blood.

Diagnostic Studies

Laboratory studies must include an assessment of hematocrit, hemoglobin, and red blood cell indices. It is important to recognize that these may all be within normal limits early in a bleeding episode, as whole blood is lost with no proportional change. Consider ordering prothrombin time and partial thromboplastin time to determine coagulation status. If the source of a bleed is an active upper gastric lesion, the aspirate from a nasogastric tube may contain obvious or occult blood. Diagnostic studies commonly used to evaluate complaints of GI bleeding include upper endoscopy, colonoscopy, barium studies, and abdominal scans, depending on the nature of the presentation and suspected cause. Endoscopies of the upper and lower GI tract are recommended as the most effective diagnostic tools because they allow for direct visualization of the mucosa, provide access for direct treatment of identified defects, and do not interfere with later studies. When the site of bleeding is not determined through the usual routes, nuclear medicine scans and arteriograms may demonstrate the site and rate of bleeding.

MALLORY-WEISS TEAR

Upper GI hemorrhage may result from a tear at the gastroesophageal junction, a Mallory-Weiss tear. A patient may develop more than one tear.

Signs and Symptoms.

These tears are most common in alcoholic patients, following an episode of vomiting or retching. If a laceration/tear of the mucosa causes GI bleeding, the patient may demonstrate alterations in hemodynamic status.

Diagnostic Studies.

Consider ordering an ethanol level, if alcohol is suspected as a contributing factor. The bleeding associated with a laceration is considerable, and the patient must be referred for evaluation and visualization of the lesion.

GASTRITIS

Although gastritis is not commonly associated with major GI bleeding, it may lead to chronic blood loss and anemia. More often, bleeding occurs after an area of gastric mucosal injury has ulcerated.

Signs and Symptoms.

Explore symptoms of epigastric and/or periumbilical discomfort. Identify potential causes of gastric mucosal injury—the most common being NSAID use and stress. Stress-related mucosal damage may follow a major surgery, burn, or severe medical illness, that is, a disorder that has caused the patient to become extremely ill, rather than a mild, transient condition. More recently, stress has become a less-common cause as patients at risk of developing stress-related injury are often prophylactically treated with agents to alter the gastric pH.

Diagnostic Studies.

See PUD section, p. 228.

MALIGNANCY

Even though cancer can cause a major bleeding episode, it more commonly causes chronic, slower bleeding. When occult blood or other signs of GI bleeding are present, a malignancy must be considered in the differential diagnosis, with a likely site dependent on the presentation.

Signs and Symptoms.

Determine the history of malignancies and risk factors for malignancy. Bleeding that is due to cancer is usually painless but may have associated symptoms, such as altered bowel patterns, fatigue, and so on. A palpable mass may be present. There is usually no tenderness on exam. Rectal examination may detect a palpable mass. Consider the patient's overall appearance, and determine whether there has been a significant weight loss.

Diagnostic Studies.

A CBC should be drawn to check for anemia that may be the first sign of a malignancy, and a chemistry profile for distant metastases.

HEMORRHOIDS

The most common cause of lower GI bleeding is hemorrhoids. The bleeding associated with hemorrhoids is usually evident as red blood on the formed stool, in the toilet bowl, or on the toilet tissue following a bowel movement.

Signs and Symptoms.

Patients with hemorrhoids often complain of rectal discomfort, as well as the contributing factors for hemorrhoid development, including constipation. Inspect the perianal, rectal tissue. Anoscopy may be indicated. Perform a digital rectal examination to assess internal hemorrhoids.

Diagnostic Studies.

No diagnostic studies are generally indicated. The patient should be reassessed following treatment of the hemorrhoids to ensure there is no continued bleeding to investigate.

DIVERTICULA

Most diverticula do not commonly cause GI bleeding; however, diverticula are quite common. Because the incidence of diverticula is so high and they do have the potential to bleed, diverticula actually account for a great percentage of lower GI bleeding that is not related to hemorrhoids.

Signs and Symptoms.

Diverticular bleeding is usually painless. Diverticula should be considered if the patient gives the history of sudden onset of bright red blood, in a large amount. Chronic, small bleeding is not associated with diverticula. The physical examination is usually unremarkable.

Diagnostic Studies.

Because the amount of bleeding is significant, the patient should be referred and a colonoscopy will likely be performed to identify the site of bleeding.

Colitis

See p. 216.

PORTAL HYPERTENSION

Patients with portal hypertension may develop GI bleeding from varices of the esophagus, stomach, intestines, or other sites.

Signs and Symptoms.

Because the incidence of esophageal and gastric variceal bleeding is greater than that associated with the intestines, it is important to assess the history of liver disease in any patient presenting with upper GI bleeding. Determine whether there have been previous episodes of variceal bleeding. Rule out risk factors for the development of liver disease and portal hypertension. Determine the presence of any signs of liver disease, including jaundice, telangiectasia, hepatomegaly, and RUQ tenderness.

Diagnostic Studies.
See previous discussion on liver disease, p. 194.

Esophagitis and Hiatal Hernia

It is rare for patients to develop a significant bleeding episode related to esophagitis or a hiatal hernia. Either may cause a chronic blood loss, with occult blood in the stool and anemia. See previous section on epigastric discomfort for further information.

Peptic Ulcer Disease

Peptic ulcer disease (PUD) causes over 50% of GI bleeding, with the most common site being the duodenum. The use of NSAIDs is the most important risk factor for the development of bleeding from PUD, although the risk can be increased further by the use of anticoagulants, by *H. pylori*, and by increased acid in such conditions as Zollinger-Ellison syndrome.

References

AGA. (2001). *The Burden of Gastrointestinal Diseases.* Bethesda, MD: American Gastroenterological Association.
CDC. (2003). *National Ambulatory Medical Care Survey: 2001 Summary.* Hyattsville, MD: CDC/National Center for Health Statistics.
CDC. (2000). United States Cancer Statistics. URL: http://www.cdc.gov/cancer/npcr/uscs/2000/index.htm.
Ebell, M.H. (2001). *Evidence-Based Medicine.* New York: Springer.

  SUGGESTED READINGS

AGA. (2001). *The Burden of Gastrointestinal Diseases.* Bethesda, MD: American Gastroenterological Association.
Bickley, L.S., & Szilagyi, P.G. (2003). *Bates' Guide to Physical Examination and History Taking.* Philadelphia: Lippincott, Williams, and Wilkins.
CDC. (2003). *National Ambulatory Medical Care Survey: 2001 Summary.* Hyattsville, MD: CDC/National Center for Health Statistics.
CDC. (2000). United States Cancer Statistics. URL: http://www.cdc.gov/cancer/npcr/uscs/2000/index.htm.
Dillon, P.M. (2003). *Nursing Health Assessment: A Critical Thinking, Case Studies Approach.* Philadelphia: F.A. Davis.
Ebell, M.H. (2001). *Evidence-Based Medicine.* New York: Springer.
Feldman, M., Friedman, L.S., & Sleisenger, M.H. (2002). *Gastrointestinal and Liver Disease.* Philadelphia: Saunders.
Friedman, S.L., McQuaid, K.R., & Grendell, J.H. (2003). *Current Diagnosis and Treatment in Gastroenterology.* New York: Lange.
Powell, D.W. (2004). Approach to the Patient with Gastrointestinal Disease. In Goldman, L. & Ausiello, D. (Eds.), *Cecil Textbook of Medicine.* Philadelphia: Saunders.
Rodney, W.M. (2001). Gastroenterology. In Rakel, R.E. (Ed.), *Textbook of Family Medicine.* Philadelphia: Saunders.
Swartz, M.H. (2002). *Textbook of Physical Diagnosis: History and Examination.* Philadelphia: Saunders.

Chapter 10
Genitourinary System

S.A. Quallich
& P. Rupp

The assessment of a genitourinary (GU) complaint should lead the practitioner to a differential diagnosis; the history of the complaint will help confirm the initial impression as to the part of the GU system that may be the cause of the symptomatology. Symptom analysis of lower urinary tract complaints can be aided by objective instruments, which can reliably reflect a change (improvement or worsening of the condition) in symptoms over time. Many of the disease entities can significantly affect a patient's quality of life, as well as the patient's overall social functioning. Genitourinary conditions can impact a variety of patient behaviors, including travel, social functions, entertainment pursuits, sexual activity, sleep, and activities around the home. This chapter focuses on groups of complaints that are unique to the GU system, and it presents the most common differential diagnoses in each category.

Throughout life, hormonal influences as well as age-related structural changes in anatomy and tissue consistency cause variance in voiding function that affect the quality of life. In infancy, the emptying of the bladder is reflexive. As we age into puberty and adulthood, unless there is a congenital anomaly, trauma, or an intervening illness or surgery that directly affects our ability to maintain urinary control, voiding function is taken for granted. Middle adulthood and later adulthood for both men and women are the times when hormonal influences and anatomical changes are noted by their effect on quality of life. At this time, the degree to which one is able to remain continent of urine, and comfortably empty the bladder, begins to affect quality of life.

In men, the prostate is under the influence of the testosterone over the entire life span. The prostate gradually undergoes hypertrophy, thus causing obstructive symptoms, as though liquid flowing though a tube were being slowly held back. An assessment of urinary function for men should include the International Prostate Symptom Score (IPSS). This is a validated, reliable instrument designed to objectively measure the amount of bother that urinary symptoms play in the overall quality of life for men (Barry et al., 1992).

In women, estrogen influences tissue elasticity and bacterial populations. Birth trauma and female surgery with the resulting scar tissue may change the anatomic relationships and musculature of the pelvis and therefore have a roll in future urinary function.

Although lower urinary tract symptoms arise from different causes in men and women, the signs and symptoms can be very similar. Over the life span, storage function and bladder outlet obstruction for both genders varies more than bladder contractility. The discussion of presentation, symptoms, and diagnostic workup are directed at the evaluation of these clinical entities in the adult or geriatric patient. Evaluation of the pediatric patient with GU complaints, although similar, does vary and is not addressed in this chapter.

HISTORY
General History
The general history for a patient who presents with genitourinary complaints should begin with questions regarding a history of any similar complaints in the past. Including a sexual history is appropriate, as well as recent changes in partners and an assessment of general sexual habits. The history should include a discussion of any recent (within the last six months) systemic illness; recent weight gain or loss; a smoking, alcohol consumption, and illicit drug use history; a history of recent nausea, vomiting, fever, or chills; a history of other constitutional symptoms; and a history of exposure to chemicals or dyes as part of the occupational and/or social history. A general history of the genitourinary tract must also include a listing of current prescription and over-the-counter, homeopathic, or naturopathic medications. The patient should be asked about what remedies have been tried prior to presentation. As each presenting complaint is listed, additional specific history-taking points will be discussed.

Past Medical and Surgical History
The past medical and surgical history specific to the GU system will include any surgeries to the GU tract or reproductive structures, prostate surgery, bladder reconstructions, and previous treatment for reproductive or GU malignancies. It is vital to elicit an accurate history of any surgery that may potentially affect the vascular or nerve supply to the urinary tract or bladder, including any pelvic surgery, retroperitoneal surgery, or back surgery. Include a previous history of stone disease or treatment for other GU conditions. For women, previous pregnancies, live births, birth trauma, and manner of delivery should be assessed.

Family History
Family history is very important, particularly because it can help establish a patient's risk for various GU conditions. Include a history of GU malignancies, prostate or bladder problems; family history of stone disease; family history of incontinence (particularly female relatives); as well as other members of the family with similar complaints, particularly first-degree relatives. It is recommended that the family history be as specific as possible, noting the relationship to the patient; this provides further insight into congenital or hereditary risk factors.

Sexual History

The degree of detail regarding sexual history will be guided by the patient's presenting complaint(s). Sexual history should include activity from adolescence through adulthood, and include the patient's sexual orientation (hetero/homo/bisexual). The number of current and lifetime sexual partners should be discussed, as well as any history of sexually transmitted diseases (STDs), including gonorrhea, chlamydia, herpes simplex, condyloma, HIV, or syphilis and the treatment received. A history of intravenous drug use and the date and results of the patient's last HIV test should also be noted.

Questions regarding safe sex and condom use (serial monogamy risk) and specifics about sexual practices are also relevant. The patient's preferred method of birth control should be noted. Questions regarding erectile dysfunction, premature ejaculation, and change in libido can also provide insight into disease pathology (see Chapter 11 for details on these topics).

PHYSICAL EXAMINATION
General History

Inspection

Look for suprapubic fullness, and fullness at the costovertebral angle (CVA). Examine for any visible striae or truncal obesity. Refer to male and female reproductive chapters for the specifics of genital inspection. The male patient should be standing and facing the examiner; there is a potential for the patient to develop an erection during the exam.

Auscultation

The examiner can auscultate the scrotum to distinguish loops of bowel vs. scrotal mass, if a hernia is suspected. Listen over the renal artery to rule out renal artery aneurysm; otherwise, perform the usual auscultation of the abdomen as described in Chapter 9.

Percussion

Perform percussion at the CVA and flank to elicit pain that may be associated with hydronephrosis or pyelonephritis. This can also help to localize or outline a suspected renal mass and to determine whether tender. The percussion of the abdomen is as indicated in Chapter 9.

Palpation

The specifics of palpation relative to the GU system pertain to the palpation of the kidneys and the palpation of inguinal regions for hernia or adenopathy, as well as the digital rectal exam (DRE) (Table 10-1).

Patterns of GU Pain

Knowledge of the potential sources of GU pain and a range of pain syndromes is important to accurately assess complaints of pains. These are reviewed in Tables 10-2 and 10-3.

Table 10-1. ■ Palpation of GU System

Procedure	Technique
Digital rectal examination (DRE)	Gloved, lubricated finger is inserted into anus. Sweep back and forth across the surface of the prostate. Sweep the anal ring and the rectal walls 360 degrees. The exam can result in a sensation of pressure, and possibly an urge to urinate. The prostate should be symmetric (but asymmetry is a normal variant), non-tender, free of nodules, approximately the size of a walnut, and have a smooth rubbery consistency. The exam also involves an assessment of anal sphincter tone and an estimate of prostate size in grams. This exam can be done with the patient standing and bent over, side lying, or in dorsal lithotomy position.
Examination for inguinal hernia	The index finger is inserted into the scrotum and invaginates the scrotum into the external inguinal ring (scrotum should be invaginated in front of testicle); fingertips of other hand should then be placed over internal inguinal canal and patient should be asked to cough. If present, a hernia will be felt as a bulge that descends against the index finger with Valsalva maneuver.
Palpation of kidneys	With the patient lying supine: for the right kidney, the examiner should place the left hand, palm up, under the 10th-12th ribs, and place the right hand on top of the abdomen, just below the right costal margin. For the left side, the examiner should reverse the hands, so the right hand is under the patient's left costovertebral angle. Ask the patient to take a deep breath. When the breath is fully drawn, ask the patient to exhale. As the diaphragm moves into the thoracic cavity, the lower pole of the kidney may be felt slipping across the fingertips of the hand beneath the 10th and 12th ribs.

DIAGNOSTIC STUDIES
Laboratory Evaluation
Urine Cultures
Laboratory cultures of the urine are indicated with suspected urinary tract infection (UTI) and are particularly important for recurrent UTIs or a UTI that seems refractory to treatment. Urine dipstick will show positive leukocyte esterase and greater than 3–5 white blood cells per high power field.

Cytology
Urine cytology is part of a routine microscopic or gross hematuria workup, and a positive cytology may indicate bladder, ureteral, or renal pelvic malignancy. This test should be sent from a patient's first voided morning urine on three separate days if possible, for the greatest degree of accuracy. Urine cytology is an inexpensive means of screening for cancer in any patient with irritative lower urinary tract complaints.

Serum Creatinine and Blood Urea Nitrogen
Serum creatinine and blood urea nitrogen (BUN) provide information regarding kidney function. They are useful with suspected disease and possible obstruction that are due to benign prostatic hyperplasia (BPH), kidney stones, or ureteral stones.

Table 10-2. ■ Sources of Pain.

Source of Pain	Spinal Level	Presentation
Kidney/renal pain	T10–12, L1	Dull, constant ache to the CVA, lateral to sacrospinalis muscle and just below 12th rib. Can spread to subcostal area toward umbilicus or LLQ. Results from distension of renal capsule.
Pseudorenal pain	T10–12	Caused by mechanical derangement of costovertebral or costotransverse joints, resulting in pressure on costal nerves. Mimics renal pain or ureteral colic. Can cause costovertebral pain. May radiate to ipsilateral LQ. Pain is positional, acute, absent on arising, and increases during the day. Pain exacerbated with heavy work.
Ureteral pain	*Upper ureter:* T11–12 *Mid-left ureter:* T12, L1	Due to acute obstruction. Pain due to hyperperistalsis and smooth muscle spasm as ureter tries to overcome obstruction. Back pain from renal capsular distension and colicky pain (from ureteral muscle and renal pelvic spasm): • Radiates to CVA, toward LQ, along the course of the ureter. • In men, also pain to bladder, scrotum, testicle. • In women, also pain to vulva. *Upper ureter stone:* pain radiates to testicle (nerve supply similar to kidney and upper ureter). *Mid-right ureter stone:* pain referred from McBurney's point and can look like appendicitis. *Mid-left ureter stone:* mimics pain to descending and/or sigmoid colon. *Stone close to bladder:* edema and inflammation to ureteral outlet, with resulting vesical (bladder) irritability.
Vesical (bladder) pain	No corresponding level	Overdistension: suprapubic pain; other suprapubic pain is likely not bladder in origin. Pain with UTI: usually referred to distal urethra (terminal dysuria).
Prostatic pain	S2–4	Pain directly from prostate is uncommon. Acute inflammation: may have discomfort or fullness to perineal and/or rectal area. Possible lumbosacral backache. Can cause dysuria, frequency, urgency.
Epididymal pain	No corresponding level	Due to acute infection. Pain in scrotum. Begins as pain in groin or LQ abdomen. Can reach costal angle and mimic stone pain. Inflammation of testicle possible.
Testicular pain	No corresponding level	Very severe, felt locally. Can radiate along spermatic cord to lower abdomen and/or costovertebral angle. Varicocele can cause dull ache that worsens after heavy exercise (see Chapter 11).

Table 10-3. ■ Pain Syndromes

Genitourinary pain syndromes	Description
Painful bladder syndrome	Complaint of suprapubic pain related to bladder filling. May be associated with other symptoms. Increased daytime and nighttime frequency, in the absence of proven urinary infection, or other pathology.
Pelvic pain syndrome	Persistent or recurrent episodic pain, associated with symptoms similar to urinary tract infection. May include complaints of sexual dysfunction, bowel, or gynecological function in the absence of proven pathology.
Perineal pain syndrome	Persistent or recurrent episodic perineal pain related to urinary voiding, or with symptoms similar to urinary tract infection. Possible sexual dysfunction (male or female).
Scrotal pain syndrome	Persistent or episodic scrotal pain of varying degree. May be associated with symptoms similar to urinary tract infection. Possible sexual dysfunction.
Urethral pain syndrome	Recurrent episodic urethral pain usually while voiding, in the absence of proven infection or other disease process.
Vulvar pain syndrome	Persistent or recurrent episodic vaginal pain associated with symptoms similar to those of urinary tract infection. Possible complaints of sexual dysfunction.

Other labs will be ordered at the clinician's discretion to evaluate the suspected cause of disease, and are discussed within the diagnosis sections of specific conditions.

Radiologic Evaluation

Uroradiologic Study

The simplest uroradiologic study is the KUB (kidney, ureters, bladder). It can be helpful as a screening or preliminary test, especially if clinical suspicion points to possible renal or ureteral lithiasis. A KUB study often shows calcified abnormalities, both within the urinary tract and the skeletal system, and it may also demonstrate large soft tissue masses. A KUB is routinely used to track the progress of ureteral stones as they are passed and to provide a rapid method for evaluating the asymptomatic stone patient for recurrence.

Red Flags in the Assessment of the Genitourinary System

- Gross hematuria needs to be referred urgently to a urologist, with accompanying studies arranged, and completed if possible, before the appointment.

- Abrupt onset or worsening testicular pain, regardless of patient age (see Chapter 11).

- Anuria/oliguria requires aggressive evaluation and/or admission for management.

- Acute urinary retention needs to be referred to the nearest emergency department immediately.

- Large kidney masses—particularly when accompanied by the classic triad of gross hematuria, flank pain, and a palpable mass—need to be referred emergently to a urologist.

- Pain associated with any GU structure that awakes the patient or prevents sleep.

- A toxic-appearing patient with poor urine output.

Urinalysis component	Interpretation
Color	Bright red if urologic or anatomic cause.
	Tea-colored or brown urine may be due to old clots, glomerulonephritis, or other medical cause.
Specific gravity	May see low specific gravity with hydronephrosis, intrinsic renal disease.
Protein	3−4+ may indicate glomerulonephritis or other decline in kidney function.
Leukocyte esterase	If positive, suggests infection within urinary tract (does not localize source of infection); 80%–90% sensitive; approximately 95% specific.
Erythrocyte casts	Indicates glomerular source for hematuria (medical hematuria).
Crystalluria	May indicate stone disease.
Nitrite	If positive, suggests infection within urinary tract (does not localize source of infection); 50% sensitive; approximately 95% specific.

Intravenous Pyelography, Intravenous Urography, and Excretory Urography
Intravenous pyelography (IVP), also known as intravenous urography or excretory urography, remains the initial and preferred study for evaluation of the renal pelvis and ureter, owing in part to its moderate cost and ease of administration. It remains the gold standard for noninvasive visualization of ureteral intraluminal filling defects and urothelial abnormalities.

This test demonstrates a wide variety of upper tract lesions and is well tolerated by most patients, although it is recommended that a patient have a serum creatinine ≤1.6. Most commonly used to screen for filling defects, IVP may miss small filling defects (such as small ureteral tumors) as a result of the bolus of dye. Because plain abdominal films are taken after the dye injection, this test requires bowel preparation to help ensure the production of high-quality images. The number of films, volume of dye injection, and speed of the injection depend on the institution, as well as on the patient's age, comorbidities, and physical condition.

Intravenous pyelography also provides a crude estimation of renal function. Its use is complicated by possible allergy to the dye (which can be treated with pre-procedure steroids), modest soft-tissue contrast resolution, possible contrast-induced renal toxicity, and potential cardiovascular issues related to the osmotic load. No special training is required for its administration, and thus IVP is widely available. Its utility, however, is coming into question with the advent of ultrasound, computerized tomographic (CT) scanning, and CT urography because it has a lower specificity, and patients who are found to have abnormalities on an IVP often proceed to a CT or ultrasound study.

Ultrasonography
Ultrasound is a noninvasive, relatively inexpensive, and widely available procedure that avoids radiation exposure and the risk of intravenous contrast. It is widely used to image all parts of the GU system. Ultrasound is superior to IVP for the evaluation of small

lesions, and it is more sensitive in the evaluation of renal masses than is IVP. It has limited utility for upper tract filling defects but can be useful for differentiating between medical and urologic renal disease. Ultrasound is also limited by the patient's body habitus and the skill of the operator.

Ultrasound is excellent for examination of the scrotum and its contents, and can definitively distinguish between extra- and intratesticular pathologies.

Computerized Tomography

Computerized tomography can also demonstrate filling defects, but it is not cost effective as a screening tool or as an initial step in the evaluation of most GU complaints, unless stone disease is highly suspected. Its main role remains in staging malignancies of the GU tract. The CT scan is a superior imaging method for the evaluation of renal and retroperitoneal pathology and is indicated when there is suspicion of bladder or renal malignancy, or when an IVP or ultrasound indicates a mass. Unenhanced helical CT scanning is also superior for the evaluation of suspected or actual stone disease because slices 3 mm thin are used. Computerized tomographic scans can be combined with angiography.

The advantages of CT include a quick scanning time, wide field of view, good cross-sectional views, and the ability to detect subtle differences in tissues. The disadvantages of CT include the radiation dose, low soft-tissue resolution, the need for contrast media, and images that are limited to the transaxial plane.

Magnetic Resonance Imaging

Magnetic resonance imaging (MRI) has wide applications in the evaluation of GU patients; it provides excellent images of the retroperitoneum, bladder, prostate, testes, and even the penis. The use of gadolinium as a contrast media has broadened the use of MRI further because it is well tolerated, even by patients with compromised renal function. An MRI with contrast can provide increased characterization of renal masses. The MRI is clearly superior when compared with CT in imaging the pelvis. When it is combined with angiography, renal vessels, renal vein thrombosis, and congenital abnormalities can be demonstrated with an MRI.

The advantages to MRI include imaging in any plane, excellent soft tissue characterization, and the lack of exposure to radiation. It does have disadvantages, which include slow scanning time, decreased imagine clarity when compared with CT, heat generation, and claustrophobia for the patient.

Computerized Tomographic Urogram

A computerized tomographic urogram (CT urography) is a CT test done with the addition of radiopaque dye, and it can image both the renal parenchyma and urothelium (the lining of the ureters, bladder, and urethra) with a single examination. It combines the sensitivity and specificity of a CT scan for urinary calculi and small renal masses with the sensitivity and specificity of intravenous urography for urothelial abnormalities (Kawashima, Glockner, & King, 2003). Some authors (Perlman et al., 1996) have reported that CT urography further characterizes masses seen on IVP and better detects small renal cell carcinomas. Its sensitivity and specificity is superior to the IVP, and it can provide a safe and more precise evaluation. It is not widely available, but it is becoming the preferred initial study in the evaluation of hematuria (Kawashima, Glockner, & King, 2003).

Magnetic Resonance Urography

Magnetic resonance urography (MR urography) is another emerging technology in the evaluation of GU pathologies. Similar to MR cholangiopancreatography, images are taken after the administration of intravenous gadolinium contrast. It is especially helpful in imaging patients with dilated tracts (Kawashima, Glockner, & King, 2003). This study is currently limited by the poor spatial resolution of the resulting images and its poor record with calculi detection. However, it does provide another method for the detection of urinary tract dilatation, ureteric obstruction, duplicated renal collecting systems, and urothelial tumors. The sensitivity of MR urography is currently considered to be similar to that of the CT urogram (Kawashima, Glockner, & King, 2003), but it is not yet widely available.

DIFFERENTIAL DIAGNOSIS OF CHIEF COMPLAINTS
General Complaints

Flank Pain and Renal Colic

The kidney is designed to make urine, and have the urine flow freely out of the kidney, down the ureter, and into the bladder. The kidney and ureters are described as the upper tracts. Symptoms in this anatomic area are a subjective indicator of change in the urinary outflow system. Upper tract symptoms arise from irritation in the kidney and/or blockage of urinary outflow (see Table 10-3). Causes of upper tract symptoms (UTS) include kidney stones, rarely renal cell carcinoma, and urothelial cell carcinoma.

History

Presentation can vary widely—the onset of complaints may be acute or insidious. Complaints can include a dull renal pain or a constant ache in CVA area that can radiate laterally to the sacrospinalis muscle and just below 12th rib. Pain can spread to the subcostal area toward the umbilicus or left lower quadrant. The patient may describe only back pain, which is the result of renal capsular distension, and/or colicky pain from ureteral muscle and renal pelvic spasm. There may also be concurrent constitutional symptoms (nausea, vomiting, fever) and associated weight loss or gross hematuria.

Signs and Symptoms

On physical exam, there may be CVA tenderness. The patient may have a palpable renal mass if the patient is thin and/or the mass large enough. Patients with complaints of flank pain can have widely varying presentations, including toxic, cachectic, or merely uncomfortable.

Physical Examination

Routine GU and abdominal exams are mandatory, with a pelvic exam as complaints warrant. As noted in Chapter 9, a pelvic examination should be included to evaluate a complaint of lower abdominal pain in a female.

RENAL MASS

Renal cell carcinomas (RCCs) have been referred to as the "internist's tumor" and as one of the great masqueraders in medicine. There is extraordinary variation in the presentation of a patient with RCC, from a small asymptomatic lesion that is found on a CT or MRI scan during an evaluation for another complaint to a full-blown paraneoplastic syndrome with liver function derangements and hypercalcemia. Renal cell carcinomas can secrete biologically active substances, such as gonadotropins and ACTH. Laboratory findings can include normochromic anemia, an elevated erythrocyte sedimentation rate, and hematuria on urinalysis. Risk factors for RCC include smoking, environmental exposure to heavy metals, and hereditary conditions, such as von Hippel-Lindau disease.

Signs and Symptoms.

The signs and symptoms are described as in the preceding history subsection. The patient may present with obvious symptoms or vague constitutional complaints.

Diagnostic Studies.

The workup will be dictated by the patient's presentation and complaints. Initial lab work can include a urinalysis, complete blood count (CBC), liver function tests, and serum electrolytes. Imaging studies can include an IVP or renal ultrasound, CT scan, or MRI; the CT scan remains the gold standard for detection of RCC. Referral to a urologist is indicated; the more symptomatic the patient, the more urgent the referral.

NEPHROLITHIASIS

Kidney stones are more common in men and rank as the third-most common condition of the urinary tract. There are several varieties of stones that can be formed, the majority of which are radiopaque, and, after an initial episode, the recurrence rate can be up to 50%. Most stones present with acute-onset pain due to the obstruction of the upper urinary tract. The symptoms associated with a kidney stone are due to the inflammation, edema, and hyperperistalsis of the GU tract, particularly the ureter (see Table 10-2, particularly in regard to ureteral pain). The number or size of the stone(s) correlates poorly with the degree of pain. Risk factors include a history of crystalluria, low fluid intake or dehydration (such as living in a hot, dry climate), socioeconomic factors (industrialized countries), and a family history of stones. Ninety percent of stones measuring 4 mm or less will pass spontaneously, 50% of stones of 4–6 mm are likely to pass spontaneously, but only 10% of stones larger than 6 mm will pass spontaneously.

Signs and Symptoms.

As in the history subsection; patients will appear uncomfortable as they try to find a resting position that is not painful. Patients may also experience nausea and vomiting; other systemic indicators of renal colic may be noted, such as tachycardia. If a patient appears septic, referral to the nearest emergency room is mandatory.

Diagnostic Studies.

The initial study can be a KUB or IVP; however, many facilities have the capability of performing a stone protocol spiral CT, which is a much more definitive test for the evaluation of kidney stones. Urinalysis will usually show some degree of hematuria, may indicate infection, and may also show crystals that can be a clue to the diagnosis of stone type. Referral to a urologist for management is indicated. Recurrent stone formers should also undergo a 24-hour urine collection for electrolytes (calcium, uric acid, phosphate, oxalate, phosphate uric acid) to evaluate for a metabolic condition that may be amenable to medical management.

UPPER URINARY TRACT OBSTRUCTION
OR HYDRONEPHROSIS

This condition could be caused by either an obstructing stone, ureteral stricture, prostatic hyperplasia, or renal or abdominal tumor that prevents the kidney from draining. The obstruction can be unilateral or bilateral, symptoms can be sudden or gradual in onset, and progressive renal damage will occur with time.

Signs and Symptoms.

Flank pain may radiate along the course of the ureter, and may be accompanied by a variety of constitutional symptoms. More severe or bilateral obstruction may cause weight loss and eventual uremia. A distended kidney may be noted on palpation and CVA pain may be present if there is infection. Genitourinary, abdominal, pelvic, and rectal exams are indicated.

Diagnostic Studies.

The workup is the same as for the evaluation of kidney stone or renal tumor. Imaging studies are the key to determining the etiology.

PYELONEPHRITIS

This is a bacterial infection of the renal pelvis and parenchyma, typically caused by *Escherichia coli* ascending from the lower urinary tract. Risk factors include vesicoureteral reflux, neurogenic bladder, stone disease of any part of the GU tract, immunosuppression, and diabetes mellitus.

Signs and Symptoms.

The patient will have bilateral or unilateral flank pain, fever, chills, nausea, and vomiting. Lower urinary tract symptoms, such as dysuria, may also be present. The patient will appear ill on presentation, with fever and tachycardia commonly noted. Palpation and/or percussion over the infected side is painful. There may be accompanying abdominal discomfort or abdominal distension.

Diagnostic Studies.

A CBC will show leukocytosis, often with a shift to the left. Urinalysis will also demonstrate leukocytosis, RBCs, protein, and bacteria. Urine culture will be positive with heavy growth. Blood cultures may be necessary. Imaging studies should be considered if the patient appears ill or does not respond to initial outpatient management (CT scan or renal ultrasound to assess for urinary obstruction). Assessment must include the determination of whether or not the patient requires inpatient management.

AUTOSOMAL DOMINANT POLYCYSTIC KIDNEY DISEASE

A family history of autosomal dominant polycystic kidney disease (ADPCKD) should raise the level of suspicion if a renal mass is palpated. Adult-onset ADPCKD is uncommon below the age of 40.

Signs and Symptoms.

Back or flank pain (60%), gross hematuria (30%), and renal stones (20%) are most common symptoms. There may be infections within the cysts, hypertension, and decreasing renal function associated with the initial presentation. A CT scan may also reveal liver cysts concurrent with renal cysts, and may begin to appear at age 30. During palpation of the abdomen, cysts on either or both kidneys may be evident.

Diagnostic Studies.

A family history of liver or renal cysts will aid in diagnosis even in the absence of palpable masses. A renal ultrasound may reveal cystic lesions; a CT examination is more sensitive in the evaluation of cysts, but also more costly. Once the diagnosis is established, imaging studies need not be routinely performed unless new symptoms require evaluation. Patients with an established diagnosis of ADPCKD should be followed by a urologist or nephrologist for monitoring pyelonephritis, nephrolithiasis, and renal function.

BLUNT RENAL TRAUMA

Blunt trauma typically causes damage in the transverse plane of the kidney. Damage to the kidney represents the most common injury to the GU tract. Trauma can be the result of a motor vehicle accident or contact sports, and is usually seen in men and boys.

Signs and Symptoms.

The patient will usually have evidence of abdominal trauma, such as fractured ribs, with complaints of pain that localize to the affected side. If the injury is severe, there may be signs of shock.

Diagnostic Studies.

History may be sufficient to establish that renal injury is likely. Urinalysis will show some degree of hematuria. The initial imaging study is the IVP, with a CT scan for evaluation if the kidney is poorly visualized on the IVP. The patient should be referred to a urologist for further evaluation and management or to the nearest emergency department if the injury appears severe.

Gross Hematuria

A sudden noticeable change in the color of his or her urine is usually quite alarming to a patient. Gross hematuria results from a sufficient number of erythrocytes in the urine for the patient or clinician to perceive a color change in the urine. It is commonly ignored, as it is typically painless, and patients may report previous episodes of gross hematuria that were ignored, thus resulting in a significant delay before presentation for evaluation. Gross hematuria is often the only indication of a urologic malignancy; a malignancy is found in up to 40% of gross hematuria cases.

Therapeutic anticoagulation should not lead to gross or microscopic hematuria. Anticoagulation does not necessarily predispose to hematuria, unless the patient becomes excessively anticoagulated. However, patients who are anticoagulated may also have coexisting urologic malignancies, and an episode of gross hematuria in the anticoagulated patient warrants an evaluation.

History

The patient will report a color change to the urine (it may be pinkish, reddish, or simply look like she or he is urinating blood). The episode is usually painless, but it can be associated with flank pain, nausea, vomiting, or generalized dysuria, with or without other lower urinary tract symptoms. There may be an extensive smoking history or history of exposure to chemicals through the patient's job. It is vital to try to establish the timing of blood in the urinary stream, as it can help predict the source of bleeding (see Table 10-4).

Physical Examination

A routine GU exam, and a pelvic exam for female patients (see Chapter 12 for pelvic exam methodology) is mandatory. The physical exam is often unremarkable, except in the case of a kidney stone or autosomal dominant polycystic kidney disease, in which case a large boggy kidney may be palpated.

Selected Causes

Box 10-1 lists many of the most common causes; gross hematuria is commonly due to anatomic causes (nonglomerular bleeding).

Diagnostic Studies

Lab studies can include CBC, urinalysis, serum electrolytes, urine electrolytes, and urine cytology and are guided by the patient's presentation, risk factors for such GU diseases as

Table 10-4. ■ Possible Significance of Timing of Blood in the Urinary Stream

Description of hematuria	Possible site	Possible cause
Microscopic hematuria	Any site within upper or lower urinary tract	UTI, prostatitis, urethritis, medical renal disease, bladder/ureteral/renal malignancy, stone disease
Initial gross hematuria	Anterior urethra	Stricture, meatal stenosis, urethritis, urethral cancer
Total gross hematuria	Source above bladder neck: bladder, kidney, ureter	Renal/ureteral/bladder stone or renal/ureteral/bladder tumor; trauma; vigorous exercise; renal tuberculosis, hemorrhagic cystitis; interstitial cystitis; sickle cell disease; nephritis; autosomal dominant polycystic kidney disease (ADPCKD); poststreptococcal glomerulonephritis
Terminal gross hematuria	Bladder neck, prostate, posterior urethra	Benign prostatic hyperplasia (BPH), regrowth BPH post-transurethral resection, bladder neck polyps, posterior urethritis, tuberculosis

bladder cancer, and comorbidities. Urine cultures are indicated with suspected urinary tract infection. Coagulation studies are performed as appropriate in anticoagulated patients. An imaging study (IVP, CT, or ultrasound) will aid in evaluating an anatomic cause for the microscopic hematuria. The patient should be referred urgently to a urologist, with the following studies completed before the visit: IVP, CT, or ultrasound; BUN and creatinine; urinalysis; and at least one urine cytology.

Box 10-1

Selected Causes of Gross Hematuria

Arteriovenous malformation
Autosomal dominant polycystic kidney disease (ADPCKD)
Benign prostatic hyperplasia (BPH)
Bladder neck polyps
BPH regrowth post transurethral resection
Contamination from menstruation
Hemorrhagic cystitis
Interstitial cystitis
Meatal stenosis
Nephritis
Posterior urethritis
Poststreptococcal glomerulonephritis
Renal tuberculosis
Renal/ureteral/bladder stone
Renal/ureteral/bladder tumor
Sickle cell disease
Trauma
Tuberculosis
Urethritis
Urethral cancer
Urethral stricture
Vigorous exercise

Suprapubic Pain

The differential for complaints of midline lower quadrant pain includes many conditions that are not specific to the GU system. The key in evaluation of this complaint is a careful history and physical examination to localize the complaints to the actual structures involved.

History

Complaints on presentation may include pain to the midline lower abdomen that is constant or intermittent. The onset of the discomfort may have been acute or gradual. There may be associated complaints of perineal fullness, irritative voiding symptoms, or urinary retention. There may also be a variety of constitutional symptoms, including fever, chills, nausea, or vomiting.

Signs and Symptoms

Physical examination may demonstrate pain on palpation of the suprapubic region, and the bladder may be palpable. There may be global abdominal discomfort if GI structures are involved. The patient may have CVA tenderness.

Physical Examination

A routine GU exam is mandatory, including a DRE. An abdominal exam, and pelvic exam in women (see Chapter 12 for pelvic exam methodology), are also suggested.

Selected Causes

Localization of the source of pain after physical examination, coupled with the history, aids in diagnosis of the potential cause. See Table 10-5 for examples.

Diagnostic Studies

The suspected cause will guide the diagnostic workup. Lab studies can include CBC, urinalysis and culture, and urine cytology. The initial imaging study, if indicated, could be either a KUB or CT scan, with any further workup dictated by initial findings of the lab studies and imaging. The patient may require urgent referral to a urologist, general surgeon, or gynecologist.

Anuria, Oliguria, and Renal Failure

Although anuria and oliguria are unusual as acute complaints, the course toward renal failure can be predicted in many patients. However, it remains important to establish the causes contributing to the renal dysfunction because many patients with severe kidney dys-

Table 10-5. ■ Selected Causes of Suprapubic Pain

Urethral	Prostate	Vesical	Distal ureteral	Large or small bowel	Gynecologic
• Urethral syndrome • Urethral stenosis	• Acute or chronic bacterial prostatitis • Nonbacterial prostatitis • Prostadynia	• Bladder cancer • Bladder stone • Interstitial cystitis • Urinary retention • UTI	• Ascending infection • Foreign body • Stone	(See Chapter 9.) • Appendicitis • Diverticulitis • Inflammatory bowel disease • Malignancy	(See Chapter 12.) • Ectopic pregnancy • Endometriosis • Pelvic inflammatory disease • Uterine fibroids

function will need a variety of support services, including dieticians and dialysis, and select patients may be candidates for a renal transplant.

History

The history is the key to evaluating the suspected cause. The patient may report decreasing urine output over time, or a recent change in medications. This can be complicated if the patient has a solitary kidney or previous renal transplant. Associated symptoms (flank pain, nausea, vomiting) must be noted, as well as a history of recent IV dye administration.

Signs and Symptoms

The signs and symptoms will be dependent on the cause and are not restricted to the GU system: flank pain, if stone obstruction; murmur, if endocarditis; palpable bladder, if BPH; generalized edema, if myocardial failure.

Physical Examination

A complete physical is required, including routine GU exam.

Selected Causes

Table 10-6 lists many common causes, categorized as prerenal vs. postrenal.

Diagnostic Studies

The suspected cause and physical presentation will guide the diagnostic workup. Lab studies can include CBC, urinalysis, serum electrolytes, and urine electrolytes. Initial imaging

Table 10-6. ■ Selected Causes of Renal Failure, Anuria, and Oliguria

Prerenal	Postrenal
Decreased vascular volume	Upper urinary tract obstruction
• 3rd spacing	• Kidney stone (unilateral vs. bilateral)
• GI losses	• Obstructing retroperitoneal mass
• Hemorrhage	• Pregnancy
• Reduced cardiac output	Lower urinary tract obstruction
• Septic shock	• Benign prostatic hypertrophy
• Severe dehydration	• Carcinoma (bladder, prostate)
• Spinal shock	• Neuropathic bladder
Myocardial failure	• Prostatitis
• Cardiomyopathy	• Urethral stricture
• Ischemic heart disease	
• Tamponade	
• Valvular heart disease	
Renal/glomerular causes	
• Acute glomerulonephritis	
• Vasculitis	
Vascular	
• Renal vein thrombosis	
• Renal artery occlusion	
Medication-related	
• Anticonvulsants	
• Antihypertensives	
• Chemotherapeutic agents	
• Diuretics	
• Radiographic contrast media	

studies can include a renal or bladder ultrasound, with any further workup dictated by initial findings of the lab studies and imaging. A patient presenting acutely with anuria, oliguria, or renal failure requires an emergent referral for further evaluation and appropriate management, based on the suspected cause.

Microscopic Hematuria

Microscopic hematuria is rarely a patient complaint, but is rather a finding on evaluation—be it a routine medical examination or when monitoring a patient's kidney function. Differing opinions exist as to the appropriate long-term follow-up of the patient with persistent microscopic hematuria, and ultimately the follow-up will be guided by the patient's overall medical conditions and medication profile.

History

Usually there is no history, although the patient may give a history of recurrent stones, recent UTI, long-standing diabetes, or other medical renal disease. The patient may be taking prescription medication that can cause renal damage when used long-term.

Signs and Symptoms

There are no signs and symptoms that are distinctly related to the microscopic hematuria. Microscopic hematuria may be found incidentally on a routine screening urinalysis.

Physical Examination

A routine GU exam is required, including pelvic exam for female patients (see Chapter 12 for pelvic exam methodology).

Selected Causes

A detailed discussion of each potential differential diagnosis is beyond the scope of this chapter, and in many cases a referral for further urologic and/or nephrology evaluation is warranted. Box 10-2 lists many common causes; microscopic hematuria is due to a physiologic process (glomerular bleeding). Small, asymptomatic stones within the GU tract can

---

Box 10-2

Selected Causes of Medical/Renal Hematuria

Arteriovenous fistula
Benign familial hematuria
Berger's disease (IgA nephropathy)
Bleeding disorder
Bleeding dyscrasias/Sickle cell disease
Diabetes mellitus
Drug-induced interstitial disease
End-stage renal disease
Exercise (marathon running)
Familial glomerulonephritis
History of analgesic abuse
HIV
Infections (e.g., hepatitis)
Mesangioproliferative glomerulonephritis
Postinfectious glomerulonephritis
Systemic lupus erythematosus
Vascular disease (e.g., renal artery embolism)

cause intermittent microscopic hematuria. Excessive anticoagulation has been known to lead to microscopic hematuria.

Diagnostic Studies

Lab studies can include CBC, urinalysis, serum electrolytes, urine electrolytes, and urine cytology. Hemoglobin and hematocrit are not routinely indicated except as part of the CBC: microscopic hematuria rarely causes significant blood loss. Urine cultures are indicated with suspected urinary tract infection. Order coagulation studies as appropriate in anticoagulated patients. An imaging study (IVP, CT, or ultrasound) will aid in ruling out an anatomic cause for the microscopic hematuria.

Prostate Nodule, Elevated Prostate-Specific Antigen, and Asymmetric Prostate

An asymmetric prostate is typically asymptomatic, and not necessarily diagnostic of prostate cancer; asymmetry can be a normal finding on DRE. A second opinion of a questionable finding on digital rectal exam is always a wise idea, whether from another practitioner in the clinic or by referral to a urologist.

An elevation in (PSA) is relative to a baseline PSA value or is a value that lies outside the established norms for race and age (see Table 10-7). Prostate-specific antigen velocity is also a valuable way to gauge the significance of the PSA value for a patient; it describes the rapidity of increase in PSA over time. Generally, a 50% increase in PSA over the previous value should trigger referral for a transrectal ultrasound–guided prostate biopsy for a histological evaluation for prostatic carcinoma.

Age-specific reference ranges for PSA (Table 10-7) should be used as a guide when there is no previous PSA for comparison. A prostatic nodule found on DRE necessitates a referral to a urologist or radiologist for transrectal ultrasound–guided prostate biopsy, and may well be the first indication of the presence of a cancer.

History

Usually there is no history. This may be a finding on routine physical. There may be a history of mild or moderate lower urinary tract symptoms with obstructive features.

Physical Examination

A routine GU exam, including DRE, is required. On exam, a normal prostate will be smooth, have a rubbery surface (posterior surface of the gland is palpated through the rectal wall), the lateral lobes and median sulcus can usually be appreciated, as well as the base and apex of the prostate. The seminal vesicles should not be palpable. Documentation should reflect the gland's size (estimated in grams), consistency, symmetry, and the presence or absence of nodules. Other abnormalities found during the digital rectal exam can include hemorrhoids, condyloma, and anal fissures.

Table 10-7. ■ Age-Specific PSA Reference Ranges

Age range	African-Americans	Asians	Whites
40–49 yr	0–2.0 ng/mL	0–2.0 ng/mL	0–2.5 ng/mL
50–59 yr	0–4.0 ng/mL	0–3.0 ng/mL	0–3.5 ng/mL
60–69 yr	0–4.5 ng/mL	0–4.0 ng/mL	0–4.5 ng/mL
70–79 yr	0–5.5 ng/mL	0–5.0 ng/mL	0–6.5 ng/mL

Adapted from the American Urology Association's Best Practice PSA Guidelines (2000).

BENIGN PROSTATIC HYPERTROPHY

Benign prostatic hypertrophy (BPH) describes a nonmalignant enlargement of the transition zone of the prostate gland; the precise etiology is unclear. Risk factors are simply advancing age and normal androgen status, although there may be an additional genetic predisposition. The terms "BPH" and "obstructive symptoms" have traditionally been used to describe a collection of complaints associated with prostate overgrowth; in 2002, the International Continence Society assigned these symptoms under the term "Lower Urinary Tract Symptoms" (LUTS; detailed under later subsection). Prostate size correlates poorly with the degree of symptoms; that is, a larger size does not automatically mean worse symptoms, in part due to the subjective impressions of the patient.

Signs and Symptoms.

Lower urinary tract symptoms associated with bladder outlet obstruction secondary to an enlarged prostate include urinary urgency, frequency, hesitation in getting the stream started, decreased caliber and force of stream, and nocturnal frequency of urination that is bothersome. This collection of symptoms has also been termed "prostatism." A patient with benign prostatic hypertrophy will evidence symmetric or asymmetric enlargement, and a firm nontender gland that is smooth.

Diagnostic Studies.

If the PSA level is found to be elevated relative to the age-specific reference, there should be referral to a urologist for discussion and management, including possible prostate biopsy or surgery to improve the urinary outlet (transurethral resection of the prostate).

PROSTATE CANCER

Early-stage prostate cancer is largely asymptomatic and is found as a result of screening for prostate cancer by digital rectal exam and PSA. Histological evaluation of biopsy specimens obtained during transrectal ultrasound–guided biopsy of the prostate provides a tissue diagnosis of prostate cancer and a Gleason score, which aids in deciding potential treatment options. Increased risk for prostate cancer is associated with more than two first-order relatives diagnosed with prostate cancer. Family members, such as grandfathers with prostate cancer, should raise the index of suspicion.

Signs and Symptoms.

An asymmetric prostate, a prostatic nodule, or an elevated PSA level may be found during a routine physical. There may be a history presented of mild or moderate lower urinary tract symptoms with obstructive features. A prostate suspicious for malignancy will demonstrate nodular areas and/or an overall hardness.

Diagnostic Studies.

Definitive diagnosis is made via prostate biopsy. Routine or urgent referral to a urologist is indicated, depending on the degree of PSA elevation and/or the degree to which it has risen since the previous value.

PROSTATITIS

This is an acute or chronic infection of the prostate gland itself. Acute bacterial prostatitis is usually the result of infection by aerobic gram-negative rods (coliform bacteria or *Pseudomonas*). *Enterococcus faecalis*, an aerobic gram-positive bacteria, can also be the cause. Routes of infection are ascent from the urethra, reflux of infected urine into the prostatic ducts, and direct extension of bacteria, and migration via the lymphatic and vascular system. It may be associated with acute cystitis and may result in urinary retention.

Signs and Symptoms.

Acute: febrile illness, low back and perineal pain, urinary urgency and frequency, nocturia, dysuria, and muscle and joint aches are common. Transrectal palpation of the prostate reveals a very tender, boggy, swollen prostate. Urine may smell strong, and be cloudy. Gross hematuria may be present. Complete blood count will be positive for leukocytosis and a shift to the left. Chronic prostatitis manifests as recurrent episodes of irritative symptoms of dysuria, nocturia, frequency, and urgency. Febrile episodes, gross hematuria, and hematospermia are rare. A tender, indurated epididymis is sometimes associated with chronic prostatic infection.

Diagnostic Studies.

In prostatitis, low back pain in the sacral area differentiates this affliction from pyelonephritis, which manifests as flank pain. A urine culture will reveal the offending pathogen. Presentation of acute onset vs. recurrent episodes differentiates chronic prostatitis from acute.

CHRONIC INFLAMMATION AND PROSTATODYNIA

The etiology of male chronic pelvic pain syndrome is still not certain, although an autoimmune process is favored. Further research is required to determine the putative auto-antigen, the immune responses of patients, the role of bacteria in the inflammatory process, and the patients' pain response to genitourinary insults. As yet no diagnostic tests (other than to eliminate other pathology) and few treatments for chronic prostatitis can be recommended on the basis of scientific evidence (Batstone, Doble, & Batstone, 2003).

Signs and Symptoms.

The signs and symptoms are often similar to those of BPH or prostatitis.

Diagnostic Studies.

Chronic inflammation can only be diagnosed via prostate biopsy. Routine referral to a urologist for biopsy is indicated.

Recent Ejaculation

Recent ejaculation has no clinically significant effect on the PSA value. Men should not be asked to abstain from sexual activities before a PSA screening test (Stenner et al., 1998).

Proteinuria

This is another clinical entity that is discovered during an evaluation, rather than as a presenting GU complaint. Proteinuria is an indicator of parenchymal disease of the kidney and is commonly seen in patients with conditions such as diabetic nephropathy, nephritic syndrome, autoimmune disease, multiple myeloma, and acute inflammation of the urinary tract. It can also be the result of prolonged use or abuse of nonsteroidal anti-inflammatory medications.

History

Proteinuria is likely to be present with no structural abnormalities found. It is almost always painless. It is important to establish the timing of proteinuria (relative to the patient's medical history): transient, intermittent, or persistent, or whether it is the initial episode.

Signs and Symptoms

There are no signs or symptoms, other than as a result of the causative medical condition (focus on peripheral exam).

Physical Examination
A routine GU exam is required. Other aspects of the exam will be guided by the suspected cause (flank bruit, pericardial rub, skin lesions, edema).

Selected Causes
The medical/renal disease is glomerular, tubular, overflow, or tissue proteinuria.

Diagnostic Studies
Proteinuria is usually found on routine urinalysis; it may be falsely positive in the context of dilute urine. No further studies are indicated unless there are new progressive symptoms, or the patient appears toxic or is manifesting other symptoms. Renal ultrasound or IVP studies can be considered in these cases (if the renal function can withstand contrast media). Referrals to a nephrologist for all persistent proteinuria and to an oncologist, as appropriate, are recommended.

Lower Urinary Tract Symptoms

Lower urinary tract symptoms (LUTS) are a variety of complaints that help in the clinical identification of a potential diagnosis. Not all patients will experience all symptoms, and the symptoms may be present in varying degrees at varying times. The symptoms are much more descriptive of lower urinary tract pathology in men and can be graded using a tool such as the American Urological Association symptom score. The following are the components of LUTS:

- Acute retention (suprapubic pain, severe urgency)
- Chronic retention (much hesitancy starting stream, reduced force/caliber of stream)
- Cystitis
- Hesitancy (strains to force urine)
- Interruption of stream (can be accompanied by pain radiating down urethra)
- Loss of force/decreased caliber of stream (urethral resistance increases despite increased intravesical pressure)
- Sense of residual urine
- Terminal dribbling
- Urgency (strong sudden desire to urinate owing to hyperactivity and irritability of the bladder)

The following presenting complaints represent common manifestations of disorders of the lower urinary tract. *As part of the diagnosis, a measurement of a postvoid residual volume can be included with each differential that follows in this section, if the clinical environment has the appropriate equipment. This will confirm that the patient is actually emptying the bladder or can provide a baseline against which to gauge interventions if the bladder is not being emptied.*

Dysuria

Complaints of dysuria—or burning, pain, or discomfort on urination—present more frequently in women than in men, largely as a result of the shorter urethral length in women. Infection is the most common cause of dysuria, and its presentation depends on which structure of the GU tract is affected. The infection can be secondary to an anatomical abnormality or abnormality of function, including postmenopausal status or prostatic hypertrophy. The patient may have undergone recent GU instrumentation or catheter placement, leading to a mechanical cause for the dysuria.

Dysuria can also be an indicator of other systemic conditions, such as diabetes mellitus, renal calculi, GU neoplasms, or depression. Debate exists over treating complaints of dysuria empirically with antibiotics, particularly when it is a recurrent complaint for a patient. The most common causes for dysuria are presented here as differentials.

History

The patient may report pain, hesitancy, urgency, frequency, and discomfort on urination and may describe bladder fullness. There is usually a negative history of fever, chills, or other constitutional symptoms. He or she may also report a color change in urine or the presence of a strong odor to the urine. The timing of pain with urination (external, initial, during, terminal) may provide clues to the cause. In the female patient, there may be associated vaginal symptoms; both men and women should be asked about their risk for sexually transmitted diseases. The patient should also be asked about any herbal, homeopathic, or vaginal hygiene remedies that have been tried since symptom onset. Male patients should be specifically queried about the presence of LUTS.

Physical Examination

A routine GU exam is required, including DRE and pelvic as indicated, based on the patient's gender. A CVA exam and general abdominal exam should also be performed. Note should be made of the patient's general appearance—whether he or she appears toxic.

UNCOMPLICATED URINARY TRACT INFECTION

Uncomplicated urinary tract infection (UTI) is one of the most common infections seen in a primary care setting and occurs among all ages of patients, but it is more commonly seen in women. The etiology of UTIs is affected by a patient's comorbidities, including age, use of catheters, or neurologic disease. The most common pathogen causing acute, uncomplicated UTIs is *Escherichia coli*, followed by *Staphylococcus saprophyticus*, and *Klebsiella*, *Enterobacter*, and *Proteus* species. Risk factors for the development of a UTI are well established and include increasing age, recent sexual intercourse, a history of UTI, use of a diaphragm or cervical cap, and anatomic abnormalities.

Signs and Symptoms.

The signs and symptoms are as described in the immediately preceding history subsection; onset is typically sudden and without other constitutional symptoms.

Diagnostic Studies.

Urinalysis will confirm the presence of a UTI; hematuria, pyuria, and/or bacteriuria will be observed. However, there exists debate as to whether the specimen must be a clean-catch specimen. The leukocyte esterase test combined with the nitrite test provide a high sensitivity and specificity for infection. In women whose symptoms suggest uncomplicated UTI, a culture of greater than 10^2 CFU/mL is indicative of cystitis (Bent & Saint, 2003). Urine cultures should be considered in the patient with recurrent UTI, refractory UTI, and the patient who appears toxic. Blood for CBC and electrolyte tests should also be drawn based on the overall clinical presentation. If anatomic causes are suspected, diagnostic imaging, such as KUB or IVP, should be arranged based on the suspected cause and patient's presentation.

INTERSTITIAL CYSTITIS

Interstitial cystitis (IC) is a poorly understood entity with a suspected cause related to a variety of factors that include autoimmune, allergic, and infectious components. Patients with IC suffer from chronic symptoms that include a combination of suprapubic pain, chronic pelvic pain, dyspareunia, and negative urine cultures in addition to dysuria. Patients may become debilitated by this disease; they may be making up to 40 trips to the bathroom in 24 hours. Interstitial cystitis is also marked by periods of remission and flare-up throughout a patient's lifetime. Interstitial cystitis is much more prevalent in women, and some authors estimate the nationwide prevalence of IC among females to be approximately one in five (Parsons et al., 2002). Typical age at onset varies from 30 to 70, and most patients visit an average of five physicians and wait four years before the correct diagnosis is made.

Signs and Symptoms.

Patients will describe a history of irritative voiding symptoms: urinary urgency, frequency, and pain. There may also be complaints of suprapubic pain, dyspareunia, and chronic pelvic pain. Symptoms may worsen in the week preceding menstruation, and have often been present for a period of several months or years.

Diagnostic Studies.

Urinalysis will eliminate a UTI as the cause of these complaints. In order to diagnose IC, all other potential etiologies should be ruled out, including such things as carcinoma or medication-induced cystitis. Confirmation of diagnosis is via bladder appearance on cystoscopy; referral to a urologist is indicated.

SEXUALLY TRANSMITTED DISEASE–RELATED URETHRITIS

Presentation of STD-related dysuria varies by gender, with females usually more affected than males.

Signs and Symptoms.

See specific signs and symptoms in male and female patients in Chapters 11 and 12, respectively. Some STDs may be accompanied by complaints of constitutional symptoms or malaise.

Diagnostic Studies.

Sexually transmitted diseases can be diagnosed with the appropriate cultures, gram stains, swabs, and serologic studies. Unless a patient appears ill and a WBC seems indicated, no additional lab work or imaging studies are indicated. Treatment is often begun before receiving the results of any diagnostic testing, remembering that it is imperative to simultaneously treat the partner(s). Many STDs must be reported to the local health department.

URETHRAL SYNDROME

This syndrome brings with it nonspecific complaints of frequency, urgency, and dysuria without objective clinical findings; it is more common in females during their reproductive years. Risk factors include a history of UTI, GU tract obstruction, and neurogenic bladder, and the condition is similar to prostatodynia in men.

Signs and Symptoms.

The signs and symptoms are similar to those of UTI and may include complaints of back or suprapubic pain.

Diagnostic Studies.

Both urinalysis and urine cultures will be negative; this is a diagnosis of exclusion. If suspected, the patient can be referred to a urologist for additional specialized testing.

COMPLICATED URINARY TRACT INFECTION

Defined as a UTI in a context that increases the likelihood of treatment failure or recurrent infection, this condition is seen in patients with abnormalities of GU anatomy (such as BPH) or functional abnormalities (such as a neurogenic bladder) and diabetes or other metabolic derangements. Other risk factors for a complicated UTI include male gender, pregnancy, extremely old or young age, or immunocompromised status. A complicated UTI can also be indicated when multiple organisms are present on culture. Complicated UTIs can evolve into more serious conditions, such as pyelonephritis.

Signs and Symptoms.

Patient complaints are typically the same as for an uncomplicated UTI, but often include constitutional symptoms. Symptom onset may be sudden or insidious. Prostatic symptoms may be present in men with prostate enlargement, or there may be symptoms of concurrent prostatitis (see BPH and prostatitis sections). Complaints may also indicate upper tract involvement (see pyelonephritis section).

Diagnostic Studies.

Initially infected urine will be noted on urinalysis. Urine culture and sensitivity are recommended, particularly if the presentation is one of recurrent UTI or refractory UTI, and appropriate lab work (CBC, serum electrolytes, blood cultures) should be ordered based on the patient's overall presentation and other comorbidities. Imaging studies will be indicated based on the suspicion for anatomy abnormalities or suspected obstruction. There is the potential for admission based on overall clinical picture, comorbidities, hydration status, and need for further evaluation.

Vaginitis

Vaginitis can be accompanied by irritation to adjacent structures as well as vaginal discharge and vulvar irritation. See Chapter 12 for additional discussion.

POSTMENOPAUSAL STATUS

Dysuria seen in women after menopause can be accompanied by stress urinary incontinence and urinary frequency. All result from the mucosal thinning of the urethra and bladder in the absence of estrogen.

Signs and Symptoms.

The signs and symptoms are similar to the complaints seen with a UTI, except without constitutional symptoms. Patients may also describe symptoms that result from vaginal dryness. Vaginal and urethral areas will appear pale owing to the diminished vascularity.

Diagnostic Studies.

A history and physical exam are usually sufficient; a urinalysis will rule out UTI.

GENITOURINARY NEOPLASM

Bladder cancer in particular can be accompanied by complaints of bladder irritability, or LUTS, along with either gross or microscopic hematuria. Symptoms of bladder irritation are also common with both BPH and prostate cancer.

Signs and Symptoms.

Patients with bladder cancer may have unremarkable physical findings, unless there is a large-volume invasive tumor, in which case there may be a palpable thickness to the bladder. Patients who have prostate cancer may also describe LUTS and general bladder irritability; other physical findings are typically unremarkable.

Diagnostic Studies.

A urinalysis is required to confirm or investigate for the presence of blood. Urine cytology is needed to evaluate for malignant cells, although this will not determine the source of the abnormal cells (bladder vs. ureter vs. renal pelvis). If malignancy is suspected or confirmed, a staging CT scan should be ordered before urgent/emergent referral to a urologist for further management.

ANATOMIC ABNORMALITY

Anatomic abnormality includes such conditions as a ureteral or urethral stricture, duplication of the collecting system, meatal stenosis, phimosis, or vesicovaginal fistula. These conditions may become apparent after surgical procedures that promote scar tissue in the urethra, prolonged catheterization, and surgeries to the pelvic region.

Signs and Symptoms.

Patients may describe a gradual onset of changes to their pattern of urination, such as spraying, painful urination, frequency, and the necessity to push in order to urinate. Physical examination includes a pelvic exam for women and special attention to the foreskin and meatal opening in men.

Diagnostic Studies.

Physical exam alone may provide the diagnosis. Urinalysis may show some degree of contamination or a UTI. Suspicion of a structural abnormality will require referral to a urologist for further evaluation; depending on the suspected location of the abnormality, a retrograde urethrogram or IVP may be considered.

Difficulty Urinating or the Inability to Urinate

Urinary difficulties often occur insidiously, with few complaints from the patient until the situation is advanced or has created a social difficulty. However, when a patient has difficulty urinating or emptying his or her bladder, there is a motivation to seek evaluation sooner rather than later.

History

A patient may describe recurrent or persistent UTIs, dysuria, varying LUTS, including difficulty starting the stream or nocturia. There may be a history of recent GU instrumentation, indwelling Foley catheter, or surgery. The patient may also describe a history of declining bladder control.

Physical Examination

A routine GU exam is required, including DRE and a pelvic exam in women.

Benign Prostatic Hyperplasia

See p. 246.

Prostatitis

See p. 246.

NEUROGENIC AND NEUROPATHIC BLADDER

This is a broad term that describes the failure of the bladder to store or the failure to empty. There may be spontaneous and uncoordinated contractions of the bladder when it is filling, or the bladder and sphincter may not work in concert, preventing the bladder from effectively emptying. Risk factors include spinal cord injury, trauma to the central nervous system, diabetes mellitus, spina bifida, multiple sclerosis, spinal disc disease, and pelvic surgery, among many others.

Signs and Symptoms.

There may be a variety of urinary complaints, including incontinence, dribbling, and retention, as well as disorders of bladder sensation. Associated complaints may reflect changes to bowel habits, sexual function, or lower extremity sensation. Physical examination involves not only a routine GU and pelvic exam, but also a full neurologic exam.

Diagnostic Studies.

Order a urinalysis to rule out UTI as a treatable cause that would be contributing to the complaints. Conduct other lab studies as suspicions dictate (such as an evaluation for diabetes). You should consider an evaluation of the upper tracts with IVP or renal ultrasound. Referral to a urologist is warranted for further specialized testing.

Postoperative Urinary Retention

The bladder may recover sluggishly after anesthesia, requiring a patient to embark on a short-term regimen of intermittent catheterization. A history of recent surgery that required bladder catheterization should be sufficient to confirm the diagnosis.

URETHRAL LESIONS

Urethral cancer is a rare condition for both men and women, but it can change the quality of the urinary stream. Some STDs can cause lesions within the urethra itself, resulting in pain and changes in the urinary stream.

Signs and Symptoms.

Complaints of a splayed or intermittent urinary stream. The symptoms may be gradual in onset. There may be a history of STD, recent urethral trauma or instrumentation, or a possible history of previous urethral stricture. Inspection may show visible lesions at the meatus.

Diagnostic Studies.

Visual inspection may be sufficient to confirm the presence of lesions. Referral to urology for cystoscopic examination of the urethral tissue is recommended because lesions may indicate a urethral carcinoma.

BLADDER CALCULI

In the United States, these are most commonly due to bladder outlet obstruction, commonly BPH. They can also be caused by an elevated bladder neck in combination with an increased postvoid residual, which results in stagnant urine.

Signs and Symptoms.

The presentation may be completely asymptomatic; there may be various complaints, including urinary retention, recurrent urinary tract infection, bladder pain, microscopic or gross hematuria, dysuria, urgency, or nocturia. The bladder may be palpable due to distension. Physical examination involves palpation of the bladder, and pelvic examination in women.

Diagnostic Studies.

Urinalysis will confirm hematuria, and possibly test positive for a UTI. A urine cytology and urine cultures may be considered. The initial imaging study can be a KUB, IVP, or pelvic ultrasound, all of which will demonstrate the presence of a stone(s). Referral to urology for management is indicated.

Decreased Force of Stream or Spraying with Urination

Any change in the pattern of urination to which a patient is accustomed can be upsetting. Some of these complaints have causes that are easily remedied and may simply be related to age and/or pelvic floor weakness.

History

The patient will give a history of decreased force and/or caliber of stream. There may be complaint of spraying with urination. Pain is not typically associated with this complaint.

Physical Examination

A routine GU exam is required, with attention to location of urethral opening, and DRE.

Benign Prostatic Hyperplasia

See p. 246.

EPISPADIAS/HYPOSPADIAS

This condition is more commonly diagnosed in infancy, and has varying degrees of severity. Severe hypospadias in the infant, male or female, can be confused with an intersex condition. In a female, leaving an epispadias untreated can result in incontinence as an adult. It is not uncommon for an adult male (hypospadias occurs in one of every 300 male births) to have a slight displacement of the urethral opening that was not surgically corrected as an infant or child. There is also an increased incidence of undescended testes with hypospadias; other consequences include infertility and upper urinary tract damage.

Signs and Symptoms.

A patient may complain of a displaced urethral opening or the inability to direct the urinary stream. Men may also complain of chordee (curvature of the penis caused by tethering of the skin and dartos fascia). A careful scrotal examination should be performed to confirm the presence of both testicles and to rule out an inguinal hernia. Rarely, the patient may present with complaints of infertility.

Diagnostic Studies.

Physical examination should be sufficient to make the diagnosis. The patient should be referred to a urologist for further evaluation and management.

Lesions Related to Sexually Transmitted Diseases

See Table 11.3 and discussions in Chapters 11 and 12.

Distorted Female Pelvic Anatomy

Cystocele, prolapse of the uterus, and failed continence surgery can all affect pelvic floor anatomy and cause urinary changes, including incontinence and changes to the quality of the urinary stream. See Chapter 12 for descriptions of these conditions.

Frequency, Urgency, and Hesitancy

Urinary complaints that involve frequency, urgency, or hesitancy can be seen by patient and provider alike as part of the aging process. However, in many cases these complaints may have treatable or even reversible causes. In some cases, a thorough history will uncover the cause, such as with radiation cystitis.

History

These complaints may have an acute or insidious onset, particularly if irritative and obstructive symptoms are involved. The patient may provide a history of some degree of incontinence or dysuria.

Physical Examination
A routine GU exam is needed; other system exams are dictated by history and accompanying complaints. Patients may have a palpable bladder on exam.
Interstitial Cystitis (IC)
See p. 249.
Urinary tract infection (UTI)
See p. 249, 251.
Benign Prostatic Hyperplasia
See p. 246.
Neurogenic and Neuropathic Bladder
See p. 252.

VOLUME OR METABOLIC-RELATED CAUSE

The kidneys receive roughly 20% of cardiac output and have a major role in the volume and electrolyte homeostasis of the body. Changes to the fluid and electrolyte balance of the body can directly affect urinary output, such as in the osmotic diuresis seen with poorly controlled or undiagnosed diabetes mellitus. Other examples include diabetes insipidus, metabolic acidosis and alkalosis, renal insufficiency, and congestive heart failure.

Signs and Symptoms.

Often this involves varying GU complaints, along with frequency, urgency, and hesitancy. There will be other systemic complaints representative of the particular endocrinopathy or underlying disease process. The physical exam will involve a routine GU exam, along with additional system exams as indicated by presentation and history.

Diagnostic Studies.

Urinalysis should be performed to rule out UTI as a treatable cause contributing to the complaints. Other lab studies can be ordered as suspicions dictate (such as evaluation for diabetes), particularly electrolytes. Referral to the appropriate subspecialty may be needed for further diagnosis and management.

DRUG-INDUCED (DIURETICS)

A patient may complain of frequency that she or he associates with a particular medication. Alternatively, this association may not be clear until a complete list of the patient's medications is available.

Signs and Symptoms.

These are primarily frequency and urgency, both of which may be complicated by coexisting GU conditions, such as BPH, some type of incontinence, or mobility issues.

Diagnostic Studies.

A review of a patient's medications and the schedule used for taking the medications should be sufficient to determine that a diuretic is a contributing cause. Consider urinalysis to rule out a UTI.

Neoplastic (Bladder or Renal Cancer)
See pp. 251–252.

Nocturia

As nocturia persists, patients become more likely to seek evaluation and treatment. They begin to suffer fatigue from sleep interruption and deprivation, as there may be 45 minutes or less between urges to urinate.

History

The actual duration of the problem may be difficult to gauge, as the onset may have occurred over several months. The patient's overall disposition and energy level should be noted. The patient should be asked to estimate the average number of episodes per night, and the presence of other associated LUTS should be queried.

Physical Examination

A routine GU exam is needed; a pelvic exam and/or full physical may be indicated by history.

Benign Prostatic Hyperplasia

See p. 246.

Interstitial Cystitis

See p. 249.

Volume or Metabolic-Related Disorder

See p. 255.

Excessive Fluid Intake in Evening

When questioned, the patient will describe a pattern of increased fluid intake later in the day. History is usually sufficient to confirm the cause.

Pharmacologically Induced

This problem can present when a patient times the administration of a diuretic late into the afternoon or evening, with consequent complaints of urinary frequency late into the night. A review of medications and their timing should be sufficient to confirm this cause.

Urinary Incontinence

Urinary incontinence (UI) is a prevalent and costly public health problem. Twenty million adults have urinary incontinence or an overactive bladder, causing urinary leakage that is bothersome. It is estimated that 15% to 30% of the adult women in the United States experience UI. Men can experience UI after pelvic surgery and also as they age owing to prostate enlargement. The prevalence of UI increases as age increases for both genders; approximately 50% of elders in extended care are incontinent of urine, and 33% are incontinent all or most of the time. Given the increase in numbers of the aging population, UI will continue to affect large numbers of the population. The Agency for Healthcare Research and Quality has determined that incontinence carries a significant financial burden to the individual for supplies and services; the overall annual cost has been estimated at about $5 billion.

As a result of the constant production of urine, and the bladder's finite storage capacity, incontinence will occur in anyone who does not have timely access to facilities, regardless of age, mobility status, or gender. There are several recognized patterns of urine loss:

1. *Mild incontinence*, or a loss of a few drops of urine.
2. *Stress incontinence*, or the loss of urine with activities that cause changes in intraabdominal pressure, such as sneezing.
3. *Urge incontinence*, or the loss of urine that results from detrusor overactivity.
4. *Mixed incontinence,* or a combination of both stress and urge incontinence.
5. *Functional incontinence,* or the inability to make it to the toilet before losing control and/or an inability to undress properly; commonly influenced by both cognitive and functional status.

6. *Overflow incontinence*, or a bladder that does not empty completely owing to outlet obstruction or neurogenic causes and subsequently spills urine when full.

7. *Total incontinence*, or a complete lack of control over urinary function, which can be the result of a variety of causes.

The bladder has a normal capacity of 400–500 mL, without resulting in an increase in intravesical pressure owing to its spheric shape. The sensation of bladder fullness is transmitted via the sacral cord reflex arc to cause detrusor contraction and urination (if voluntary control is lacking). The bladder has several functional features that contribute to normal continence: its normal capacity of 400–500 mL; the fullness sensation; the ability to accommodate various volumes without changes in intraluminal pressure; the ability to initiate and sustain contraction until the bladder is empty; and a response to the voluntary inhibition of voiding, despite the inherent involuntary nature of the organ.

The bladder receives afferent and efferent innervation from both the autonomic and somatic nervous system. Parasympathetic innervation arises from sacral segments 2–4 and projects to the pelvic plexus, supplying both the bladder and sphincter. Sympathetic control originates at the T10–L2 level. Somatic innervation originates from S2–3 and travels via the pudendal nerve to the external urethral sphincter and permits the sensation of fullness, inflammation, or pain depending on the specific pathway. Damage or other pathologies that affect these areas of the spine (herniated disc, spinal stenosis, degenerative changes in the vertebrae, or metastatic disease) can result in changes to bladder function and/or sensation. Diseases that result in neuropathies (such as diabetes mellitus or multiple sclerosis) can contribute to the dysfunction of bladder sensation and function.

Gender-specific anatomy, in males and females, may explain some of the difference in the incidence of UI. Female gender greatly increases the risk for urinary incontinence, as does childbearing. Age is a risk factor but is not causative; there are normal age-related changes associated with the urinary tract. The most significant age-related changes in women are related to decreased estrogen influence. As estrogen levels decline, the epithelium and supporting tissues of the pelvis atrophy, resulting in friable mucosa and possible prolapse of the pelvic structures. The change in relationship of the pelvic structures results in hypermobility of the bladder base, pelvic muscle weakness, and urethral weakness, resulting in stress urinary incontinence in women. The decreased glycogen content of the vaginal epithelium causes decreased lactic acid metabolism by Döderlein's bacillus, an increased pH of vaginal secretions, and therefore an increased risk for urinary tract infection.

There are a variety of history and assessment points that aid in narrowing the etiology of a patient's specific complaints.

History

The patient will report some pattern of involuntary loss of urine; this may occur under specific circumstances or be nearly continuous. Detailing the context in which the urine loss occurs will aid with diagnosis. Existing comorbidities and surgical history will provide additional clues to the etiology of the incontinence.

Signs and Symptoms

The signs and symptoms involve the loss of urine involuntarily; descriptions will vary based on the underlying etiology.

Table 10-8. ■ Selected Causes of Urinary Incontinence

Female	Male	Male or Female
• Childbirth • Cystocele • Estrogen deficiency (atrophic vaginitis or urethritis) • Failed previous surgery to correct incontinence • Hysterectomy • Rectocele • Vesicovaginal fistula	• Prostatic hypertrophy • Prostatitis • Post radical prostatectomy	• Anatomic (constipation; urinary retention; pelvic, back, or retroperitoneal surgery) • Irritative (interstitial cystitis, urinary tract infection) • Metabolic (diabetes mellitus, diabetes insipidus, aging) • Neurologic (dementia, peripheral or autonomic neuropathy, spinal cord trauma or lesions, multiple sclerosis, diabetes) • Pharmacologic (diuretics, sedatives, anticholinergics, alpha-adrenergic blockade • Vascular (stroke)

Physical Examination

A routine GU exam, including DRE, is needed—a pelvic exam in women.

Selected Causes

See Table 10-8.

Diagnostic Studies

The initial evaluation should include a urinalysis to rule out reversible causes of incontinence, such as a UTI. Consider a urine culture based on urinalysis results, BUN and creatinine as history and comorbidities indicate, and measurement of a postvoid residual volume to help distinguish the type of incontinence. If an imaging study seems needed, the initial choice would be an IVP or renal ultrasound. Consider referral to a urologist or urogynecologist as needed, for specialized testing and concerns regarding an anatomic basis for the incontinence.

References

Barry M.J., Fowler, F.J. Jr., O'Leary, M.P., Bruskewitz, R.C., Holtgrewe, H.L., Mebust, W.K., Cockett, A.T. (1992). The American Urological Association symptom index for benign prostatic hyperplasia. *Journal of Urology*, 148(5), 149–157.

Batstone, G., Doble, A., & Batstone, D. (2003). Chronic prostatitis. *Current Opinions Urology*, 13(1), 23–29.

Bent, S., & Saint, S. (2003). The optimal use of diagnostic testing in women with acute uncomplicated cystitis. *Disease-A-Month*, 49(2), 83–98.

Kawashima A., Glockner, J.F., & King, B.F. (2003). CT urography and MR urography. Radiologic Clinics of North America, 41(5), 945–961.

Parsons, C.L., Dell, J., Stanford, E.J., Bullen, M., Kahn, B.S., Waxell, T., & Koziol., J.A. (2002). Increased prevalence of interstitial cystitis: Previously unrecognized urologic and gynecologic cases identified using a new symptom questionnaire and intravesical potassium sensitivity. *Urology*, 60(4), 573–578.

Perlman, E.S., Rosenfield, A.T., Wexler, J.S., Glickman, M.G. (1996). CT urography in the evaluation of urinary tract disease. *Journal of Computer Assisted Tomography*, 20(4), 620–626.

Stenner, J., Holthaus, K., Mackenzie, S., & Crawford, E. (1998). The effect of ejaculation on prostate specific antigen in a prostate cancer-screening population. *Urology*, 51(3), 455–459.

SUGGESTED READINGS

Abrahams, P., Cardozo, L., Fall, M., Griffiths, D., Rosier, P., Ulmsten, U., van Kerrebroeck, P., Victor, A., & Wein, A. (2002). The standardization of terminology of lower urinary tract function: Report from the standardization sub-committee of the international continence society. *American Journal of Obstetrics and Gynecology*, 187(1), 116–126.

Agency for Health Care Policy and Research. (1992). *Clinical practice guideline: Urinary Incontinence in Adults*, U.S. Department of Health and Human Services.

Brownlee, N. (1999). Taking the mystery our of ureteroscopy. *Association of Operating Room Nurses (AORN)*, 69(1), 162–171.

Fielding, J., Silverman, S., Samuel, S., Zou, K., & Loughlin, K. (1998). Unenhanced helical CT of ureteral stones: A replacement for excretory urography in planning treatment. *American Journal of Roentgenology*, 171(4), 1051-1053.

Grossfeld, G.D., Litwin, M.S., Wolf, J.S., Hricak, H., Shuler, C.L., Agerter, D.C., & Carroll, P.R. (2001). Evaluation of asymptomatic microscopic hematuria in adults: The American Urological Association best practice policy—Part I: Definition, detection, prevalence, and etiology. *Urology*, 57(4), 599–603.

Grossfeld, G.D., Litwin, M.S., Wolf, J.S., Hricak, H., Shuler, C.L., Agerter, D.C., & Carroll, P.R. (2001). Evaluation of asymptomatic microscopic hematuria in adults: The American Urological Association best practice policy—Part II: Patient evaluation, cytology, voided markers, imaging, cystoscopy, nephrology evaluation, and follow-up. *Urology*, 57(4), 604–610.

Lehmann, S., & Dietz, C. (2002). Double J stents: They're not trouble free. *RN*, 65(1), 54–60.

Ouslander, J. (1997). Aging and the lower urinary tract. *American Journal of the Medical Sciences*, 314(4), 214–218.

Prostate-Specific Antigen (PSA). *Best Practice Policy*, American Urological Association, 2000.

Sachs, H., and Stone, A. (2003). Benign prostatic hypertrophy: How and when to treat it. *Consultant*, 43(3), 297–305.

Wyndaele, J. (1999). Normality in urodynamics studied in healthy adults. *Journal of Urology*, 161(3), 899–902.

Chapter 11
Male Reproductive System

Knowledge of the anatomy and the ability to focus the history on the presenting complaint are the keys to accurately assessing complaints that relate to the male reproductive system (see Figure 11-1). The majority of the information needed to arrive at an accurate diagnosis will be gained through inspection, palpation, and a very precise history. Because not all assessment points are relevant to every complaint, taking a problem-focused history is vital.

HISTORY
General History
In order to confirm normal physiologic male development, the general history of a male patient relative to reproductive or genital complaints should first establish that puberty started in his early or middle teens. The history should include any past reproductive complaints; a discussion of any recent (within the last six months) systemic illness; recent weight gain or loss; and a smoking, alcohol consumption, and illicit drug use history. It must also include a listing of current prescription and over-the-counter medications. As each complaint is discussed in this chapter, additional general and specific history-taking points will be discussed.

Past Medical History
The evaluation should then proceed to discuss a history of any condition that would affect the penis, testes, or hormones (including cryptorchidism, hypothyroidism, pituitary malfunction); any history of genitourinary surgeries (such as orchidopexy; YV plasty to bladder neck; inguinal hernia repair as infant, small child, or adult; epispadias or hypospadias repair, prostate surgery, bladder reconstructions, bladder surgeries, testicular surgeries); previous treatment for testicular or genitourinary malignancies; and a history of vasectomy and when it was performed.

S.A. Quallich

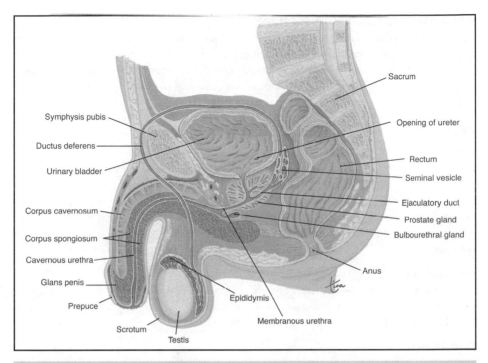

Figure 11-1. ■ Anatomical structures of the male reproductive system. (From Scanlon, V.C. & Sanders, T. Essentials of anatomy and physiology, 4th ed. Philadelphia: F.A. Davis, 2003, p. 438. Reprinted with permission.)

Family History

The family history should include a discussion of testicular or other genitourinary (GU) malignancies—specifically, a history of any other cancers; prostate or bladder problems in other family members (including female relatives with bladder conditions); other members of the family with complaints similar to the patient's presenting complaint; a history of maternal medication or drug use while pregnant, if known.

Sexual History

A sexual history is particularly relevant when the main complaint involves the GU system. The history should include recent changes in sexual partners; the overall pattern of sexual activity; history of having previously fathered any children; libido; erectile function; and evaluation and treatment of a partner that may have preceded the patient's current visit.

Habits

This discussion will include any activity that would put the groin area at risk for trauma (such as football, hockey, marathon cycling, motocross, or riding three- or four-wheeled vehicles). It also includes any potential exposure to environmental toxins.

PHYSICAL EXAMINATION

Examination of the male patient is best done in a warm room, in order to avoid any exaggeration of the cremaster reflex. A "routine genital exam" for the purposes of this chapter involves inspection and palpation of the male genitalia. A "routine GU exam" for the purposes of this chapter involves the routine genital exam and digital rectal exam. Specialized examination maneuvers will be indicated as needed.

Order of the Examination

Inspection

Look for age-appropriate development of male secondary sex characteristics; lesions or scarring of the penis/scrotum/groin; discoloration of the penis/scrotum/groin; asymmetry of testicles; gynecomastia; hirsutism; location and size of the opening of the meatus, presence of scars in the abdomen, groin, or inguinal areas. The tone of the dartos muscle will govern the size of the scrotum; in a cool environment, it will cause the scrotum to contract.

Auscultation

Auscultate the abdomen as indicated; refer to Chapter 9. Auscultation is rarely indicated in the evaluation of male reproductive complaints, except with a suspected herniation of bowel into the scrotum or as part of a complete physical.

Percussion

Percuss the abdomen as indicated; refer to Chapter 9. Percussion is rarely indicated in the evaluation of male reproductive complaints, except as part of a complete physical.

Palpation

Palpation is the most important part of the physical. This requires palpation of all suspected intrascrotal masses, that is, masses that may arise from the surface of testicle, or adjacent to or separate from testes. Table 11-1 reviews the palpation of the male reproductive structures.

Special Maneuvers

There are several physical examination points that are specific to the assessment of male reproductive complaints. See Table 11-2.

Red Flags in the Assessment of the Male Reproductive System

- Sudden onset of acute testicular pain
- Cellulitic or necrotic changes to the skin of the scrotum, penis, perineal region
- Erection lasting >60 minutes after cessation of sexual activity
- Inability to urinate
- New painful mass in the scrotum

Table 11-1. ■ Palpation of Male Reproductive Structures

Male Reproductive Structure	Normal Findings on Palpation	Abnormalities and Possible Significance
Penis	• Soft and pliable along length of shaft • Meatus midline and central to glans • Foreskin should retract and draw forward easily	• Areas of fibrous plaque along shaft—Peyronie's disease • Tenderness—possibly secondary to a urethral stricture • Difficulty with foreskin retraction—phimosis, edema, balanitis, balanoposthitis • Difficulty moving foreskin forward—paraphimosis, edema • Entire shaft of penis fibrous and with reduced pliability—previous priapism • Meatus not midline or central to glans—hypospadias, epispadias
Scrotum	Loose sac of skin partially covered with hair	• Areas of erythema or nodularity—infected sebaceous glands or hair follicles • Unilateral, uncomfortable swelling of the scrotum—hydrocele, hematoma, varicocele
Testes	• Two testes, freely movable within the scrotum • Palpate between thumb and 1st two fingers of the hand • Firm, smooth, rubbery consistency • Average 6 cm × 4 cm in size • Symmetrical • Right testicle may be slightly anterior to left • Separate from epididymis	• Mass associated with testicle—tumor, hydrocele, spermatocele • Solitary testes—nondescent of testicle or previous surgical removal • Small, soft testicle(s)—Klinefelter's disease, history of infection, late orchidopexy
Epididymis	• Soft ridge of tissue longitudinally posterior to the testicle • Separate from testicle	• Cystic or nodular—spermatocele, previous or current infection, history of vasectomy • Large and fluctuant—spermatocele • Localized pain—epididymitis, postvasectomy pain syndrome
Vas deferens and spermatic cord	• Soft, rubbery consistency • Smooth along its length • Able to trace vas deferens from epididymis to inguinal canal	• Absence of vas bilaterally or unilaterally—cystic fibrosis or a variant • Sperm granuloma—S/P vasectomy • Congested veins unilaterally or bilaterally—varicocele • Beading/nodularity of the cord—obstruction of epididymis, tubercular infection of the epididymis

Table 11-2. ■ Physical Examination Maneuvers for Assessment of Male
Reproductive Complaints

Maneuver	Description
Cremasteric reflex	Brushing or touching the skin of the scrotum in a downward direction will result in the prompt elevation of the testicle on the same side. This reaction can be aggravated by a cool room—the reflex may have engaged before any contact with the examiner.
Digital rectal examination (DRE)	Gloved, lubricated finger is inserted into the anus and swept across the surface of the prostate; prostate should be symmetrical, non-tender, free of nodules, approximately the size of a walnut, and have a smooth, rubbery consistency. Exam also involves estimation of anal sphincter tone.
Examination for hernia	Index finger is inserted into the scrotum and invaginated into the external inguinal ring (scrotum should be invaginated in front of the testicle); fingertips of other hand should then be placed over the internal inguinal canal and patient should be asked to Valsalva. A hernia will be felt as a bulge that descends against index finger with Valsalva maneuver.
Neurologic examination	Testing of superficial anal reflex (perianal sensation)—stroking the anus with a cotton swab will result in reflexive contraction of the external anal sphincter ("anal wink"). Testing of bulbocavernosus reflex—insertion of a gloved finger into the anus and squeezing the glans penis will result in contraction of the anal sphincter and bulbocavernosus muscles. (These tests are most helpful when evaluating complaints of erectile dysfunction and ejaculatory dysfunction.)
Transillumination of hydrocele	Light source shined through mass; hydrocele will glow reddish; may feel as though it surrounds testicle; may feel turbid or tense.
Transillumination of spermatocele	Light source shined through mass; should palpate testicle as separate from the spermatocele, and note that the epididymis may not be palpated separately from the spermatocele; the mass feels connected to testicle at testicle's superior aspect.
Valsalva maneuver to evaluate for varicocele	Performed with patient standing, and in a warm room; having patient perform Valsalva will reverse the flow into the pampiniform plexus and result in palpable distention of the vessels ("bag of worms" if varicocele is of sufficient size).

DIFFERENTIAL DIAGNOSIS OF CHIEF COMPLAINTS
General Complaints
Testicular or Scrotal Pain

Complaints of pain in the testicles or scrotum can take many forms, including an acute, nauseating pain after trauma to the area; a dull ache with a progressive onset; and the sharp, focused pain associated with an infection. A focused history and targeted examination will often provide the necessary clues to diagnosis.

History

Trauma may precede the complaint of pain in the testes or scrotum; it is important to establish the mechanism of injury, if possible. The patient may report acute pain or progressive pain and tenderness after the insult. There may be a history of a sudden onset of acute pain and elevation of the affected testicle. The onset of the discomfort also may have occurred over time and could be associated with lesions or drainage from the scrotum; in such a case, the patient may also provide a history of recurrent scrotal infections and current constitutional symptoms, such as fever, chills, malaise, and nausea.

Examination

A thorough examination of the genitals is vital, despite the fact that it may cause additional discomfort to the patient. Exam may reveal generalized tenderness of the scrotum and its contents, unilateral scrotal swelling, localized tenderness to one or more of the scrotal structures, or painful and edematous genitalia. If mild or moderate trauma has been involved, ecchymotic areas or abrasions may be observed.

TESTICULAR TORSION

This is most commonly seen in early puberty and results in the loss of blood flow to the affected testicle. This compromised blood flow results in swelling and tissue necrosis after 6 to 8 hours. There are no established risk factors, but this is more common during adolescence due to the rapid growth of the testes.

Signs and Symptoms.

Patients experience an acute and sudden onset of pain that localizes in the affected testicle, but it may also radiate to the inguinal areas or abdomen. This pain is often accompanied by abdominal discomfort, nausea, and vomiting. Asymmetric scrotal swelling will be apparent on physical exam, with the affected testicle being somewhat elevated. The affected testicle may also have a somewhat horizontal lie. Traditional landmarks within the scrotum may be difficult to assess because of edema, and the cremaster reflex may be absent on the affected side.

Diagnostic Studies.

This is a true urologic emergency that must be identified quickly. If testicular torsion is suspected, the patient must be immediately referred to the closest emergency department for evaluation and probable surgery in attempts at preserving the testicle.

FOURNIER'S GANGRENE

This progressive necrotizing fasciitis of the genitals and perineum is most commonly seen in males in their sixth decade and is usually caused by a combination of aerobic and anaerobic organisms. It can progress to involve the entire perineal area, abdominal wall, and buttocks. Risk factors for its development include poor personal hygiene, phimosis, diabetes, alcoholism, malnutrition, chemotherapy or radiation treatment, perirectal or perianal infections, and local trauma to the genitals or perineal area (such as surgery).

Signs and Symptoms.

There may be a prodromal period of generalized discomfort, followed by erythema and edema in the affected areas. Cellulitic changes are apparent on physical exam and may be accompanied by crepitus, dark purple coloration, necrosis, eschar, and a foul odor. Often there are constitutional complaints of fever, chills, nausea, and vomiting, and the patient may progress to frank sepsis. Specific urologic complaints may be noted as well: dysuria, urethral discharge, or urethral obstruction.

Diagnostic Studies.

If Fournier's gangrene is suspected, the patient must be immediately referred to the closest emergency department for evaluation and likely admission: this is a true urologic emergency that must be identified quickly. A scrotal ultrasound can be helpful in defining areas of crepitus, but this should not delay referral.

Incarcerated Inguinal Hernia

See Chapters 9 and 10.

TESTICULAR MASS OR TUMOR

Malignant tumors of the testes are uncommon, usually present between the ages of 15 and 35, are slightly more common on the right side, and arise from germ cells. The greatest risk factor for the development of a testicular tumor is cryptorchidism, with an overall incidence of 7%–10% in the patient with a history of unilateral or bilateral undescended testes. Increased screening and early detection have significantly decreased the mortality from this malignancy, but up to 10% of patients will present with pain, constitutional, or pulmonary complaints that indicate metastasis.

Signs and Symptoms.

A patient may have noticed a painless swelling of the testicle or a distinct nodule on self-examination; there may have been some minor trauma to the affected side that initiated the onset of pain and/or swelling. The testicle gradually enlarges over time, with some associated heaviness. Patients will rarely complain of acute pain as their presenting symptom, but rather of a dull ache or heaviness that localizes to the affected side. Physical examination will reveal a distinct mass or diffuse enlargement of the affected testicle; the mass may be firm, smooth, nodular, or fixed. Palpation of the inguinal, supraclavicular, and axillary areas may show evidence of enlarged lymph nodes; examination of the abdomen may also demonstrate bulky retroperitoneal disease. In advanced disease, gynecomastia resulting from hormonal changes and wheezing due to lung metastasis may be observed.

Diagnostic Studies.

A scrotal ultrasound will quickly and accurately distinguish a tumor from other intrascrotal pathologies and the ultrasound is considered an extension of the physical exam in the case of a suspected testicular mass. The biochemical markers that are helpful in the diagnosis and classification of testicular masses, in addition to routine chemistries and white blood cell (WBC) count, are alpha-fetoprotein (AFP) and beta human chorionic gonadotropin (beta-hCG). A chest x-ray and CT scan of the chest, abdomen, and pelvis complete the metastatic workup. The patient should be referred urgently to a urologist for further management because in many cases the removal of the testicle and prompt treatment of the associated adenopathy can be curative, depending on the stage of the disease. Removal of the testicle is also necessary for an accurate pathologic diagnosis.

EPIDIDYMITIS

This is inflammation or infection of the epididymis and is caused by the spread of an infection from the bladder or urethra, owing to an alteration in the urethral closure mechanism. Uncircumcised men, men with indwelling catheters, benign prostatic hypertrophy (BPH), recent GU instrumentation, or prostatic surgery create a risk for epididymitis. In heterosexual men younger than 35, the causative organisms are likely to be *Neisseria gonorrhoeae* and *Chlamydia trichomatis*. In homosexual men, the causative organism is usually *Escherichia coli*. In cases where an organism associated with a sexually transmitted disease is suspected, the exposure to the organism can significantly predate the development of epididymitis. If epididymitis is left unrecognized and untreated, it can progress to an abscess or chronic infection, with resulting fibrosis, chronic scrotal pain, and infertility.

Signs and Symptoms.

Complaints usually involve a sudden onset (over 24–48 hours), painful swelling in the scrotum, which can be unilateral or bilateral. Pain may decrease with elevation of the scrotum (Prehn's sign). There may be an associated urethral discharge and/or fever, and complaints of urethritis, cystitis, or prostatitis are possible. On physical exam, the pain will localize to the affected epididymis with palpation, which will be swollen and indurated. The spermatic cord is usually tender and swollen, and pain may radiate to the inguinal canal and/or flank.

Diagnostic Studies.

An ultrasound will differentiate between testicular torsion and epididymitis, and can be helpful in establishing the correct diagnosis in cases of the acute onset of pain. Lab work is not usually necessary, although the patient may exhibit an elevated white count with a fever. If a sexually transmitted disease (STD) is suspected, a gram stain of a urethral smear can be ordered, and the partner must also be treated to prevent recurrent episodes.

ORCHITIS

This is usually caused by the extension of an infection from the epididymis to the testicle itself, and rarely exists independent of epididymitis. The risks and causative organisms are the same as for epididymitis. Orchitis may also occur as a sequela of mumps and occurs in up to 30% of prepubertal male patients with mumps.

Signs and Symptoms.

The signs and symptoms are the same as those for epididymitis. On physical exam, the pain will localize to the affected testicle, and it may not be possible to distinguish the separation between the epididymis and testicle owing to inflammation. A reactive hydrocele may also form.

Diagnostic Studies.

The diagnostics are the same as those for epididymitis, although an ultrasound is not typically needed.

HYDROCELE

A hydrocele is a collection of fluid between the layers of the tunica vaginalis, which surrounds the testicle, or fluid along the spermatic cord. It often occurs unilaterally, and its origin is idiopathic in adult males, although there appears to be some decreased absorption of this fluid by the tunica itself. The fluid collection may be large enough to completely encompass the testicle, and the composition is primarily water with some albumin.

Signs and Symptoms.

Hydroceles are not usually painful, and they typically present as a unilateral swelling of the scrotum that may extend into the inguinal canal. There may be associated heaviness or discomfort during specific activities, such as prolonged sitting or bicycle riding. If the hydrocele is large enough, it is possible for the scrotal skin to suffer excoriation and erythema. It may not be possible to feel the testicle during a physical exam if the hydrocele is large enough. A hydrocele can be confirmed with transillumination. A large hydrocele can distort the position of the other scrotal structures, particularly the epididymis, and make their identification challenging.

Diagnostic Studies.

A scrotal ultrasound is not necessary but will definitively confirm a hydrocele and rule out any testicular pathology, if the testicle cannot be palpated.

VARICOCELE

A varicocele is a palpable or visible dilation of the vessels of the pampiniform plexus in the scrotum; retrograde reflux of venous blood in the internal spermatic vein dilates the pampiniform plexus. Varicoceles are more common on the left owing to the greater distance the internal spermatic vein must traverse to the left renal vein when compared with the right. The etiology of varicoceles remains unclear, and there are no specific risk factors. It is unusual for males to exhibit a varicocele before adolescence, and most varicoceles are asymptomatic. Varicoceles are commonly diagnosed during a male infertility evaluation (semen parameters are often decreased; varicoceles represent a common cause of secondary male infertility) or, less commonly, during an evaluation for scrotal pain or a scrotal mass. If a varicocele is painful, the pain may increase with prolonged standing, exertion, or sitting; pain is rare after prolonged recumbency or sleeping. A varicocele will typically present unilaterally, on the left side. The acute onset of a painful varicocele may indicate obstruction of the spermatic or renal vein.

Signs and Symptoms.

Most are asymptomatic, but the patient may complain of a dull ache, fullness, pain that does not radiate, or pulling to the affected side of the scrotum. If the varicocele is large enough, it typically results in scrotal swelling that is noticeable to the patient, along with a bluish discoloration beneath the scrotal skin. Primary or secondary male infertility may be the presenting symptom. The varicocele can be exaggerated during physical exam by asking the patient to perform Valsalva's maneuver while standing; any distention of the pampiniform plexus will disappear when the patient lies down. A long-standing varicocele may cause testicular atrophy. If the varicocele is large, it may be visible during inspection ("bag of worms").

Diagnostic Studies.

A scrotal ultrasound is not necessary, but will definitively confirm a varicocele and rule out any testicular or scrotal pathology. If the patient presents with only a right-sided varicocele, this can be a sign of right renal vein obstruction and an abdominal CT scan should be ordered to rule out any pathology. The patient can be routinely referred to a urologist for further assessment and management, particularly if there are fertility concerns.

SPERMATOCELE

A spermatocele is usually a painless mass in the head of the epididymis that contains fluid and sperm. Since sperm are not produced until puberty, this lesion is never seen in preadolescents. Patients may complain of a scrotal mass that feels like "a third testicle."

Signs and Symptoms.

The spermatocele usually presents as a non-tender mass that is clearly distinct from and above the testicle on palpation. Larger spermatoceles may present as a turbid mass; smaller lesions may feel more nodular. A spermatocele can be transilluminated.

Diagnostic Studies.

History and physical exam are usually enough to confirm the diagnosis. A scrotal ultrasound is not necessary but will definitively confirm a spermatocele and rule out any testicular pathology. Lesions as small as 2 mm can be detected by ultrasound.

Testicular Mass

Any complaint of a testicular mass is considered cancer until proven otherwise.

History

The patient may report a painful or tender testicle, with a sudden or acute onset. Most patients are unable to report the length of time the lesion has actually been present. If a palpable mass is present, the patient may give history of increasing size and/or tenderness over a period of weeks or months.

Physical Examination

A thorough examination of the genitals is vital, despite the fact that it may cause discomfort to the patient. Pain or tenderness may be noted on the exam, and may localize to the testicle where a palpable mass can be felt, either continuous with the testicle or adjacent to it. There may or may not be inguinal adenopathy associated with the testicular pain.

Testicular Tumor

See p. 266.

Testicular Torsion

See p. 265.

Hydrocele

See p. 267.

Spermatocele

See p. 268.

Varicocele

See p. 268.

HEMATOMA

The patient describes a steadily enlarging, firm, and possibly painful mass located unilaterally in the scrotum. The mass can be of varying sizes. The key point is a recent history of some invasive procedure, such as a vasectomy, hydrocelectomy, spermatocelectomy, or trauma sustained during sports activities or a motor vehicle accident.

Signs and Symptoms.

The patient will complain of an enlarging mass that became noticeable within a few days after his surgical procedure. Physical exam will usually show a unilateral firm mass that is non-tender on palpation. Any complaints of pain are due to distortion and displacement of the surrounding structures.

Diagnostic Studies.

History is usually sufficient. A scrotal ultrasound is not necessary but will definitively confirm a hematoma and rule out any other pathology. Small hematomas can be expected to resolve over time as they are reabsorbed. Large hematomas may need to be drained; the patient should be referred back to the physician who performed the procedure.

Scrotal Mass

A scrotal mass can cause great concern for patient and clinician alike and may be detected by self-examination or during a routine physical. The key to diagnosing the mass is a thorough examination of the scrotal contents in an attempt to localize the mass and identify any associated structures.

History

The patient presents with complaints of a painful or nonpainful mass in the scrotum. He may provide a long history of its presence in the scrotum or a history of recently increasing size. There may also be discomfort associated with the mass, and it may worsen with activities such as running, weight lifting, or the Valsalva maneuver.

Physical Examination

A routine genital exam is required, with additional special maneuvers based on findings and the suspected cause.

Inguinal Hernia

See Table 10-1 and discussions in Chapter 10.

Hydrocele

See p. 267.

Varicocele

See p. 268.

SPERM GRANULOMA

After a vasectomy, sperm can leak from the testicular end of the vas, causing an inflammatory reaction and granuloma formation. This granuloma helps to vent the pressure that can build up in the epididymis after a vasectomy, as sperm production does not cease. It is commonly apparent on physical exam and can be mistaken for other scrotal pathology. It may also indicate that the patient has formed antibodies against his own sperm, which can complicate attempts at pregnancy after a vasectomy reversal.

Signs and Symptoms.

Usually no signs or symptoms are evident, other than a non-tender, firm mass at the end of the proximal vas deferens that can range in diameter up to 1 cm. In some cases, the granuloma may be tender on palpation.

Diagnostic Studies.

Diagnosis is based partly on the physical exam; a scrotal ultrasound is not necessary or indicated based on the history of a vasectomy, but it will definitively confirm a granuloma at the proximal end of the vas and rule out any other pathology.

Spermatocele

See p. 268.

Penile or Genital Lesions

Complaints of lesions on the genitals are a common presentation of otherwise healthy males. These lesions may be the result of a communicable disease or simply razor burn. Any sort of genital lesion is often a cause of significant anxiety to the patient. There are many additional, albeit less common, lesions that are not discussed in this section. If there is any uncertainty about the identification of a lesion, a referral to a urologist or dermatologist is appropriate.

History

The male patient may give a history of transient, recurrent, or nonhealing lesions to the penis or scrotum; there may also be a urethral discharge. The lesions may be described as small or moderately sized, or as blisters or papules. The patients may describe progressively worsening and increasingly painful lesions. There may be complaints of dysuria, urethral itching, or malaise.

Physical Examination

A thorough inspection is mandatory, including examination of the scrotal contents, distal urethra, and inguinal regions for adenopathy. The exam may also reveal scars that indicate previous lesions from sexually transmitted diseases. Examination and culture of lesions or discharge also may cause additional pain to the patient.

PENILE CANCER

Relatively rare in the United States, cancer of the penis is usually a squamous cell lesion that presents on the prepuce, glans, shaft, or base of the penis. If the lesion involves the glans, prepuce, or penile shaft, it is called erythroplasia of Queyrat; if it presents on the other aspects of the male genitalia or perineal region, it is called Bowen's disease. Risk factors include not being circumcised, a history of sexually transmitted diseases, particularly condyloma acuminatum, or a history of balanitis xerotica obliterans (BXO), which is discussed later in the chapter.

Signs and Symptoms.

Patients may complain of a nonhealing ulcer, erythema that does not resolve, induration of the skin, or a lesion with a warty appearance. Patients may also report a history of difficulty with foreskin retraction—the lesion being concealed by the foreskin.

There may be associated itching and/or burning with the lesion, and there may be visible ulceration of the penile tissue. Lesions are most common on the glans. On physical exam, the presentation of a lesion has a variety of appearances, including flat and erythematous or papillary, but is typically a well-marginated lesion. The tissue surrounding the lesion may feel less pliable than unaffected areas, and the foreskin of an uncircumcised male may be difficult to retract. The entire penis must be palpated to assess the possible extent of the lesion into the corpora and deeper tissues. There may be palpable inguinal adenopathy, and the lesion may show evidence of a secondary bacterial infection. A digital rectal exam (DRE) is necessary to evaluate for prostatic or urethral involvement.

Diagnostic Studies.

Definitive diagnosis is via biopsy; the patient should be referred urgently to a urologist for diagnosis and management. If inguinal adenopathy is present, the patient can be started on oral cephalosporins in advance of the urology appointment to attempt to treat any superimposed bacterial infection. A CT scan may be required to assess the extent of any inguinal adenopathy.

SEXUALLY TRANSMITTED DISEASE–RELATED LESIONS

There are many ways in which an STD can present in the male patient. Any complaint of lesions on the genitals should be thoroughly evaluated, including questioning the patient regarding his sexual conduct and frequency of new partners.

Signs and Symptoms.

Some STDs may be accompanied by complaints of constitutional symptoms or malaise. Refer to Table 11-3 for details of the lesion presentation on physical examination.

Diagnostic Studies.

Sexually transmitted diseases can be diagnosed with the appropriate cultures, gram stains, swabs, and serologic studies. Unless a patient appears ill and a WBC seems indicated, no additional lab work or imaging studies are indicated. Many STDs must be reported to the local health department. For complex, extensive, or refractory cases of genital warts, the patient can be referred to a urologist or dermatologist.

BALANITIS

Generally seen only in uncircumcised males, this is in inflammation of the glans, commonly caused by a *Candida albicans* infection. Men with poorly controlled diabetes mellitus are at particular risk for balanitis.

Table 11-3. ■ Sexually Transmitted Diseases and Their Presentation in the Male

Sexually Transmitted Disease	Clinical Presentation in the Male
Chancroid	Tender ulcer with deep undermined border, may be soft or indurated; friable base with ragged edges; purulent exudate possible; painful lymphadenopathy.
Chlamydia	Scant mucoid or mucopurulent urethral discharge; may be accompanied by mild dysuria and urethral itching.
Genital *Herpes simplex*	*1st episode:* Fluid-filled painful vesicles that may coalesce, with erythema to surrounding skin, and that eventually rupture, resulting in painful ulcerative lesions with erythematous edges; tender adenopathy, fever; dysuria also common. Lesions typically last 2–3 weeks, possibly up to 6 weeks.
	Recurrences: Prodromal pain, burning, tingling at site where vesicles will erupt with shorter course of constitutional symptoms; lesions usually resolve after 7–10 days.
Genital warts (human papillomavirus)	Soft, fleshy, exophytic lesions with raised granular surfaces; commonly seen on glans and prepuce; also present as small papular lesions on the skin or nonhealing penile lesion(s). The majority of lesions are subclinical and can be detected by using 3%–5% acetic acid.
Gonorrhea	Urethral discharge may be yellowish or gray-brown, purulent, and accompanied by itching and dysuria; may be accompanied by epididymal or testicular pain; asymptomatic in 5%–10% of cases; rare superficial lesions to the penile shaft.
Nongonococcal urethritis	Mild to moderate clear or white urethral discharge; or thin mucoid urethral discharge; accompanied by mild dysuria and urethral itching.
Pediculosis pubis	Severe pruritus; observation of ectoparasites on hair and/or skin in the genital area.
Scabies	Papular or linear burrow-like lesions.
Syphilis	*Primary:* Solitary, painless, non-tender, and rubbery ulcer (chancre), superficial or deep, with indurated edge and no exudate.
	Secondary: Papulosquamous or maculopapular rash that is indicative of systemic infection.
Trichomoniasis	Usually asymptomatic, may cause urethritis.

Signs and Symptoms.

The patient may present with a combination of symptoms that include edema, erythema, and pain of the glans; dysuria; urethral discharge; and a history of a discharge from between the foreskin and glans. Physical exam will confirm the edema, erythema, and exudates; there may be a cracked appearance to the prepuce. Palpation should always be done to the affected area to evaluate for changes in the consistency of the tissue. The patient should also be examined for any inguinal adenopathy.

Diagnostic Studies.

Any exudates should be cultured for STDs, and for other viral and fungal organisms; KOH (potassium hydroxide) and Tzanck preparations should also be included.

BALANOPOSTHITIS

This condition is generally seen only in uncircumcised males and is an inflammation that involves both the glans and foreskin.

Signs and Symptoms.

The presentation and physical exam are similar to those for balanitis but can include an edematous and painful foreskin that may not retract.

Diagnostic Studies.
Same as for balanitis.

BALANITIS XEROTICA OBLITERANS

This is a variation of lichen sclerosus et atrophicus, which is common in middle-aged men and is a painful condition associated with patches of white, thinned skin. Uncircumcised and diabetic males have an increased risk, and the patient with long-standing BXO has a higher risk for squamous cell carcinoma of the penis.

Signs and Symptoms.

Patients may complain of localized penile discomfort, painful erections, or urinary obstruction. On physical exam, there can be a whitish patch or patches on the prepuce or glans, and the meatus may become involved. The meatus itself may become edematous and indurated. As the condition progresses, there can be erosions, fissures, or meatal stenosis, and the foreskin may adhere to the glans.

Diagnostic Studies.

Diagnosis can be made only via biopsy. If suspected, a referral to a urologist is mandatory, particularly because meatal stenosis or urinary obstruction can occur over time.

TRAUMA

The patient may present with a history of some manner of trauma (including robust sexual activity or the use of an unlubricated condom) to the genitalia, with some resulting lesions. In the case of bruising to the genitals, the causative trauma may have happened a few days earlier. The patient may also admit to the use of some kind of penile enlargement device, with resulting trauma to the penis.

Signs and Symptoms.

Examination of the genitalia reveals ecchymotic areas on the penile shaft, scrotum, or glans. There may also be abraded areas on the genitalia.

Diagnostic Studies.

No lab work or imaging studies are indicated; the history should be sufficient to provide the diagnosis. If the resulting lesions are severe, or there is evidence of infection, a referral to a urologist is recommended.

The Inability to Retract or Advance the Foreskin

Complaints of difficulty manipulating the foreskin will occur only in males who have not been circumcised. These complaints are often accompanied by a history of chronic irritation or poor personal hygiene.

History

The patient will report difficulty at retracting the foreskin, possibly as complicated by a history of poor personal hygiene and/or a recent groin skin infection. Alternatively, there may be a history of pain and progressive difficulty with retraction. There may be complaints of the inability to advance the foreskin over the glans, possibly after a prolonged period of retraction. Pain may also be associated with any of these complaints.

Physical Examination

A thorough genital inspection is required, along with a gentle attempt to retract or advance the foreskin.

PHIMOSIS

This condition is seen only in males who are uncircumcised. The patient will often present with a history of progressive difficulty at retracting the foreskin and, in some cases, urinary obstruction. This is commonly preceded by poor personal hygiene, chronic balanitis or balanoposthitis, or poor control of diabetes mellitus. Long-standing phimosis will create a risk for chronic inflammation and squamous cell cancer of the penis.

Signs and Symptoms.

The patient may complain of pain when retracting or attempting to retract the foreskin, and possibly a "ballooning" of the foreskin when voiding. If the patient reports a complete inability to retract the foreskin, physical examination may show that the opening of the foreskin has contracted to the point at which the actual opening is quite small. There may be evidence of balanitis or balanoposthitis.

Diagnostic Studies.

History and presentation are usually sufficient to confirm the diagnosis. The patient should be referred to a urologist for further evaluation and management, as a dorsal slit or circumcision may be required.

PARAPHIMOSIS

This condition is one in which the foreskin has been retracted and cannot be advanced forward to it normal position over the glans. This is due to chronic inflammation under the foreskin and is also commonly preceded by poor personal hygiene, chronic balanitis or balanoposthitis, or poor control of diabetes mellitus. Over time a tight ring of tissue forms when the foreskin is retracted, resulting in additional edema to the glans with retraction of the foreskin.

Signs and Symptoms.

The patient may present with complaints of pain, swelling, and possible discoloration of the glans. Physical examination will reveal a foreskin that cannot be retracted or can be retracted with some difficulty; the shaft of the penis and glans may be tender/painful on palpation. There may be evidence of balanitis or balanoposthitis.

Diagnostic Studies.

History and presentation are usually sufficient to confirm the diagnosis. Any exudates should be cultured for STDs, and for other viral and fungal organisms; KOH and Tzanck preparations may also be included. *However*, this is a urologic emergency; the patient should be referred to a urologist for further evaluation and management because arterial occlusion and necrosis of the glans and distal urethra may result if the paraphimosis is not reduced.

Balanitis

See p. 271.

Balanoposthitis

See p. 272.

GENERALIZED EDEMA

The patient who suffers from generalized edema, such as that seen in cardiovascular or congestive heart failure patients, may also experience difficulty with advancing or retracting the foreskin.

Signs and Symptoms.

The complaints are similar to those for phimosis or paraphimosis. Physical examination shows a swollen glans; there may be discolored skin if this condition has persisted; the glans, penile shaft, and foreskin may be painful to palpation. Physical exam should also yield evidence of edema of the feet, legs, and possibly trunk, along with findings consistent with the causative condition(s).

Diagnostic Studies.

History and presentation are usually sufficient to confirm the diagnosis. The patient should be urgently referred to a urologist for management if paraphimosis is noted; otherwise, a routine referral to urologist for consideration of dorsal slit or circumcision in the case of phimosis, if personal hygiene becomes an issue (although any elective surgical intervention will be delayed by persistent edema).

The Absence of One or Both Testes in the Scrotum

The male may present at any age with the complaint of the absence of one or both testes in the scrotum. Evaluation of the testes is a required physical assessment point in male infants. But it is not uncommon that adolescent or adult males will present with this complaint in the absence of a surgical history that indicates a testicle was removed.

History

The patient (or possibly a parent if the patient is a minor) will complain of the absence of one or both testicles in the scrotum. If the patient is an adult, he may provide a history of difficulty conceiving with his female partner or a history of semen analysis abnormalities. If there is a failure of both testicles to descend, the patient may report late, or failure of, puberty onset. There may also be a history of inguinal or lower abdominal pain.

Physical Examination

Physical exam involves a genital exam that notes the absence of one or both testicles in the scrotum. It is vital to note the stage of development of secondary male characteristics. The patient may have a testicle that is palpable in the inguinal canal that can be tender on exam. There may be age-appropriate secondary sexual characteristics, particularly with one descended testicle.

CONGENITAL CRYPTORCHIDISM OR ECTOPIC TESTICLE(S)

This is the condition in which one or both testes have failed to descend normally into the scrotum. Descent may have stopped at any point between the renal and scrotal areas, but most commonly the undescended testes will be found in the inguinal canal. In male infants with undescended testes, more than half will descend into the scrotum during the first month after birth. There are no genetic abnormalities associated with this condition, and many males with a unilaterally undescended testicle do not have trouble initiating a pregnancy, despite decreased sperm counts. There is an increased risk of infertility owing to damage to the seminiferous tubules, depending on the length of time after birth the testes were brought down into the scrotal sac. The majority of patients with bilateral cryptorchidism become appropriately androgenized as adults but are at increased risk for inguinal hernias.

Signs and Symptoms.

There can be complaints of pain, as the testes may be in a position that is uncomfortable. The patient may complain of infertility. On physical exam, the scrotum on the affected side will be atrophic. The testes may be felt in the inguinal canal or not palpable at all. If the testicle is palpable, it cannot be manipulated into the scrotum. An inguinal hernia may also be present on the affected side. The stage of development of secondary sexual characteristics should be noted in postpubertal males.

Diagnostic Studies.

Ultrasound is usually successful if the suspected testis is in the groin; a CT scan or MRI will detect an intraabdominal testis in a postpubertal male. Lab work can include testosterone, follicle-stimulating hormone, and luteinizing hormone (FSH and LH, which may help differentiate intraabdominal from bilateral anorchia because both are significantly elevated in anorchia). A routine referral to a urologist for further evaluation and management should also be made.

SEVERE ATROPHY OF ONE OR BOTH TESTICLES

This can be the result of a mumps infection in the prepubertal male, although it is rare in this era of a successful mumps vaccine. The patient will give a history of mumps before puberty and will often relate a history of profound swelling of one of the testicles. Orchitis will result in approximately 30% of males who contract mumps, with approximately one-third of those developing testicular atrophy.

It is also possible to encounter severe atrophy of a testicle as the result of a varicocele that has been present for many years (see previous section on varicoceles for details).

Signs and Symptoms.

Possible signs include complaints of size differential between the testicles, or altered semen analysis. On physical exam, there will be pronounced testicular atrophy when compared with the unaffected side. The affected testicle is non-tender on exam and has a softer consistency.

Diagnostic Studies.

History and examination are usually sufficient. A scrotal ultrasound is not necessary but will definitively confirm the size differences and rule out any additional pathology.

KLINEFELTER'S SYNDROME

This is the most common abnormality of sexual differentiation, occurs in approximately 1 in 500 live births, is one of the most common causes of primary hypogonadism, and is the most common sex chromosome abnormality seen in infertile men. Patients will present with the typical triad of small, firm testes; gynecomastia; and elevated urine gonadotropins. Variants of Klinefelter's may also result in increased height, diabetes mellitus, obesity, and decreased intelligence. Although testicles are not absent, their small size may lead to lack of recognition as the testes.

Signs and Symptoms.

Patients complain of delayed completion of puberty and delayed virilization. There are usually few physical complaints associated with Klinefelter's disease, other than concern regarding testicle size in this context. There will be a lack of development of secondary sexual characteristics on physical exam (small [<3.0 cm] atrophic testes, small phallus, diminished body hair, diminished muscle bulk), and a feminine, or truncal, rather than male, fat distribution that often includes gynecomastia. Patients will be tall, due to a delay in the fusion of the epiphyseal plates in the long bones.

Diagnostic Studies.

Clinical suspicion will lead to diagnosis via karyotype analysis, which will show 47, XXY or a mosaic 46, XY/47, XXY. Hormone studies will demonstrate decreased or normal testosterone, decreased free testosterone, elevated estradiol, normal or elevated LH, and elevated FSH. A scrotal ultrasound is unnecessary, but would confirm the presence of and small size of the testes. If fertility is an issue, the patient should be routinely referred to a urologist specializing in male infertility, as semen analysis will show azoospermia.

PHYSIOLOGIC RETRACTILE TESTICLES OR MIGRATORY TESTES

The rare male patient may present with a history of one or both of his testicles "climbing into his belly" or inguinal canal. This is a normal variant due to a hyperactive cremasteric reflex. Usually it can be demonstrated in children and into puberty, at which point it resolves. Occasionally it can persist into adulthood. The patient will demonstrate normal male physiologic development.

Signs and Symptoms.

As stated, the patient will report that one or both testicles retract to the point that they are no longer palpable or visible in the scrotum. The important point of the physical examination is to locate the testicle(s) and gently manipulate it (them) into usual anatomic position(s). This does not usually cause the patient pain. The scrotum will also be normally developed, with no sign of atrophy.

Diagnostic Studies.

The history and examination is typically sufficient. A scrotal ultrasound will aid in the diagnosis. If there is any doubt or trouble locating a testicle, the patient may be referred to a urologist.

Erectile Function Complaints

Erectile Dysfunction

Male erectile dysfunction (ED) is an extremely common problem (Laumann, 1999) and may have far-reaching effects on the self-esteem and relationships of those involved. Some estimates give men with complete ED as numbering as many as 10–20 million in the United States alone; this number increases to an excess of 30 million men, if moderate to complete erectile dysfunction is also included. The worldwide incidence of ED is projected to rise to greater than 322 million men by 2025 (Ayta, 1999).

There are several underlying causes that contribute to ED: arteriogenic, venogenic, endocrinologic, neurologic, psychologic, and medicinal. Vascular disease is one of the most common causes of organic ED. Many epidemiological studies have shown that not only does ED coexist with hypertension, but also that as the severity of hypertension increases, so do reports of ED severity from patients. The incidence of ED in diabetic men has been quoted at 35% (Sullivan, 2001), but other investigators have reported this incidence ranging from 20% to 85%, with the incidence rising with age and degree of glycemic control. But many men will complain of erectile problems in the absence of any other currently diagnosed pathologies, and ED may provide a clue to the subtle onset of many systemic diseases. This is particularly true in patients who proceed to formal diagnoses of hypercholesterolemia, hypertension, or diabetes mellitus. However, a complete discussion of ED is beyond the scope of this chapter.

Erectile dysfunction can be successfully treated without knowing the precise nature of its cause.

History

The patient will often give a history of declining erectile function, usually insidious and progressive, and that may span the course of several years. Alternatively, he may provide a history of the relatively rapid or recent onset of decline in erectile function, perhaps associated with the history of recently starting new medication. Some degree of ED is a frequent complaint after prostate, bladder, rectal, or other retroperitoneal surgery.

The history should include several points specific to the patient's sexual functioning: the precise nature of the dysfunction (i.e., whether the problem is attaining or sustaining an erection, insufficient rigidity, penetration, or ejaculation); whether ED occurs with all sexual partners or only specific partners; psychosocial factors, including the nature of current relationship(s); the presence or absence of nocturnal and morning erections and their quality; and any treatments (pharmacologic and nonpharmacologic) that the patient has tried.

An assessment of the degree to which this condition has impacted the patient's quality of life is also important. This can be assessed using the Sexual Health Inventory for Men (SHIM), a short questionnaire that has been validated for the assessment of ED.

Physical Examination

If this is a complaint in a man with no other recognized medical conditions, a full physical examination is necessary. In the patient with recognized chronic conditions, the focus should be on the routine genital exam, along with a cardiovascular examination for cardiovascular risk assessment (Debusk et al., 2000).

Categories of Erectile Dysfunction

See Table 11-4, which is representative and is not all inclusive. Systemic disease–induced causes for ED are usually a combination of other etiologic categories. Medications that contribute to erectile dysfunction are listed in Table 11-5.

Diagnostic Studies

Based on the clinical suspicion for undiagnosed underlying disease, common causes of ED should be screened for with a testosterone level, urinalysis, CBC, glucose, BUN, serum

Table 11-4. ■ Categories of Erectile Dysfunction and Selected Examples

Category of ED	Examples of Causes
Arteriogenic	Atherosclerosis, hypertension, hyperlipidemia, smoking, pelvic trauma, diabetes mellitus
Cavernosal (venogenic)	Vascular disease, diabetes mellitus, Peyronie's disease, insufficient trabecular smooth muscle contraction, age
Endocrinologic	Hypogonadism, hyperprolactinemia, hyperthyroidism, hypothyroidism, diabetes mellitus, orchiectomy
Medication-induced	Antihypertensives, antidepressants, antipsychotics, EtOH abuse, smoking, antiandrogens, alpha-adrenergic blockers, beta-blockers, tranquilizers, thiazide diuretics, centrally acting sympatholytics, cimetidine, estrogens, polypharmacy, marijuana use, chemotherapy
Neurologic	Retroperitoneal surgery, SCI, MS, diabetes mellitus, pelvic trauma, spina bifida, CNS tumors, EtOH abuse, Parkinson's disease, Alzheimer's disease, CVA, pelvic irradiation
Psychologic	Performance anxiety, depression, psychological stress, relationship issues, psychotic disorders, misinformation or ignorance of normal anatomy/function
Systemic disease-induced	CRF, coronary heart disease, COPD (fear of inducing exacerbation), CHF, hepatic failure, recent MI, cirrhosis

Table 11-5. ■ Selected Medications That Have Been Reported to Contribute to Erectile Dysfunction

Medication Class	Selected Examples
Antiandrogenic medications	alpha-5 reductase inhibitors, LHRH analogues, leuprolide acetate
Anticholinergics	Diphenhydramine
Antihypertensives	Diuretics (thiazides), vasodilators, central sympatholytics (methyldopa, clonidine), beta-blockers, calcium-channel blockers, angiotensin-converting enzyme inhibitors
Benzodiazepines	Diazepam, clonazepam
Lipid-lowering agents	Lovastatin, pravastatin sodium
Miscellaneous medications	Cimetidine, lithium, baclofen
Monoamine oxidase inhibitors	Phenelzine, procarbazine
Recreational drugs	Alcohol, marijuana, barbiturates, opiates, nicotine
Tranquilizers	Haldol
Tricyclic antidepressants	Nortriptyline hydrochloride, amitriptyline hydrochloride

creatinine, and cholesterol profile. A free testosterone may also be considered, particularly if hypogonadism is suspected. If these tests are inconclusive, the patient can be referred to a urologist for further evaluation with specialized diagnostic testing, as well as management if first-line pharmacologic management is not sufficient. If the history and physical appear to suggest a stronger psychological than organic component to the complaints of ED, it can be suggested that a referral to a sexual counselor or therapist would be helpful.

Prolonged Erection

Priapism is the presence of a prolonged erection that occurs in the absence of sexual stimulation or that remains after orgasm. This condition usually affects only the corpora cavernosa of the penis. It is uncommon, and, although it can occur in any age group, it is more common from ages 20 to 50. Priapism is usually painful, and it is a urologic emergency. Failure to reverse the erection can result in scarring of the penile corpora and permanent erectile dysfunction owing to tissue ischemia. Unfortunately, there can be a significant time delay between the onset of priapism and the patient's presentation for evaluation and treatment.

History

The patient will complain of a persistent erection that did not resolve with cessation of sexual activity or after orgasm. The erection may have occurred spontaneously. He may complain of pain, depending on length of time penis has remained erect (pain does not usually occur until after 6–8 hours). He may also provide a history of the use of injectable erectogenic agents, sickle-cell disease, or a history of similar episodes that resolved painlessly after a couple of hours. It is vital to establish as accurately as possible the duration of the erection.

Signs and Symptoms

The patient will complain of a painful prolonged erection (does not have to be a 100% erection to be considered priapism), possible discoloration of skin, and pain on palpation of the penis. Sexual activity may or may not have preceded the onset of the priapism.

Physical Examination

A routine genital examination will establish the presence of an erection; the corpora will be partially to fully rigid, depending on the etiology of the priapism. The penis may be tender on exam. The penis feels somewhat tense and congested, but the corpus spongiosum and glans are of normal consistency. A DRE, abdominal exam, and neurologic exam should also be performed.

Selected Causes

See Table 11-6.

Diagnostic Studies

None: the history and presentation are usually sufficient. Priapism requires immediate referral to the nearest emergency department, and often requires evaluation by a urologist.

Curvature of the Penis

Male patients of any age may present with the complaint of curvature of the penis, which is usually noticeable only when the penis is erect. As men present at older ages, the likelihood that the curvature is congenital decreases, especially if they report that the erection was previously straight. The proper course of care for these patients is referral to a urologist for further examination and treatment, particularly in a case such as congenital penile corporal disproportion. Most complaints of curvature (in the absence of a clinically apparent plaque) are amenable to some type of surgical correction.

History

The patient will report a progressive curvature of the shaft of the penis with erection; the curve can occur at any site along the shaft of the penis. There may be a concurrent history of a decline in erectile function with the onset of curvature, as well as pain with erections. Some patients are able to relate a history of some sort of trauma to the shaft of the penis with resulting bruising and pain that preceded the onset of the curvature. Alternatively, the patient may give a history that curvature has "always" been present, with no pain associated with erections, no impact to erectile function, and merely cosmetic concerns.

Physical Examination

A routine genital exam is necessary, and a palpable plaque may be felt anywhere along the shaft of the penis. Plaque can also be absent, particularly if the history indicates that the curvature may be congenital.

PEYRONIE'S DISEASE

Although the precise cause of Peyronie's disease is not known, current belief regarding its etiology is that the plaque formation results after disordered wound healing, often with

---

Table 11-6. ■ Selected Causes of Priapism

Causes of Priapism	Explanation
Idiopathic (primary) priapism	Accounts for up to 60% of cases
Medication-induced priapism	Resulting after penile injection treatment for ED, some recreational or psychotropic drugs (cocaine, EtOH)
Priapism caused by other medical condition	Sickle cell disease, leukemia, pelvic tumor, spinal cord trauma, thromboembolic event, neoplastic causes due to metastases
Priapism due to trauma	Perineal or penile trauma can lead to high-flow (arterial) priapism

calcium deposition in the plaque (Levine & Elterman, 1997). During regular sexual activity, susceptible patients may suffer nonpainful minor trauma to the penis that leads to both a decrease in the elasticity of the tissue and fibroblast formation, eventually resulting in a plaque. The plaque is present in the tunica albuginea of the corpora cavernosa, which leads to shortening and curvature of the shaft of the penis. The resulting curvature can be in any direction: lateral, ventral, or dorsal. Often the quality of erection distal to the plaque is poor and prevents adequate penetration during sexual activity. Peyronie's disease is most commonly seen between the ages of 45 and 60, and complaints of erectile dysfunction may predate any curvature. Peyronie's disease can go into spontaneous remission, and there is a 30% association with Dupuytren's contracture of the tendons of the hand.

Signs and Symptoms.

The patient complains of curvature of the penis, noticeable with erections. The curve may be progressive or may have stopped curving. If it is painful, it is only while the penis is erect. Physical exam may yield evidence of a palpable plaque that involves the tunica albuginea; the plaque is commonly located at or near the dorsal midline of the shaft.

Diagnostic Studies.

History and physical exam are usually sufficient to confirm the diagnosis. A routine referral to a urologist can be considered for further treatment and possible surgical intervention.

PENILE CORPORAL DISPROPORTION

This is a relatively rare congenital condition in which the corpora cavernosa of the penis are not of identical length. This leads to painless curvature with erection; there are no associated erectile function complaints. The curvature will cause some distress to the patient, and he will seek evaluation to correct the curvature.

Signs and Symptoms.

The patient will describe curved erections, without a history of having previously had straight erections. On physical exam, the difference in between the corpora may be palpable. The patient will demonstrate age-appropriate development of secondary sexual characteristics.

Diagnostic Studies.

Diagnosis is typically through history and physical. Routine referral to a urologist is recommended; this condition can be corrected with surgery.

PENILE FRACTURE

This results in an acquired curvature of the penis and is the result of trauma during intercourse that causes a rupture to the tunica albuginea of one of the corpora cavernosa of the penis. The patient will present with a history of a lateral buckling of the penis and a "snap" heard during intercourse, typically when the woman is in the superior position. This is followed by possible bleeding from the urethra, loss of penile rigidity, and eventual ecchymosis of the penis. The trauma may also be less severe and result in a gradual curvature over time. Often there is an accompanying complaint of loss of rigidity or pain with subsequent erections. There may also be some disruption of the urethra.

Signs and Symptoms.

The patient will complain of decreased and/or painful erections. On physical exam (including GU, rectal, and lower abdominal exams), there may be a palpable indentation or scar at the site of the corporal rupture, and possibly ecchymosis of the scrotum. If the patient presents acutely, there may be blood at the meatus. Physical findings depend on the length of time since the injury.

Diagnostic Studies.

History and physical exam are usually sufficient to confirm the diagnosis. An urgent consult to a urologist should be made if the patient presents acutely. A routine referral to a urologist can be considered for further evaluation, treatment, and possible surgical intervention if the patient presents after the acute period.

Low Testosterone

Low testosterone is less a direct patient complaint than representative of a combination of symptoms. There may be discussion of moodiness, loss of interest in usual activities, loss of libido, fatigue, and even complaints of diminished muscle bulk. The key in its evaluation is establishing the cause of the low level of testosterone.

History

There is likely to be an insidious onset of some degree of ED, loss of libido, depressed mood, and fatigue. If this has been progressing over a significant length of time, there may also be decreased muscle mass and strength and loss of facial and body hair.

Physical Examination

A complete physical is necessary, including routine genital exam and DRE.

HYPOGONADISM

This is defined as failure of the testes to produce normal levels of testosterone (and/or sperm). Primary causes of hypogonadism are due to testicular failure; secondary causes are due to pituitary or hypothalamic causes. Combined hypogonadism is due to the decreased pulsatility of gonadotropins plus decreased testicular Leydig cell response. Hypogonadism is estimated to affect four to five million men in the United States alone; in aging males, the causes are more likely to be secondary causes. Hypogonadism represents the only cause of male infertility that can successfully be treated with hormone therapy, although the response is largely dependent on the length of time of the hypogonadism. However, a complete discussion is beyond the scope of this chapter. Table 11-7 summarizes several causes of hypogonadism.

Table 11-7. ■ Selected Causes of Hypogonadism

Primary Hypogonadism	Secondary Hypogonadism	Combined Hypogonadism
• Aging	• Aging	• Aging
• Chemotherapy/irradiation	• Hemochromatosis	• Cirrhosis
• Cryptorchidism	• Hypertrophic hypogonadism	• Sickle cell disease
• Chromosome abnormalities (e.g., Klinefelter's syndrome)	Kallmann's syndrome	
• Myotonic dystrophy	• Medication-induced (e.g., antiestrogens for treatment	
• Orchitis (e.g., mumps)	of prostate cancer)	
• Testicular loss from trauma, tumor	• Obesity	
	• Pituitary mass lesions	
	• Prolactinoma	
	• Psychological stress	
	• Uremia	

Signs and Symptoms.

In the adult male, hypogonadism is manifested by changes in sexual function, behavior, muscle mass, and some loss of secondary sexual characteristics. The patient may report mood and behavioral symptoms (depression, irritability, loss of motivation) in addition to complaints of lethargy or loss of energy. Physical exam may demonstrate some regression of secondary sexual characteristics such as hair loss and possible loss of muscle bulk. There is no change to penis or prostate size.

Diagnostic Studies.

Hypogonadism can be confirmed by checking a testosterone level; morning values are superior to afternoon blood samples because testosterone is secreted in the morning. If the patient is not available for morning lab draws, at least three afternoon values at close to the same time of day can provide an average testosterone value. If the total testosterone is low, a free testosterone level should be checked; a free testosterone level is the most accurate measurement of a significant deficiency. Additional hormones can also be evaluated (LH, FSH, estradiol, prolactin, thyroid profile) if secondary causes are suspected. An MRI is necessary if pituitary lesions are suspected. A semen analysis will show oligospermia or azoospermia in the patient with hypogonadism.

Congenital Hypogonadism

The most common variant of this is Klinefelter's syndrome. See p. 276.

OBESITY

Obesity can lead to the aromatization of testosterone in fatty tissue to estradiol, leaving lowered amounts of testosterone available for maintenance and virilization functions.

Signs and Symptoms.

The patient is a clinically obese male, with possible evidence of feminization or regression of secondary male sex characteristics found on physical exam.

Diagnostic Studies.

Testosterone and free testosterone levels, along with estradiol, LH and FSH levels should be done. Routine referral to an endocrinologist or urologist, preferably one with expertise in male infertility (if this is an issue) and andrology, is recommended.

ANDROPAUSE

This is a symptom complex in the presence of low levels of testosterone that can include a decline in libido and erectile function, as well as irritability and loss of the ability to concentrate. As males age, there is both decreased production of testosterone and decreased clearance beginning at age 40, but it is not analogous to menopause in women because men retain reproductive capacity, and not all men decline below the normal limits for serum testosterone. Many of the complaints that accompany the aging male have shown a weak correlation with plasma testosterone levels (Vermeulen, 2001).

Signs and Symptoms.

The patient may have a variety of complaints, including fatigue, truncal obesity, atrophic testes, loss of facial and pubic hair, and decreased muscle bulk. Additional complaints are similar to those for hypogonadism. Physical examination supports these complaints.

Diagnostic Studies.

Testosterone and free testosterone will confirm lowered levels, but should be drawn as early in the morning as possible. Androgen replacement is not without risk of reproductive malignancies; referral to a urologist or endocrinologist for management can be considered.

Complaints Related to Male Fertility and Sexual Function

Infertility

In 30% of all couples being evaluated for infertility, there is a clear, significant male factor alone involved; both male and female factors are present in approximately 20% of couples seeking an infertility evaluation (Sigman, Lipshultz, & Howards, 1997). Many of these male factors can be corrected, or improved, to the point at which the couple is able to conceive naturally or take advantage of less-expensive assisted reproductive technologies. An infertility evaluation is usually initiated after a 1-year history of unprotected intercourse that fails to achieve a pregnancy, although this length of time can be shortened as the female partner's age increases.

History

The patient may give a history of trying to achieve pregnancy for a lengthy period of time. It is vital to carefully detail the duration of the couple's infertility, previous pregnancies for either partner, the regularity of the female partner's menstrual cycle, the timing of intercourse in relation to ovulation, and the use of lubricants. Inquire about any established abnormal semen analysis that may have been ordered by the female partner's clinician. There may also be a history of male or female siblings (or members of extended family) who have had trouble conceiving. Several aspects of the male's medical history are particularly important: any specific childhood illnesses (e.g., mumps, orchitis), a history of cryptorchidism, the timing of puberty, and any GU or abdominal surgeries as an infant or child.

It is possible for a couple to present with a history of little difficulty achieving a first pregnancy and yet be unsuccessful in establishing a second pregnancy (secondary infertility).

Physical Examination

A complete physical examination may demonstrate that the male has failed to attain secondary male sex characteristics, lacks the vas deferens, or is obese. A careful GU examination is required. The physical examination may be completely normal.

Varicocele

See p. 268.

Hypogonadism

See p. 282. See also sections on cryptorchidism, testicular atrophy, and Klinefelter's disease.

CONGENITAL BILATERAL ABSENCE OF THE VAS DEFERENS

Congenital bilateral absence of the vas deferens is a genetic abnormality that is seen with cystic fibrosis (CF) and its variants. If not previously diagnosed with cystic fibrosis, the patient may present with a history of chronic bronchitis requiring hospitalization, recurrent respiratory infections as a child and adolescent, or asthma or an asthma-like condition. There are usually no other physical complaints. There may be a family history of infertility or persistent respiratory illnesses.

Male CF patients frequently demonstrate malformation of the epididymis; the vas deferens, seminal vesicles, and ejaculatory ducts are atrophic or absent. However, spermatogenesis is usually normal. It is possible that the patient has a much more rare unilateral absence of the vas deferens.

Signs and Symptoms.

Usually there are no signs and symptoms other than infertility, if the patient has not been previously diagnosed with CF. Physical examination may show complete absence of the vas deferens unilaterally or bilaterally, or a palpable gap in the vas deferens. Testes are usually of normal size and consistency, and the patient will demonstrate normal libido and secondary sexual characteristics.

Diagnostic Studies.

Physical examination is usually sufficient to confirm the absence of the vas deferens. Testosterone levels will be normal. Because this is a genetic abnormality, referrals to a urologist with expertise in male infertility, a reproductive endocrinologist, and a medical genetics consultation to discuss genetic analysis of the couple should be encouraged, as establishing a pregnancy will require high-level assisted reproductive technologies.

EXOGENOUS TESTOSTERONE SUPPLEMENTATION OR ANABOLIC STEROID USE

Supplementation with testosterone or with testosterone-like substances can result in decreased endogenous testosterone and decreased LH, and result in hypogonadotropic hypogonadism and suppressed spermatogenesis. Hypogonadism induced by exogenous steroid use is usually temporary, and endogenous hormone production and spermatogenesis rebounds after approximately 4 months.

Signs and Symptoms.

The patient may complain of increased or decreased libido and possible erectile dysfunction. Patients using anabolic steroids may also have skeletal muscle hypertrophy, acne, gynecomastia, and striae. There may be some noticeable testicular atrophy on exam.

Diagnostic Studies.

Semen analysis will show oligospermia or azoospermia, and total testosterone will be above the normal range (or supraphysiologic with anabolic use) (Table 11-8). Levels of LH and FSH will be decreased. Routine referral to a urologist, preferably one with expertise in male infertility and andrology, is recommended.

Ejaculatory Dysfunction

In some cases of ejaculatory dysfunction, the cause is idiopathic, and may be caused by a failure of bladder neck closure. Men with diabetes can develop retrograde ejaculation. Neurologic disease, such as multiple sclerosis and spinal cord injury, can lead to retrograde

Table 11-8. ■ Normal Values in Semen Analysis

Semen Parameters	Normal Values
• Morphology	≥15% normal forms
• Motility	≥50%
• Total concentration	≥20 million
• Volume	2.0–5.0 ml

Adapted from Rowe, P.J., et al. (2000). WHO Manual for the Standardized Investigation, Diagnosis and Management of the Infertile Male. Cambridge: Cambridge University Press.

ejaculation or anejaculation. Genitourinary infections can also contribute to ejaculatory dysfunction, commonly owing to obstruction of the vas deferens or ejaculatory ducts.

History

The patient may present with complaints of cloudy urine after ejaculation, hematospermia, possible recent-onset anejaculation, oligospermia or azoospermia with a low-volume ejaculate on semen analysis, and a history of retroperitoneal or bladder neck surgery or neurologic disease. There may also be complaints related to a decreased amount of ejaculate, a decreased volume of ejaculate, or the inability to ejaculate. It is possible that ejaculatory dysfunction will present during a male infertility evaluation.

Physical Examination

A routine GU exam is needed, which is usually benign, as well as a careful inspection of the abdomen to examine for surgical scars.

SELECTED CAUSES

Refer to Table 11-9.

Signs and Symptoms.

The signs and symptoms are as described in the preceding history subsection; a normal exam is obtained, with the exceptions relevant to the preceding differentials.

Diagnostic Studies.

Order a semen analysis—antegrade and retrograde semen analysis if retrograde ejaculation suspected. The evaluation of the semen sample will show a fructose-negative, acidic pH, azoospermic sample if obstructed. Routine referral to a urologist for further evaluation and treatment is necessary.

Painful Ejaculation

Male patients may occasionally complain that they experience pain with or following ejaculation. This can be distressing, and over time may cause avoidance of sexual activity, which in turn can affect the quality of the relationship with the partner.

History

The patient will describe pain on ejaculation, usually of relatively recent onset. The pain may localize to a specific scrotal structure or radiate into the testes. There also may be complaints of a decreased volume to the ejaculate, hematospermia, or difficulty with bowel movements.

Table 11-9. ■ Selected Causes of Ejaculatory Dysfunction

Selected Causes	Example
Anatomic	Congenital bilateral absence of the vas deferens, obstruction of seminal vesicles, bladder neck abnormalities, retrograde ejaculation
Functional	Premature ejaculation
Medical	SSRIs, MAOIs, alpha-blockers, antipsychotics, benzodiazepines, EtOH, methadone
Neurologic	Diabetes mellitus, spinal cord injury, multiple sclerosis
Surgical	Bladder reconstructive surgery, retroperitoneal lymph node dissection, radical prostatectomy, TURP, cystoprostatectomy

Physical Examination

The exam will include a careful inspection and palpation of the scrotal contents and a DRE.

EJACULATORY DUCT OBSTRUCTION

In this condition, one or both of the ducts leading from the seminal vesicles into the prostate become partially or completely blocked. This causes only prostatic fluids to contribute to the ejaculate volume, thus resulting in decreased volume, possible hematospermia, and possible azoospermia, if both ducts are blocked. There is an increased risk of obstruction associated with recent GU instrumentation or repeated urinary tract infections.

Signs and Symptoms.

Testes are usually normally sized. If the obstruction is long-standing, there may be evidence of epididymal induration on physical exam. A digital rectal exam may demonstrate distended seminal vesicles, but this condition is often difficult to distinguish.

Diagnostic Studies.

The ejaculate will be of low volume, acidic, and with no sperm, fructose, or coagulation factors on a semen analysis. Routine referral to a urologist is indicated, particularly if fertility is an issue.

Epididymitis/Orchitis

See pp. 266 and 267.

Prostatitis

See Chapter 10, p. 246.

Hematospermia

Changes to the ejaculate can cause concern for the male patient. Although this is a relatively uncommon complaint, it does have some common causes.

History

If the patient or patient's partner complains of blood in the ejaculate; it may have been present intermittently for several months preceding the patient's presentation. The ejaculate will be pink, reddish (new blood), or brownish tinged (old blood). The presence of blood may be intermittent or with each ejaculate, there may be a history of recent GU instrumentation, or the patient may describe some sense of pressure with ejaculation.

Physical Examination

A routine GU exam is necessary, including DRE.

Ejaculatory Duct Obstruction

See p. 287.

Prostatitis

See Chapter 10, p. 246.

Benign Prostatic Hyperplasia

See Chapter 10, p. 246.

RECENT GU PROCEDURE

It is possible to have several episodes of hematospermia after a prostate biopsy, resection of the prostate, incision, or other procedure that involves trauma to the prostate. In this case, the hematospermia will be transient and self-limited and is usually not associated with pain.

Signs and Symptoms.

The patient will complain of blood in the ejaculate.

Diagnostic Studies.

History of recent procedure involving the prostate will confirm the diagnosis.

References

Ayta, I.A., McKinlay, J.B., & Krane, R.J. (1999). The likely worldwide increase in erectile dysfunction between 1995 and 2025 and some possible policy consequences. *BJU International,* 84(1): 50–56.

DeBusk, R., Drory, Y., Goldstein, I., et al. (2000). Management of sexual dysfunction in patients with cardiovascular disease: Recommendations of the Princeton Consensus Panel. *American Journal of Cardiology,* 86: 175–81.

Laumann, E.O., Paik, A., & Rosen, R.C. (1999). Sexual dysfunction in the United States: Prevalence and predictors. *Journal of the American Medical Association,* 281: 537–544.

Levine, L.A., & Elterman, L. (1997). Peyronie's disease and its medical management. In Hellstrom, W.J.G. (Ed.), *Male Infertility and Sexual Dysfunction.* New York: Springer.

Rowe, P.J., Comhaire, F.H., Hargreave, T.B., & Mahmoud, A.M.A. (2000). *WHO Manual for the Standardized Investigation, Diagnosis and Management of the Infertile Male.* Cambridge: Cambridge University Press.

Sigman, M., Lipshultz, L.I., & Howards, S.S. (1997). Evaluation of the subfertile male. In Lipshultz, L.I., & Howards, S.S. (Eds.), *Infertility in the Male* (3rd ed.) St. Louis: Mosby.

Sullivan, M.E., Keoghane, S.R., & Miller, M.A.W. (2001). Vascular risk factors and erectile dysfunction. *BJU International,* 87: 838–845.

Vermeulen, A. (2001). Androgen replacement therapy in the aging male: A critical evaluation. *Journal of Clinical Endocrinology and Metabolism,* 86(6): 2380–2390.

Chapter 12

Female Reproductive System

G
ynecological complaints account for more than 65,000 visits annually, and more than 8% of the total yearly office visits (Center for Health Statistics, 2004). Endometrial cancer is the most common genital cancer in women. For the year 2000, there were more than 36,000 new cases, accounting for 6,500 deaths (Dorigo & Goodman, 2003). The fifth most common cancer and fifth most frequent cause of death in women is ovarian cancer, with the highest incidence in postmenopausal women (Dorigo & Baker, 2003). Cervical cancer accounts for over 4,000 deaths annually with approximately 13,000 new cases of diagnosed annually (Holschneider, 2003).

Laurie Grubbs

ANATOMY AND PHYSIOLOGY

Figures 12-1 and 12-2 show the major structures of the female reproductive system. Figure 12-3 depicts the menstrual cycle.

Reproductive Hormones

- Estrogen—a group of estrogenic hormones, termed the female hormones, produced by the ovary. Estrogens are responsible for the development of secondary sexual characteristics in the female and for cyclic changes in the vaginal epithelium and uterine endometrium.
- Progesterone—a steroid hormone secreted by the corpus luteum and placenta that is responsible for changes in the endometrium in the luteal phase of the menstrual cycle making implantation possible. It is used in combination with estrogen in oral contraceptives.
- Follicle-stimulating hormone (FSH)—a hormone produced by the anterior pituitary that stimulates the graafian follicles of the ovary for follicular maturation and secretion of estradiol.
- Luteinizing hormone (LH)—a hormone produced by the anterior pituitary that stimulates ovulation, which involves rupture of the

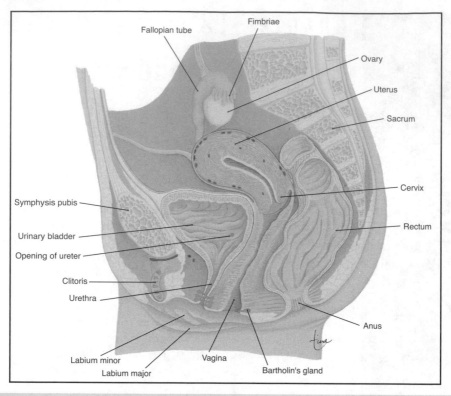

Figure 12-1. ■ Internal female genitalia. (From Scanlon, VC, and Sanders, T. Essentials of Anatomy and Physiology, 4th ed. Philadelphia, FA Davis, 2003, p. 441. Reprinted with permission.)

mature ovarian follicle, transformation of the follicle into the corpus luteum, and secretion of progesterone and estrogen by the corpus luteum.

- Prolactin level (PRL)—a hormone produced by the pituitary gland that stimulates breast development and lactation during pregnancy, in conjunction with estrogen and progesterone. In the postpartum period, sucking by the infant stimulates prolactin so milk continues to be produced. Elevations in prolactin in the female can cause amenorrhea, galactorrhea, and infertility, and in the male, impotence. These symptoms in a patient should alert the examiner to the possibility of a pituitary tumor.
- Estradiol—a steroid produced by the ovary that is a component of estrogen. It is found in large quantities in pregnant women. In the body, it is converted to estrone, another of the estrogenic hormones.
- Testosterone—an androgen and principal hormone produced by the testicle. Some testosterone is also produced by the adrenal cortex in both males and females. It is responsible for the development of secondary sexual characteristics and for sexual function in the male. It also accounts for the larger muscle mass in men compared with women, and for distribution of fat in the male. It affects blood flow and other metabolic activities.

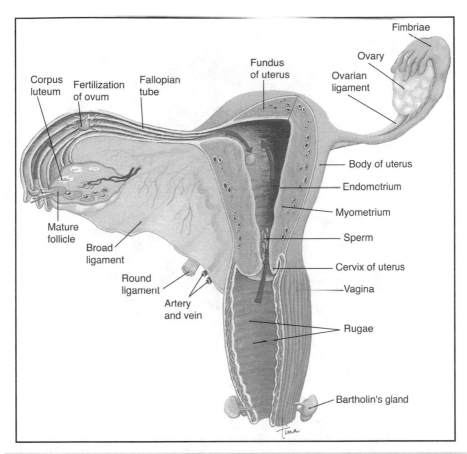

Figure 12-2. ■ Internal structures of adnexa. (From Scanlon, VC, and Sanders, T. Essentials of Anatomy and Physiology, 4th ed. Philadelphia, FA Davis, 2003, p. 442. Reprinted with permission.)

- Thyroid-stimulating hormone (TSH)—a hormone produced by the anterior pituitary that stimulates the thyroid gland to secrete thyroxine and triiodothyronine.

HISTORY
General History

The gynecological history is complex, and complaints should not be treated lightly. The gynecological cancers may present with vague, nonspecific complaint and an index of suspicion is necessary for early diagnosis and treatment. Last menstrual period is one of the most important questions to ask, particularly when prescribing medications because many are contraindicated in pregnancy. If menstrual cycles are not regular, pregnancy should be ruled out first, and then other diagnoses can be considered. The menstrual history includes any episodes of amenorrhea, menorrhagia (excessive bleeding at the time of the menstrual cycle), metrorrhagia (bleeding at irregular noncyclic intervals), dysmenorrhea, and

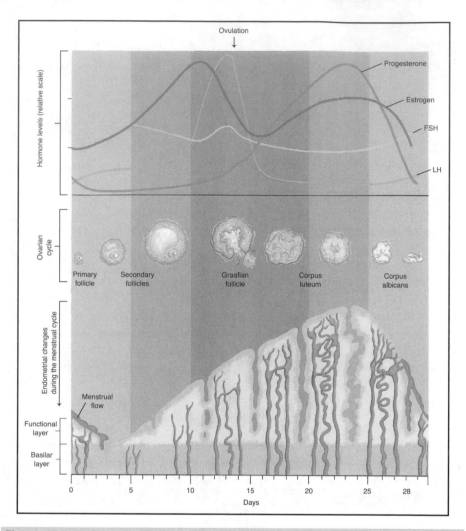

Figure 12-3. ■ The menstrual cycle. (From Scanlon, VC, and Sanders, T. Essentials of Anatomy and Physiology, 4th ed. Philadelphia, FA Davis, 2003, p. 447. Reprinted with permission.)

postmenopausal bleeding. Amenorrhea has many causes, including pregnancy; anorexia nervosa; excessive exercise; low body fat; and disorders or tumors of the hypothalamus, pituitary gland, ovary, uterus, and thyroid gland. Menorrhagia is most commonly caused by uterine fibroids, but hematologic disorders should be considered. Metrorrhagia can be caused by anovulation, intrauterine devices (IUDs), and ovarian and uterine tumors. Primary dysmenorrhea is common and generally does not indicate pathology, particularly in the young population. It is most severe in the first few days of the menstrual cycle. Secondary amenorrhea can occur with fibroids, IUDs, cervical stenosis, and pelvic inflammatory diseases. The pain is more persistent with menstrual flow and, occasionally, nausea, vomiting, or fever accompanies the pain. Bleeding that occurs after menopause has been established is cause for concern. It may indicate endometrial cancer and referral for endometrial biopsy, or D and C is warranted. If the patient is menopausal, ask about age of menopause, symptoms of menopause, and past or current use of hormone replacement therapy (HRT).

Ask the patient about the type of birth control being used, if any. If the patient is not in a monogamous relationship, ask about condom use. Be sure to inquire as to the consistency with which they use birth control methods. Often patients deny the use of birth control, deny the desire for pregnancy, and yet admit to being sexually active. This definitely indicates the need for health teaching and counseling.

Inquire about any masses or lesions that the patient may feel on the external genitalia, which could indicate infection, sexually transmitted disease (STD), vulvar malignancy, Bartholin's or Skene's gland infection/inflammation, uterine prolapse, cystocele, or rectocele.

If the patient complains about vaginal discharge, inquire as to the amount, color, consistency, odor, itching, burning, inflammation, or lesions, and history of STDs.

Dyspareunia is one symptom that patients may be reluctant to mention or discuss, so specific inquiries should be made by the practitioner. Dyspareunia may accompany infections that are due to the inflammation of the vaginal mucosa, uterus, or pelvic structures, vaginal dryness or atrophy usually seen in postmenopausal women; fibroids; endometriosis; sexual difficulties; or psychosomatic illnesses.

Infertility may be caused by anovulation, decreased function of the corpus luteum, or blocked or scarred fallopian tubes. Any of these can occur, in spite of the fact that the patient may be having menstrual cycles. A history of menstrual irregularities may suggest anovulation or thyroid disease, either of which can cause infertility. A history of STDs could lead to scarring of the tubes. If the patient has not already done so, ask her to chart her menstrual cycles and basal body temperatures for 3 months to determine if, and when, ovulation is occurring.

Past Medical History

Past medical history includes age at menarche, menstrual irregularities, gynecological surgeries or procedures, history of ovarian cysts or uterine fibroids, endometriosis, infertility, STDs, and chronic diseases that might impact hormonal or menstrual function—the most common one being thyroid disease. Ask the patient about past or present use of medications, such as oral contraceptives, hormone replacement therapy, fertility drugs, or thyroid medicine. An obstetrical history should be obtained that includes pregnancies, live births, miscarriages, and abortions.

Habits

The matter of sexual activity and sexual partners is one of the more important areas to inquire about, especially with the high risk of HIV and other STDs. Multiple sexual partners, even in the absence of STDs, puts women at risk for infection with human papilloma virus (HPV). Smoking may also be a contributing factor in the development of HPV infection. Exercise habits, if extremely rigorous or excessive, can contribute to menstrual irregularities. Stress, if significant and prolonged, can cause menstrual irregularities. The use of drugs or alcohol may put women at risk for promiscuous behavior, unsafe sexual practices, or even "date rape."

PHYSICAL EXAMINATION

Patients are often uncomfortable with the gynecological exam, so it is important to spend a sufficient amount of time taking the history and establishing a rapport before beginning the exam. A thorough explanation of the exam both before and as you are doing the exam will help allay the patient's fears. Be sure to have the patient empty her bladder before beginning. The exam should start with an abdominal exam, then examination of the external genitalia, and followed by the speculum and bimanual exam.

Order of the Examination

Inspection

Inspect the abdomen for any signs of masses, visible pulsations, peristaltic waves, or swelling, which might indicate ascites. Inspect the lower extremities for edema, which can be attributed to many things, one of which is lymphedema secondary to a malignancy. Inspect the external genitalia for lesions, ulcerations, inflammation, warts, swelling, discharge, or nodules. Inspect the perineum and anal areas for fissures, hemorrhoids, inflammation, lesions, ulcers, warts, or nodules. Assess the support of the vaginal outlet by asking the patient to bear down while you look for bulging at the introitus, suggesting a cystocele, rectocele, or prolapsed uterus. Observe the Bartholin's and Skene's glands for inflammation or swelling.

Auscultation

Auscultate the abdomen before beginning the gynecological examination. Listen for bowel sounds and bruits. Note any abnormalities in the bowel sounds. Gynecological malignancies can cause abnormalities of bowel sounds owing to peritoneal inflammation, infection, ascites or gastrointestinal obstruction.

Percussion

Percuss the abdomen, paying particular attention to the suprapubic area and the right and left lower quadrants. An enlarged uterus will percuss dull in the suprapubic region. Other masses or inflammation will cause dullness or rebound tenderness as a result of peritoneal irritation. Percuss for shifting dullness in the abdomen, indicating ascites, which may be the first sign of ovarian cancer.

Palpation

Palpate the abdomen for rebound tenderness, ascites, or masses. Palpate the inguinal lymph nodes for swelling or tenderness. Sexually transmitted diseases often cause inguinal lymphadenopathy with tenderness. Ovarian cancer that has metastasized to the lymph system will cause inflammation and swelling of the lymph nodes in the inguinal area.

Speculum Examination

In addition to the Pap smear samples, the standard of practice generally includes cervical samples for gonorrhea and chlamydia, and these should be taken first. Next obtain the Pap smear samples from the endocervix, cervix, and vaginal pool. If the patient has had a hysterectomy, obtain samples from the vaginal cuff, and be sure to mark the cytology slip accordingly.

Observe the cervix for inflammation, lesions, growths, nodules, discharge, or bleeding. A parous cervix will be more open and may show healed lacerations. The cervix of a pregnant woman will be purplish in color. Cervical polyps are common and appear as pedunculated, teardrop growths from the cervical os.

Observe the vaginal walls for inflammation, discharge, color changes, or ulcers. Infection can cause discharge and redness of the vaginal walls. Menopause causes the vaginal walls to be pale and smooth as opposed to the normal pink and rugose. Varicose veins may be seen on the sides of the vaginal walls mostly in pregnant and obese women.

Bimanual Examination

The bimanual exam is performed to determine the position, size, shape, consistency, and mobility of the uterus and ovaries. It is also used to assess tenderness that might be associated with inflammation, infection, or cysts.

The uterus should be pear-shaped, smooth, mobile, non-tender, and firm, but not hard. Malignancies may occur causing the uterus to be hard and fixed. Fibroids present as firm, nodular growths. Ultrasound or a computerized tomographic (CT) scan is needed to determine whether the growths are benign fibroids or malignant growths. Tenderness with movement of the cervix and uterus occurs in pelvic inflammatory disease, termed cervical motion tenderness.

Variations in the position of the uterus are not considered abnormal, but significant variations may be related to back pain especially during menses or childbirth, and, occasionally, to infertility. Figure 12-4 shows the common uterine positions (normal, retroverted, retroflexed, anteverted, anteflexed). The uterus can be situated in the midline, posteriorly toward the sacrum, or anteriorly toward the abdominal wall, termed normal, retroverted, or anteverted, respectively. The long axis of the uterus can also be bent over on itself either backward or forward, termed retroflexed or anteflexed. A digital rectal examination is useful for indirect palpation of the uterus. It is particularly helpful if the uterus is retroverted or retroflexed.

The ovaries are small and almond-shaped, smooth, mobile, non-tender, and firm. Ovaries are more difficult to palpate because of their small size and anatomical location. Ovaries are normally slightly tender on palpation. Ovarian cysts or inflammation cause a significant increase in tenderness that is easy to diagnose. Unilateral adnexal pain and tenderness in an early pregnant woman should alert you to the possibility of a tubal pregnancy, considered a surgical emergency. Malignancies may result in nodular, enlarged, hard, and fixed ovaries, but the cancer may have been present for some period of time before the physical exam signs are detected. Any masses or abnormalities on palpation of the uterus or ovaries warrant prompt ultrasound or CT.

DIFFERENTIAL DIAGNOSIS OF CHIEF COMPLAINTS
Mass and/or Swelling at the Introitus

Vaginal infections or malignancies may lead to irritation and swelling of the external genitalia. Swelling and/or infection of a Bartholin's gland is common and presents as a very painful, inflamed, tender cyst on either side of the introitus. Non-tender masses include uterine prolapse, cystocele, and rectocele. Occasionally, pregnant women develop painful, varicose veins in the vagina that appear swollen and purplish in color. Inspection and

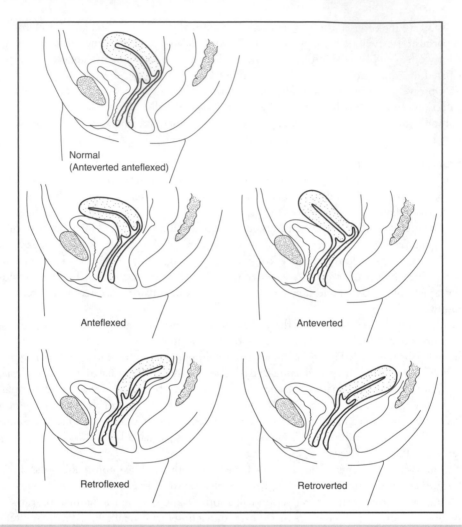

Normal
(Anteverted anteflexed)

Anteflexed

Anteverted

Retroflexed

Retroverted

Figure 12-4. ■ Common uterine positions. (From Swartz, M.1998, Textbook of Physical Diagnosis, 3rd ed. Philadelphia, WB Saunders, 1998, p 442. Reprinted with permission.)

palpation are most helpful in the diagnosis. Laboratory and diagnostics are usually not necessary for initial diagnosis. Referrals to the surgeon or gynecologist are necessary for treatment in most cases.

History

A childbirth history is important in patients with this complaint because difficult or numerous childbirths may lead to problems with the pelvic support structures or damage to the bladder or rectal wall. Any change in elimination patterns is one of the most important questions to ask this group of patients. Ask about urinary incontinence or more frequent urinary tract infections. Uterine prolapse and cystocele can cause frequency,

Red Flags for Examination of the Female Reproductive System

- Significant unilateral adnexal pain in an early pregnant female
- Frank uterine bleeding in a pregnant female
- Frank uterine bleeding in a postpartum or postabortion patient for more than 7 days
- Fever or significant abdominal pain in a postpartum or postabortion patient
- Free fluid in the peritoneal cavity (ascites)
- Uterine bleeding in a postmenopausal patient
- A uterus or ovaries that are fixed, hard, or nodular on palpation

incontinence, and residual urine, thus increasing the risk for urinary tract infections. Ask about changes in bowel movements, such as constipation, difficulty with evacuation, and rectal fullness, which could be symptoms of a rectocele. Ask about recurrent infections in the Bartholin's gland, which are sometimes, but not always, related to STDs.

Physical Examination

A thorough pelvic exam including a speculum and bimanual exam are necessary. Assess for support of the vaginal outlet. It may be possible to visualize a mass or swelling in the vaginal area on inspection. If not, ask the patient to strain down while you insert your finger into the vaginal opening. Feel for the mass to come to meet your finger when the patient bears down. Palpate superiorly, inferiorly, and on the sides over the Bartholin's glands for swelling and tenderness.

UTERINE PROLAPSE

Uterine prolapse is a downward placement of the uterus into the vaginal canal. It occurs more in older, multiparous women as a result of injury, weakening, and stretching of the pelvic musculature and ligaments. Prolapse can be due to traumatic vaginal delivery, multiple births, chronic straining, pelvic tumors, and obesity. It may take years for the prolapse to develop, which partly explains why it is seen more often in older women. Prolapse of the uterus is often accompanied by cystocele and rectocele.

Signs and Symptoms. Early on, the patient may complain of a full feeling in the vaginal area or may be unaware that the uterus is prolapsed until it is discovered on physical exam. As the uterus prolapses further, the patient will feel a mass at the introitus or even protruding from the vagina. The patient may also have complaints of urinary frequency or incontinence owing to pressure on the bladder from the uterus. Kegel exercises and estrogen therapy, either oral or vaginal, can be used as prevention or treatment of mild prolapse. The use of a pessary will hold the uterus in place and lessen symptoms. Surgical intervention may be required, particularly when cystocele and rectocele are present.

Diagnostic Studies. The diagnosis is made by physical exam, although pelvic ultrasound may help to rule out other conditions. The degree of prolapse depends on the degree of weakness of pelvic support.

- In 1st-degree uterine prolapse, the uterus partially descends into the vagina.
- In 2nd-degree uterine prolapse, the uterus descends into the introitus.
- In 3rd-degree uterine prolapse, the uterus can be visualized outside of the vagina, and often the vagina becomes inverted.

CYSTOCELE

A cystocele occurs when a portion of the bladder herniates into the vagina. Similar to uterine prolapse, it is the result of weakness of the supporting muscles and ligaments, and cystocele often accompanies uterine prolapse.

Signs and Symptoms.

Although a cystocele can contribute to urinary frequency, urgency, and infection, it is not the only cause of stress incontinence, and surgical repair of the cystocele may not resolve the incontinence. The bimanual exam reveals a smooth, soft, bulge of the anterior vaginal wall that may be more pronounced with straining. Kegel exercises may be helpful, but surgical repair may be needed.

Diagnostic Studies.

Pelvic ultrasound, CT scan, or magnetic resonance imaging (MRI) of the abdomen and pelvis, and videocystourethrography are all useful tools for the diagnosis of cystocele.

RECTOCELE

A rectocele occurs when a portion of the connective tissue of the rectal wall herniates into the vagina. As in uterine prolapse and cystocele, rectocele occurs more often in multiparous women as they age. Breech deliveries and episiotomies also may contribute to the development of a rectocele.

Signs and Symptoms.

Patients are often asymptomatic but may complain of difficulty defecating, constipation, incomplete evacuation, or a feeling of rectal fullness. Rectovaginal exam reveals a soft bulge in the posterior vaginal wall.

Diagnostic Studies.

Along with the history, MRI and cystoproctography can aid in the diagnosis of rectocele. Tumors often give rise to symptoms similar to those of rectocele, and must be ruled out. Surgical repair is indicated when it obstructs and impairs fecal evacuation.

BARTHOLIN'S CYSTS

The two Bartholin's glands are mucus-secreting glands located one in each lateral wall of the vagina at the introitus. They can become abscessed in acute or chronic inflammatory processes usually as a result of STD infection or from other bacteria that are prevalent in the vaginal and perineal area, but also by thickened mucus or congenital narrowing of the duct. In postmenopausal women, a malignant cause should be considered in the differential diagnosis.

Signs and Symptoms.

Acutely, Bartholin's abscesses are extremely painful, in part due to their anatomical location, which makes sitting difficult. The area becomes swollen, with the presence of a tender, inflamed, fluctuant cyst that is easily visualized. Systemic symptoms are usually absent. The cysts generally require incision and drainage (I & D), and a Word catheter may be necessary to keep the cyst open and draining until it is completely cleared. In addition to I & D, an oral antibiotic is necessary to clear the infection. Marsupialization is often adequate to treat the abscess, but, in recurrent cases, removal of the entire gland may be necessary. The cysts often become chronically inflamed, in which case surgery may be indicated. Occasionally, solid malignant tumors can occur in the Bartholin's glands and will need prompt referral. Other considerations include vaginal wall cysts (Gartner's duct cysts), Skene's gland cysts, or urethral diverticulum although the latter two are located superiorly to the Bartholin's gland. As previously mentioned, malignancy should always be considered in the postmenopausal woman.

Diagnostic Studies.

The diagnosis is made by physical examination. A culture and sensitivity (C & S) of the fluid drained from the cyst will identify the causative organism so that proper antibiotic therapy can be instituted. If malignancy is suspected, prompt referral and biopsy are necessary.

Vaginal Discharge

A complaint of vaginal discharge is one of the more common complaints in both primary care and women's health. The history and physical exam are often sufficient to give a diagnosis, but, in some cases, further laboratory testing may be necessary before a definitive diagnosis can be reached. If the history, physical exam, and any vaginal smears or cultures lead to a diagnosis of a sexually transmitted disease, further serology is indicated and patient education is of utmost importance in treatment and future prevention. "Where there's smoke, there's fire." There are several diagnoses to consider when the patient presents with a complaint of vaginal discharge. These include yeast, trichomoniasis, chlamydia, gonorrhea, bacterial vaginosis, cervicitis, gynecological cancer, pelvic inflammatory disease (PID), and pregnancy.

History

The history includes the length of time the patient has had the discharge, the color and consistency of the discharge, presence of itching or odor, unusual bleeding, abdominal pain, or fever. Abdominal pain or fever suggests inflammation in the fallopian tubes and ovaries rather than just being confined to the vaginal area. It is imperative to obtain a menstrual and sexual history as well as method of birth control and history of STDs. Many health care agencies require a pregnancy test on all patients presenting with a complaint of vaginal discharge to aid in diagnosis, but also to be sure that prescribed medication is not contraindicated.

Physical Examination

A thorough gynecological exam is necessary, including a speculum exam to observe the discharge, and presence of inflammation of the vaginal mucosa or cervix; a wet prep to examine the discharge microscopically, cervical cultures if necessary to rule out STDs, and a bimanual exam to rule out tenderness or enlargement of the uterus or ovaries. See Table 12-1 for differentiation of vaginal discharge.

MONILIA (CANDIDIASIS)

Monilia, otherwise known as yeast vaginitis, is one of the more common vaginal infections in young women and is caused by the fungus *Candida albicans*. It is not considered an STD and, therefore, transmission to or from sexual partners is unlikely. Since the advent of over-the-counter (OTC) preparations to treat yeast vaginitis, it is not seen in office practice as frequently. There should be a high index of suspicion in patients who complain of

Table 12-1. ■ Differentiation of Vaginal Discharge

Characteristic	Yeast	Trichomonas	Bacterial Vaginosis	Chlamydia	Gonorrhea
Color	White	Grayish	White/Yellow	Yellowish	Yellowish
Odor	Absent	Foul	Fishy	Absent	Absent
Consistency	Thick, curdy	Frothy	Creamy	Purulent	Purulent
Location	Adheres to vaginal walls	Pooled in vagina	Introitus, vagina	Introitus, vagina, cervical os	Introitus, vagina, cervical os
Vulva	Erythematous and pruritic	Edematous	Normal	Normal	Normal
Vaginal Mucosa	Erythematous	"Strawberry spots"	Normal	Normal	Normal
Cervix	No discharge	"Strawberry spots"	Normal	Purulent discharge	Purulent discharge
Wet Prep	Hyphae, yeast buds	Motile protozoa	Clue cells + whiff test	Numerous white cells	Numerous white cells

failure with OTC preparations because they have most likely misdiagnosed their problem or perhaps have more than one infection occurring. Patients who have documented recurrent yeast vaginitis should be screened for diabetes because this type of infection is common in the diabetic population. The high concentration of glucose in the blood offers a favorable medium for yeast to flourish. In addition, HIV is a concern because yeast is more prevalent in immunocompromised individuals. Other causes include medications, particularly antibiotics, but also oral contraceptives and corticosteroids.

Signs and Symptoms.

The discharge associated with yeast vaginitis can be differentiated from other infections by symptomatology and wet prep examination. The discharge is very thick, curdlike, and adheres to the vaginal walls. There is intense vulvar itching that accompanies the discharge. Because the discharge is thick, patients often give a history of only itching and no discharge since it adheres to the vaginal walls and may not be seen by the patient. In most cases, inflammation and swelling around the labia and introitus occur. This inflammation causes dyspareunia and, also, burning of the labia with urination. Partners generally do not have any related complaints.

Diagnostic Studies.

A high suspicion of yeast can be made on physical exam with a wet prep to confirm the diagnosis of *C. albicans*. A 10% KOH prep is most helpful for visualizing budding yeast and hyphae microscopically. A saline prep should also be done in looking for alternative causes of the discharge. The presence of *C. albicans* may be reported on a Pap smear.

BACTERIAL VAGINOSIS

Although it is believed that the gardnerella bacteria can be transmitted through sexual contact, it is not strictly considered an STD. A change in the vaginal pH to a value >4.5 and a change in the bacterial flora with a decrease in lactobacilli gives rise to increases in aerobic and anaerobic bacteria. *Gardnerella vaginalis* is the most prevalent vaginal infection, although many of the women with this infection are asymptomatic. It is considered a risk factor for preterm labor, and pregnant women should always be treated. Also, women who are undergoing pelvic surgery are believed to benefit from treatment before surgery.

Signs and Symptoms.

Of those women who are symptomatic, the overwhelming complaint is of a malodorous discharge. The odor of *G. vaginalis* is a distinct, fishy odor. The odor is usually noticeable during the pelvic exam, but a few drops of 10% KOH solution on the wet prep slide augments the odor. The discharge is fairly thick and white. Patients do not complain of itching and, generally, there is no inflammation of the vaginal mucosa. Male partners do not complain of discharge, odor, or dysuria although it is believed they may harbor the bacteria without being symptomatic. The higher pH of semen may be related to the higher vaginal pH that triggers the overgrowth of anaerobes and aerobes. Antibiotics, either oral or in vaginal creams, are the treatment of choice. In pregnancy or preoperatively, intravenous antibiotics may be warranted.

Diagnostic Studies.

The diagnosis is made on symptomatology and wet prep. Microscopically, the wet prep shows the characteristic clue cells (epithelial cells embedded with bacteria), and the odor of *G. vaginalis* is unmistakable.

TRICHOMONAS

A sexually transmitted disease, *Trichomonas vaginalis* is a unicellular, flagellate protozoan. It is associated with an increased incidence in the transmission of HIV; therefore, women with trichomoniasis should be screened for other sexually transmitted diseases including HIV, gonorrhea, chlamydia, and syphilis. *Trichomonas vaginalis* has also been associated with perinatal complications.

Signs and Symptoms.

The presenting complaints with trichomoniasis are discharge and itching. It can be differentiated from yeast by the discharge, which is thin and frothy rather than the thick, curdlike discharge of yeast. It can also be differentiated from *G. vaginalis* by the fact that there is vulvar itching and inflammation with trichomoniasis, but no complaint of odor, as there is with *G. vaginalis*. Inflammation with petechiae of the vaginal walls, known as "strawberry spots," is diagnostic of *T. vaginalis*. Male partners are usually asymptomatic but harbor the organism, and they must be treated along with the patient; intercourse should be avoided or condoms used until treatment is completed. A single, large dose of antibiotics for the patient and partner is the recommended treatment.

Diagnostic Studies.

Trichomonas vaginalis is easily seen on a wet prep in the majority of cases as a flagellate protozoan. If they are present, it is diagnostic. If protozoa are not seen on wet prep and trichomoniasis is suspected, a culture is recommended. Pap smears may also show the presence of *T. vaginalis* but are only 60%–70% accurate for diagnosis.

CHLAMYDIA

Chlamydia is a sexually transmitted disease caused by the bacteria *Chlamydia trachomatis*. It is thought to be the main cause of salpingitis and scarring of the fallopian tubes, thus leading to ectopic pregnancy or infertility. It can also cause conjunctivitis in the neonate if present during delivery.

Signs and Symptoms.

Patients are often asymptomatic with chlamydia infections, but may present with mucopurulent discharge, dysuria, abdominal pain, fever, and abnormal vaginal bleeding. Cervicitis and cervical motion tenderness on physical exam indicate pelvic inflammatory disease. It is the causative organism in the majority of non-gonococcal urethritis in both women and men, and in most cases of cervicitis. Reiter's syndrome, a serious systemic complication of chlamydia infection that occurs more commonly in men, is characterized by urethritis, arthritis, and conjunctivitis or uveitis.

Diagnostic Studies.

Often accompanied by gonorrhea, a Gynprobe cervical culture will screen for both chlamydia and gonorrhea. A PCR (polymerase chain reaction) nucleic acid amplification is more sensitive than a cervical culture, but is currently not routinely done except in cases of recurrent salpingitis or cervicitis with a negative culture. Because it is a sexually transmitted disease, both the patient and partner should be screened and treated with antibiotics. Patients should abstain from intercourse during treatment, and repeat cultures should be performed at 3 weeks and 3 months.

GONORRHEA

Gonorrhea is a sexually transmitted disease caused by *Neisseria gonorrhoeae* that can present in any degree ranging from asymptomatic to severe infection. Initially, symptoms are mild and usually begin within 7–21 days after exposure, although women may remain asymptomatic for weeks or months after infection. In addition to cervical or higher reproductive organ infection, *N. gonorrhoeae* can affect the urethra, rectum, and Skene's and Bartholin's glands. In spite of continued public education on STDs, the incidence of gonorrhea is increasing.

Signs and Symptoms.

Patients may be asymptomatic or present with complaints of mucopurulent discharge, fever, abdominal pain, lymphadenopathy, and joint pain. Be suspicious of infection with *N. gonorrhoeae* in a young patient who complains of abrupt onset of polyarthritis. Clinically evident vaginal infection is only transitory, but infection with *N. gonorrhoeae* can persist, leading to salpingitis, abscess, and peritonitis. As with chlamydia, long-term complications include scarring of the fallopian tubes, ectopic pregnancy, and infertility. In addition, *N. gonorrhoeae* can cause conjunctivitis in the newborn in infected mothers.

Two more serious complications of gonorrhea are disseminated gonococcal infection (DGI) with bacteremia and gonococcal arthritis. In DGI, symptoms of genital infection may be absent. The patient presents instead with systemic complaints, such as fever, malaise, migratory polyarthralgias, and pustular skin lesions on the limbs. The bacteremia occasionally can lead to pericarditis, endocarditis, and meningitis; therefore, prompt diagnosis and treatment are necessary. Gonococcal arthritis presents with more severe and localized joint symptoms. The patient is usually febrile with severe joint pain, limited range of motion, redness, tenderness, and effusion of a few joints rather than disseminated as seen in DGI. Prompt treatment is required to avoid articular destruction.

Diagnostic Studies.

A cervical culture, Gynprobe, is the standard diagnostic tool. It detects the presence of both *N. gonorrhoeae* and *C. trachomatis*. As with chlamydia, a PCR nucleic acid amplification can be performed and is more accurate, but also more expensive and usually not necessary. Uncomplicated infections can be treated with single-dose intramuscular or oral antibiotics. A repeat culture for cure should be repeated in 2–3 months. If DGI is suspected, blood cultures or synovial fluid cultures should be drawn. In gonococcal arthritis, joint aspirate will show pus and the presence of gonococci.

PELVIC INFLAMMATORY DISEASE AND SALPINGITIS

Pelvic inflammatory disease is defined as an infection of the uterus, fallopian tubes, and adjacent pelvic structures. It is often secondary to a sexually transmitted disease or other infection of the lower reproductive tract that migrates upward into the uterus and tubes. *Neisseria gonorrhea* and *Chlamydia trachomatis* are two of the commonly offending organisms. Pelvic infections can also occur postsurgery, postpartum, or postabortion but are generally caused from other organisms, such as staphylococcus or streptococcus.

Signs and Symptoms.

Abdominal pain, mucopurulent cervical discharge, and often fever are the more common presenting symptoms. Rebound tenderness indicates peritoneal irritation. Dysuria may also be present, as well as nausea and vomiting. The abdominal pain is midline and often accompanied by right and left lower quadrant pain, particularly when accompanied by salpingitis. During the pelvic examination, there is pain with cervical motion, and with palpation of the uterus and ovaries. Risk factors include a history of PID or STDs, multiple sexual partners, douching, and IUDs. Infertility may occur as a complication owing to scarring and occlusion of the fallopian tubes. Antibiotic therapy is necessary for treatment.

Diagnostic Studies.

The diagnosis is based mostly on history and physical exam. A positive culture of the cervical discharge identifying a bacterial organism is helpful. An elevated white blood cell count will be present. Surgical emergencies, such as ectopic pregnancy or appendicitis must be ruled out. Culdocentesis, endometrial biopsy, and laparoscopy can be performed if the diagnosis is unclear or to isolate the causative organism.

ATROPHIC VAGINITIS

Although atrophic vaginitis is not an infection and does not cause a discharge, its signs and symptoms can mimic the *C. albicans* yeast vaginitis. It occurs in postmenopausal women as a result of a lack of estrogen. It can occur with surgical or natural menopause, and occasionally in lactating women.

Signs and Symptoms.

The vaginal mucosa thins and becomes smooth and pale. The complaint most often heard from patients is itching owing to dryness and atrophy of the vaginal tissue. It is often mistaken for *C. albicans* by patients because of the pruritus, but the physical exam shows no similarity. Systemic or topical estrogen is recommended for symptomatic relief.

Diagnostic Studies.

The diagnosis is made by pelvic examination. A vaginal scraping can be obtained and placed on a slide for cytological evaluation, and a maturation index can be ordered for confirmation.

Labial Lesions

The common causes of labial lesions include the herpes simplex virus (HSV); condyloma acuminatum; cancer of the vulva; syphilitic chancre; and, just inferior to the labia, a Bartholin's cyst. Although HSV is the most common cause of this complaint, it depends somewhat on the age and sexual history of the patient.

History

As with most gynecological complaints, a thorough sexual history is imperative. The number of partners, type of birth control, condom use, history of STDs, length of time in current relationship, perceived monogamy of the relationship, last Pap smear, and history of abnormal Pap smears. Ask the patient to describe the location and characteristics of the lesion and whether it is a single lesion or multiple lesions. Inquire about accompanying symptoms, such as pain, tenderness, burning, itching, excoriation, redness, swelling, or discharge. Herpetic lesions usually burn or itch in the prodromal stage and then become painful and tender, condyloma often itch but are not painful, syphilitic chancres are usually not tender, labial lesions are neither tender nor pruritic, Bartholin's cysts present with severe discomfort and tenderness especially with sitting. The age of the patient can play a part in prioritizing differential diagnosis because labial cancer rarely occurs in women less than 50 years of age.

Physical Examination

The physical exam includes a thorough visualization of the skin over the entire body to look for other lesions or skin changes, particularly in the anal area, mouth, palms of the hands, and soles of the feet. Labial lesions caused by STDs may also be present in the mouth or anus depending on sexual practices. Syphilis may manifest itself with pigmented or light-red macules or papules on the soles or palms.

Examine the abdomen for tenderness, and perform a lymph node examination, especially in the inguinal area. A thorough gynecological exam is necessary, including a speculum exam, wet prep, viral and/or bacterial cultures, and Pap smear if necessary. A scraping or biopsy of the lesion may be necessary if cancer is suspected. A blood sample for the Venereal Disease Research Laboratory (VDRL) is needed if syphilis is suspected.

HERPES SIMPLEX VIRUS

The majority of labial herpes infections are due to HSV2, and approximately 10% are due to the HSV1 virus that has been transferred to the labial area either by genital or oral contact. Although blood tests can be done to determine the presence or absence of antibodies to HSV1 and HSV2, it is mostly academic because the symptoms, transmission, and treatment are the same regardless of type.

Signs and Symptoms.

Although antibodies to the herpes virus can be found in the majority of patients 3 weeks after exposure, the symptoms may be absent or mild enough to go unnoticed by the patient. Approximately 10%–15% of persons who carry the virus are asymptomatic, but they can still shed the virus—thus, referred to as "asymptomatic shedders." This, among other things, contributes to the spread of the herpes virus. The lesions begin with a slightly reddened area on the labia that is pruritic and tingling. There may be systemic symptoms, such as fever, headache, malaise, lymphadenopathy, and urinary frequency/dysuria. After a few days, a patchy lesion appears containing several small vesicles. The vesicles then rupture and a painful, tender ulcerated area remains for 10–14 days. Lesions may be single or multiple. They may also occur on the cervix, perianal area, and mouth depending on contact area. Lesions can reoccur as frequently as once a month, often with menstruation, or as infrequently as once a year or longer. The virus may remain dormant for years until a stress or illness causes a recurrence. Treatment with antiviral medication can lessen and sometimes prevent recurrence.

Diagnostic Studies.

A viral culture of the active lesion will yield positive results in the acute phase. Additionally, about 85% of patients will develop antibodies within 21 days of exposure and a blood test will be positive for IgM antibodies. Type-specific assay tests are available to distinguish Type I from Type II.

CONDYLOMA ACUMINATUM

Condyloma is one of the manifestations of the human papilloma virus, which is the most common STD. Approximately 30%–60% of the American population has had HPV infection, and it is estimated that 50% of college women have the disease. The peak age range for HPV is 20–24 years. It is diagnosed more often in women, not necessarily because they have a greater incidence, but because they are more likely to get regular checkups. There are over 70 types of HPV, 20 of which commonly affect the anogenital region. The virus is categorized by DNA pattern (genotype) rather than by host antibodies to the virus (serotype). Types 6, 11, 42, 43, and 44 are most commonly associated with condyloma. There is an increased incidence of cervical cancer in women infected with HPV, with neoplasias being associated with types 16, 18, 31, 33, and 35. Previous chlamydia infection was shown to be an independent and cofactor with HPV for cervical cancer risk. The incubation time is 1–6 months. It is highly contagious and can be transmitted through intercourse, oral/anal sex, and mother to infant. Human papilloma virus can affect the respiratory or reproductive tract of newborns, termed "respiratory papillomatosis." Condyloma grow more rapidly in pregnancy; therefore, early treatment is recommended so healing can occur before delivery. However, the presence of lesions during delivery is not always a contraindication to a vaginal delivery. Those who are immunocompromised are also at greater risk for infection or proliferation of condyloma.

Signs and Symptoms. The incubation period for appearance of clinical disease is at least 3 months. Visible manifestations of HPV occur in less than a dozen genotypes, estimated at only 1% of those infected. Of those who develop condylomas, the presentation is variable. The patient may complain of itching in the area, or the condylomas may only be an incidental finding during a routine gynecological examination. Lesions are white with a rough, granular appearance with fingerlike projections often containing capillaries or a mosaic pattern. Condyloma may be single or multiple, and can occur on the vagina, cervix, vulva, perineum, and perianal areas.

Diagnostic Studies. In women, diagnosing condyloma through physical exam can be a challenge. Lesions are often very small, even microscopic, and the rugae of the vaginal mucosa may mask the lesion. Applying white vinegar to a suspected lesion helps to distinguish it from normal tissue. Condyloma will turn white against the surrounding tissue when the vinegar is applied. Many of the small lesions can only be seen on colposcopy.

Although there are many topical preparations for treatment, patients should be referred for colposcopy because of the microscopic condyloma that may be present. If dysplasia is seen on the Pap smear, biopsies should be taken to rule out intraepithelial neoplasia because >90% of the cervical neoplasias are caused by HPV. Unfortunately, barrier contraceptives offer only limited protection against the spread of HPV infection.

SYPHILIS

Syphilis is an STD caused by the spirochete *Treponema pallidum*. It is transmitted through intact or abraded mucous membranes and rapidly spreads to the lymph nodes and throughout the body. The incidence of syphilis has risen dramatically in the last 30 years with the increase in HIV and other STDs. In response, state and federal agencies put forth massive campaigns for prevention of all STDs and, in the last few years, have been able to show a decrease in newly reported cases of syphilis.

Signs and Symptoms.

The primary chancre lesion occurs anywhere from 10 to 90 days after exposure. It appears as a firm, indurated, painless papule that erodes into an ulcer with raised or reddened borders. Chancres are usually single lesions and can occur on any mucous membrane or skin area. Non-tender lymphadenopathy is present in the regional nodes. Genital lesions are most commonly seen in women on the external genitalia. Symptoms may be mild enough to go unnoticed, especially when they are in areas other than the genitalia, and they heal without treatment in 4–8 weeks.

If the primary infection is not treated, secondary syphilis develops and is characterized by more systemic symptoms, such as diffuse lymphadenopathy, malaise, fever, headache, anorexia, joint pain, and rash, which appears most commonly on the soles and palms, but can also be present on the trunk. The rash can be macular, papular, or pustular, making the differential diagnosis variable. Erosion of the mucous membranes occurs, mostly in the mouth, forming grayish-white patches. Alopecia also may occur in patches. In secondary syphilis, anemia, jaundice, albuminuria, neck stiffness, and syphilitic meningitis may develop, causing cranial nerve lesions and deafness. If secondary syphilis is untreated, a latent stage develops. Approximately one-third go on to develop tertiary syphilis, although it may not manifest for many years. Tertiary syphilis affects the skin, bones, and cardiovascular and neurological systems.

Diagnostic Studies.

Serum for VDRL is the necessary laboratory test for diagnosis and it will generally convert to positive 3–6 weeks after infection or 3–4 weeks after appearance of the primary lesion. False-positive serologic reactions are common, transient, and usually with a low titer. The fluorescent treponemal antibody absorption test (FTA-ABS) and the micro-hemagglutination assay for *T. pallidum* are more specific and will assist in differentiating true from false positives. These tests remain positive regardless of treatment. *Treponema pallidum* can be detected by dark-field examination of specimens from skin and mucous membrane lesions, but serologic testing is more reliable. Polymerase chain reaction is very specific for detecting *T. pallidum* in serum, spinal fluid, and amniotic fluid.

CANCER OF THE VULVA

Vulvar carcinoma accounts for <5% of gynecologic cancers. It occurs more commonly in women over 50 years of age. Over 90% of these cancers are squamous cell carcinomas;

about 4% are basal cell; and the remaining are melanomas, Paget's disease, and Bartholin's adenocarcinoma.

Signs and Symptoms.

The lesions of vulvar carcinoma are easily seen and palpated by the patient, but are not recognized as serious and often do not bring the patient into the office for many months. They are often pruritic, white, macerated lesions initially on the vulva that may extend to the vagina, urethra, and anal area. They begin superficially but can become quite extensive in depth and breadth if left untreated. They may become infected, ulcerated, and necrotic.

Diagnostic Studies.

Biopsy is the definitive diagnostic procedure and, for squamous cell carcinoma, radical vulvectomy with inguinal and femoral lymph node dissection is the definitive treatment. Patients should be followed closely for at least 5 years for early detection of recurrences. Prognosis depends on the depth of the lesion.

Abnormal Pap Smear

The Pap smear is designed to detect cancer cells in the cervix and vagina. It was developed in the 1940s and, since then, the incidence of cervical cancer has declined more than 70%. The technology for the interpretation of Pap smears has improved greatly over the years, with computer-generated procedures now being used. The recommendations vary some, but for most women, a Pap smear is recommended by age 18 or sooner if the woman is sexually active. Pap smears should be repeated every 1–3 years depending on the age and history of the patient.

History

Ask the patient about a history of abnormal Pap smears, cryosurgery, colposcopy, or cervical/endometrial biopsy. Ask about any history of STDs, especially HSV and HPV, both of which can be a reason for an abnormal Pap smear. Ask about the use of diethylstilbestrol (DES) by the patient's mother during pregnancy. Before the 1970s, the drug DES was widely used in pregnant women with threatened abortion. Subsequently, it was found to cause abnormalities and malignancies of the reproductive tract in the children of those mothers. Its use was banned in the United States in 1971, and in Europe, in 1978.

Physical Examination

While obtaining the Pap smear, a thorough gynecological exam should be performed and notations made of any cervical inflammation (cervicitis), discharge, STDs, or other reproductive abnormalities. It is important to continue Pap smears in postmenopausal women for cervical and endometrial cancer screening. Surprisingly, 25% of cervical cancers occur in women >65 years of age, and the peak incidence of endometrial cancer occurs in postmenopausal women between 50 and 60 years. In patients who have had hysterectomies, a smear of the vaginal cuff is still suggested as well as inspection of the vaginal mucosa and external genitalia looking for signs of malignancy.

Signs and Symptoms

Patients rarely exhibit symptoms of an abnormal Pap smear unless it is due to infection or inflammation, in which case vaginal discharge is commonly present.

Table 12-2. ■ Bethesda System for Reporting Abnormal Pap Smears

Negative for Intraepithelial Lesion or Malignancy	Epithelial Cell Abnormalities	Other
Organisms • Trichomonas • Fungal • Bacterial • Herpes simplex virus	Squamous Cell • Atypical cells of undetermined significance (ASCUS) • Low-grade intraepithelial lesion (LSIL); includes HPV/mild dysplasia/CIN 1 • High-grade intraepithelial lesion (HSIL); includes moderate-severe dysplasia, CIS/CIN 2 and CIN 3 • Squamous cell carcinoma	Other Malignant Neoplasms
Other Non-Neoplastic Findings • Reactive cellular changes, such as inflammation, radiation, IUD • Glandular cells S/P hysterectomy • Atrophy Other—Endometrial cells in a woman ≥40 years	Glandular Cell • Atypical cells of undetermined significance (AGCUS); includes endocervical, endometrial, glandular • Endocervical adenocarcinoma in situ • Adenocarcinoma, includes endocervical endometrial, extrauterine, NOS	

Diagnostic Studies

Diagnosis is made solely through the Pap smear cytology report from the sample taken of the endocervix, cervix, and vaginal pool, or the vaginal cuff in the case of hysterectomy. The Bethesda system is the standard for reporting cervical cytology (National Cancer Institute, 2001). See Table 12-2 for an outline of the Bethesda System. If the Pap smear changes are due to infection or a reparative process, appropriate treatment should be instituted and the Pap smear repeated in 3–6 months. For other abnormalities, referral should be made to a specialist for colposcopy and/or biopsy.

Dysfunctional Uterine Bleeding

Abnormal uterine bleeding is much more common in the younger population especially during the teen years when menstrual patterns are becoming established. Also, during the early reproductive years, malignancies are much less likely to be the cause. Most cases of dysfunctional uterine bleeding are due to organic causes and to dysfunction of the hypothalamic-pituitary-ovarian axis. Bleeding after menopause has been established is cause for concern, and referral for endometrial biopsy is a must.

History

Start with the date of the last menstrual period and reconstruct as much of the menstrual history as possible, including age at menarche, menstrual patterns, and episodes of amenorrhea or abnormal bleeding in the past. Ask for a complete description of the current problem with abnormal bleeding. Important things to know include the time of onset; the pattern of bleeding (intermittent or constant); the amount and frequency of bleeding; the color of the blood (bright red or dark); and any history of trauma, vaginal discharge, recent STDs, abdominal pain, fever, or missed periods. Inquire about type of birth control and sexual activity. Determine whether there is a history of abnormal Pap smears. In postmenopausal women, ask about the use of unopposed estrogen replacement, which is a risk factor for endometrial cancer. Bleeding disorders can arise, so it is important to ask the patient about easy bruising or any recent gum or nosebleeds.

Physical Examination

Both an abdominal and a pelvic exam should be done to assess for masses or tenderness and the size, consistency, and mobility of the uterus and ovaries. During the pelvic exam, a Pap smear should be obtained to rule out cervical cancer. An endometrial biopsy might be needed to rule out endometrial cancer, especially in middle-aged and older women, but it is wise to wait for the results of the Pap smear before proceeding with a biopsy. A pelvic ultrasound or MRI should be considered to rule out pelvic mass. An hCG measurement should be performed to rule out pregnancy, as well as a CBC and platelet count to rule out hematologic causes.

ENDOMETRIAL CARCINOMA

Endometrial cancer can follow atypical hyperplasia or can arise de novo. It occurs twice as much in white compared with black women. The peak incidence is between 60 and 70 years but has been reported in patients as young as 20 years old. Although it is the most common pelvic genital cancer in women, a complaint of dysfunctional uterine bleeding assists in early detection. Patients with hyperestrogenism that is due either to altered estrogen metabolism or to the use of unopposed estrogen are at increased risk. Patients taking tamoxifen for breast cancer are also at increased risk.

Signs and Symptoms.

Abnormal bleeding occurs in the majority of women with endometrial cancers. Spotting or bleeding of any kind in a postmenopausal woman is a red flag, and endometrial biopsy is warranted. A small number of women complain of lower abdominal pain or cramping. Physical examination is usually not helpful in the early stages, but in later stages, may reveal an enlarged, fixed uterus. It is necessary to refer the patient to a gynecological surgeon for hysterectomy.

Diagnostic Studies.

A Pap smear should be part of the routine examination and may show abnormal cytology indicative of endometrial carcinoma. For definitive diagnosis and histological typing, an endometrial biopsy or D and C is necessary. The three histological types are adenocarcinoma (most common), adenocarcinoma with squamous differentiation, and adenosquamous carcinoma. Serum Ca-125, a tumor marker for ovarian cancer, is also elevated in endometrial cancer, with the more advanced stages more likely to have elevations. A complete metabolic profile, CBC, urinalysis, and chest x-ray should be performed at the time of diagnosis to identify or rule out metastases.

Hormonal Imbalances

Irregular bleeding occurs more frequently early in menarche, before the body establishes a regular pattern, as well as during the perimenopausal period, when hormones are changing. Other causes of hormonal imbalances are discussed throughout this chapter.

Oral Contraceptives

If the progesterone component of the pill is not sufficient to maintain the lining of the uterus, metrorrhagia may occur in the luteal phase of the cycle. If a patient complains of spotting or bleeding during this time, a different pill with a stronger or different type of progesterone should be prescribed. If the bleeding continues, consider stopping the pill temporarily to determine whether that is the aggravating factor. There are enough choices of pills available to find one that most all patient can take without unwanted side effects.

FIBROIDS

Uterine leiomyomas, more commonly known as uterine fibroids, are benign growths consisting mostly of smooth muscle. The etiology is unknown, but their growth is hormone dependent; therefore, they are seen in approximately 25% of women during their reproductive years. They generally do not originate after menopause and, if present, will decrease in size after menopause. A tumor that arises in a postmenopausal woman should always have a high suspicion for malignancy, rather than benign leiomyoma. Leiomyomas are more common in black women, occurring in as many as 50%. They can be single or multiple, usually measuring <15 cm. A very small percentage (0.1%–0.5%) may undergo malignant transformation to become a leiomyosarcoma requiring prompt surgical intervention.

Signs and Symptoms.

Heavy menstrual bleeding (menorrhagia) and irregular bleeding (metrorrhagia) are the most common presenting symptoms although a large percentage of patients are asymptomatic. Other symptoms include heaviness or fullness in the lower abdomen, pelvic pain, backache, dysmenorrhea, and urinary complaints. The pain can be severe if caused by torsion of a pedunculated fibroid. Fibroids are thought to contribute to infertility and spontaneous abortion, as well as preterm labor and problems with labor and delivery. Most leiomyomas can be palpated on bimanual examination and some larger fibroids can be palpated through the abdomen. The uterus may feel enlarged, irregular, or nodular; pedunculated fibroids can be difficult to differentiate from other pelvic or abdominal masses. A retroverted uterus may obscure palpation.

Diagnostic Studies.

A pregnancy test should be performed to rule that out as a cause of the symptoms. A CBC is needed in cases of heavy bleeding to determine whether anemia or platelet disorder is present. Pelvic ultrasound or MRI should be performed if symptoms of leiomyoma are present or for any palpable pelvic mass detected on physical examination. Imaging will assist in differentiating ovarian cancer, leiomyosarcoma, endometrial cancer, or other neoplasms. An endometrial biopsy, D and C, laparoscopy, or laparotomy may be necessary to rule out malignancies.

ANOVULATION

The causes of chronic anovulation are numerous, with some resulting in dysfunctional uterine bleeding and some resulting in amenorrhea. The main categories for causes are as follows.

- Inappropriate feedback, including polycystic ovary syndrome; neoplasms that produce excess androgens, estrogens, or human chorionic gonadotropin; excess estrogen production associated with obesity or liver disease.

- Pituitary dysfunction related to tumors or hypopituitarism.
- Hypothalamic dysfunction associated with stress, exercise, malnutrition, or anorexia nervosa.
- Endocrine or metabolic dysfunction, including thyroid disease, adrenal hyperfunction as seen in Cushing's disease, and prolactin or growth hormone excess.

Signs and Symptoms.

Anovulation may present with amenorrhea, but also may present with dysfunctional uterine bleeding, polymenorrhea, or menorrhagia. The symptoms vary with the cause. Overweight may be seen with several of the causes, including hypothyroidism, polycystic ovary syndrome, and pituitary and adrenal dysfunction. Underweight is seen in anorexia nervosa, excessive exercise, hyperthyroidism, or stress-induced anovulation. Hirsutism, acne, and other skin changes can be seen with imbalances in LH, FSH, and androgens, as seen in polycystic ovary disease. Delayed puberty or regression of sexual characteristics is seen in hypopituitarism; galactorrhea can be the presenting symptom in pituitary tumors.

Diagnostic Studies.

Appropriate laboratory and diagnostic testing depends on the history and physical exam and on the preliminary differential diagnosis. Thyroid-stimulating hormone (TSH), LH, FSH, estradiol, and testosterone levels will give information about sex and thyroid hormone levels, and ovarian function. If polycystic ovary disease is suspected, a pelvic ultrasound is necessary although it may be normal even with the disease. If pituitary or adrenal dysfunction is suspected, tests include glucose, cortisol, growth hormone, TSH, adrenocorticotropic hormone (ACTH), prolactin, LH, and FSH. Abnormalities in any of these studies may warrant MRI or CT scanning of the head.

PERIMENOPAUSE

Generally, there is no objective way to determine when the perimenopausal period begins, but from subjective data gathered from patients, menstrual changes begin to take place in the fourth decade of life.

Signs and Symptoms.

Follicle-stimulating and luteinizing hormones remain normal, but patients who had regular menstrual cycles all of their lives begin to complain of more-frequent periods with more dysmenorrhea or, conversely, missed periods. Patients may also begin to have sleep disturbances, decreased energy, increased weight, urinary frequency, and other complaints that are usually associated with menopause.

Diagnostic Studies.

Pregnancy and pathology must be ruled out. The following labs and diagnostics are recommended: hCG; urinalysis; Pap smear with bimanual exam to rule out fibroids or a malignancy; CBC to rule out anemia, which can cause menorrhagia; and FSH and LH to ensure that the patient is not menopausal. A pelvic ultrasound is indicated if fibroids or malignancy is suspected. If the symptoms are established to be benign perimenopausal symptoms, then no treatment is really necessary because the symptoms are bothersome but not dangerous. However, they can be managed with low-strength birth control pills as long as there are no contraindications.

Amenorrhea

The four main causes of primary amenorrhea are disorders of the outflow tract, disorders of the ovary, disorders of the anterior pituitary, and disorders of the hypothalamus. Secondary amenorrhea can occur for many reasons: pregnancy, oral contraceptives, high prolactin due to a pituitary microadenoma, stress, rapid weight change, anorexia nervosa, menopause, vigorous exercise, hypothyroidism, chronic disease, and polycystic ovary disease.

History

It is necessary to determine whether the amenorrhea is primary or secondary. Primary amenorrhea is defined as the absence of menarche by age 16. Secondary amenorrhea is the absence of menstruation for >3 months in a woman with past menses. If there is no past history of menses, consider the age and Tanner stage of the patient. Constitutional delay occurs in teenagers whose family has a history of late growth. These teens can experience late, but normal, sexual maturation. In the case of no menstrual cycle, consider also the disorders of the outflow tract, and hypoestrogenic amenorrhea. If the patient has had menstrual cycles in the past, inquire as to age of onset, duration, amount of flow, regularity, and date of last menstrual period. Irregular menses is very common in adolescents and does not necessarily indicate pathology. Ask the patient about lifestyle, exercise and eating habits, and weight gain or loss that might indicate thyroid disease, polycystic ovary disease, or an eating disorder. It is necessary to know about prescription or OTC medication; use of oral contraceptives; birth control method, if any; and sexual activity that might indicate pregnancy or oral contraceptive–induced amenorrhea. Major stresses or life-changing events, and/or chronic illness that can cause physical and emotional stress have been shown to cause amenorrhea. Ask the patient about the presence of galactorrhea, indicating the possibility of a pituitary tumor.

Physical Examination

A height and weight are a good start and give you an idea about several possible explanations for the amenorrhea. Short stature, obesity, or underweight are associated with both primary and secondary causes of amenorrhea. Inspect for webbing of the hands and neck that accompany the short stature of Turner's syndrome. Assess the skin for dryness and the hair for signs of dryness, thinning, or brittleness indicating hypothyroidism or altered nutritional state. Inspect the patient for hirsutism, which can occur in pituitary and hormonal abnormalities. The gynecological exam includes inspection for patency of the introitus and cervix; inspection of the vaginal mucosa for dryness or atrophy, which accompanies a lack of estrogen; a bimanual exam to determine uterine size, which can be enlarged in pregnancy or tumors; and palpation of the ovaries for cysts.

Diagnostic testing is necessary in most cases because a cessation of menses may be the only symptom, and physical exam findings may be absent. The initial step should be to rule out pregnancy with a urine or serum hCG analysis. If negative, a TSH and prolactin level should be drawn to rule out thyroid disease or pituitary tumor. A decreased TSH, indicating hyperthyroidism, can result in hypomenorrhea or amenorrhea. Hyperprolactinemia can lead to lower FSH and LH levels, and hypogonadism. If the prolactin is normal and galactorrhea is absent, a pituitary tumor can be ruled out, and, likewise, a normal TSH rules out thyroid disease. Before ordering other expensive or extensive laboratory studies, a progesterone challenge should be given. If the patient experiences menstrual bleeding after

7 days of oral progesterone, it can be assumed that the endometrium is sufficiently prepared by endogenous estrogen and that there is, at least, minimal function of the ovary, pituitary, and central nervous system. This rules out primary ovarian failure and tells you that the patient has some circulating estrogen. In this case, the patient is likely not ovulating and, therefore, is not getting the postovulatory rise in progesterone needed for menses. Polycystic ovary disease is the most common cause of anovulation, and an increase in LH, estrogen, and androgen levels along with a decreased FSH can help to confirm this. Although in polycystic ovary syndrome (PCOS) the ovaries are not always enlarged or cystic, a pelvic ultrasound may assist in the diagnosis. Adrenal dysfunction plays a part in ovarian and menstrual function, although in the case of adrenal dysfunction, menstrual irregularities are only one of many other more serious symptoms related to the action of adrenocortical hormones.

If bleeding does not occur with the progesterone challenge, estrogen should be added to the progesterone challenge to differentiate a disorder of the outflow tract from hypoestrogenic amenorrhea. An ultrasound will also assist in the diagnosis of an outflow tract disorder. In the case of no menses with the combination estrogen and progesterone challenge, an FSH and LH test, as well as an MRI of the sella turcica, are needed to determine gonadal failure versus hypothalamic amenorrhea caused by pituitary adenoma or other hypothalamic/pituitary abnormalities.

Figure 12-5 provides a flowchart for the evaluation of amenorrhea.

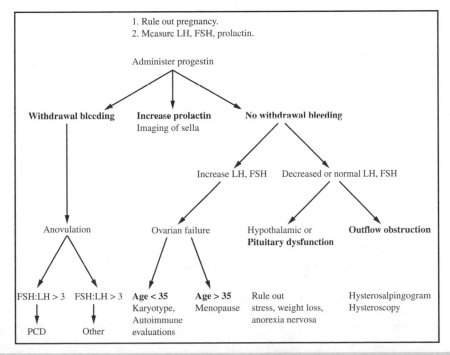

Figure 12-5. ■ Evaluation of amenorrhea. (From Kiningham, R.B., Apgar, B.S., & Schwenk, T.L. Evaluation of amenorrhea. *American Family Physician, 53* (4), 1185-94, 1996. Reprinted with permission.)

POLYCYSTIC OVARY SYNDROME

Formerly called Stein-Leventhal syndrome, polycystic ovary syndrome is a hypothalamic-pituitary-ovarian axis disorder resulting in high levels of LH, low levels of FSH, a high nonfluctuating level of estrogen, and an overproduction of androgens. It occurs in 5%–10% of the female population.

Signs and Symptoms.

Polycystic ovary syndrome is characterized by anovulation, amenorrhea, and hirsutism, although some women with PCOS have menorrhagia or dysfunctional uterine bleeding rather than amenorrhea. It also has been associated with infertility, insulin resistance, truncal obesity, and dyslipidemia. Enlarged ovaries are usually present, but are not required for diagnosis. Other physical findings associated with PCOS include acne, alopecia, and acanthosis nigricans.

Diagnostic Studies.

No one test can give a definitive diagnosis of PCOS. There are several tests that assist in the diagnosis. Elevated androgen values (free testosterone, dehydroepiandrosterone sulfate [DHEAS], total testosterone) are seen in many women, most commonly free testosterone. If elevated androgen levels are present, adrenal tumors need to be ruled out. Elevated levels of LH, and an elevated LH-to-FSH ratio may be present, although results vary widely depending on the timing of the laboratory testing. Prolactin and TSH levels are normal but will assist in ruling out pituitary tumors or thyroid disease as a cause of the amenorrhea. Cushing's disease should be ruled out because PCOS has many similar signs and symptoms. Ultrasound of the ovaries may assist in the diagnosis, but many women who have cystic ovaries do not have PCOS. If PCOS is suspected, a glucose tolerance test, insulin levels, and a lipid profile should be done to monitor other health problems associated with PCOS. Management includes hormone therapy, insulin-sensitizing drugs, and weight loss. Weight loss will help to prevent diabetes, dyslipidemia, and cardiovascular disease and will also reduce circulating testosterone.

Menopause

Menopause is defined as the absence of menses for at least 6 months. See Box 12-1 for physiological changes that occur with menopause.

HISTORY

In addition to inquiring about the typical menopausal symptoms as mentioned above, ask the patient about recent major life changes, as stress has been shown to affect menstrual regularity. Age of menopause varies greatly although age 50–55 is the typical range of onset.

Box 12-1

Physiological Changes with Menopause

- Hot flashes, fatigue, insomnia, urinary frequency and incontinence, nervousness, decreased libido, and depression
- Increased bone resorption especially in the first 5 years of menopause leading to osteopenia and osteoporosis
- Increased incidence of atherosclerosis
- Vaginal and urethral dryness and decreased integrity
- Decreased skin turgor

Diagnostic Studies.

Although the absence of menses in a woman around the age of 50 years is diagnostic for menopause, measurement of FSH, LH, and estradiol levels are helpful in confirming the diagnosis. In menopause, FSH rises first and then LH, both greater than 100 mU/mL. A fall in estradiol is the last hormonal change that occurs with the decline of ovarian function. An estradiol level of <30 pg/mL indicates loss of ovarian function.

Dysmenorrhea

Dysmenorrhea is the most common gynecological complaint, particularly in the adolescent and young adult population. Primary dysmenorrhea is due to a rise in prostaglandins that occurs at the onset of menses, and it has been found that prostaglandins are higher in women with dysmenorrhea. Recently, increased leukotriene levels have been found to contribute to dysmenorrhea. Other psychosocial variables may contribute, such as response to pain, anxiety, stress, and attitudes about menstruation.

Secondary dysmenorrhea is most often caused by endometriosis. Other causes include chronic pelvic inflammatory disease, adhesions, IUDs, cervical stenosis, and uterine fibroids.

History

Take a menstrual history including age at menarche, menstrual patterns, and the qualitative and quantitative factors of the dysmenorrhea. Important things to know include the time of onset in the menstrual cycle; pattern (intermittent or constant); regularity with the cycles; severity and duration of the pain; amount of lost work/school time; and medications taken for relief. Also ask about any history of trauma, vaginal discharge, recent STDs, fever, history of endometriosis, infertility, or missed periods. Inquire about the type of birth control and sexual activity. Determine whether there is a history of abnormal Pap smears.

Physical Examination

Both an abdominal and a pelvic exam should be done to assess for masses or tenderness. During the pelvic exam, a Pap smear should be obtained, along with cultures for chlamydia and gonorrhea. Assess for size, consistency, mobility, and tenderness of the uterus and ovaries.

PRIMARY DYSMENORRHEA

Primary dysmenorrhea is often used to describe menstrual cramping but strictly speaking the term should be used only to describe pain with menses that interferes with normal daily living, and requires pain medicine, either narcotic or nonnarcotic.

Signs and Symptoms.

The pain is in the pelvic area and begins with the onset of menses or shortly thereafter. The pain can be so severe as to be accompanied by nausea, vomiting, and diarrhea. It is short in duration, usually lasting only the first day or two of the menstrual cycle. If pain worsens over time or occurs between cycles, secondary causes should be suspected.

Diagnostic Studies.

In primary dysmenorrhea, diagnosis is by history because menstrual pain is a subjective complaint and cannot be measured objectively. However, if a secondary cause is suspected, an exam should be done to inspect for vaginal discharge that might indicate infection, and cervical cultures are needed to test for gonorrhea and chlamydia. A bimanual exam should be done to palpate for tenderness that might indicate infection or fibroids. Laboratory tests and diagnostics to consider include a serum hCG for pregnancy, a pelvic ultrasound to rule out fibroids or endometriosis, an endometrial biopsy, and possibly laparoscopy if endometriosis is suspected in order to determine the extent of disease. Oral contraceptives will diminish the severity of the dysmenorrhea along with NSAIDs or other pain medication.

ENDOMETRIOSIS

Endometriosis is characterized by a proliferation of endometrial tissue in sites other than the lining of the uterus. It typically grows on the outside of the uterus, tubes and ovaries, broad ligament, uterosacral ligaments, large and small bowel, bladder, ureters, vagina, and cul-de-sac. It is almost exclusively found in premenopausal women and is estimated to cause as much as 50% of infertility in women. Several theories exist, but the exact cause is unknown. Theories include retrograde menstruation with transport of endometrial cells, lymphatic transport of endometrial cells, metaplasia of coelomic epithelium, or immune response resulting in endometrial hyperplasia. In addition, there seems to be a genetic predisposition, with a 6%–10% increase in patients with first-degree relatives who have endometriosis.

Signs and Symptoms.

The main symptom of endometriosis is dysmenorrhea, which sometimes makes it difficult to differentiate from primary dysmenorrhea. Other presenting symptoms include dyspareunia, infertility, and constant pelvic and low back pain that occurs before menses. Adhesions may cause chronic pelvic pain unrelated to menstrual cycle. The physical exam may reveal a fixed uterus as a result of adhesions, thus causing pain on uterine movement; nodules on the posterior vaginal fornix; and tenderness in the adnexal area. In many patients, the physical exam is unremarkable.

Diagnostic Studies.

The history and physical exam generally lead you to suspect endometriosis, but the definitive diagnosis is made through laparoscopic surgery and biopsy. The lesions seen in endometriosis, termed endometrial implants, appear as dark red to dark brown lesions that give the appearance of a powder burn from a gunshot. They appear on the peritoneal, bladder, uterine, and ovarian surfaces. Over time they become thickened and produce scar tissue. Ultrasound may give information about the extent of the disease but should not be used as the sole diagnostic tool. Various hormonal treatments are helpful, as well as laparoscopic ablation of extrauterine endometrial tissue, and lysing of adhesions with the goal of restoring pelvic anatomy.

Uterine Fibroids

Along with dysfunctional uterine bleeding, leiomyomas can cause dysmenorrhea, which is often one of the presenting complaints. See the section on fibroids under dysfunctional uterine bleeding.

Ovarian Cancer

Although patients do not come in with a chief complaint of ovarian cancer, the symptoms and physical findings are usually vague or nonexistent, thereby making it a differential diagnosis or a diagnosis of suspicion, rather than one based on history or physical. Ovarian cancer has the highest mortality of the gynecological malignancies because as much as 85% of cases have metastases outside the ovaries at the time of diagnosis, and the cancer is usually widespread before the patient has signs or symptoms. It occurs most often in post-menopausal women, and in women with a positive family history.

History

The history should include both abdominal and gynecological complaints, as many patients with ovarian cancer present with vague GI complaints. A menstrual history is nec-essary because some of the patients have dysfunctional uterine bleeding. A positive family history of ovarian cancer is a red flag, as well as a history in the patient of other gyn-ecological or breast malignancies.

Physical Examination

In the premenopausal female, 95% of ovarian masses are small (<8 cm), cystic, and benign, although ovarian malignancies do occur in this population. In the postmenopausal female, there should be a high index of suspicion for ovarian cancer. Early symptoms are vague and include mild lower abdominal discomfort, feelings of fullness, bloating, disten-tion, nausea, dyspepsia, constipation, and urinary frequency if the tumor is large. Abnormal uterine bleeding is uncommon. Pelvic pain, anemia, ascites, and cachexia are seen in late disease.

The characteristics typical of a malignant ovarian mass include solid, fixed, nodular, non-tender, and bilateral. The abdominal exam is essential looking for distention, changes in percussion, or ascites. As the cancer metastasizes, lymphadenopathy occurs, especially in the inguinal and supraclavicular areas. The cancer spreads by direct extension to the abdominal and pelvic peritoneum, and through lymph nodes. Laboratory and other diag-nostics are needed for a definitive diagnosis.

Pelvic examination has been shown to have a low sensitivity and specificity for ovarian cancer, with many tumors <10 cm being missed. Several diagnostic studies are useful for detecting ovarian cancer. The Ca-125 blood test by immunoassay is used as a tumor marker for treatment decisions, but can also be used as a diagnostic tool. False-positive elevations do occur with endometriosis and pelvic surgeries; therefore, tests should be interpreted with caution, and followed up with an ultrasound. Transvaginal ultrasound will show a solid, irregular mass that may be adhered to adjoining structures. A pap smear may contain malignant cells. X-rays may show metastatic lung or bone lesions. Prognosis is poor, with a mean survival of 18 months. Surgery is necessary for staging and also as the mainstay of treatment, along with chemotherapy and possibly radiation.

OVARIAN CYSTS

There are several differentiating factors that separate ovarian cysts from ovarian cancer. The primary factor is that cysts are fluid-filled sacs and cancer is a solid tumor. Ovarian cancer is much more prevalent in women over 50 years of age, although it can occur in younger women. Ovarian cysts are common in the younger population and tend to occur in the latter half of the menstrual cycle. Many spontaneously resolve. Others may need sur-gical intervention, if they become twisted, owing to the risk of gangrene.

Signs and Symptoms.

Right or left lower quadrant pain is usually the presenting complaint. Pelvic exam reveals significant tenderness in the affected adnexal area. Rebound tenderness may be present. Follicular cysts are most common, and the pain typically occurs in the second half of the menstrual cycle. These cysts usually resolve with menses and require no further treatment. Other cysts—including corpus luteum cysts, inflammatory cysts occurring with tubo-ovarian abscess, and endometriotic cysts—may require surgical intervention.

Diagnostic Studies.

Tubal pregnancy must be ruled out immediately with a urine and/or serum hCG. Transvaginal ultrasound will give the best information for differentiating a blood- or fluid-filled cyst from a solid mass.

HYDATIDIFORM MOLE AND CHORIOCARCINOMA

These solid tumors are part of a category of gestational trophoblastic neoplasias. In the United States, the incidence is 1:1500 pregnancies. Risk factors include low socioeconomic status, and age <18 or >40 years (Crombleholme, 2004).

Signs and Symptoms.

Clinical signs are those of a missed abortion, that is, uterine bleeding, nausea, vomiting, and enlarged and/or tender uterus and ovaries. Collapsed vesicles from the mole may pass through the vagina.

Diagnostic Studies.

A quantitative hCG should be done as these values may differ from those of a normal pregnancy. Grapelike clusters within an enlarged uterus in the absence of a fetus and placenta are diagnostic for hydatidiform mole. In partial hydatidiform mole, pelvic ultrasound may show an embryo or gestational sac. These partial moles are slow growing, but are more likely to become choriocarcinomas. A solid mass on ultrasound is suspicious for choriocarcinoma and requires biopsy for diagnosis.

Uterine Fibroids

See Dysfunctional Uterine Bleeding, p. 308.

GI, Liver, Pancreatic Cancers

See Chapter 9.

Irritable Bowel Syndrome

See p. 216.

Sexual Dysfunction

There are many causes of sexual dysfunction that may have a physical or psychological origin or a combination of both. Dysfunction generally stems from decreased desire, decreased arousal, orgasmic dysfunction, and physical discomfort.

History

A sexual history should be part of the gynecological review of systems, although it is often omitted as a result of examiner discomfort or a failure to view it as an integral part of the exam. If problems exist, the examiner should explore with the client her relationships, life circumstances and changes, medical conditions, surgeries, sexual activity and behaviors, sexual development, and fertility issues.

Physical Examination

There are no special examinations to be done for sexual dysfunction, although hormonal assessment may be helpful. A thorough gynecological examination is adequate to determine whether there is a physical cause for the problem. If dyspareunia is part of the complaint, a pelvic ultrasound may assist in the diagnosis of structural pathology.

LOSS OF LIBIDO AND DECREASED SEXUAL RESPONSE

Decreases in libido and sexual response are not uncommon with aging although it is an erroneous stereotype to assume that sexual desire or functioning automatically declines with age. Inhibited or decreased sexual desire has many causes, including aging, marital discord, drug or alcohol abuse, pregnancy, physical illness or discomfort, depression, history of sexual abuse, sexual phobias, and anxiety.

Signs and Symptoms.

The diagnosis of inhibited sexual desire is primarily a subjective one based on patient history. If organic causes, such as illness and physical discomfort are ruled out, a thorough psychological evaluation is recommended. As previously mentioned, desire and response may slow with aging, but a good history should be able to discern when a psychological evaluation is warranted. In the aging client, lubricating agents may be helpful to deal with decreased or uncomfortable stimulation due to loss of lubrication.

Diagnostic Studies.

Although a thorough history is most helpful, serum for free testosterone will show an androgen deficiency, which has been blamed for decreased libido, particularly in the postmenopausal woman.

DYSPAREUNIA

The causes of dyspareunia are numerous and include vaginal infection or irritation, PID, endometriosis, pregnancy, atrophic vaginitis, decreased lubrication, episiotomy, labial lesions, Bartholin's cysts, adhesions from previous gynecological or abdominal surgeries, and psychological causes.

Signs and Symptoms.

The age of the client should be considered because decreased estrogen can cause atrophic vaginitis and thus decreased lubrication leading to dyspareunia. The history can give information about pregnancy or delivery difficulties, past surgeries, and the possibility of adhesions. The history should include a thorough sexual history to uncover any psychological issues. A pelvic exam should be done looking for vaginal discharge, inflammation, or lesions.

Diagnostic Studies.

Structural abnormalities should be ruled out, and transvaginal ultrasound may be helpful. If vaginal discharge is present, wet prep and cultures should be obtained to rule out infection. Blood samples for hormonal testing may be necessary, particularly if mucosal atrophy is evident on physical examination.

VAGINISMUS

Vaginismus is defined as a painful contraction of the lower vaginal and thigh adductor muscles that occurs unconsciously in a woman who does not desire penetration. It most often occurs in young women who have been molested, sexually abused, or raped, or secondary to gynecological trauma or medical procedures.

Signs and Symptoms.

The physical or psychological causes can be uncovered during history and physical exam. A good history, inquiring specifically about sexual abuse, is necessary. Involuntary vaginal spasm can be observed during the pelvic examination, and the patient often exhibits avoidance behavior in response to the examiner and the pelvic exam.

Diagnostic Studies.

Once structural and other physical causes have been eliminated, vaginismus can be treated with gradual dilation techniques. In many instances, psychotherapy is necessary.

Infertility

The workup for infertility is complex and will need to be referred to a gynecologist specializing in infertility. The causes are numerous but generally fall into the categories of anovulation, implantation failure, hormonal failure, chromosomal abnormalities, or low sperm count in the male partner. Preliminary tests that can be initiated by the nurse practitioner include the following.

- Pelvic exam to ensure that the cervix is open and that there are no uterine abnormalities.
- Basal body temperature charts to plot monthly ovulation and menstrual patterns.
- Laboratory testing including TSH, FSH, LH, and estradiol.
- Ultrasound—shows the position of the uterus, the presence of fibroids or other growths, and the thickening of the endometrium that may occur in endometriosis, all of which can affect fertility.
- Hysterosalpingography—radiography of the uterus and fallopian tubes to assess patency and the presence of any structural abnormalities.
- Sperm count for the male partner—this is one of the first things that should be done in an infertility workup.

References

Center for Health Statistics. (2004). Centers for Disease Control and Prevention *Faststats*. Accessed online at URL *www.cdc.gov/nchs/*.

Crombleholme, W.R. (2004). Obstetrics. In Tierney, L.M., McPhee, S.J., & Papadakis, M.A. (Eds.), *CURRENT: Medical Diagnosis & Treatment* (43rd ed.). Stamford CT: Appleton & Lange Medical Books.

Dorigo, O., & Baker, V.V. (2003). Premalignant and malignant disorders of the ovaries and oviducts. In DeCherney, A.H., & Nathan, L. (Eds.), *CURRENT: Obstetric and Gynecological Diagnosis & Treatment* (9th ed.). New York: Appleton & Lange Medical Books.

Dorigo, O., & Goodman, A. (2003). Premalignant & malignant disorders of the uterine corpus. In DeCherney, A.H., & Nathan, L. (Eds.), *CURRENT: Obstetric and Gynecological Diagnosis & Treatment* (9th ed.). New York: Appleton & Lange Medical Books.

Holschneider, C.H. (2003). Premalignant & malignant disorders of the uterine cervix. In DeCherney, A.H., & Nathan, L. (Eds.), *CURRENT: Obstetric and Gynecological Diagnosis & Treatment* (9th ed.). New York: Appleton & Lange Medical Books.

Kiningham, R.B., Apgar, B.S., & Schwenk, T.L. (1996). Evaluation of amenorrhea. *American Family Physician,* 53(4): 1185–1194.

National Cancer Institute (2001). *The Bethesda System for Reporting Cervical Cytology.* Accessed online at URL http://bethesda2001.cancer.gov/terminology.html.

Chapter 13

Musculoskeletal System

S. Turner

The bones and muscles provide the infrastructure for the stability and movement of the body. Individual abilities and limitations in strength, movement, ease, and grace are defined by the abilities of this system to respond to stimuli. Limitations are a result of disease, injury, metabolic disorders, and lack of conditioning, which can lead to temporary or permanent disability. Complaints related to the musculoskeletal system are common across the lifespan. The types of problems vary between age groups.

Over 100 rheumatologic problems can cause musculoskeletal pain, swelling, and/or stiffness. There are over 33 million persons in the United States with arthritis; the majority are women. In fact, arthritis is the leading cause of disability in the United States. Even though the incidence of several of the chronic joint disorders increases with age, approximately two-thirds of patients with arthritis are under 65 years old.

As with all systems in the body, the musculoskeletal system is closely linked with other systems. The neurological and circulatory systems and the skin are most often associated with problems that also affect the musculoskeletal system. Problems affecting one system often produce associated problems in others. Problems with the musculoskeletal system most often relate to the joints but the examination must also include the bone and the associated muscles and joints to obtain a complete picture of the problem.

ANATOMY AND PHYSIOLOGY

The musculoskeletal system consists of a framework of bones that come together at joints. Ligaments attach them. Muscles are attached to the bones by tendons. Cartilage acts as cushioning between bones. This system provides for support, structure, and movement. They protect the internal organs and support the system through the production of red blood cells.

Bones and Joints

There are three types of joints: synovial, cartilaginous, and fibrous. The degree of movement differs by type of joint. Synovial joints are characterized by being freely moveable, covered by articular cartilage and separated by a synovial cavity. The bones involved in synovial joints, therefore, do not come into direct contact with each other. Examples of synovial joints are the hip, knee, shoulder, and elbow. Fingers and toes are also synovial joints. Bursae develop in spaces formed by joint articulation and serve as a cushion to ease motion between tendons, ligaments, and bones.

Cartilaginous joints have less mobility, and the bones are in closer proximity with one another. Fibrocartilaginous discs separate the bones and provide a cushioning support system that interlinks the vertebral bodies of the spine. Fibrous joints have nearly no movement between bones and are held together with a small amount of cartilage. The sutures in the skull, in adulthood, are immobile examples of these joints.

Bones and muscles are affected by genetics as well as environment. Activity will affect size as well as flexibility. Individual muscles are also dependent on innervation from the neurovascular system for function.

ASSESSMENT OF MUSCULOSKELETAL COMPLAINTS

Patients who have musculoskeletal problems usually present with pain, deformity, or weakness. Joint pain is the most common problem and backache is the most common disorder for which patients seek health care. The examination is often centered on the joints that are the focus of the pain, but often muscles and nerves are also a focal point of the examination.

A number of presentations are indications of urgent problems, requiring immediate recognition and definitive treatment. It is essential that the history and physical be directed to identify any of these symptoms or signs.

HISTORY

General Musculoskeletal History

It is important to complete a thorough symptom analysis for any musculoskeletal complaint (see chief complaint sections below). When a musculoskeletal disorder is suspected,

---

Red Flags in the Assessment of the Musculoskeletal System

- History of major trauma
- Hot and/or swollen joint(s)
- Systemic/constitutional symptoms
- Focal or diffuse weakness
- Neurogenic pain
- Claudication
- Unrelenting night-time pain
- Poorly localized pain

the review of that system should be complete. Ask about the history of associated pain, discomfort, swelling, redness, stiffness, crepitus, limitation, and weakness. The onset of symptoms is important, as certain traumatic or acute problems result in sudden onset of symptoms, whereas chronic diseases become evident over time. The musculoskeletal history should be appropriate to the patient's age because many problems are more likely to occur at certain times in one's life than others.

Past Medical History

Identify any history of musculoskeletal trauma, injuries, disorders, and procedures. The history of both remote and recent trauma and/or other injuries should be determined. When investigating previous injury, it is essential that the patient describe exactly what happened to result in injury to the muscles, bones, joints, or accessory structures. Disorders to ask about include recent infections, which could explain symptoms such as polyarthritis, monoarthritis, or generalized aches. A history of rheumatoid arthritis (juvenile and adult onset), osteoarthritis, osteoporosis, gout, or other musculoskeletal problems should be noted. The treatment and response related to any identified musculoskeletal problem(s) should be noted. Develop a profile of all medications that are currently or recently taken. In addition to the potential that information about recently taken drugs may shed light on disorders omitted from the overall medical history, it may also identify the etiology of complaints. Table 13-1 identifies medications that are commonly associated with musculoskeletal effects. Previous treatments from physical therapists, chiropractors, and practitioners of other disciplines are important to note relative to musculoskeletal complaints.

In addition to specific musculoskeletal disorders, also determine whether the patient has a history of any skin disorders that might suggest a cause for the musculoskeletal complaint, such as gonococcal arthritis, Lyme disease, systemic lupus erythematosus, or other systemic disorder. Several endocrine disorders may result in musculoskeletal symptoms, including hyperparathyroidism, hyper- and hypothyroidism, and diabetes. History of any neurological problems should be established.

Family History

Identify the family history of various types of arthritis, osteoporosis, gout, and other musculoskeletal disorders. Also determine the history of related systems.

Habits

Identify all nonprescription drugs the patient takes, as well as any herbal remedies. Determine the patient's normal activity level and any limitations realized since the pre-

Table 13-1. ■ Medications with Musculoskeletal Effects

Medications	Possible Musculoskeletal Side Effects
• Diuretics	• Secondary hyperuricemia
• Chemotherapies for malignancies	• May increase hyperuricemia
• Hydralazine, procainamide, chlorpromazine, methyldopa, isoniazid, and oral contraceptives	• Triggers for SLE

senting complaint was first noticed. Have the patient identify all occupational, social, and recreational physical activities. Identify any use of devices such as crutches, cane, walker, splint, or sling. Any activities that require repetitive motions and/or stressors to the musculoskeletal system should be identified. Environmental issues, such as where the patient works, lives, and spends his or her time in the present or past should be explored. Exposure to such toxins as Agent Orange or to the toxins that military personnel in the First Gulf War were exposed to, as well as any toxic substance exposure in the patient's work place should be explored.

PHYSICAL EXAMINATION
Order of the Examination

The musculoskeletal examination is primarily limited to inspection and palpation. After an initial observation of the patient's general appearance, gait, and gross range of motion (ROM), the remainder of the exam is usually performed in a head-to-toe sequence. However, depending on the presentation, the general survey may be followed by a more focused exam of the affected area, with comparison to the opposite side/structures. Regardless, although assessment involves both inspection and palpation, there are specific procedures used to assess individual joints that combine inspection with palpation as muscle tone, muscle strength, range of motion, and joint stability are determined.

General Survey

As the history is obtained, observe the patient's general appearance, including body build, posture, obvious deformities, general gait, movement, and any assistive aids used (crutches, walker, cane, bracing, etc). A limp, guarding, or obvious weakness can provide a valuable indication of a musculoskeletal or neurological problem and how the patient is compensating. Notice whether the patient appears comfortable in the current position, guards a particular extremity or region during the initial portion of the visit, and so on. Observe the patient's general skin condition. Note the vital signs.

Inspection

The focused musculoskeletal examination begins with inspection. For overall assessment, it is essential that the patient disrobe, usually to his or her underwear. When examination is limited to a specific region, it is essential that the region be completely free of clothing to allow adequate observation. Once the patient is disrobed, the general posture should again be noted, as well as any deformities, limited motion, and asymmetry of bony pairs or muscle groups. Identify any skin lesions, scars, bulges, and areas of redness or swelling. The patient should be directed through a variety of maneuvers intended to demonstrate range of motion and general ability to control movement. These include a variety of gaits (normal, heel-toe, on-toes, on-heels, etc.), as well as full range of motion of all joints without resistance. In addition to general inspection, more focused attention should be paid to any area of complaint.

Palpation

For complete musculoskeletal examination, palpation involves assessment of each joint, as well as the major muscle groups and accessory structures, such as ligaments and tendons. Joint assessments are complex. During palpation, note any palpable deformities, nodularities, areas of tenderness, and swelling or warmth/inflammation. Muscles should be palpated for tone, size, and tenderness. Any palpable crepitus should be identified. As specific complaints are assessed, the problem can be further identified by having the patient point to the specific region or site that is most painful and by more carefully assessing that area.

Range of Motion

Active motion of the major joint groups is determined. If there is any abnormality or complaint, active ROM should be followed by passive and/or assisted movements, comparing the findings in each. Noting that the patient's response to active ROM also provides clues as to how the examiner should best support the limb through passive motion. A goniometer provides an objective measure of ROM. Although a loss of motion will occur to some degree in most adults as they age, it is usually minimal. Substantial loss should be considered an abnormal finding, except in the distal finger joints. An injured or diseased joint will likely be painful on motion, and active ROM may be limited to a greater degree than passive ROM. Motion in an abnormal plane may indicate looseness in ligaments. Roughness in the surfaces of articulating bones may produce crepitus or grating on movement. Clicks can occur from previous injuries to the joints, abnormalities of a meniscus, or merely from soft tissue sliding over bone.

Ligamentous Tests

When a patient complains of pain or injury to a joint, the stability of the joint should be determined. Ligamentous tests involve applying stress to the ligaments by a variety of maneuvers that typically involve the examiner flexing or extending the joint while applying pressure in a particular direction and determining the "feel" of the resulting movement, including any laxity, crepitus, or pain. Ligamentous stressing of any particular joint should start with only gentle pressure and then repeated with increasing amounts of pressure/stress so that the test remains within the patient's pain tolerance, yet provides information on the degree of laxity in a joint with any particular amount of stress.

Muscle Strength and Tone

Muscle strength is determined by flexing the muscle (shortening it) and asking the patient to resist movement from the examiner. Alternatively, the patient can be asked to fully extend or flex against the examiner's resistance. Muscle strength is graded 0 (no evidence of strength) to 5 (complete or full resistance). Pain, contracture, and disease can all affect muscle strength. Table 13-2 depicts a rating scheme for muscle strength.

Joint and muscle pain typically increase when the muscle is stretched and the joint is extended. For instance, an injured hamstring muscle is more painful when the leg is straightened/ extended and the muscle pulled tight. Joint and tendon pain also increase when the area of injury is stressed.

Assessment of the muscle tone helps to determine nerve supply. A relaxed muscle should retain a slight residual tension when palpated. This is muscle tone. To assess muscle tone, passively stretch the muscle, ask the patient to relax, and then palpate the muscle, comparing side to side. It takes practice on the part of the examiner to develop a smooth motion when performing passive stretching. Assessment of muscle tone can be combined with a determination of the patient's resistance to passive movement. Tense patients, those

Table 13-2. ■ Muscle Strength Assessment

Muscle Strength Assessment	Grade Notation	% Normal
No muscle contraction noted when resistance applied.	M0	0
A slight muscle contraction seen or palpated but insufficient for joint movement.	M1	10
Weak contraction when the joint is held in position. Full passive range of motion.	M2	25
Contraction weak but there is full active movement against resistance.	M3	50
Some muscle strength against resistance.	M4	75
Normal strength is present.	M5	100

with increased muscle tone, will have increased resistance to passive movements. Marked floppiness indicates flaccid or hypotonic muscles. Decreased resistance may indicate peripheral nervous system disease, cerebellar disease, or spinal cord problems. A spastic muscle has increased resistance and may vary as the limb is moved, as in "cogwheeling," such as that found in patients with Parkinsonism. Resistance with both flexion and extension is called lead-pipe rigidity.

Special Maneuvers
There are a variety of special maneuvers indicated during the assessment of specific muscle, ligament, and/or joint groups. Some of the major maneuvers are described in subsequent sections on specific complaints.

DIAGNOSTIC STUDIES
Depending on the extent of the problem and the initial evaluation, it may be necessary to order additional testing to obtain a more complete evaluation of the injury. Radiographs, magnetic resonance imaging, and arthroscopic procedures may be necessary for a complete evaluation. Joint swelling may suggest a need for aspiration of fluid to determine pyogenic or gouty arthritis. These procedures are done only when necessary and by persons well qualified to perform them. The risk of contamination of the joint space or rupture of a ligament is a major consideration. Doppler studies may be helpful in determining problems with blood flow, clotting, and inflammation in the veins. Blood work to determine the presence of infectious, metabolic, or rheumatologic, or other disorders may also be needed.

DIFFERENTIAL DIAGNOSIS OF CHIEF COMPLAINTS
Pain is a common complaint associated with musculoskeletal disorders. Any complaint of musculoskeletal pain requires further symptom analysis. The analysis is very similar, regardless of the specific joint or region involved. Box 13-1 identifies the basic symptom analysis for musculoskeletal pain. The subsequent sections of this chapter will refer to this box.

Box 13-1

Musculoskeletal Symptom Analysis

Questions to determine what causes and/or relieves the pain:

- What, if anything, has the patient done to relieve the pain? What was the response?
- Is there any situation or activity that relieves the pain or causes it to diminish?
- What, if anything, triggers the pain or makes it worse?
- Is the pain worse at any particular time of day?

Questions to identify the type or quality of the pain:

- How can the pain be described?
- Is it burning, cramping, aching, sharp?
- Is it constant, throbbing, shooting?
- How bad is the pain on a scale?

Questions to determine the location and radiation of the pain:

- Where exactly does it hurt the most? (Can the patient point to the area where the pain is the worst?)
- Where does the pain radiate? Where else has there been pain?

Questions about associated symptoms:

- What other symptoms have been noticed since the pain first occurred?
- Have any other unusual sensations been noticed? Any tingling, numbness?
- Has there been any weakness, fatigue, swelling, redness, limited motion, popping?
- Have there been any other generalized symptoms? Any fever, malaise, decreased energy, ...?

Questions about the temporal sequence of the symptoms:

- Exactly when was the pain first noticed? What was the patient doing at the time?
- Since the pain was noticed, has it been persistent? Intermittent?
- Has the pain gotten worse? Stayed the same?

Joint Pain

The assessment and differential diagnosis for joint pain, or arthralgia, is determined by whether the pain is limited to only a few joints or is more widespread, involving several joints. Arthralgia is differentiated from arthritis, in that arthralgia simply indicates joint pain/discomfort, whereas arthritis indicates associated joint inflammation. Therefore, one can have arthralgia with or without accompanying signs of arthritis.

The causes of joint pain are often categorized by the number of joints involved. Monoarthralgia involves only one joint, oligoarthritis involves a small number of joints (for instance, two to four), and polyarthralgia involves several (five or more) joints. The following content on joint pain assessment is categorized by polyarthralgia and mono/oligoarthralgia.

Polyarthralgia

The differential diagnosis for polyarthralgia is broad and includes infections, rheumatic conditions, noninflammatory degenerative disorders, malignancies, and endocrine disorders, for example. For this reason, it is important that the history and physical obtain the necessary data to narrow the differential diagnosis.

History

Essential components of the history include determination of the nature of symptom onset and progression, as well as the presence of extraarticular symptoms. Establish whether the pain and any other symptoms have been constant, progressive, and/or intermittent and whether the same joints are consistently involved or the pain "migrates" among differing joints. Family history is important, particularly for autoimmune disorders, rheumatoid arthritis, and osteoarthritis.

Physical Examination

When examining a patient who complains of pain in multiple joints, it is important to determine the distribution of the involved joints, noting the degree of symmetry and the types of joints (large weight-bearing versus small joints) affected. The presence of inflammatory signs helps to differentiate arthritic conditions from noninflammatory arthralgias. Other important signs include the presence or absence of nonarticular signs, including abnormalities of the integumentary, cardiac, gastrointestinal, genitourinary, neurologic, and/or lymphatic system.

Diagnostic Studies

There are many diagnostic studies used to evaluate musculoskeletal complaints. Imaging studies are commonly used to evaluate the structure and integrity of affected joints. The range of relevant imaging studies is broad, although plain films are generally the first images indicated. Depending on the presentation, appropriate laboratory studies include a complete blood count, a metabolic profile, a urinalysis, and a variety of rheumatologic tests. Analysis of synovial fluid is often warranted to differentiate among potential etiologies.

RHEUMATOID ARTHRITIS

Rheumatoid arthritis (RA) is a progressive, inflammatory, and erosive condition that usually affects multiple joints. In addition to the articular changes associated with RA, there is a range of systemic effects. Rheumatoid arthritis is an autoimmune condition.

Signs and Symptoms.

The joints are typically affected symmetrically. Symptoms may wax and wane, but the effects are cumulative and progressive. Although RA can affect any joint, it commonly affects the small joints of the hands and feet, and this is often helpful in diagnosis. Affected joints are often tender, swollen with effusions, warm, and inflamed. Nodules and deformities are common to RA. Rheumatoid arthritis most commonly affects metacarpophalangeal and proximal interphalangeal joints. Over time, a variety of typical RA deformities develop, including subluxation of the metacarpophalangeal joints and ulnar deviation and hyperextensions of the proximal interphalangeal (swan neck) joints.

Diagnostic Studies.

A variety of laboratory tests are used to diagnose RA, including the rheumatoid factor, which is positive in up to 80% of persons with rheumatoid arthritis, but not specific to this disorder. It is often falsely positive in patients with other diseases, including lupus, sarcoidosis, and syphilis. Rheumatoid arthritis is often associated with normocytic, hypochromic anemia, as well as elevations in sedimentation rate and C-reactive protein.

OSTEOARTHRITIS

Osteoarthritis (OA) is another common cause of polyarthralgia. This progressive disorder is associated with age and with wear and tear. Osteoarthritis causes a loss of cartilage and progressive erosion of bone.

Signs and Symptoms.

Compared with RA, OA has a higher likelihood of affecting larger joints, such as the hips and knees. Like RA, OA also frequently involves the small joints of the hands, although it tends to occur at the distal interphalangeal joints (Heberden's nodes) and proximal interphalangeal joints (Bouchard's nodes). Most frequently, the second and/or third digits are involved, as well as the base of the thumb. The distribution is asymmetrical. The pain and stiffness associated with OA often improves with moderate use and is worst after extended periods of rest. If three or more metacarpophalangeal joints are swollen, the differential should include rheumatoid arthritis.

Diagnostic Studies.

Plain films reveal progressive changes, including diminishing joint space, sclerosis, and osteophyte formation. The sedimentation rate is negative and the rheumatoid factor is negative.

FIBROMYALGIA

The etiology of fibromyalgia is not known. This complex, multifactoral disorder affects approximately 2% of the population and occurs primarily in females. Although patients may present with complaints of multiple joint pain, the disorder does not actually involve joints. Instead, it is a noninflammatory soft tissue disorder.

Signs and Symptoms.

The most common symptoms are generalized pain, stiffness, decreased range of motion, with multiple point tenderness. In fact, the diagnostic criteria currently rest on a patient being identified with point tenderness in at least 11 of 18 specified sites. The most common tender sites are in the neck, shoulders, spine, and hips. Other common symptoms include morning stiffness, anxiety, sleep disturbances, and irritable bowel syndrome.

Diagnostic Studies.

There are no definitive diagnostic studies for fibromyalgia, which is often a diagnosis of exclusion and based on the presence of painful trigger points.

SYSTEMIC LUPUS ERYTHEMATOSUS

Systemic lupus erythematosus (SLE) is a chronic autoimmune disorder that has widespread effects. The prevalence is much higher in women, particularly in the childbearing years, than in men.

Signs and Symptoms.

Systemic lupus erythematosus has many potential symptoms. The classic findings include a malar rash. Patients often have arthralgias, myalgias, fever, fatigue, and neuropathy. Systemic lupus erythematosus effects depend on the organs involved. Cardiovascular, renal, pulmonary, hematologic, neurological, and musculoskeletal symptoms are possible.

Diagnostic Studies.

The diagnostic findings depend on the organs involved, and diagnosis can be difficult. A positive ANA (antinuclear antibody) occurs at some point in the condition in the majority of patients but is neither consistent nor specific for SLE. Positive anti-DNA and lupus erythematosis prep are also common to SLE. The sedimentation rate and C-reactive protein level are increased.

SARCOIDOSIS

Sarcoidosis is an inflammatory disorder in which patients develop granulomas and a wide range of symptoms, including arthritis. It is most commonly diagnosed in persons between ages 20 and 40.

Signs and Symptoms.

Although the disorder may be asymptomatic, it often is accompanied by multiple symptoms, including joint pain. Arthralgias occur in approximately 3% of patients with sarcoidosis, and the most commonly affected joints include the ankles, feet, and hands. The patient may complain of constitutional symptoms, including fatigue, fever, and altered appetite. Respiratory symptoms, including cough, wheezing, and shortness of breath are primary symptoms. Others include lymphadenopathy, rash, eye changes, and palpitations.

Diagnostic Studies.

Appropriate diagnostic studies depend on the symptoms and involved organs. However, definitive diagnosis involves biopsy of involved organs. Other laboratory abnormalities depend on involved organs. There is often an elevated sedimentation rate and normocytic, normochromic anemia.

REITER'S SYNDROME

This syndrome is described by several terms, including seronegative arthritis and reactive arthritis, and is the most common cause of migratory arthritis in young males. The complex of symptoms develops following an infection, usually of chlamydia. However, other associated causes include shigella, salmonella, and clostridia.

Signs and Symptoms.

Multiple joints are involved, primarily those of the lower extremities, as well as the vertebrae. The arthritis is migratory, involving varied joints. In addition to the arthritis pain, often present are urethritis, conjunctivitis, and/or iritis, as well as diarrhea and fever.

Diagnostic Studies.

There are no studies specific to Reiter's syndrome, although the sedimentation rate and C-reactive protein are often elevated.

GONOCOCCAL ARTHRITIS

This polyarthritis is also common in young men and follows infection with gonorrhea. Gonococcal arthritis occurs as part of disseminated infection.

Signs and Symptoms.

The polyarthritis is often migratory and affects lower extremities, as well as the hands. In addition to the arthritis, the syndrome usually includes a nonpruritic dermatitis and tenosynovitis. Generalized muscle aches and fever are also common.

Diagnostic Studies.

The sedimentation rate and C-reactive protein are often elevated. Plain films will reveal joint distention, which can later progress to joint destruction. Synovial fluid with increased polymorphonuclear leukocytes and positive culture occur in fewer than 50%.

GOUTY ARTHRITIS

Gout is a form of arthritis that results from the deposition/collection of microcrystals within a joint space. The offending agents are usually urate crystals. The condition usually occurs after middle age and is associated with an elevated uric acid level.

Signs and Symptoms.

Gout is a classic cause of monoarthritis but more rarely affects multiple joints. It should be considered when polyarthritis occurs recurrently over a long period of time. Even though most cases involve a joint in the lower extremities, others may be affected. Acute pain usually develops in one joint, with swelling, redness, and warmth, and the severity of the pain increases rapidly. Range of motion of the affected joint(s) is limited by pain and there is significant tenderness to the site. Patients who have had gout for an extended time often have gouty tophi, which are soft-tissue nodules, containing urate crystals. The olecranon bursa is a common site for tophi development, and the tophi themselves are often painful.

Diagnostic Studies.

Plain films are generally negative, unless the condition has persisted for a long period of time. In this case, films may reveal "punched-out" lesions of the bone. The uric acid level is elevated. Joint aspirate will reveal crystals. There may be a mild increase in white blood cells, and sedimentation rate is increased.

LYME DISEASE

Lyme disease was recognized in 1977 and is caused by the bacterium *Borrelia burgdorferi,* which is transmitted by a bite from a deer tick. Whereas the incubation period ranges from 3 to 30 days, the onset of symptoms typically appears in 7 to 14 days.

Signs and Symptoms.

Although the disorder can be asymptomatic, the patient generally develops migratory polyarthralgia, as well as myalgia and neurological findings, including meningitis and/or neuropathy. An early finding is a solitary target lesion that may be followed by multiple lesions.

Diagnostic Studies.

The diagnosis is often made based on the physical findings. Definitive diagnosis is based on laboratory studies, including ELISA, indirect immunofluorescent IgG antibody, and/or Western blot.

ACUTE RHEUMATIC FEVER

Acute rheumatic fever is becoming more rare in the United States. However, this disease should be considered when children and young adults develop polyarthralgia. This complex of symptoms occurs following an infection with streptococci, typically following streptococcal pharyngitis.

Signs and Symptoms.

There is typically a history of recent sore throat. Initially, pain develops in the larger joints and the pain is often migratory. Cardiac symptoms may be present, including heart failure, murmur, or pericarditis. Other signs include fever, rash, and subcutaneous nodules.

Diagnostic Studies.

There may be elevations of sedimentation rate and C-reactive protein, as well as a prolonged PR interval on electrocardiogram. Throat culture is positive in approximately 25% of patients.

Neck Pain

Neck pain is a common complaint and may originate from the neck structures or radiate from another region. Many of the potential causes are benign and self-limiting. Neck pain may also be an indication of a rheumatologic disorder, traumatic injury, or neurological disorder.

History

When a patient complains of neck pain, it is important to obtain a thorough history of the complaint, as well as any associated symptoms. The questions in the general pain symptom analysis (Box 13-1) should be explored. Determine whether there is any accompanying pain in other areas, including the head, shoulders, back, and upper extremities. Identify any stiffness or decreased ability of motion, as well as whether certain motions increase the discomfort. Mechanical problems are more likely to be aggravated by certain position changes. Determine the patient's normal activities during work or recreation, as well as any unusual exertion/activities. Always determine whether there is a history of recent injury or trauma.

Physical Examination

The examination relevant to neck pain will vary depending on the presentation. For recent trauma, a brief examination to determine stability may be performed and then radiographs obtained prior to proceeding with further examination. Otherwise, the examination should be thorough, with the patient undressed from the waist up. It can be helpful to observe the patient as he undresses, noting movement, which actions appear to aggravate the discomfort, dexterity, and the like. Observation should begin with the patient's general posture, head placement, cervical curve, and symmetry of movement. The neck structures should be observed and palpated, noting any deformity, tenderness, muscle spasms, or other abnormalities. Active ROM of the neck should be performed in all planes (flexion, extension, rotation, lateral flexion) within the patient's tolerance, followed by passive movement if there is any limitation suspected. Pain associated with movement is noted. Range of motion of the upper extremities should also be determined. The strength and tone of the neck and upper extremities should be determined, as should reflexes.

Diagnostic Studies

The history and clinical findings should guide the determination of when to order diagnostic studies. Patients with a recent onset of neck pain but no neurological symptoms and no history of trauma do not necessarily require imaging, and the selection of diagnostic studies is guided by clinical judgment. However, any patient with a history of trauma and neck discomfort should have a minimum of a three-view radiograph ordered: anteroposterior, lateral, and open mouth views. With any neurological signs, altered sensorium, or abnormal radiographic findings, a CT scan should be obtained as well. Patients with history of chronic neck pain should have plain cervical films, including anteroposterior, lateral, and open mouth views. Oblique views are often obtained. When patients have neurological symptoms, an MRI should be ordered as well. Alternatively, if the patient cannot tolerate or has other contraindications to the use of an MRI, a CT scan should be obtained and followed by a myelogram, as necessary. Electromyography and nerve conduction studies are helpful in identifying level of involvement.

CERVICAL DISC DISEASE

Cervical disc disease results from compression associated with herniated cervical discs. When cervical disc disease is identified or strongly suspected, the patient should be referred for specialist evaluation and definitive treatment.

Red Flags in the Assessment of the Patient with Neck Pain

- History of injury/trauma preceding onset of pain
- Associated neck stiffness (nuchal rigidity) with fever
- Neck pain in a child
- Pain that is unrelenting and/or worsening in patients who have tried and failed conservative treatment
- Acute, severe pain upon awakening in the morning, with or without radicular symptoms
- Pain relieved by elevating the arm above the head on the side of the pain
- Severe pain on flexion or extension of the neck, with or without radicular symptoms
- Chronic neck pain with weakness of upper or lower extremity(ies), stumbling, muscle atrophy, bowel or bladder incontinence
- Pain with a history of malignancies

Signs and Symptoms. Cervical disc disease is frequently manifested by morning tightness, stiffness, and/or pain. Coughing and straining can increase the pain, which may radiate to the shoulder and arm. Elevating the arm may provide relief. Numbness along the medial border of the scapula is a common finding. There may be radicular sensations, including paresthesias or pain that is sharp or burning in the shoulders, arms, or back. The actual distribution of radiating symptoms will depend on the affected nerve root. Neurologic findings including altered upper extremity deep tendon reflexes can be present, as well as weakness of the extremities and diminished sensation. If disc rupture is due to trauma, the onset of symptoms will typically be acute.

Spurling's sign is tested for by lightly pressing downward on the top of the patient's head, while tilting back and towards the side of pain. A positive Spurling's sign is noted if this maneuver reproduces neck and radicular pain, suggesting herniated disc. Another helpful maneuver is to assess for Lhermitte's sign by having the patient flex the neck in a chin-to-chest motion. A positive Lhermitte's sign, indicated by an electric shock–like sensation down the spine when the neck is flexed, also supports suspicion of herniated disc. The sign may also be positive in a number of other conditions, including spondylosis and Chiari I malformation.

Diagnostic Studies. Plain films will often identify the diminished disc space. An MRI is indicated for chronic neck pain with diminished disc space and/or neurological findings.

CERVICAL SPONDYLOSIS

Cervical spondylosis results from bone spur development associated with degenerative arthritis. The term cervical stenosis is used when the degenerative changes are more focal than diffuse. In both instances, the bony osteophytes compress the spinal cord so that both motor and sensory neurological symptoms may result. Patients in whom cervical spondylosis is identified should also be referred to specialty evaluation and treatment.

Signs and Symptoms. Neck tenderness is a common finding of cervical spondylitis. The neurological symptoms and clinical findings are specific to the affected nerve root. These can include radicular pain and dysesthesias, abnormal deep tendon reflexes, and weakness. *Diagnostic Studies.* Plain radiographs identify osteophyte formation and may suggest narrowing of spaces. An MRI will identify the site(s) and degree of compression.

NECK STRAIN

Neck strain is a common problem, which can be caused by positioning or overuse/ repetitive use of neck and related structures. Acceleration injury, or "whiplash" (typically seen following a car accident), is also a form of neck strain.

Signs and Symptoms.

The most common symptom of neck strain, regardless of the cause, is neck pain. However, there is often associated occipital, shoulder, and/or upper back pain, as well. The history usually identifies the source of the strain. With more severe strain, such as is seen with acceleration injuries, other common complaints include paresthesias of the upper extremities. The general strength and reflexes of the upper extremities should be within normal limits and the patient should be neurologically intact.

Diagnostic Studies.

Radiographs should exclude cervical fractures and subluxation if trauma has occurred or any neurological findings are present. If spasm is present, the only radiologic finding may be loss of the lordotic curve.

ANKYLOSING SPONDYLITIS

Ankylosing spondylitis is one of the spondyloarthropathies, which have genetic predispositions and are inflammatory disorders. The incidence is higher in men than women, and onset is generally in young adulthood. Neck pain is a late symptom and often occurs some time after the development of lower back pain.

Signs and Symptoms.

Early symptoms include low back pain and stiffness, which gradually become persistent and increase in severity. Later, the pain may again become intermittent. Other symptoms can include bony tenderness, malaise, loss of appetite, fever, and fatigue. There is loss of spine mobility, and posture gradually changes with flexion of the neck, increased kyphosis of the thoracic region, and loss of the lumbar curve. Although chest expansion is affected, respiratory function usually remains intact.

Diagnostic Studies.

The gene *HLA-B27* is present in most patients. Most have elevations of ESR and C-reactive protein, as well as some degree of anemia. Radiographs show sacroiliitis, with progressive erosion of joints.

MENINGITIS

Meningitis is a meningeal infection caused most often by virus or bacteria. Other causes include atypical organisms and inflammatory disorders.

Signs and Symptoms.

Neck pain and nuchal rigidity are common symptoms of meningitis. Other common symptoms include headache, altered mental status, nausea and vomiting, seizures, generalized aching/myalgia, and fever.

Diagnostic Studies. Examination of the cerebrospinal fluid provides definitive diagnosis. If bacterial infection is present, the organisms will be identified. In viral meningitis, viral cultures may not isolate the organism. However, there is typically an elevated protein level and increase in polymorphonuclear neutrophils. A CBC is ordered to assess white blood cell count. Scans (either MRI or CT) of the head exclude tumor and other space-occupying lesions.

SYRINGOMYELIA (SYRINX, HYDROSYRINGOMYELIA)

Syringomyelia is a fluid cavity in the spinal cord that can occur in the cervical and/or thoracic areas. The most common cause of syringomyelia is Chiari malformation (see Chiari malformation in the headache section of Chapter 14). Other, less common causes include spinal tumor, arachnoiditis, trauma, or idiopathology.

Signs and Symptoms. The patient often describes burning pain in the neck or thoracic area, as well as parasthesias or numbness in the neck or thoracic areas, as well as in the extremities. Progressive weakness of the extremities may occur, as well as limited range of motion of the neck and/or back. Other possible symptoms include bladder retention or incontinence. Sensation may be diminished. Reflexes and strength may be impaired. The gait may be altered.

Diagnostic Studies. The test of choice for diagnosis of syringomyelia is an MRI of the cervical, thoracic, and lumbar spine with and without contrast. The area of the spine that is imaged should depend on the area of symptoms reported by the patient.

Pathologic Fracture and Metastatic Tumor

Any spontaneous fracture should be explored for possible relation to carcinoma, either metastatic or multiple myeloma, in an older adult.

Fibromyalgia

See p. 329.

Low Back Pain

Low back pain (LBP) is extremely common. Nearly three-fourths of the world's population will have at least one disabling episode of LBP in their lives. It is the most common cause of limited activity and most common reason for office visits for patients under 45 years of age in the United States. Although most episodes are self-limited and resolve in less than 3 weeks, the longer an employee is absent from work owing to LBP, the lower the chance the employee has of returning to the workplace. The cause of LBP can be difficult to differentiate/diagnose, and the condition may be poorly treated. Moreover, many patients forgo standard medical assessment and treatment in favor of chiropractic care.

History

As with all pain syndromes, it is important to obtain a detailed history of the onset and of the progression of the pain since onset. A thorough pain history should be completed, noting the quality, location, radiation, and intensity of the pain, as well as any exacerbating and relieving factors. A thorough review of systems is necessary to identify any associated symptoms that may indicate an urgent problem. These include altered bowel and/or bladder function, fever, weight loss, and/or weakness. The medical history should identify previous episodes of back pain and other musculoskeletal disorders and should include the treatment and responses for them. Specifically ask about a history of malignancy, arthritis, recent infection, and neurological disorders. Family history should be obtained. The patient's recreational and occupational activity patterns should be determined. A history of all medications, both over the counter and prescription, should be identified.

Physical Examination

The physical examination should begin by noting the patient's posture and level of comfort. The standing patient should be directed through a series of maneuvers, including bending forward (back flexion), backward (hyperextension), and to each side (lateral flexion) and also twists at the waist (rotation), as the examiner notes smoothness of motion, range of motion, any obvious signs of discomfort. Then the examiner should palpate along the spinal column with the patient standing and then bending forward. Whether or not natural curvature is present should be noted. The patient should be observed walking on heels and on toes, observing for signs of weakness.

Next, the patient should rest supine on the exam table, and the straight leg maneuver should be performed. This test is often misinterpreted. However, as the patient rests supine with both legs extended, the examiner should passively elevate one leg at a time. A positive test is indicated if the patient experiences discomfort with the initial elevation, rather than once the hip has been hyperflexed beyond 50 degrees. It should be noted whether any pain is experienced on the side of the raised leg or contralaterally. The results of the straight leg test should be considered in combination with the rest of the physical examination, including neurosensory and reflex testing. If the results indicate nerve impingement or disc injury, further radiographic testing is then indicated.

Throughout the assessment, the examiner should always be attentive for signs of serious diseases associated with low back pain, including malignancy, abdominal aortic aneurysm, fracture, and bone infection.

Diagnostic Studies

The following diagnostic tests should be considered, based on history and presentation.

Red Flags in the Assessment of the Patient with Low Back Pain

- Pain is associated with neurologic deficits (weakness, altered sensation, bowel/bladder changes
- Pain in a child
- Pain is associated with fever and/or stiff neck
- Pain is associated with unexplained weight loss, with or without a previous history of malignancy
- Pain is worse at rest
- Pain is associated with radiation to the abdomen or stomach area
- Pain is related to history of urinary tract infections, drug use, or other infections (including AIDS)
- Pain increases with coughing/sneezing or straining

- Lumbar x-rays with anteroposterior/lateral and flexion/extension views will provide information about bony abnormalities. Acute fractures and subluxation are often discernable on plain x-rays.
- An MRI of the lumbar spine with and without contrast is the test of choice for diagnosis of herniated discs, intra- or extradural mass lesions, spina bifida occulta, and cauda equina syndrome.
- A CT scan with myelogram is not commonly used because MRI is a more sensitive test for determining tissue abnormalities. However, for those in whom MRI is contraindicated, a CT myelogram is useful. This is an invasive test and the patient should understand the risks and benefits before proceeding.
- Electromyography and nerve conduction tests may help to determine the exact nerve root involved in the setting of radiculopathy associated with low back pain.

MECHANICAL LOW BACK PAIN

Mechanical low back pain is extremely common, and most individuals experience some type of mechanical back pain at least once in their life. The causes are varied.

Signs and Symptoms. Pain in the back, buttocks, and thigh may be severe. The onset occurs after new or unusual exertion. There is no history of major trauma, systemic infection, or malignancy. Pain relief is achieved when lying down. Physical exam reveals paravertebral tenderness/spasm, scoliosis, or loss of natural lumbar lordosis with no neurological signs or radiculopathy.

Diagnostic Studies. None are needed.

Herniated Intervertebral Disc

Herniated discs are most common after age 30. Symptoms are dependent on the degree of disc protrusion and are often referred to as *sciatica.*

SIGNS AND SYMPTOMS.

A flexion injury or trauma may precede the onset of symptoms. Lying with hips flexed provides pain relief. Associated paravertebral tenderness and spasm often result in awkward posture. The acute phase is associated with radicular irritation and symptoms, including diminished reflexes and muscle strength. Major prolapse may be associated with bilateral weakness and bowel and bladder dysfunction. Pain associated with chronic irritation is usually dull and unilateral.

DIAGNOSTIC STUDIES.

The diagnostics include MRI, CT, or myelogram. Electromyography (EMG) may give supporting documentation regarding the nerve damage.

Spinal Stenosis

Caused by progressive degenerative spine changes, spinal stenosis is most common at middle age or later.

SIGNS AND SYMPTOMS.

Spinal stenosis pain is usually worst during the day. It is aggravated by standing and relieved by rest. The pain veries from severe to mild. The level of neurologic findings varies and can include weakness and bowel or bladder dysfunction. Osteoarthritis signs may be present.

DIAGNOSTIC STUDIES.
Radiologic findings may indicate extensive vertebral osteophytes and degenerative disc disease. An MRI or CT scan can be helpful if initial x-rays are inconclusive.

Osteoarthritis
See p. 329.

MALIGNANCY
When assessing the complaint of back pain, it is important to consider the potential that the complaints and findings are suggestive of a malignancy.

Signs and Symptoms. The patient is often over 50 years of age and presents with the complaint of dull pain that has gradually increased in intensity. There are often neurological findings, which vary by the level of involvement. A fever may be associated. The potential increases with a history of another malignancy.

Diagnostic Studies. When malignancy is suspected, plain films should be ordered, followed by CT, MRI, and/or bone scan.

SPINAL INFECTION
Vertebral osteomyelitis is rare, but it should be considered, particularly with at-risk patients. These include persons with advancing age, history of IV drug use, and compromised immune systems.

Signs and Symptoms. The history includes fever and chills, with possible weight loss. There is pain, which is often worst at night. There are usually no neurological complaints; this is dependent on the degree and level of involvement. There is point percussive tenderness and elevated temperature.

Diagnostic Studies. After the infection is advanced, plain films will reveal vertebral destruction. An MRI with enhancement is more diagnostic. Bone scan could be used for patient who cannot tolerate MRI, but it is not specific. Blood cultures should be obtained. The sedimentation rate and C-reactive protein are elevated.

COMPRESSION FRACTURE
Compression fractures are most commonly associated with osteoporosis and have a higher incidence with age.

Signs and Symptoms. The patient presents with complaints of back pain that may range from mild to severe. Onset can be gradual or acute. With acute onset, the patient can often describe a precipitating injury. There is a loss of height. Kyphosis results from thoracic fracture and lordosis from lumbar fracture. Depending on the degree of deformity associated with the fracture(s), the patient can have pulmonary symptoms.

Diagnostic Studies. Plain films reveal compression deformity, with loss of vertebral height and/or wedge deformity.

Isolated or Limited Joint Pain
A common complaint involves pain of an isolated joint or a limited number of joints. The conditions associated with joint pain can be categorized broadly into four major groups: mechanical problems, soft tissue conditions, inflammatory diseases, and noninflammatory diseases. Conditions that are frequently associated with pain in one or a few joints include

osteoarthritis, tendonitis, bursitis, infection, gout/pseudogout, and, more rarely, rheumatoid arthritis. This is true regardless of which joint(s) are affected. For this reason, the assessment for pain affecting only one or several joints is similar, regardless of the joints involved. This section will provide an overview of the assessment for limited joint involvement, and then problems specific to individual joints will be addressed.

History

Even when pain is limited to one or a few joints, a thorough history is warranted. It is important to quickly identify any recent trauma—both major and minor trauma. A standard symptom analysis should be performed relevant to the chief complaint, including the questions identified earlier.

Physical Examination

The physical exam should follow the general musculoskeletal exam described earlier. For any abnormality, a more detailed and focused assessment is necessary. For range of motion, palpation, strength testing, and so on, start with joint(s) that are not involved and then compare these to the joints of interest. If the patient's history includes major trauma, an x-ray should be obtained of the area to rule out fracture, displacement, or other mechanical problems. Consider an x-ray early if the patient presents with constitutional symptoms and/or focal bone pain, which could indicate malignancy.

If an effusion, bulging, redness, and/or warmth are detected, the cause is more likely gout, infectious arthritis, or another inflammatory condition, such as rheumatoid arthritis, systemic lupus erythematosus, or Lyme disease. These can be differentiated by serum tests and/or joint aspiration. If an infectious joint is suspected, an aspiration is necessary to obtain a synovial fluid specimen for culture.

Point tenderness in the absence of inflammatory signs suggests bursitis or tendinitis. Both tendinitis and bursitis are typically limited to one joint and have similar complaints (pain, point tenderness), regardless of the joint involved.

When pain is present in a limited number of joints with few or no signs of inflammation or effusion, the cause is often osteoarthritis. Other considerations should include localized derangement or strain, injury of the surrounding soft tissue, and viral infection. The potential for referred or neuropathic pain must be considered as well.

Shoulder Pain

Shoulder pain arises both from disorders affecting the shoulder structures as well as conditions involving other structures, such as the neck. Many of the conditions have very similar symptoms and physical findings. Shoulder pain in young patients (under 45 years old) is often related to trauma. Shoulder pain in older patients (over 45) is more often related to degenerative disease. Biomechanical trauma to the shoulder accentuates degenerative changes, causing degenerative changes to become more symptomatic as a result of mechanical stress. Shoulder syndromes frequently arise from inflammation. Most frequently, the capsule of the glenohumeral joint, supraspinatus tendon, and the subacromial bursa are involved.

TRAUMA

Trauma to the shoulder can result in a range of injuries, including brachial plexus injury, acute rotator cuff tear, acromioclavicular injury, and fractured clavicle.

Signs and Symptoms.

The history should identify the traumatic event, for instance a direct blow, fall on the shoulder, or twisting injury. Physical findings will be consistent with the degree of trauma and involvement of the shoulder and other structures. Whereas rotator cuff injuries (see next subsection) typically result from chronic impingement, they can result from acute trauma. A fall or blow to the shoulder area may result in a fractured clavicle, which is often associated with an obvious deformity at the site of the fracture and significant pain when pressure is applied over the fracture site. Another common injury associated with shoulder trauma is acromioclavicular separation or strain. The presence of an obvious deformity depends on the severity of separation/displacement. Acromioclavicular injury typically results in pain over the joint, which increases when the arm is elevated. A brachial plexus injury with trauma to C5–7 is indicated by paresthesia and/or sharp pain that radiates to the arm. The exam will identify significant weakness and decreased sensation.

Diagnostic Studies.

An x-ray should be ordered for any complaint of shoulder pain following an acute trauma.

ROTATOR CUFF SYNDROME AND IMPINGEMENT SYNDROME

The rotator cuff consists of the supraspinatus, infraspinatus, subscapularis, and teres minor.

Injury to the rotator cuff is typically due to chronic impingement, with degenerative changes over time. It is most common in persons over 40 years of age. Impingement results in rotator cuff tendinitis and/or bursitis of the subacromial bursa. As the structures thicken, increased mechanical injury occurs.

Signs and Symptoms.

The patient will typically complain of anterior and lateral shoulder pain that increases with arm elevation and reaching overhead. The pain is usually progressive and may be associated with repetitive activities. Pain at night may cause sleep disturbance. Range of motion is typically preserved. There may be point or diffuse tenderness to the shoulder area. Crepitus and/or arm weakness suggest an acute tear.

Diagnostic Studies.

Plain films are often normal, but may show subacromial spurs.

ROTATOR CUFF TEAR

Injury to the rotator cuff usually follows chronic impingement and degenerative changes over time. Injury to the structures may also result from trauma.

Signs and Symptoms.

Pain associated with a tear of the rotator cuff is sudden in onset and may be worst at night. Associated weakness and atrophy of surrounding structures occurs and range of motion is limited. The limitation is sometimes connected with the pain, as it will be painful for the patient to lift the arm; however, weakness of the periarticular structures also contributes to weakness. With a large tear, the patient will be able only to shrug the shoulder, but not lift the arm. Tenderness is greatest at the supraspinatus insertion, and pain may radiate to the deltoid region. Crepitus is often noted with rotation at 60–120 degrees of abduction, as this maneuver compresses the injured tissue. To compensate, the patient may rotate the palm up (supination) during abduction, which rotates the shoulder and widens the rotator cuff, decreasing the pain on movement.

Diagnostic Studies. Plain films are usually not helpful unless the injury has been long-standing, in which case some sclerosis may be noted. Diagnosis can be confirmed by arthrogram, which should be considered if shoulder pain persists or the onset of pain was preceded by trauma.

BICEPS TENOSYNOVITIS

Inflammation of the biceps tendon is another frequent cause of shoulder pain. The patient is usually middle aged or is an athlete with repeated injuries related to the throwing motion.

Signs and Symptoms. Tenderness is noted with active and passive motion as well as with palpation of the tendon sheath. The tendon becomes inflamed in the bicipital groove that can be felt on palpation. A positive Yergason test suggests this problem: with the elbow flexed, the patient supinates the arm against resistance from the examiner. The test is positive if pain is produced at the bicipital groove.

Diagnostic Studies. No radiologic testing is indicated.

ADHESIVE CAPSULITIS ("FROZEN SHOULDER")

"Frozen shoulder" refers to a variety of conditions that are associated with shoulder stiffness and limitation of motion. Although many other terms are used to refer to this condition, the most commonly accepted term is adhesive capsulitis. There is controversy regarding the etiology.

Signs and Symptoms. The patient is unable to abduct the affected arm beyond 90 degrees, with the scapula on that side stabilized/immobilized. A period of pain without limited motion often precedes the loss of motion. Then, there may be progressive stiffness associated with the pain, until the patient recognizes inability to perform certain tasks requiring elevation of the arm or reaching behind the head/back. At the point that passive and active range of motion are affected, there is generally diffuse tenderness.

Diagnostic Studies. Plain films may be helpful in identifying other disorders that cause secondary adhesive capsulitis, such as osteoarthritis, fracture, avascular necrosis, and calcific tendinitis.

GLENOHUMERAL INSTABILITY

Unlike the other conditions affecting the shoulder, glenohumeral instability is most common in young patients who are physically active. The instability can result in displacement of the humeral head in various directions.

Signs and Symptoms. The patient will experience sudden onset of pain and be unwilling to move the arm. The displacement may follow an acute injury/trauma, or may be associated with specific movements or overuse.

Diagnostic Studies. Plain film will identify the direction of instability and may show a defect of the humeral head that is associated with the instability.

Cardiac Pain

When patients present with complaints of exertional pain in the shoulder region, it is important to maintain a level of suspicion for referred cardiac pain. The presentation would likely include exertional shoulder pain, which is relieved with rest, and history of cardiac risk factors. See Chapter 6.

Pulmonary Pain

Pulmonary disorders can be associated with pain that is referred to the shoulder region. See Chapter 7.

Referred Abdominal Pain

Certain abdominal conditions, such as gallbladder disease, may result in pain that refers to the shoulder. See Chapter 9.

Elbow Pain

Pain related to the elbow is commonly mechanical in origin. The elbow is a very complex joint, with articulations between the humerus and radius, the humerus and ulna, and the ulna and radius. The innervation is also complex and at risk for entrapment between the various soft tissue and bony structures. Overuse and repetitive movement is responsible for many causes of elbow pain. However, rheumatoid, gouty, and septic arthritis can also affect the elbow.

Trauma

As with other joints, the elbow is at risk for acute trauma, which can result in fracture or dislocation or which can trigger reactive tendinitis. The presentation will be specific to the trauma experienced.

EPICONDYLITIS

Epicondylitis involves inflammation of the tendon/tendon insertion of the forearms. This tendinitis results in either lateral elbow pain associated with overuse of the wrist extensors (tennis elbow) or in medial elbow pain associated with overuse of involving wrist flexion and rotation (golfer's elbow).

Signs and Symptoms. Point tenderness is noted at the medial or lateral epicondyle. The onset and severity of pain is usually gradual and progressive, but may have relatively acute onset following an activity involving significant repetitive use. The pain may be referred to the forearm and is increased by the offending motion (wrist flexion, extension, or rotation). Pain is usually greater when the motion is made against resistance. There may be a locking sensation with motion and the area of point tenderness may be swollen.

Diagnostic Studies. Plain films are often normal, but may reveal spurs, loose bodies, and/or loss of joint space. Imaging is indicated particularly if there is a history of trauma.

OLECRANON BURSITIS

The olecranon bursa is superficial and at risk for repeated trauma. Olecranon bursitis can result from repetitive overuse, trauma, and infection.

Signs and Symptoms. The patient will usually complain of swelling and tenderness at the "tip" of the elbow, over the olecranon. Point tenderness is common although found most frequently in patients with septic bursitis. Septic bursitis is also often associated with a skin lesion either over the bursa or distal to the elbow and/or an elevated body temperature.

Diagnostic Studies. Plain film will be negative. An aspiration of the bursa should be performed for culture (septic bursitis), as well as determination of whether there is a collection of crystals (gouty bursitis) and/or elevated white cell count (greatest in septic bursitis).

Gout

Whereas gout typically involves a lower extremity joint, it is a frequent cause of elbow inflammation.

Rheumatoid Arthritis

Rheumatoid arthritis is a systemic condition, but may affect individual joints. See p. 328.

Osteoarthritis

See p. 329.

Wrist and Hand Pain

Pain and numbness of the hand and wrist may be unilateral or bilateral, but they are usually associated with biomechanical injuries related to overuse. The hands are common sites of both osteoarthritis and rheumatoid arthritis.

CARPAL TUNNEL SYNDROME

The carpal tunnel is a space located on the anterior aspect of the wrist, between the carpal bones and a ligamentous band. The carpal tunnel provides a "route" through which the median nerve and several tendons traverse. Often with overuse and repetitive movements, the various tissues hypertrophy, cause a loss of space, and impinge upon the median nerve, thereby resulting in the symptoms associated with carpal tunnel syndrome. The types of activities that are associated with carpal tunnel syndrome include computer use and painting.

Signs and Symptoms. Carpal tunnel syndrome causes a range of neurological symptoms, including pain, paresthesia, and weakness. Frequently, nighttime pain is an early symptom. There may be a swelling at the wrist related to inactivity or flexion at night. The pain and/or paresthesias typically involve the anterior aspects of wrist, medial palm, and first three digits on the affected hand. However, pain may radiate up the forearm to the shoulder with numbness and tingling along the median nerve. Over time, hand weakness often develops. Pain and paresthesia are often relieved by the patients "shaking" the affected hand in a downward fashion; this is called the flicking sign. A positive Tinel's sign is elicited by tapping on the median nerve at the carpal tunnel, thus causing pain and tingling along the median nerve. Phalen's maneuver reproduces the pain after 1 minute of wrist flexion against resistance.

Diagnostic Studies. Nerve testing, including nerve conduction studies, is indicated to determine the location and extent of the compression.

DE QUERVAIN'S TENDONITIS/TENOSYNOVITIS

De Quervain's tenosynovitis involves irritation of a tendon located on the radial side of the wrist, near the thumb. With overuse, the tissues surrounding the tendon sheath hypertrophy, causing pressure on the tendon and making it difficult to move.

Signs and Symptoms. The pain is usually limited to the radial aspect of the wrist and area immediately around the base of the thumb. Pain increases with use of the hand. Other symptoms include swelling at the site, decreased sensation, limited ROM, including a sensation of locking or catching with thumb motion. The Finkelstein maneuver is used to diagnose De Quervain's disease. This maneuver involves the patient making a fist, with the fingers flexed over the thumb, which is flexed/placed against the palm of the hand. Holding this position, the patient then flexes the wrist toward the ulnar surface. The test is positive when pain is reproduced. The pain associated with this maneuver is often very severe.

Diagnostic Studies. Plain films of the wrist are normal.

GANGLION CYSTS

Ganglion cysts are very common soft tissue abnormalities involving the wrist and/or hand. The fluid-filled cyst typically occurs in an area adjacent to a tendon sheath. The etiology is not clear, but ganglia are believed to be associated with some degenerative or traumatic damage to tendon sheaths.

Signs and Symptoms. The most obvious sign involves the swollen defect over the fluid-filled ganglion cyst. The area often becomes inflamed and is painful. However, the presence and severity of discomfort is variable and may be mild and/or limited to hand motion. The size of the ganglion cyst may vary over time, becoming smaller and larger intermittently. The cyst should transilluminate.

Diagnostic Studies. Plain films will be negative. Ultrasound will reveal the cystic structure.

Osteoarthritis
See p. 329.

Rheumatoid Arthritis
See p. 328.

Hip Pain
There are many potential causes of hip pain. Among adults, the most common cause is OA, with degenerative changes. In younger patients, the cause is often strain of the muscles or tendons. In comparison to other joints, the hip is often difficult to assess, in part because much of the joint and its periarticular structures lie much deeper than those of other joints.

Osteoarthritis
Osteoarthritis causes degenerative hip changes and is a frequent cause of hip pain in adults, becoming more prevalent after age 50. In younger patients, it may be secondary to trauma or congenital problems, such as a congenital hip dislocation or slipped capital femoral epiphysis. See p. 329.

TROCHANTERIC BURSITIS

Trochanteric bursitis involves a presumed inflammation or irritation of the gluteus maximus bursa or the bursa surrounding the greater trochanter. Other problems that result in changes in the patient's gait tend to increase the stress on the joint.

Signs and Symptoms. The patient presents with pain from the lateral hip and thigh to the knee or numbness. Pain is precipitated by walking, climbing, or prolonged standing. There is point tenderness at the greater trochanter, with increased pain on resisted abduction and external rotation.

Diagnostic Studies. X-rays are usually not helpful and may show no abnormalities.

ASEPTIC/AVASCULAR NECROSIS OF THE FEMORAL HEAD

This condition involves bone deterioration associated with diminished circulation stemming from trauma or other disorders, such as malignancy, sickle cell disease, lupus, infections, or Legg-Calve-Perthes disease. It is also associated with the use of corticosteroids and radiation treatment. Avascular necrosis can also affect other structures, such as the humeral head and knee.

Signs and Symptoms. The patient presents with complaints of hip pain and difficulty bearing weight. There is a history of an offending medication, trauma, or condition. Actual onset of pain can be very sudden or gradually recognized. In addition to weight bearing, other activities, such as coughing and other non-weight-bearing movements, often increase pain and the pain often persists at rest and occurs at night. Range of motion is significantly limited. Pain often radiates down the thigh.

Diagnostic Studies. Early in the progression, plain films may be normal or reveal increased bone density. As collapse of the affected bone occurs, the density will increase. However, these changes may not be evident until the disorder is very advanced. For this reason, definitive diagnosis is made with MRI, which is more sensitive than plain films. Bone scan will show increased uptake in the region surrounding the necrotic bone.

TENDONITIS

This typically follows overuse activities, with strain and/or inflammatory changes.

Signs and Symptoms. The patient will usually be able to identify recent activities that included repetitive motions and/or risk for straining tendon structures related to hip. The onset of pain is delayed, rather than first being noted during the repetitive activity. The pain is localized and increases with further activity. There is often a snapping or catching sensation. Point tenderness may be accompanied by swelling.

Diagnostic Studies. The diagnosis is typically made on physical findings and history alone. Plain films will be normal. Even though MRI or ultrasound may reveal the injury to tendon, these studies are not usually indicated or ordered.

Inflammatory Arthritis

Rheumatoid arthritis and other forms of inflammatory arthritis, such as gout and Reiter's syndrome, should be considered in assessment of hip pain. See elsewhere in this chapter.

SLIPPED FEMORAL CAPITAL EPIPHYSIS

This condition causes hip pain in adolescents. It is more common in overweight male adolescents during a time of rapid growth.

Signs and Symptoms.

There is usually a gradual progression of symptoms, with stiffness progressing to pain, and later development of a limp. There is usually no history of preceding activity or trauma. Pain often involves the buttocks and/or groin and can radiate to the medial knee. The presentation may be knee pain, with normal knee exam. Comfort is increased with external rotation of the hip and passive internal rotation of flexed hip increases pain. If advanced, avascular necrosis may occur, resulting in collapse of the femoral head. The condition is often bilateral, although complaint may be limited to one hip.

Diagnostic Studies.

Plain films with anteroposterior and lateral frog leg views reveal widening of the epiphyseal line and/or femoral displacement.

Knee Pain

The knee is vulnerable to injury from recreational and occupational activities, as well as from a variety of conditions. Assessment of the knee requires skill and practice in performing special maneuvers, such as the McMurray's test and tests of ligament integrity, including the drawer test and Lachman's test.

This section does not address knee fractures. However, the Ottawa knee rules provide a set of evidence-based criteria by which to determine when radiographs of the knee are warranted, following trauma. The criteria have been shown to have 100% sensitivity and 49% specificity for fracture of the knee. According to the findings, films should be ordered only if at least one of the following criteria are met: patient at least 55 years of age, tenderness present at tibial head, isolated tenderness present at the patella (i.e., no other knee tenderness), patient unable to flex knee to 90 degrees, or patient is unable to bear weight four steps (i.e., two steps on each foot), even with limping.

MENISCUS (LATERAL, MEDIAL) TEAR

Tears or disruptions of the meniscus sheath of cartilage are associated with osteoarthritis in older persons and with athletic activities in younger persons.

Signs and Symptoms.

There is typically a sudden onset of pain and swelling over the lateral or medial joint line as well as locking and painful popping. Onset often follows a twisting injury. There is point tenderness over the joint line, with mild effusion. A positive McMurray's test is often present (See Figure 13-1). To test the medial meniscus, the hip is flexed and the knee externally rotated as the examiner moves the knee from full flexion to extension. To test the lateral meniscus, the knee is internally rotated during the procedure. A snap may be heard or felt during this maneuver suggesting a tear of the medial meniscus.

Diagnostic Studies.

If meniscal tear is suspected, plain films are of little use, as they are usually negative. An MRI will reveal the defect in most cases. Arthroscopy can be performed alternatively or as a follow-up to the MRI.

LIGAMENTOUS INJURIES

The anterior, medial, and lateral knee ligaments are vulnerable to injury in athletic activities. The mechanism through which the anterior cruciate ligament (ACL) is typically injured involves deceleration combined with sudden turning or pivoting. The medial collateral ligament (MCL) is most prone to injury through motions that place valgus stress on the knee. Compared with ACL and MCL injury, damage to the lateral collateral liga-

Figure 13-1. ■ McMurray's Test (From Dillon, P.M. *Nursing health assessment: A critical thinking, case studies approach.* Philadelphia, F.A. Davis, 2003. Reprinted with permission.)

Figure 13-2. ■ Drawer sign. (From Starkey, C, and Ryan, JL. *Orthopedic and Athletic Injury Evaluation Handbook.* Philadelphia, F.A. Davis, 2001. Reprinted with permission.)

ment (LCL) is much rarer but typically occurs when sudden varus stress is placed on the knee.

Signs and Symptoms.

The patient often relates history of an acute trauma, followed by onset of pain, swelling, and limited mobility. Often patients recall hearing or feeling a "pop" at the moment of injury. Anterior cruciate ligament injury is identified through positive drawer and/or Lachman's test. The drawer sign (Figure 13-2) is elicited by the examiner holding the patient's leg at the level of the tibial tubercle and pulling anteriorly on the lower leg as the patient's knee is flexed at 90 degrees. The test is positive for ACL injury when there is laxity and forward motion and for posterior cruciate ligament injury if there is laxity in posterior movement. Lachman's test (Figure 13-3) is performed similarly, with the patient's

Figure 13-3. ■ Lachman's test. (From Starkey, C, and Ryan, JL. *Orthopedic and Athletic Injury Evaluation Handbook.* Philadelphia, F.A. Davis, 2001. Reprinted with permission.)

knee flexed to 30 degrees, noting laxity in anterior and posterior movement of the lower leg with the maneuver. Laxity of the MCL is assessed by placing valgus stress on the knee first with the leg extended and next with it flexed at 30 degrees. Laxity of the LCL is assessed by placing varus stress on the knee with the leg both extended and flexed.

Diagnostic Studies.

Radiographs are generally not indicated. If there is an ACL injury, plain film may reveal the presence of a tibial avulsion fracture. Tears are revealed with MRI.

CHONDROMALACIA PATELLA

Chondromalacia patella is seen in young active persons of either gender. The condition is also commonly called patella-femoral syndrome and runner's knee. In some cases, this problem is associated with other problems, such as congenitally high-riding patellae and tight hamstrings.

Signs and Symptoms.

The pain involves anterior knee, often develops gradually, and is moderate in intensity. For some, there is sudden onset of patellar pain. The pain is often noticed when rising to stand after sitting for a prolonged time. Runners sometimes indicate that their discomfort was first noticed when running downhill or walking up and down stairs. The pain is relieved during rest. Pain can be reproduced by pressing the patella against the femoral condyles, and there is tenderness around the patella. Other maneuvers that will reproduce the pain include applying pressure against the patella as the patient extends the lower leg, flexing the quadriceps, as well as moving the patella from side to side. Crepitus and effusion are often present.

Diagnostic Studies.

Diagnostic studies are not necessarily warranted. However, sunrise x-rays may reveal irregular surfaces of the patella.

PATELLAR TENDONITIS

Tendonitis can develop in any of the knee tendons but is most common with the patellar tendon. It most commonly affects boys during their teens and is also referred to as jumper's knee.

Signs and Symptoms.

The patient complains of pain inferior to the patella, at the site of the patellar tendon. The pain is often vague and increases with walking stairs or jumping. There is point tenderness over the tendon and pain can be reproduced by having the patient extend the knee against resistance. There is usually no effusion or crepitus.

Diagnostic Studies.

None indicated.

PREPATELLAR BURSITIS

Bursitis often accompanies tendinitis and is also associated with mild trauma. The term housemaid's knee is also used to refer to this problem, which is common to persons whose occupations requires extended periods of kneeling, such as plumbers and carpet layers. This bursitis can also be caused by an infection.

Signs and Symptoms.

The patient complains of pain in the area inferior to and over the patella, and there is swelling and inflammation of the bursa. The swelling and pain can occur suddenly and there is point tenderness over the affected area. The pain is worse with activity and does not bother the patient at night. The problem can become chronic.

Diagnostic Studies.

No diagnostic studies are generally performed. However, aspiration of the bursa can be performed to assess for crystalline deposits (gout) or signs of infection.

OSGOOD-SCHLATTER DISEASE

This self-limited condition occurs in adolescents and involves inflammation of the site where the patellar tendon inserts on the tibia.

Signs and Symptoms.

The patient complains of pain centered 2 to 3 inches inferior to the patella. The pain ranges from very mild to severe. Patients with mild pain often notice discomfort only on extensive activity, which resolves after a period of rest. Patients with severe pain often complain of persistent pain, regardless of their level of activity. Some patients develop swelling at the insertion site over the tibial tubercle, where there is also point tenderness.

Diagnostic Studies.

Images are not necessary, as the diagnosis is made on history and physical findings. However, if plain films are ordered, they often reveal an area of ossification over the tibial tubercle.

BAKER'S CYST

This is a popliteal cyst that often arises secondary to some other knee condition or injury.

Signs and Symptoms.

Baker's cysts can cause mild-to-moderate discomfort in the posterior knee/popliteal space. The cyst is palpable as an area of fullness. Other physical findings will depend on associated knee problems, such as meniscal tear.

Diagnostic Studies.

Diagnosis is typically made based on physical finding of the palpable cyst. However, an ultrasound of the popliteal space will provide definitive diagnosis.

Osteoarthritis

See p. 329.

Inflammatory Arthritis

Knee pain is often associated with inflammatory forms of arthritis. See p. 328.

Ankle and Foot Pain

Although this section does not address fractures, the Ottawa ankle and Ottawa foot rules provide evidence-based criteria to determine when, following acute trauma/injury, radiographs are warranted. These are summarized in Table 13-3. The identified specificity and sensitivity are based on adequate training in application of the rule.

SPRAINS

Sprains are the most common of all ankle injuries. Most ankle sprains involve the lateral ligament complex and are caused by forceful inversion and plantar flexion.

Signs and Symptoms.

The patient relates the history of an injury, followed by sudden onset of pain. Pain is noted in the region of the strained muscles or ligaments with local tenderness on palpation.

Table 13-3. ■ Ottawa Ankle and Foot Rules

Ankle Rule: Order film if one of following met	Foot Rule: Order film if one of following met
Inability to bear weight four steps (both immediately and in emergency department)	Inability to bear weight four steps (both immediately and in emergency department)
Bone tenderness at posterior edge or tip of either malleolus	Bone tenderness at navicular or base of 5th metatarsal
Sensitivity = 100%, Specificity = 79%	Sensitivity = 100%, Specificity = 79%

Ankle stability is assessed in a manner similar to that used to test the ligaments of the knee. By immobilizing the lower leg, grasping the foot while applying anterior and posterior stress, a drawer test is achieved. Valgus and varus pressure can also be applied, with inversion and eversion of the foot. Sprains can be classified using the Ottawa guidelines to provide information concerning the degree of disability and requirements for treatment. Table 13-4 depicts the classification for strains.

Diagnostic Studies.

Unless indicated by the presence of one of the findings described by the Ottawa ankle rule, no diagnostic imaging is warranted.

PLANTAR FASCIITIS

Plantar fasciitis is often incorrectly referred to as heel spur pain. In fact, this condition can occur in the absence of a calcaneal spur. It involves inflammation of the plantar fascia, associated with biomechanical tension on the fascia, most commonly involving the site of insertion at the calcaneal tubercle.

Signs and Symptoms.

The history includes pain on the undersurface of the heel, worse upon weight bearing after periods of rest or dorsiflexion of the toes. It can be present in one or both feet, but bilateral problems may represent an early symptom of gout, rheumatoid arthritis, or ankylosing spondylitis. There is point tenderness at the fascia insertion site.

Diagnostic Studies.

Images are not warranted. The absence of a calcaneal spur does not rule out the condition. However, plain films can rule out stress fracture.

Table 13-4. ■ Classification of Strains

Grade	Degree of Injury
I	Partial tear but no instability, or opening of the joint on stress maneuvers
II	Partial tear with some instability indicated by partial opening of joint on stress maneuvers
III	Complete tear with complete opening of joint on stress

ACHILLES TENDINITIS

Chronic overuse of the muscles of the calf or extreme stress on the Achilles tendon from activities such as jumping can lead to inflammation.

Signs and Symptoms.

Passive stretching of the tendon by dorsiflexion of the ankle will reproduce this pain. The patient will be unable to stand on the ball of the foot and will have tenderness and hemorrhage at the site of rupture (ruptured tendon). The patient will be unable to flex the foot. Thompson's test will be positive. There is a loss of movement in the foot when the calf is squeezed. This maneuver will result in plantar flexion of the normal foot.

Diagnostic Studies.

X-ray can be helpful to rule out fracture.

HALLUX VALGUS, OR BUNION

This is an enlargement of the metatarsophalangeal joint of the great toe resulting in lateral deviation.

Signs and Symptoms.

Pain and deformity are the initial complaints with soft tissue tenderness and redness.

Diagnostic Studies.

X-rays will rule out degenerative changes and differentiate soft tissue injuries from deformity.

Gout

The great toe is the most common site of gouty arthritis, which can also affect other areas of the foot or ankle. See p. 330.

Osteoarthritis

See p. 329.

Rheumatoid Arthritis and Other Forms of Inflammatory Arthritis

See p. 328.

Myalgia

Myalgia is a nonspecific complaint, accompanying many conditions. The history and physical are essential in arriving at a definitive diagnosis. Whereas many conditions do have myalgia as one finding, others include myalgia as the central complaint. The latter are described in the following.

Fibromyalgia

Myalgia is often the primary complaint in fibromyalgia. See the section on polyarthritis, p. 329.

POLYMYALGIA RHEUMATICA

Polymyalgia rheumatica is usually identified in adults aged 60 or older. The actual etiology of this condition is unknown. Giant cell arteritis occurs in about 15% of those with polymyalgia rheumatica, and the two conditions may be different expressions of the same etiology.

Signs and Symptoms.

The patient typically complains of sudden onset of widespread pain. Commonly affected sites include the neck, shoulders, and pelvis. Pain is accompanied by fatigue and stiffness. The stiffness is most profound in the morning. There is no actual muscle weakness. Unlike RA, there is no small joint inflammation and effusion.

Diagnostic Studies.

The C-reactive protein and sedimentation rate are often elevated. Biopsy and EMG are normal.

Rheumatoid Arthritis

Although RA typically affects multiple joints, it is not unusual for patients to present with complaints of muscle aches. See p. 328.

Infection

A variety of infections cause varying degrees of myalgia. Myalgia is a common component of viral syndrome.

Signs and Symptoms.

The patient describes acute onset of symptoms, which often includes complaints more specific to the infectious agent. There is often an increased temperature and signs of infection.

DRUG-INDUCED MYALGIA

Myalgia is associated with several medications. Drugs associated with myalgia include diuretics, anticonvulsants, lipid-lowering agents, hydralazine, chloroquine, and procainamide.

Signs and Symptoms.

The signs and symptoms are dependent on the medication taken.

Diagnostic Studies.

In general, no diagnostic studies are ordered. However, when drug-induced myalgia is present, there is often eosinophilia. For drug-induced SLE, ANA is positive.

CONCLUSION

All evaluations of muscle and joint problems should be made with concern for the patient's optimal function and pain reduction. The possibility of systemic disease should be ruled out and x-rays should accompany the examination. Injury may result in an insurance claim that will need clear and concise documentation, which should always be a result of detailed and follow-up examinations.

 SUGGESTED READINGS

Bickley, L.S., & Szilagyi, P.G. (2003). *Bates' Guide to Physical Examination and History Taking*. Philadelphia: Lippincott, Williams, and Wilkins.

Dillon, P.M. (2003). Nursing Health Assessment: A Critical Thinking, Case Studies Approach. Philadelphia: F.A. Davis.

Greene, W.B. (2001). *Essentials of Musculoskeletal Care* (2nd ed). Rosemont, IL: American Academy of Orthopaedic Surgeons.

McRae, R. (1999). *Pocketbook of Orthopaedics and Fractures*. Edinburgh: Churchill Livingstone.

Mercier, L.R. (2000). *Practical Orthopedics*. (5th Ed.). St. Louis: Mosby.

Swartz, M.H. (2002). *Textbook of Physical Diagnosis: History and Examination*. Philadelphia: Saunders.

Chapter 14
Neurologic System

D. Mueller

Neurological conditions are commonly encountered in primary care settings. Often neurological problems result in nonspecific symptoms, which require careful investigation for timely diagnosis. Some of the content described in this chapter overlaps that in others. For instance, dementia and delirium are described here in detail but are also addressed in the chapters addressing mental health (Chapter 16) and elderly patients (Chapter 19). Headaches are also addressed in the chapter on assessment of the head, face, and neck (Chapter 3).

HISTORY
Chief Complaint and the History of Present Illness
The history of present illness should include the primary symptom or constellation of symptoms, the associated factors, and the onset and duration of the symptoms. Ask the patient to describe the chief complaint in his or her own words. Inquire about whether an injury or traumatic event precipitated the onset of symptoms. If an injury was involved, explore the mechanism of injury, any associated loss of consciousness, and emergent treatments at the time of injury. Ask whether the primary symptom began acutely, or was the onset gradual and worsening over time. Ask whether there has been any change in the character, severity, location, or duration of the symptoms. Determine whether the patient has ever had the same or similar symptom in the past and, if so, what treatment was rendered. Identify measures that make the symptom better or worse (e.g., lying down, movements, Valsalva, medications).

General History and the Review of Systems
The general history should include a review of all body systems because symptoms of neurological diseases often overlap with other systems. For example, endocrine disorders may manifest themselves with symptoms of lethargy, fatigue, dizziness, or paresthesias; musculoskeletal disorders may manifest as weakness, muscle atrophy, and

balance or gait problems; and psychiatric disorders may mimic signs of neurological dysfunction. Therefore, a thorough review of systems is recommended. Specific to the neurological system, the review should include questions to determine whether the patient has experienced headaches or other pain, sensory changes, motor disturbances, confusion or other altered thought processes, dizziness, syncope, or altered speech.

Medical and Surgical History

The medical history should include all disorders for which the patient has been treated in the past. This includes both recent and remote history. If the patient is a child or adolescent, inquire about common childhood illnesses and immunizations. Ask whether the patient has ever been treated for the same or a similar complaint. If so, identify what diagnosis was made at that time, what treatments were rendered, and the response. The history should include conditions that have potential neurological effects, including cardiovascular disorders, such as atherosclerosis or hypertension; endocrine disorders, such as diabetes or hypothyroidism; or malignancies. Also include any history of blood transfusions and allergy or adverse reaction to medications or treatments. Explore the history of surgery or interventional procedures and experience with anesthesia. Identify any serious injuries in the past, such as head trauma, back injury, or whiplash. Document all medications, including over-the-counter and herbal agents, as well as the patient's understanding of their indication.

General Neurologic History

The neurologic history should include any past neurological disorders, excluding the presenting chief complaint. This includes stroke, carotid artery disease, head or spine trauma, altered level of consciousness, exposure to toxins or infectious diseases (such as tick bites, spider bites, mononucleosis, insecticides), seizures, or psychiatric disorders.

Social History

Ask about the current and past use of tobacco (cigarette, cigar, pipe, smokeless), alcohol, or drugs, including the quantity and duration of each. Document the amount of caffeine the patient consumes per day (include coffee, tea, caffeinated beverages, chocolate). If the patient participates in a regular exercise program, identify the type and frequency of activity performed. Document the patient's highest level of education and current and former occupations, including any possible occupational hazards.

Family History

Inquire about the immediate family history, including parents, siblings, and children. Of particular importance would be any family history of neurological diseases, including familial tremor, stroke, cerebrovascular disease, and neuromuscular disorders. Establish whether there is a family history of cardiovascular, endocrine, or other conditions with neurological effects. Also include any family history of substance abuse or mental illness.

PHYSICAL EXAMINATION

The neurological examination should start with a review of the patient's vital signs and general survey. A comprehensive neurological examination includes the following components:

- General appearance and affect
- Mental status
- Cranial nerve exam
- Motor function
- Reflexes
- Cerebrovascular
- Funduscopic
- Sensory

The breadth of the actual examination will depend on the patient's presentation. However, familiarity with each aspect is important and these are described below.

General Appearance and Affect

Observe the patient while entering the room and during the interview. General appearance considerations include nutrition, body habitus, cleanliness, attention to grooming, and affect. Note physical appearance of the skull, identifying any asymmetry or gross lesions. Note fluidity of movements, gait, and facial expressions. Abnormalities that may be detected during the assessment of general appearance include obesity, cachexia, poor grooming, sullen or flat affect, involuntary movements, hyperactivity, jocularity, and obvious craniofacial deformities.

Mental Status

A good screening tool for use in the outpatient setting is the Mini-Mental State Exam, described in detail in Chapter 19. Ask the family or significant other whether there has been any change in behavior patterns. If the patient does not speak or write English, have an interpreter available during exam. Box 14-1 describes the components of the mental sta-

---

Box 14-1

Mental Status Components

Orientation—the patient should normally be aware of person, date, and place. Ask the patient his or her full name, current date, and place in which the exam is being done.

Memory—recent and remote memory should normally be intact. Ask what the patient had for lunch yesterday (recent) and where they graduated from elementary school (remote).

Fund of knowledge (take into consideration the patient's level of education)—ask about any recent news events or significant upcoming or past holiday.

Attention span—ability to focus on the interviewer, without being easily distracted. Ask the patient to repeat a short list of numbers (e.g., 7-8-9-3-0-2). Inability to repeat six or more numbers indicates attention deficit.

Concentration—ability to concentrate on a question or task. Ask the patient to remember three unrelated words (*red*, *happy*, and *five*) and then to repeat them in 5 minutes, or ask the patient to count backward from 100 by 7.

Language—use and understanding of language. Ask the patient to write a full sentence, or spell *world* backward. Distinguish between dysphonias or dysarthrias, as these indicate mechanical disturbances, often due to cranial nerve dysfunction. Assess fluency of speech by asking the patient to repeat "no ifs, ands, or buts about it." Dysfluent speech is Broca's aphasia. Speech that is devoid of content indicates Wernicke's aphasia.

Abstract thoughts—ask the patient to interpret a common proverb (e.g., a stitch in time saves nine), or ask the patient to answer an abstract question (e.g., is my sister's brother a man or a woman?).

tus examination. Mental status abnormalities include confusion, inability to recall recent or remote events, inability to concentrate on conversation or exam, confabulation, inappropriate crying or laughter, slurred speech, word-finding difficulty, jocularity, or difficulty with abstract reasoning.

Cranial Nerve Examination

Examination of the cranial nerves (CNs) offers information about localization of the abnormality. Table 14-1 summarizes the CN exam.

Motor Function

Begin the assessment of motor function as the patient walks into the room and becomes seated. Note the strength of handshake. Observe posture, resting movements of limbs, blinking frequency, and facial movements. More-detailed assessment involves attention to

Table 14-1. ■ Cranial Nerve Examination

Cranial Nerve	Technique
CN I, Olfactory	After establishing patency of nostrils, assess the ability to recognize the smell of an alcohol swab, soap, or coffee (never ammonia); test one side at time. (Abnormalities: inability to discriminate between odors, asymmetric sense of smell.)
CN II, Optic	Check visual acuity, visual fields; observe optic disc (diminished vision, optic disc pallor, papilledema, see Chapter 4).
CN II, Optic CN III, Oculomotor	Test pupil responses to light and accommodation. (Abnormalities: asymmetry of pupil size or reaction, ptosis; see Chapter 4)
CN III, Oculomotor CN IV, Trochlear CN VI, Abducens	Observe relative position of each eye and eye movements. (Abnormalities: asymmetrical gaze, nystagmus, limited movement of either eye or both eyes.)
CN V, Trigeminal	Assess facial and corneal sensation, and masseter muscles tone/strength. (Abnormalities: asymmetric facial sensation, inability to blink upon threat, inability to clench jaw, jaw pain.)
CN VII, Facial	Observe facial symmetry during conversation, at rest, during exaggerated expressions, assess strength of eyelids, taste on the anterior $^2/_3$ of the tongue, sensation of the palate, elevation of the palate. (Abnormalities: decreased or absent taste, palate numbness, facial asymmetry or droop, asymmetric facial sensation.)
CN VIII, Vestibulocochlear	Assess hearing, perform Rinne and Weber tests, assess balance. (Abnormalities: positive Romberg, poor balance, altered acuity of hearing, tinnitus)
CN IX, Glossopharyngeal CN X, Vagus	Assess swallowing and gag reflex, note quality of voice, observe palate elevation, taste and sensation. (Abnormalities: absent gag reflex, dysphagia, asymmetry or deviation of uvula, asymmetric decreased/absent taste or numbness of the tongue, hoarseness/altered voice quality.)
CN XI, Spinal accessory	Assess head movement, strength of sternocleidomastoid (SCM) and trapezius muscles. (Abnormalities: asymmetric movements or weakness.) Note: Both central and peripheral lesions cause ipsilateral SCM weakness: central lesions cause ipsilateral trapezius weakness, whereas peripheral lesions cause contralateral trapezius weakness.
CN XII, Hypoglossal	Observe tongue position and movement. (Abnormalities: fasciculations, atrophy, tongue or palate deviation.) The tongue will deviate *toward* the side of the lesion.

> ## Box 14-2
> ### Strength Grades
>
> - 5/5 normal strength, full range of motion (ROM) against resistance
> - 4/5 full ROM against gravity, with some effort at resistance
> - 3/5 ROM against gravity
> - 2/5 ROM without gravity
> - 1/5 trace joint or muscle contraction
> - 0/5 no movement

isolated muscle groups, noting strength, tone, bulk, and contour of muscles. Box 14-2 provides the scale for grading muscle strength. Abnormalities include a lack of muscle tone, rigidity, cogwheel rigidity, atrophy, asymmetric strength, spasticity, flaccidity, fasciculations, and tremor.

Reflexes

Test deep tendon reflexes in all extremities. Some patients will have diminished or absent reflexes, which is a normal variant providing that the finding is symmetrical. If necessary, reinforcement can be accomplished by having the patient clench the jaws or tighten muscles of extremities not being tested. The grading scale for reflexes is provided in Box 14-3. The nerves related to each of the reflexes are listed in Box 14-4. Special reflex maneuvers include the Babinski reflex, assessing for upper motor neuron lesions of the lower extremities and the Hoffman response, and assessing for upper motor lesions of the upper extremities. Abnormalities of the deep tendon reflexes include hyperreflexive responses, with clonus. Diminished or absent reflexes are particularly important if limited to specific sites, while others remain intact.

Coordination

Test fluidity of movements. Inability to coordinate volitional movements suggests cerebellar dysfunction. Also note any involuntary movements, such as tremors, or an inability to perform tests. Box 14-5 lists coordination tests.

Cerebrovascular

Auscultation of the carotid arteries is an important portion of the neurologic examination, particularly for elderly patients, or those with a history of tobacco abuse. The patient should be asked to hold his or her breath during auscultation. A bruit in the carotid artery

> ## Box 14-3
> ### Reflex Grades
>
> 0 = absent
> 1+ = hyporeflexia
> 2+ = normal
> 3+ = hyperreflexia
> 4+ and 5+ = abnormally strong contractions with clonus

> **Box 14-4**
>
> Deep Tendon Reflexes
>
> Biceps: C5, C6
> Brachioradialis: C5, C6
> Triceps: C6, C7
> Patellar: L3, L4
> Achilles: S1

may be an indicator of potential stroke or carotid artery stenosis and should be followed by further tests, such as carotid duplex and carotid ultrasound.

Funduscopic Examination
The funduscopic exam is fully described in Chapter 4.

Sensory Examination
The sensory examination should be the final portion of the neurologic examination. The sensory exam indicates the patient's ability to interpret cutaneous sensory information. The test is performed with a clean, unused safety pin, the end of a cotton swab, and a tuning fork. Test each dermatome individually for sharp/dull and vibratory discrimination. Asymmetry of sensation implies impaired sensory distribution to the particular dermatome being tested.

DIFFERENTIAL DIAGNOSIS OF CHIEF COMPLAINTS
Headache or Cephalalgia
Headache is one of the most prevalent presenting complaints in the outpatient clinical setting, as well as a leading cause of missed days of work. The occasional headache sufferer accounts for the expenditure of billions of dollars annually for over-the-counter symptom remedies. Those who suffer headaches at a rate of one or less per month are unlikely to seek professional advice; however, those who suffer chronic pain of two or more episodes per month are more likely to consult their health care provider.

The considerable frequency of headache in the general population has led to the development of the International Headache Society (IHS) classification of headaches (IHS,

> **Box 14-5**
>
> Coordination Tests
>
> **Finger to nose testing**—ask the patient to touch your index finger with his or her index finger, then touch their nose repeatedly. Poor coordination of movement indicates dysmetria.
> **Rapid alternating movements**—ask the patient to perform rapid pronation and supination of the hand on his or her thigh or on the examining table.
> **Heel to shin testing**—ask the patient to take the heel of one side and repeatedly move up and down the shin of the opposite leg.
> **Romberg**—ask the patient to stand with feet together, arms abducted outward with palms up, and eyes closed. Positive Romberg is observed as a swaying motion, or inability to maintain balance, and indicates cerebellar dysfunction.

2004). This classification is useful for appropriate diagnosis and treatment of headaches. Headaches are broadly categorized as primary (for instance, migraine, tension, or cluster) and secondary (associated with space-occupying masses, infection, trauma, or substances). In addition to the detailed discussion in the following, head pain is addressed briefly in Chapter 3.

History

The headache history should follow the basic history format, with an emphasis on the head pain episode(s). Key elements of the history should include full symptom analysis. Have the patient describe the pain in his or her own words (throbbing, aching, pressure, sharp, stabbing), rate the severity (pain on scale of 1 to 10), and point to the area of pain. An account of activities preceding the onset of the headache(s) may help to identify potential triggers, such as straining, exertion, coitus, foods, substances, and the like—although the relationship may be coincidental rather than causative. Temporal considerations include whether the pain was acute or gradual in onset and its duration. If headaches of similar character have been previously experienced, ask what, if any, treatment was rendered and the response and tolerance to the treatment. Identify any associated symptoms, such as nausea, vomiting, confusion, stiff neck, or vision changes, as well as the history of any pro-dromal symptoms or aura. Determine whether the patient has recently altered any habits, such as caffeine intake. Identify all recently used over-the-counter or prescribed drugs, illicit/recreational drugs, tobacco, and alcohol. Determine whether the patient has recently experienced or been exposed to a viral or bacterial infection, traveled out of the country, or had exposures to any environmental toxins. Ask about any recent trauma, specifically a fall or blow to the head. Explore with the patient their occupation, habits, family stressors, marital relationship, sexual factors, social relationships, hobbies, and coping strategies. A thorough psychosocial investigation should precede additional testing.

For recurrent headaches, a headache diary is helpful in arriving at a definitive diagnosis. Although details can be simply recorded on a calendar, a number of headache diaries are available and downloadable via the Internet. Regardless of the format used, the diary

---

Red Flags in the Assessment of Patients with Headaches

- Headaches that are acute in onset, severe, and described as *"the worst headache of my life"* in a patient who has no history of headache. This patient should be referred *immediately* to a local emergency department for triage and treatment.

- Headaches that are unrelenting and unrelieved with conservative treatments, or pain that steadily worsens.

- Headaches that are of new onset in patients over 50 years of age, without previous history of headache.

- Headaches that are severe and associated with a stiff neck and/or fever.

- Headaches that are significantly different in pattern or severity in patient with a longstanding chronic headache history.

- Headaches that are persistent following trauma to the head or neck.

should provide a space for the patient to identify daily whether or not a headache was experienced. When headache is experienced, the form should allow the patient to identify the type, severity, and duration of pain experienced, accompanying symptoms, treatment and response, and any suspected triggers.

Physical Examination

The neurological examination for headache should include all of the basic elements, with an emphasis on the cranial nerves. Vital signs should be recorded, noting blood pressure and heart rate to assist in determining possible vascular components of the headache and any fever, which may indicate an inflammatory or infectious process. The physical exam should include examination of the eyes/fundi, neck, throat, sinuses, and nose. Palpate the head and temporal arteries for any gross abnormalities. The remainder of the neurological examination should be conducted to detect any sensory or motor dysfunction, difficulty with coordination, diminished reflexes, or altered mental status. Lesions/tumors of the brain, in particular, may cause symptoms that are subtle or insidious in nature, requiring a thorough examination and strict attention to detail.

Patients exhibiting any of the red flags noted previously require immediate definitive diagnosis. For example, any patient with an acute, severe headache, described as "the worst headache of my life," with or without associated symptoms should be referred immediately to the emergency department because this type of complaint may indicate an intracranial bleed. Any patient with headache associated with fever and stiff neck should be referred to the emergency department for evaluation of possible meningitis. Any patient over the age of 50 with new onset of headache that is unrelieved by medication and without previous history of headache should trigger suspicion of a space-occupying lesion and imaging studies should be obtained to further assess the complaint.

Diagnostic Studies

The following list provides a brief discussion of diagnostic studies relevant to the assessment of headache:

- Magnetic resonance imaging (MRI) with and without contrast is the test of choice for the diagnosis of occult lesions and organic disorders, unless contrast is otherwise contraindicated. The MRI should be performed in the sagittal, axial, and coronal planes.
- A computerized tomographic (CT) scan of the brain is useful as a screening tool for the emergent detection of expanding mass lesions, such as subdural or epidural hematoma, hemorrhagic stroke, or large mass lesions. The CT scan with contrast will help to visualize mass lesions, although it provides less-sensitive images than an MRI. A CT scan of the brain can also help to determine evidence of hydrocephalus.
- Plain skull x-rays are helpful in determining bony, extracranial abnormalities, such as skull fractures and skull lesions; however, they are not sensitive enough to diagnose intracranial abnormalities.
- Lumbar puncture (LP) is an invasive test that should be performed only if the symptoms warrant, and no expanding mass lesion is found on contrast MRI of the brain. The patient should be fully informed of the risks and benefits of the procedure. The risks of an LP include, but are not limited to, spinal fluid leak, post LP headache, infection, and pain.
- Complete blood count, erythrocyte sedimentation rate (ESR), and basic metabolic

profile are used to detect infectious processes, anemia, and metabolic abnormalities. Thyroid function tests may help to discover hypothyroidism.

MIGRAINE HEADACHE

Migraine is one of the most common vascular headache types and accounts for a significant percentage of clinic and emergency department visits per year. They occur more frequently in women, with the typical onset at approximately age six through adolescence. The majority of patients report a family history of migraine. Onset of migraine is very uncommon after the age of 40 years. Thus, patients with an onset of headache beyond this age should be evaluated for other head pain etiologies. Migraines often subside or completely resolve during pregnancy and menopause. The International Headache Society defines migraine as a recurring, idiopathic headache that generally lasts 4–76 hours. They generally do not occur daily and are often associated with the menstrual cycle. The frequency of episodes can be one to four times per month or only several times per year. Migraines can occur with or without aura.

Signs and Symptoms.

Typical migraine pain begins unilaterally but may become generalized, may lateralize to the opposite, and/or may radiate to the face or neck. The pain ranges from a dull ache to a throbbing or pulsatile pain. The pain is often severe and/or incapacitating and is often aggravated by movement, light, and noise. The pain may be accompanied by nausea, vomiting, photophobia, phonophobia, osmophobia, dizziness, chills, and/or ataxia. There may be tenderness to palpation of the temporal arteries. For those who do experience auras, they commonly include blurred vision and scotoma, and other prodromal symptoms can include anorexia, irritability, restlessness, or parasthesias, lasting from 30 minutes to 3 hours before the onset of migraine pain. The patient may be able to identify headache trigger(s); common migraine triggers are listed in Box 14-6.

Diagnostic Studies.

Further diagnostic studies may not be necessary, but should be based on the history and physical examination, if necessary to rule out other conditions. These tests can include CBC, ESR, metabolic profile, CT scan with contrast, MRI of the brain with and without contrast. An LP is generally not useful in the diagnosis of migraine. It is often helpful to ask the patient to keep a headache diary and record any factors precipitating the headache.

CLUSTER HEADACHE

One of the most severe and incapacitating forms of headache is the cluster headache. The condition is called "cluster" because the pain occurs in episodic clusters of attacks. The

---

Box 14-6

Migraine Triggers

- Stress
- Caffeine
- Change in sleep pattern (too much or too little sleep)
- Specific foods, or missing meals
- Menses
- Alcohol
- Hormone supplements

pain of cluster headache can be so intense as to precipitate suicidal thoughts or actions in order to find relief. Cluster headache is more common in men, with onset in the second to third decades of life. Specific cases have been reported in children as young as 1 year of age, although this is a rare occurrence. One of the most distinguishing characteristics of cluster pain is that the patient will appear extremely restless and anxious, instead of the quiet composure of the migraineur.

Signs and Symptoms.

There is usually complaint of headaches that are episodic and unpredictable in nature and that may be cyclic. Episodes often occur more frequently in spring and autumn. Cluster periods last, on average, 2 to 3 months and may remit for months to years. Remissions are typically shorter than 2 years. Unlike migraines, the pain is not preceded by aura. Cluster headaches have rapid crescendo patterns, peaking in approximately 10–15 minutes and often lasting 30–60 minutes per episode (rarely lasting over 2 hours each). Attacks occur as frequently as two to three times per day. The pain is generally in the area of the trigeminal nerve and is described as unilateral, penetrating, sharp, excruciating, and unrelenting in nature. The pain is often associated with unilateral lacrimation, nasal congestion or rhinorrhea, pallor, flushing, conjunctival redness, ptosis—all on the *same side* as the pain. Some people may experience bradycardia during the episode. During an episode, the patient is restless, may hold the head, and is often anxious and unable to sit still. Cluster headache triggers are listed in Box 14-7.

Diagnostic Studies.

Diagnostic studies and workup are not definitive, but should be selected if needed to rule out other disorders. These include MRI or CT scan of the brain with contrast, dental examination for possible trigeminal neuralgia, ESR, CBC, and basic metabolic profile. An ophthalmologic examination with dilation may help to rule out ocular causes of the pain.

TENSION HEADACHE

Tension headaches are quite common. Whereas many with episodic tension headaches do not seek treatment, those who suffer from frequent or chronic tension headaches may enlist the help of their provider. Other terms to describe tension headache include: stress headache, essential headache, idiopathic headache, and muscle contraction headache. Tension headaches can occur with equal frequency among men and women, in any age group, and within any socioeconomic group.

Signs and Symptoms.

Typical symptoms of tension headache include mild to moderate, nonthrobbing, pressure, or squeezing pain that can occur anywhere in the head or neck. The pain often starts

---

Box 14-7

Cluster Headache Triggers

- Smoking
- Alcohol
- Vasodilators
- Seasonal changes
- Altitude changes

slowly as a dull and aching discomfort that progresses to holocranial pain and pressure. The pain lasts from minutes to hours, usually remitting with rest or removal of the stressful trigger. The pain can recur intermittently. Unlike migraines, there is usually no associated nausea and vomiting. Although patients may report photophobia and phonophobia, it is less severe than those associated with migraines. Tension headaches are not aggravated by movement or activity. The neck muscles are often tight to palpation. Tension headache triggers are listed in Box 14-8.

Diagnostic Studies.

Diagnostics and further workup should be ordered only if necessary to rule out other conditions.

SUBDURAL HEMATOMA

Subdural hematomas can be either acute or chronic. Acute subdural hematomas are usually associated with an acute head injury and can cause a range of symptoms, including headache and loss of consciousness. A chronic subdural hematoma in the elderly population may enlarge significantly before the patient begins to notice head pain.

Signs and Symptoms.

The headache associated with subdural hematoma is generally dull and aching in nature, and may be transient. The history often includes a blow to the head, fall, or other injury, which preceded the pain. The pain will gradually worsen over days to weeks. In the elderly, the history of head trauma may be more remote than in younger patients. A change in mentation may precede pain in the elderly population. The physical findings vary depending on the severity of the trauma but may include progressive neurologic deterioration, which may advance to include coma.

Diagnostic Studies.

A CT scan of the brain is the test of choice in the acute setting and will show both acute and chronic subdural hematoma. An MRI of the brain with and without contrast will demonstrate any associated abnormalities.

SUBARACHNOID HEMORRHAGE

Head trauma is the most common cause of subarachnoid hemorrhages (SAHs). However, a SAH can be spontaneous, stemming from a ruptured aneurysm, vascular malformations, uncontrolled hypertension, or hemorrhagic disease. Persons who smoke have a significantly higher risk of SAH. Subarachnoid hemorrhage most typically occurs in adults 50–60 years of age. *This type of headache represents a true medical emergency and necessitates immediate referral or transfer to a local emergency department for triage and treatment.*

Signs and Symptoms.

The head pain associated with SAH is generally described as severe and acute in onset. The onset is often described as a thunderbolt or lightening. The severity is described as "the

Box 14-8
Tension Headache Triggers
• Stress, fatigue, lack of sleep, anxiety, depression • Overuse of caffeine or tobacco • Latent hostility toward self or others

worst headache in my life." It is generally made worse by lying down. There is often associated nausea and/or vomiting, and possible rapid deterioration in neurologic function.

Diagnostic Studies.

A noncontrast CT scan of the brain is the test of choice in the acute setting. An LP is generally not recommended in the acute phase, as this may result in increased bleeding or herniation. If a vascular abnormality is found, magnetic resonance angiography or conventional angiogram is generally recommended to determine the exact etiology.

VIRAL OR BACTERIAL MENINGITIS

Meningitis involves inflammatory central nervous system disease generally caused by either viral or bacterial infection. The etiology of meningitis includes community acquired, posttraumatic, aseptic, carcinomatous, or transferred from another bodily source. The most common organisms belong to such genera as *Streptococcus, Neisseria (meningitides), Haemophilus (influenzae), Listeria, Staphylococcus (aureus)*—as well as gram-negative bacilli and gram-positive cocci. Meningitis can affect persons of all ages, including children. Patients with meningitis represent a medical emergency and should be referred to an emergency department for treatment.

Signs and Symptoms.

The headache associated with meningitis is described as diffuse and throbbing and is often severe or intense in nature. There is usually associated fever, photophobia, phonophobia, nausea/vomiting, and nuchal rigidity. Patients can rapidly decline to delirium, seizures, and, if untreated, coma. On neurologic examination, the patient may be lethargic and febrile, and have altered mentation, along with nuchal rigidity and/or guarding, contracted and sluggish pupils, and a generally "toxic" appearance. Brudzinski's and Kernig's signs are helpful in assessing potential meningeal conditions (see Box 14-9). Delirium or acute confusion necessitates immediate transfer to an emergency department for treatment, as the patient can rapidly deteriorate to coma.

Diagnostics Studies.

Diagnostic tests should include CBC, ESR, C-reactive protein, and CT scan or MRI to rule out a mass lesion. An LP (to obtain cerebrospinal fluid [CSF] for cell count, protein, glucose, and cultures) is generally performed *only after* ruling out a mass through imaging.

CHIARI MALFORMATION

Chiari malformation is an unusual and often insidious brainstem malformation that is defined as 3–5 mm or more of tonsillar herniation below the level of the foramen magnum. There are three types of Chiari malfunction. Chiari type I is generally seen in the adult pop-

---

Box 14-9

Meningeal Tests

Brudzinski's Test—with patient lying on exam table, gently flex the patient's neck to a chin-to-chest position. The test is positive if the patient attempts to lift legs and flex hips to relieve pain caused by the maneuver.

Kernig's Test—with patient resting on exam table, hold leg with hip and knee flexed. Without moving the upper leg, slowly extend the knee, straightening the leg. The test is positive if the maneuver results in pain, with the patient flexing the neck in attempt to relieve the pain.

ulation but can also be diagnosed in infants and children and is most commonly associated with an occipital headache. Symptoms of Chiari type I may be very vague and transient, and it is often misdiagnosed as multiple sclerosis or another neurologic degenerative disease. Young children with Chiari type I often present with swallowing difficulty and/or head pain. Infants with Chiari type I often present with swallowing difficulty, with a related failure to thrive. Chiari type II malformation is generally diagnosed in infants or children and is associated with myelomeningocele or other open neural tube defects. Chiari type II in adults is most often associated with undiagnosed spina bifida occulta or tethered cord. Chiari type III malformation is rare, only diagnosed in infants, and is associated with cervical myelomeningocele or pseudomeningocele. Chiari type III carries a very poor prognosis.

Signs and Symptoms.

The typical presentation of Chiari malformation includes a persistent headache that occurs most often in the occipital area and may radiate diffusely or behind the eyes. The headache is triggered or worsened by the Valsalva maneuver or by flexion/extension of the neck. There is often complaint of neck or skull base pain, as well as dizziness or disequilibrium, also worsened by movement or flexion/extension of the neck. Other complaints may include tinnitus and decreased hearing; weakness, numbness, paresthesias, and extremity pain; extreme fatigue, difficulty sleeping, and generalized body weakness; difficulty swallowing and voice hoarseness (often with diminished or absent gag reflex); and altered memory or concentration.

Diagnostic Studies.

The test of choice for the diagnosis of Chiari malformation is an MRI of the brain and brainstem with and without contrast.

BRAIN ABSCESS

Brain abscess can be caused by an extension of an existing extracranial infection, extension of a blood-borne infection, intracranial procedures, or penetrating head injury. Infections of the lung, heart, ear, or sinus are the most common sources of abscess transference. During the history taking, it is important to focus on any other sources of recent infection, particularly sinus, throat, tooth, and ear infections. The cause is idiopathic in approximately 25% of the cases. Inquire about recent visits to developing countries because abscess is more common and easily spread in these geographic areas, and inquire as well about recent or remote consumption of poorly cooked meats or unwashed vegetables. The most common vector is streptococcus.

Initially, the infection may be insidious, with little to no symptom constellation. The abscess generally only causes head pain after the lesion has enlarged enough to result in mass effect on the brain tissue. *Treatment for brain abscess requires immediate transfer to an emergency department for neurosurgical and infectious disease consultation.*

Signs and Symptoms.

If the condition represents an extension of a preexisting problem, the history will be consistent with that condition, as well as the symptoms specifically related to the abscess. The history usually includes a gradual onset of symptoms that progress as the inflammatory process increases. These symptoms include headache, nausea (with or without vomiting), lethargy, and fever. Over time, if the lesion expands, the symptoms progress to include seizures, lethargy, hemiparesis, and altered mental status. If left untreated, the patient can rapidly decline to seizures and coma.

Diagnostic Studies.

Diagnostic tests to be performed for patients suspected of brain abscess include CBC (may be normal in the early stage, or in the elderly population), ESR, C-reactive protein, and blood cultures (may be negative). An MRI of the brain with and without contrast will show enhancing lesions, and this is the test of choice for localization. Magnetic resonance (MR) spectroscopy may also help in determining the activity of the abscess. Lumbar puncture is not recommended in the initial workup for intracranial abscess.

TUMOR

An intracranial malignancy can result in a wide range of complaints and findings, depending on the size and location of the mass, as they commonly stem from the increased pressure on tissues, obstruction of the circulation, and/or increased intracranial pressure. Because the brain tissue does not feel pain, most patients do not present with headache as a cardinal symptom until the lesion is large enough to significantly increase intracranial pressure. Meningioma is the most likely tumor to cause headache. Brain tumors include benign, primary malignant, and metastatic lesions.

Signs and Symptoms.

Progressive neurological deterioration is one of the most common symptoms of an intracranial mass lesion. Many elderly patients may show slow progressive mental decline over months to years and may be misdiagnosed as depressed or demented. Head pain generally overlies the area of the mass lesion. Tumors of the sella generally refer pain to the vertex. The pain associated with tumors is often described as dull, aching, and transitory. New-onset seizures in the adult population should be considered the result of a mass lesion until proven otherwise. Vomiting without nausea implies increased intracranial pressure. Some persons will report improvement in their symptoms for a brief time after vomiting. Unilateral extremity numbness/paresthesias and weakness may be either slowly or rapidly progressive. Mass lesions of the cerebellum may cause disequilibrium or gait disturbance. Acute unilateral hearing loss or tinnitus may imply a lesion of the acoustic nerve. Unilateral visual disturbances may imply a lesion or compression on the optic nerve. The physical exam may reveal alterations in vital signs, particularly new-onset hypertension. The neurological exam may be normal until the lesion exerts enough mass effect to increase intracranial pressure or obstruct the flow of CSF. Focal neurological findings may include anisocoria, unilateral hearing loss, nystagmus, visual field defects, extremity weakness, numbness or paresthesia of the extremities, tongue deviation, and papilledema.

Diagnostic Studies.

An MRI of the brain with and without contrast is the imaging study of choice for assessment of intracranial lesions. Magnetic resonance spectroscopy will help to assess cell activity within the tumor. If suspicious for metastasis, imaging of the suspected area may aid in evaluation of the tumor type. If a lesion is found in the cerebellum, an MRI of the cervical spine will help to assess for any drop lesions. Surgical biopsy of the intracranial tumor is the test of choice for definitive diagnosis of tumor type.

TEMPORAL ARTERITIS

Temporal arteritis is also referred to as giant cell arteritis or cranial arteritis. It is characterized by chronic inflammation and the presence of giant cells in large arteries, usually the temporal artery, but can occur in the cranial arteries, the aorta, and coronary and peripheral arteries. It affects the arteries containing elastic tissue. The chronic inflammation causes the intima of the artery to thicken, resulting in narrowing and eventual occlusion of the lumen. It occurs more among persons over 50 years of age and is slightly more common in females than males. The cause is unknown but there seems to be a genetic predisposition.

Signs and Symptoms. The most common chief complaint is bitemporal, frontal, or vertex head pain that is lancinating, sharp, or "ice pick" in nature. The pain can be quite severe and debilitating. Patients will often complain of visual changes, including amaurosis (complete loss of vision with no apparent eye pathology), diplopia, blurred vision, visual field cuts, eye pain, periorbital edema, and intermittent unilateral blindness. Patients who present with acute vision loss should be *referred immediately* to a neurologist or neuroophthalmologist for visual field testing and fundoscopic examination with attention to the optic nerve. *If left untreated, arteritis can rapidly lead to blindness that is often irreversible.*

Other common presenting symptoms include scalp and/or jaw tenderness, facial pain, and tenderness to palpation over the affected artery. The pain is generally hemicranial but can be bilateral or diffuse. There may be eye pain, which is usually bilateral, and periorbital edema may be present. Other potential associated symptoms include an intermittent fever (generally low grade), nausea, and/or weight loss.

Diagnostic Studies. In temporal arteritis, the white blood cell count may be elevated, although often normal in the elderly population, who usually develop the condition. The ESR may be elevated, as well as the C-reactive protein. An MRI of the brain with and without contrast will help to rule out other structural causes; however, its use is not definitive for the diagnosis of arteritis. Definitive diagnosis of arteritis is determined by temporal artery biopsy. In order to prevent blindness from ischemic optic neuropathy, which occurs in approximately 20% of patients, treatment with corticosteroids should be started immediately while diagnostic studies are completed.

MEDICATION-OVERUSE HEADACHE, OR ANALGESIC REBOUND HEADACHE

Susceptible patients who take analgesic or abortive medications on a frequent basis for recurrent headaches may develop medication-overuse headaches. In addition to the susceptibility of the individual patient, the regularity with which the particular agent is taken is an important variable. This diagnosis should be considered in patients who develop chronic, daily headaches during therapy for primary headaches. Although this discussion is specific to the development of chronic headaches following overuse of headache agents, chronic headaches can also be associated with overuse of or withdrawal from a variety of other agents, as well as an adverse effect of a wide range of substances.

Signs and Symptoms.

The headache is usually described as migrainelike. History reveals that the patient has taken the analgesic or abortive agent (acetaminophen, aspirin, compounds, codeine, triptans, etc.) regularly, 15 or more times a month, usually for a period of 3 or more months. The diagnosis is supported when the chronic daily headache resolves or reverts to the earlier pattern of frequency when the patient is successfully withdrawn from the associated drug for a period of 2 months. Withdrawal may require inpatient detoxification.

Diagnostic Studies. None warranted, unless to exclude other potential causes. Urine and/or serum toxicity screens may aid in determining the levels of certain medications.

Altered Mental Status

Alteration in mental status is generally a chief complaint of the elderly population. However, some unusual forms of dementia can be diagnosed as early as the second decade of life. The causes of mental status changes include, but are not limited to, Alzheimer's disease, multi-infarct state, stroke, central nervous system infections, neurodegenerative disorders, head injury, mass lesions, metabolic disorders, and hydrocephalus. It is estimated that approximately 10%–20% of mental status changes are due to treatable causes, such as vitamin B deficiency, polypharmacy, intoxication or drug abuse, and infectious processes. Chapters 16 (on mental health) and 19 (on older patients) include additional content on altered thought processes. It is important to consider psychiatric conditions in the differential diagnosis for altered mental status.

History

A thorough history of the chief complaint should emphasize the mental status baseline and changes that have occurred. It is best if a family member or a significant other can be present when taking the history because the patient may not have full awareness of the mental status changes. *Key elements* of the history should include the patient's age and when the mental status change was first noted by the patient or the significant others. Determine whether the confusion is an acute change or has developed over time; ask whether the changes are most notable at any particular time of day. Identify the patient's baseline level of function and cognition. Determine the highest level of education, current or previous occupation, and daily routine, including whether the patient has been able to perform activities of daily living independently. It is important to determine whether the patient is aware of any functional change, as patients in the early stages of dementia often have insight into their functional capacity changes. Note whether the patient is easily frustrated with any lack of abilities or cognition. Ask whether the patient's interpersonal relationships have changed in any way. Identify any history of excessive use of alcohol or drugs, any exposures to environmental toxins (lead, ammonia, carbon monoxide, heavy metals), or recent trauma. Review all current medications because polypharmacy, especially in the elderly population, can cause states of confusion. Review recent or remote exposure to any infectious disease, such as AIDS, herpes, meningitis, mononucleosis, or syphilis. Explore psychosocial factors, such as depression, anxiety, or the loss of a loved one.

Physical Examination

The neurological examination should focus on assessment of cognition and mental status by using the Mini-Mental State Exam or another validated screening instrument. *Observation* of the patient is a key element in the neurological exam for the patient with mental status changes. Observation should include the patient's dress and personal grooming, affect, any obvious agitation or frustration, and reliance on a significant other for assistance during the history or examination. Note the fluidity of speech and speech content, and note whether the speech reveals a flight of ideas, confabulation, or echolalia, as well as whether it suggests hallucinations during the interview. Orientation is one of the basic assessments that provides information about the patient's awareness of self and environment. Ask the patient to recite his or her full name, current place (clinic, hospital, home, etc.), and the date (may include the day of the week, month, or year). Knowledge of time is generally impaired first, followed by place. The inability to recite or recognize one's name implies a significant deficit in mental status. All of the areas addressed in Box 14-1 (see p. 356) should be considered during the mental status examination.

Diagnostic Studies

- Basic metabolic profile to determine metabolic abnormalities with particular attention to electrolytes, BUN, creatinine, calcium, and liver functions
- Urinalysis to rule out urinary tract infection (particularly in older patients)
- CBC with differential to determine evidence of infectious process or anemia
- ESR to assess inflammatory process (may be normal in the elderly)
- Serum vitamin B_{12} and folic acid levels
- Thyroid function tests to discover hypothyroid states
- HIV, fluorescent treponemal antibody absorption test (FTA-ABS) for tertiary syphilis, and Lyme serology
- Pulse oximetry or blood gas to rule out hypoxia
- Chest x-ray
- Electrocardiogram (EKG)
- An MRI of the brain with and without contrast to assess for any intracranial mass lesion, infarctions, or demyelinating disease
- Electroencephalogram to determine the presence of subtle seizure activity or localization of slow wave activity.

Also consider the following.

- Toxicology screen if indicated by the history; alcohol level or drug screen panel
- 24-hour urine for heavy metals
- Lumbar puncture for CSF studies if central nervous system (CNS) infection is suspected.

DELIRIUM

Delirium can be observed in both elderly and younger patients and is generally defined as an *acute* confusional state, affecting all aspects of cognition and mentation and often

---

Red Flags in the Assessment of Patients with Mental Status Changes

- Changes that are acute and associated with fever, stiff neck, or headache. The patient should be evaluated for possible meningitis, CNS infection, or intracranial bleed.

- Changes that are acute in the elderly (particularly women). The patient should be worked up for a possible infectious process (especially urinary tract infections).

- Changes that are acute and associated with any type of head trauma. The patient should be evaluated for possible expanding mass lesion.

- Changes that are progressive and associated with gait disorder and/or incontinence. The cause should be considered hydrocephalus until proven otherwise.

- Changes that are gradual but significant. The patient can be referred to a neurologist or neuropsychologist for specific testing.

related to a treatable disorder. These include an almost endless list of potential causes, such as, but are not limited to the following: intoxication, substance abuse, medication overdose, polypharmacy, infectious processes, mass lesion, intracranial bleed, thyroid imbalance, metabolic disturbances, encephalopathy, anemia, hypoxia, acute obstructive hydrocephalus, vitamin B deficiency, nutritional deficiency, and environmental exposures.

Signs and Symptoms.

The signs and symptoms of delirium generally have a more acute or rapidly progressive onset, as opposed to the slow gradual decline noted in the organic dementias. The acute mental status change is often associated with other signs or symptoms—such as hallucinations, illusions, incoherent speech, and constant aimless activity—that help to narrow the differential diagnosis. Table 14-2 describes some of the associated findings for several of the causes of treatable delirium or confusion. The history may reveal trauma, exposure to toxins, or medications, if these are responsible for the mental status changes. In spite of the confusion, the patient's sensorium is usually intact, although some conditions (such as intoxication and severe metabolic derangements) result in altered level of consciousness as well.

STROKE

Stroke is one of the leading causes of death in the United States. Patients with stroke often have a history of hypertension, diabetes, cardiac disease, hyperlipidemia, smoking, drug or EtOH abuse, and family history of stroke. Strokes are divided into two main categories: thrombotic and hemorrhagic; however, the two can be difficult to differentiate using clinical signs and symptoms.

Signs and Symptoms.

The onset is usually an abrupt altered level of consciousness, accompanied by hemiparesis or hemiplegia. Patients may experience confusion, memory impairment, and aphasia. Signs and symptoms vary with the location and the severity of the stroke. Mentation and cognitive changes may be temporary or permanent depending on the extent of injury. Communication alterations stemming from fluent or receptive aphasia may be mistaken as dementia.

Diagnostic Studies.

A CT scan, without contrast, is the preferred imaging study in early stroke because hemorrhage may be difficult to determine on an MRI in the first 48 hours. In studies of ischemic stroke patients, researchers have shown the reversibility of abnormalities on CT/MRI through the use of thrombolytic therapy. The current time window is 3 hours. The hope is that with better imaging (perfusion-weighted imaging) the window can be

Table 14-2. ■ Select Treatable Causes of Symptoms Associated with Delirium/Confusion

Condition	Findings
Vitamin B Deficiencies	Depending on the particular deficiency, peripheral neuropathy, skin and/or mucous membrane changes, fatigue, constipation.
Hypothyroidism	Fatigue, depression, skin/hair changes, cold intolerance, constipation, anemia.
Infections	Highly dependent on the condition. For meningitis, nuchal rigidity and fever.
Nutritional Deficit	Weight loss, nausea/vomiting, anorexia, weakness, electrolyte imbalances.

expanded and more accurate decisions can be made between irreversible damage and salvageability.

PARKINSON'S DISEASE

Although altered mental status is usually not the first manifestation of Parkinson's disease (PD), mild cognitive dysfunction is often seen. Because of the flat affect and facies that patients with PD exhibit, these symptoms may be mistaken for psychosis, depression, or dementia, which can often coexist. Parkinson's disease occurs in all ethnic groups, with approximately equal sex distribution, and usually begins between 45 and 65 years of age. In patients younger than 50, also strongly consider Huntington's chorea (an inherited disease with progressive dementia and bizarre movement and posture) or Wilson's disease (the accumulation of copper in various vital organs). Another form of PD, known as posttraumatic parkinsonism—termed dementia pugilistica—is a combination of dementia and parkinsonism that develops in boxers or persons sustaining repeated blows to the head.

Signs and Symptoms.

Tremor, rigidity (cogwheeling), bradykinesia, and postural instability are the hallmark features of PD (Tierney, 2003). Unilateral pill-rolling tremor at rest is usually the first symptom. The tremor is maximal at rest but absent during sleep. It can be differentiated from essential tremor (ET) in that ET is absent at rest and worsens with voluntary movement. Essential tremor frequently affects the head, and patients have animated facies and normal rates of movement with no bradykinesia or rigidity.

The bradykinesia of PD is probably the most disabling and affects gross and fine motor movement, speech volume, swallowing, and blinking. There is generally no muscle weakness and deep tendon reflexes are normal. Although Alzheimer's disease can manifest with rigidity, bradykinesia, and gait disorders, no resting tremor is seen with Alzheimer's.

Secondary manifestations are nonspecific and include cognitive dysfunction, sleep disturbances, constipation, dysphagia, blurred or double vision, nocturia, frequency, urgency, autonomic dysfunction (such as erectile dysfunction), dizziness, and drooling.

Because some medications may cause parkinsonian symptoms (neuroleptics, phenothiazines, antiemetics, metoclopramide, methyldopa, and reserpine), a thorough medication history is imperative.

Diagnostic Studies.

A metabolic profile should be done to look particularly for thyroid or hepatic disease. Profound hypothyroidism can cause slowness of movement, and liver disease can cause tremor (asterixis). An MRI is recommended to rule out a vascular etiology or intracranial infarct. Toxicology screens should be performed, as several toxins can cause parkinsonian symptoms, such as carbon monoxide, cyanide, manganese, herbicides, carbon disulfide, methanol, lacquer thinner, and the club drug Ecstasy, which is structurally similar to amphetamine and mescaline and promotes the release of dopamine and serotonin.

NORMAL PRESSURE HYDROCEPHALUS

The etiology of normal pressure hydrocephalus is not fully understood. It is seen primarily in persons over 60 years of age and involves enlargement of the ventricles, often without increased CSF pressure; intraventricular pressures may be high or normal. One of the theorized causes includes intermittent pressure increases. It is slightly more common in men than women.

Signs and Symptoms.

The patient often first notices some degree of gait disorder, followed by the onset of a "clouding" of thought processes, which gradually progress. The typical picture is a patient who has a triad of gait disturbance, altered thought processes, and urinary incontinence. Strength and sensation are usually within normal limits. However, focal neurological findings are present and include increased deep tendon reflexes, the inability to tandem walk, positive Babinski, and/or positive Romberg.

Diagnostic Studies.

Imaging (MRI/CT) should be completed to provide definitive diagnosis.

Tumor
See p. 367.

Brain Abscess and CNS Infection
See p. 366.

ORGANIC, PROGRESSIVE DEMENTIAS

Whereas dementia generally affects persons over 60 years of age, persons in the fourth and fifth decades of life can show mental status changes as a result of some offending cause. Although Alzheimer's dementia is a frequent cause of progressive organic dementia, other causes with similar findings include Pick's disease, alcoholism-related dementia, and the causes discussed separately in the previous entries. This section is related to those types of dementias that have an organic (nonpsychiatric) basis and that can be treated conservatively, but with limited improvement. It is placed last as a reminder that they must be differentiated from reversible forms, including progressive hydrocephalic dementia, which can be corrected. Chapters 16 and 19 also include brief discussions of progressive dementia of this type.

Signs and Symptoms.

Unlike delirium, most organic dementias develop in a progressive manner, over months to years. There are typically no physical motor or sensory alterations until the condition is advanced. Progressive mental status changes associated with focal motor or sensory findings should not be attributed to Alzheimer's or Pick's diseases.

Memory impairment is the predominant symptom. There may be impairment in another area of cognitive functioning, such as with aphasia (producing language as well as understanding it), agnosia (perceptual impairments not due to dysfunction of the primary sensory organ), apraxia (inability to perform complex motor acts), and impairment in executive functioning (inability to plan, organize, sequence, and think abstractly).

Diagnostic Studies.

The studies listed above for altered mental status should be considered here, based on the history and presentation. It is crucial to rule out any correctible cause of confusion or altered mental status in a timely manner.

Dizziness and Vertigo

Patients interpret the subjective complaint of dizziness differently. Therefore, it is important to determine a true vertigo, during which the patient experiences a spinning sensation, from lightheadedness, which typically has a different etiology. Lightheadedness can be caused by a variety of things, including dehydration, hypotension, hypoglycemia, heart block, hypoglycemia, infection, fever, vasovagal response, blood loss, metabolic disturbances, medication, or anxiety. Vertigo, on the other hand, is generally vestibular in nature and related to disorders or infections of the middle or inner ear or cerebellum. It is important in the history to determine what the patient considers "dizziness" and to explore any past history of the disorders listed above.

History

The typical dimensions of the symptom are important—particularly onset and duration—because many cases of dizziness are paroxysmal, short, and self-limiting. Dizziness that is not vertigo is often associated with quick movement or bending over, and is often worse upon first arising in the morning, or when rising from a recumbent position. Vertigo, by contrast, describes the sense of spinning. It can occur at any time of the day or night. Many people will report vertigo associated with listing to one side while walking, often running into walls or door jams while walking. Nystagmus is often associated with vertigo, but rarely with dizziness. Nausea and vomiting can be associated with both dizziness and vertigo.

Dizziness that becomes frequent or lasts extended periods of time deserves closer investigation. Sustained periods of dizziness with near fainting can be a precursor to syncope or stroke and may have a neurovascular or cardiac etiology. Recently, neurocardiogenic syncope, also called vasovagal syncope, has drawn attention as a common cause of dizziness and fainting. It is due to a sudden decrease in blood pressure and heart rate after prolonged standing, with stress or from dehydration. It is due to sympathetic sensitivity causing a reflexive response that suddenly causes bradycardia and venous dilation. Hypotension and dizziness result.

Dizziness can also be a precursor (or aura) of seizures. Dizziness that leads to disequilibrium can result in inability to drive, falls, and injuries, and can be quite disabling for some persons. Lightheadedness in the elderly, or persons with vascular insufficiency is not uncommon. It is crucial to identify any associated symptoms, specifically, nausea, vomiting, fevers, vision changes, speech disturbances, and numbness or weakness of the face or extremities.

The history of head or ear trauma should be determined, as well as exposure to infections. A thorough review of the patient's current medications must be included because polypharmacy can cause dizziness in many patients. Social and recreational history is important. Activities such as scuba diving, high elevation hiking, or air travel can contribute to the development of dizziness, as can dehydration related to exercising in the heat. Other potential causes include alcohol or substance abuse. Because dizziness can be associated with hyperventilation or anxiety, ask about a history of anxiety or panic attacks. Review the family history of stroke, seizures, Ménière's disease, or other conditions that are associated with dizziness or vertigo.

Physical Examination

The neurological examination should focus on vital signs, gait, station, and cranial nerve function. Blood pressure should be taken both lying and standing, looking for orthostatic changes. Measure the rate and regularity of the pulse and obtain an EKG if necessary. Note fever that might indicate infection. The exam should include an assessment of gait, including tandem walking. Gait ataxia is noted when the patient is so uncoordinated that they are unable to walk a straight line without stumbling. The Romberg test should be performed; a positive Romberg test is noted when the patient is unable to maintain an upright posture with feet together and arms extended, and sways or falls to the side. The finger-to-nose test should be performed, observing for dysmetria, and rapid alternating movement is tested, observing the smoothness of motion.

Cranial nerve (CN) testing is important, particularly CNs II, III, IV, and VI. The eye nerves are particularly sensitive to increases in intracranial pressure. Note any vision or pupillary changes. Note decreases in visual fields, and note nystagmus on upward, downward, or lateral gaze with extraocular movements. Assess any asymmetry in facial sensation or movements (CN VII), which could indicate a transient ischemic attack or cerebrovascular accident, or pressure on the nerve from a tumor. Cranial nerve VIII is the most sensitive to tests for vestibulocochlear abnormalities. Always perform Rinne and Weber tests to localize hearing loss or tinnitus.

Diagnostic Studies
- An MRI of the brain with and without contrast will help to rule out evidence of a mass lesion or demyelinating process. An MRI of the internal auditory canal is sensitive for mass lesions on the inner ear and acoustic nerve.
- An audiogram is useful for assessing inner ear and hearing damage. This can also be helpful in assessing inflammatory disorders.
- An Electronystagmogram is useful for determining eye movements in relation to a stimulus, and helps with localizing the lesion to the nerve.
- Carotid ultrasound or duplex will determine vascular insufficiency.
- Brainstem and auditory evoked potentials help with determining whether the defect lies with the nerve or within the inner ear.
- The tilt table test can be performed to rule out neurocardiogenic syncope.
- Home blood pressure monitoring may be helpful for those patients with hypo- or hypertension–induced dizziness.

CENTRAL NERVOUS SYSTEM LESIONS

The causes of CNS vertigo include brain stem vascular disease or tumor, arteriovenous malformations, cerebellar tumor, multiple sclerosis, and vertebrobasilar migraine (Tierney, 2003).

Signs and Symptoms.

The findings will depend on the location and progression of the lesion. Most patients will present with disequilibrium or dizziness. Children may present with gait disorders.

Red Flags in the Assessment of Patients with Dizziness/Vertigo

- Associated with near fainting or fainting.
- Associated with slurred speech, numbness of the face or limbs, or loss of limb movement.
- Visual changes, particularly diplopia.
- Acute onset, associated with nausea/vomiting.

Vertigo from central lesions is constant and thus causes difficulties with the activities of daily living. Other symptoms may be present, such as cranial nerve dysfunction, motor and sensory dysfunction, and cerebellar dysfunction.

Diagnostic Studies.

An MRI of the brain with and without contrast is the test of choice for diagnosis of central lesions. An MRI of the internal auditory canal is sensitive for mass lesions on the inner ear and acoustic nerve.

CENTRAL AUDITORY AND VESTIBULAR SYSTEM DYSFUNCTION

Diseases in this category include acoustic neuroma, vascular compromise, and multiple sclerosis (MS). Acoustic neuromas are benign and are one of the most common intracranial tumors. Due to their location, they affect hearing and speech discrimination.

Vertebrobasilar insufficiency is seen mostly in the elderly and is exacerbated by extension of the neck or changes in head position. Migraines and vascular loops may cause vascular compromise and vertigo. Multiple sclerosis can also cause chronic imbalance and unilateral hearing loss. See under Weakness in Chapter 15, p. 386.

Signs and Symptoms.

The vertigo from central lesions is more likely to be persistent and chronic rather than intermittent, as is seen with other causes of vertigo. The dizziness may be described as a constant sense of disequilibrium rather than a true vertigo. Unlike benign positional vertigo, central and vestibular nystagmus is "often nonfatigable, vertical rather than horizontal in orientation, without latency, and unsuppressed by visual fixation" (Tierney, 2003). Unilateral hearing loss should be suspect for acoustic neuroma or MS. A history of migraines may suggest vascular compromise.

Diagnostic Studies.

An MRI with and without contrast of the internal auditory canal is necessary for a definitive diagnosis of acoustic neuroma. Magnetic resonance angiography or a cerebral angiogram is used to diagnose vascular abnormalities. An LP and MRI with and without contrast are necessary for a diagnosis of MS.

Ménière's Disease
See Chapter 5, p. 93.

VIRAL (SEROUS) OR BACTERIAL (SUPPURATIVE) LABYRINTHITIS

Labyrinthitis is caused by the invasion of the ear by bacteria or a virus. The bacterial is more serious because it may lead to meningitis. Prompt treatment with antibiotics is necessary.

Signs and Symptoms.

Labyrinthitis is characterized by severe vertigo, nystagmus, and hearing loss. Suppurative labyrinthitis may be secondary to bacterial otitis media or other bacterial infection. Serous labyrinthitis can be secondary to a variety of viral illnesses, including measles, mumps, chickenpox, influenza, mononucleosis, and adenovirus.

Diagnostic Studies

The diagnosis is mainly made by history and physical examination. A CBC or mono spot can assist in the diagnosis, and a culture of the fluid from the middle ear will differentiate a bacterial from a viral cause.

Cholesteatoma

See Chapter 5, p. 89.

PERILYMPHATIC FISTULA

A fistula may form from a blow to the head or from barotraumas significant enough to cause a rupture of the round or the oval window.

Signs and Symptoms.

Vertigo, ataxia, nausea, vomiting, and hearing loss can result from this fistula. A medical history would give you the necessary information for an index of suspicion for this cause of dizziness.

Diagnostic Studies.

In addition to a good history, a CT or MRI of the head can assist in the diagnosis. Surgical repair is necessary.

CUPULOLITHIASIS

Also referred to as benign paroxysmal positional vertigo, cupulolithiasis is a common condition resulting from particles or debris into the posterior semicircular canal. It can occur spontaneously with motion or position change or as a result of vascular or labyrinth trauma.

Signs and Symptoms.

Characterized by sudden-onset dizziness lasting less than 30 seconds and following a head position change. It may be accompanied by nystagmus. It usually subsides, but may recur at any time.

Diagnostic Studies.

In addition to the history, a provocative test for positional nystagmus can be performed, although it is not always positive. The provocative test involves moving the patient quickly from a sitting position to a lying position with the head turned to the side and the head dependent over the side of the exam table. After a few seconds, vertigo and nystagmus occur. This response fatigues with immediate repetition of the test. A CT or MRI may be necessary to rule out CNS lesions; however, the vertigo associated with CNS lesions is not as severe, does not have a latency period, and does not fatigue. The Epley repositioning maneuver, also called vestibular exercises, can assist in alleviating the problem.

References

IHS. (2004). International classification of headache disorders, 2nd edition. *Cephalalgia*, 24, Supplement 1.

Tierney, L.M., McPhee, S.J., & Papadakis, M.A. (Eds.). (2003). *CURRENT Medical Diagnosis & Treatment*. New York: Lange Medical Books/McGraw Hill.

SUGGESTED READINGS

Beers, M., Berkow, R., & Burs, M. (Eds.). (1999). *Merck Manual of Medical Therapeutics* (17th ed). Rahway, NJ: Merck & Co., Inc.

HeartCenterOnline for Physicians and Patients www.heartcenteronline.com/myheartdr/common Retrieved November 21, 2004.

IHS. (2004). International classification of headache disorders, 2nd edition. *Cephalalgia, 24*, Supplement 1.

International Headache Society. *Classification of Headaches*. Accessed online at URL www.w-h-a.org/wha2/Newsite/resultsnav.asp?color=C2D9F2&idContentNews=381 on February 10, 2005.

Tierney, L.M., McPhee, S.J., & Papadakis, M.A. (Eds.). (2003). *CURRENT Medical Diagnosis & Treatment*. New York: Lange Medical Books/McGraw Hill.

Weiner, W.J., & Goetz, C.G. (2004). *Neurology for the Non-Neurologist*. Philadelphia: Lippincott, Williams, & Wilkins.

Chapter 15

Nonspecific Complaints

Laurie Grubbs

HISTORY AND PHYSICAL EXAMINATION

Some of the more challenging chief complaints for any healthcare practitioner are those "generic" complaints that have a multitude of causations, such as fatigue, weakness, dizziness, numbness/tingling, headache, and so on. Deciding on which system to start with is often difficult. Because there are so many possibilities for the origin of these complaints, all systems should be considered, although the neurological and cardiac systems are often a good place to start. Proceed with the history in the typical format because the complaint may be related to a past health problem, a medication, a familial or genetic predisposition, or simply a new-onset problem. Be sure to include in your review of systems the questions under the general assessment, such as weight loss, changes in appetite, fevers, chills, night sweats, lethargy, weakness, inability to perform the activities of daily life, changes in mental status, and nutritional patterns. Pay attention to the general appearance and behavior of the patient, including personal hygiene, dress, grooming, speech patterns, mood, and affect. Patients who are depressed or ill may show signs of poor hygiene and flat affect.

DIFFERENTIAL DIAGNOSIS OF CHIEF COMPLAINTS

Fatigue

History

A complaint of fatigue has strong psychological overtones, making it extremely important to consider a psychological as well as a physical cause. It is important to take a thorough psychosocial history as part of the review of systems. Ask about living arrangements, relationships with family and significant others, environment, occupational history, economic status (including job satisfaction), daily profile (rest–activity patterns, exercise habits, social activities), and patterns of health care. In today's society, it is not uncommon for a person to be working, caring for children, and caring for elderly parents, possibly as a single parent and sole family support. People are often not aware of the physical toll that long-term stress can take on the body and immune system. A thorough medication history, including over-the-counter drugs is, of course, imperative. Ask about tobacco, alcohol, and other drug use. Investigate a past history or family history of cardiac, respiratory, endocrine, gastrointestinal (GI), or hematologic disease. A family history of Type 2 diabetes mellitus (DM) presents a significant risk for the patient developing it as well. Thyroid disease seems to show a family predisposition. A history of anemia in a patient should raise the index of suspicion for chronicity. One always needs to ask the date of the last menstrual period for young women, whether they are using oral contraceptives or not. Other common causes, particularly in the elderly, include arrhythmias, congestive heart failure (CHF), infection, and malignancy. Two uncommon causes of fatigue could be adrenal dysfunction (Addison's and Cushing's diseases), but patients might describe weakness rather than fatigue, especially in the case of Cushing's disease, where there is muscle wasting.

Physical Examination
The physical exam should follow most closely with the system suspected as causing the fatigue, although other systems should be included. The practitioner's index of suspicion involves many variables, including the age of the patient, current health, past history, and presenting symptoms. As usual, vital signs are a good place to start. Hypotension, bradycardia, tachycardia, or fever could indicate a cardiac or infectious cause, as well as Addison's disease. Unexplained weight loss might indicate a thyroid disease, DM, Addison's disease, malignancy, or depression. In the head, ears, eyes, nose, and throat exam, particular attention should be paid to examination of the thyroid, and lymph system. Significant findings in the cardiac exam include an arrhythmia or murmur, which might be compromising cardiac output; or ventricular hypertrophy, which could indicate heart failure. Electrocardiogram (EKG) changes may demonstrate the ventricular hypertrophy seen in heart failure or the conduction delays as seen in Addison's disease. Shortness of breath, tachypnea, or adventitious sounds may indicate a cardiac or respiratory cause of the fatigue. Masses in the abdomen might indicate a malignancy. Bruits, particularly over the renal arteries, could affect blood flow to the kidneys, thus giving rise to renal impairment and fatigue. Skin changes may be seen in thyroid disease, with dry skin seen in hypothyroidism and moist skin in hyperthyroidism, or in Addison's disease, which causes hyperpigmentation. A thorough neurological assessment is also in order especially in the elderly since depression and dementia are more common and could present as fatigue or lethargy. The remainder of the assessment involves laboratory or other diagnostics, which are discussed under each differential diagnosis.

STRESS, ANXIETY, DEPRESSION, AND DYSTHYMIA

Psychiatric disorders may be responsible for as much as 50% of the complaints of fatigue (Tierney, 2003). With the increased acceptance and recognition of depression as an illness, and with the treatment choices now available, patients are much more likely to seek help for depression. Often they are not aware of being depressed and they present with somatic symptoms such as fatigue.

Signs and Symptoms.
Subjectively, patients admit to feelings of sadness, hopelessness, and worthlessness with diminished interest in both work and recreation. There may be cognitive complaints, such

as difficulty thinking and concentrating, obsessive ruminations, and difficulty making decisions. There may be difficulty sleeping, appetite changes, loss of energy, and decreased libido. Often depression is accompanied by anxiety or agitation, as well as by various somatic complaints, such as fatigue, headache, nausea, and irritability.

Diagnostic Studies.

There are many diagnostic tools to evaluate depression and other psychiatric problems. The Beck Inventory of Depression is widely used. In clinical family practice, abbreviated "bedside questionnaires" can be used to evaluate the patient for referral to a mental health counselor. Antidepressant medication can be prescribed, but a thorough mental health evaluation should be done by trained personnel.

TYPE 2 DIABETES MELLITUS

The incidence of Type 2 DM in the United States has risen dramatically in the last decade mainly owing to the rise in obesity, and it was estimated that 6.3% of the population in 2004 had diabetes (CDC, 2004). Patients who are overweight and sedentary, with a positive family history, are at high risk for developing Type 2 DM.

Signs and Symptoms.

Polydipsia, polyphagia, and polyuria are the hallmark signs of diabetes, but fatigue, weight loss, and blurred vision are often the symptoms that bring patients into the office.

Diagnostic Studies.

A fasting glucose level of >110 mg/dL is considered diagnostic for diabetes. A glucose tolerance test can also be done to look for fluctuations in glucose metabolism. A test of the hemoglobin A1c level gives an estimation of blood glucose over the previous 3 months.

HYPOTHYROIDISM

Primary hypothyroidism is the most common form and is thought to be autoimmune in origin. The incidence of hypothyroidism is greater in women and more common in people over 40 years.

Signs and Symptoms.

Because the onset of hypothyroidism can be insidious, patients may not be aware that their thyroid levels have diminished. Common signs and symptoms include fatigue or lack of energy, puffy face, constipation, intolerance to cold, hypotension, bradycardia, dry skin, menorrhagia, modest weight gain, diminished deep tendon reflexes (DTRs), and dulled cognition. In the elderly, the presenting symptom may be CHF. Also see the subsection on goiter in Chapter 3.

Diagnostic Studies.

Whereas the physical examination may raise the index of suspicion, the measurement of the thyroid hormones, T_3 and T_4, and thyroid-stimulating hormone (TSH) confirms the diagnosis. Because thyroid function requires a feedback loop between the pituitary gland and the thyroid gland, in hypothyroidism, the T_3 and T_4 levels are below normal and the TSH is above normal.

MALIGNANCY

A malignancy in any place in the body may cause the patient to feel fatigued. It is often an indirect cause of fatigue stemming from anemia, shortness of breath, decreased appetite, nausea and vomiting, decreased renal function, or a variety of other symptoms caused by the malignancy.

Signs and Symptoms.

The signs and symptoms depend on the system where the malignancy exists. If a patient presents with a primary complaint of fatigue, an index of suspicion for a malignancy should alert you to ask about other signs or symptoms that patient might have noticed. If malignancy is advanced enough to cause fatigue, there are usually other symptoms present.

Diagnostic Studies.

The diagnostics also depend on the system thought to be involved. A complete blood count (CBC), urinalysis, and general chemistries are helpful, as well as liver functions and a chest x-ray. Depending on the age of the patient, a mammogram and/or colonoscopy may be warranted. New-onset anemia, especially in an older person should be thoroughly investigated, as it may be secondary to blood loss or decreased red blood cell (RBC) production as a result of colon cancer or a hematologic malignancy.

ANEMIA

The anemia may be primary or secondary to a hematologic disease or a malignancy. It is important to determine whether the anemia is due to decreased production or increased destruction of RBCs owing to diseases affecting the bone marrow, blood loss, or other hemolytic conditions. A patient with a history of anemia should alert the practitioner to start there with the differential diagnosis of fatigue. Ask about the cause or type of anemia, and any past or current treatments.

Signs and Symptoms.

Fatigue and decreased activity tolerance may be the symptoms that bring the patient to the clinic. The degree of fatigue is often proportional to the degree of anemia; however, patients with long-standing anemia compensate and may be asymptomatic, even with a significant anemia. Along with fatigue, the patient may appear pale, with pale conjunctivae and mucous membranes. There may be neurological symptoms, such as paresthesias or decreased proprioception, as is the case in B_{12} deficiency. Cardiac functioning may be affected with severe, long-standing anemia.

Diagnostic Studies.

A CBC with differential is the first laboratory test to obtain. A reticulocyte count will assist in differentiating whether the anemia is due to increased destruction of RBCs, resulting in a high reticulocyte count, versus decreased production of RBCs, resulting in a low reticulocyte count. Bilirubin in the urine or an elevated serum bilirubin suggests RBC destruction. Serum iron, total iron-binding capacity, ferritin, and B_{12} tests give important information about the specific type of anemia. Positive Hemoccult tests alert the practitioner to the need for a GI consultation to determine the source of bleeding.

CHRONIC RENAL FAILURE

The main causes of chronic renal failure are diabetes and hypertension (>50%). Polycystic kidney disease and glomerulonephritis account for another 25%, and the remaining causes are unknown (Tierney, 2003). There are three stages of chronic renal failure: diminished renal reserve, renal insufficiency in which azotemia develops and is reflected in elevations of plasma urea and creatinine, and uremia, which is accompanied by fluid and electrolyte imbalances.

Signs and Symptoms.

Patients with mild renal dysfunction are generally asymptomatic, but as the disease progresses vague symptoms appear. Fatigue and weakness are early signs, as well as decreased cognitive functioning and irritability. Patients may complain of nocturia, which is due to the kidney not concentrating the urine at night. Many of these early signs are nonspecific, and patients often pass them off as a normal part of aging. Gastrointestinal complaints, such as nausea, vomiting, and anorexia, are common and contribute to the muscle wasting and fatigue. Patients may complain of a metallic taste in the mouth. Hypertension may develop from fluid overload and can result in CHF. Pericarditis may develop, producing a friction rub. Neurologic symptoms include muscle cramps and twitching, peripheral neuropathy, difficulty concentrating, and sleep disturbances. Pruritis is a common and very uncomfortable symptom and, as patients become more uremic, crystals may appear on the skin, termed uremic frost. The skin often takes on a yellowish-brown tone with easy bruisability.

Diagnostic Studies.

The abnormal laboratory values are numerous. A blood chemistry will reveal an elevated BUN and creatinine. Metabolic acidosis, hyperphosphatemia, hypocalcemia, and hyperkalemia are present. A normocytic, normochromic anemia is present. Imaging studies of the kidney may be helpful if the chronic renal failure is due to a structural problem in the kidney; otherwise, imaging may not be helpful.

ARRHYTHMIAS

Both atrial and ventricular arrhythmias may cause fatigue. They may be secondary to age, coronary artery disease, valvular heart disease, or endocrine diseases. Atrial fibrillation is very common in the elderly, with an increased incidence that is due to the aging population. Other atrial and ventricular arrhythmias can occur in any age with or without the presence of other disorders. Supraventricular tachycardia is usually paroxysmal in nature and results from an abnormal pathway within or around the atrioventricular node. Intraventricular conduction delays may be seen in Addison's disease, in which fatigue is a common symptom. The only ventricular arrhythmias that might present with a complaint of fatigue are bigeminy or trigeminy. Ventricular tachycardia or ventricular fibrillation are life threatening and the patient generally does not remain conscious for any length of time after the onset of the arrhythmia.

Signs and Symptoms.

In atrial fibrillation, the symptoms generally depend on the ventricular response rate. The patient may be very symptomatic, with shortness of breath, decreased exercise tolerance, and fatigue, or he or she may be completely asymptomatic. In supraventricular tachycardia, the rate is usually quite high, up to 200 bpm, and the patient is aware of palpitations. There may be accompanying complaints of shortness of breath and fatigue, particularly if the arrhythmia persists for any length of time. With bigeminy and trigeminy, patients will usually be aware of palpitations or the sensation of missed beats. They may complain of shortness of breath and probably have more of a complaint of weakness or lightheadedness rather than fatigue.

Diagnostic Studies.

An EKG is a simple way to quickly and definitively diagnose an arrhythmia, as long as it is occurring when the patient presents to the office, clinic, or emergency department.

CONGESTIVE HEART FAILURE

Congestive heart failure, commonly occurring in the elderly or in patients with past myocardial infarctions or cardiomyopathy can often present with complaints of fatigue, decreased activity tolerance, and/or shortness of breath.

Signs and Symptoms.

A detailed discussion of CHF can be found in Chapter 6, but the common symptoms include shortness of breath, orthopnea, crackles at the lung bases, peripheral edema, fatigue, decreased exercise tolerance, enlarged heart on x-ray, and other cardiac abnormalities depending on history.

Diagnostic Studies.

The diagnosis is made primarily by history and physical exam as you look for the foregoing signs and symptoms. A chest x-ray is helpful. A blood test for pro–brain natriuretic protein (pro-BNP) can differentiate CHF from bronchitis, which can sometimes be difficult in a patient with chronic obstructive pulmonary disease (COPD).

CHRONIC OBSTRUCTIVE PULMONARY DISEASE

Chronic obstructive pulmonary disease covers a myriad of respiratory conditions, including chronic asthma/bronchitis, bronchiolitis, and emphysema. It is characterized by obstruction to flow owing to destruction of the alveolar wall. It is often related to smoking but also results from a genetic predisposition or exposure to environmental toxins. The effect is damage to the alveoli resulting in poor gas exchange.

Signs and Symptoms.

Common signs and symptoms include shortness of breath, exertional dyspnea, easy fatigability, cough, wheezing, prolonged expiration, barrel chest, weight loss, recurrent respiratory infections. Exertional dyspnea, rather than fatigue, is usually the presenting symptom.

Diagnostic Studies.

Pulmonary function tests are most helpful in diagnosis. Chest x-ray findings are variable depending on the underlying disease.

PREGNANCY

Females of child-bearing age should always be asked the date of their last menstrual period, and some index of suspicion should be present for any young female who presents with a complaint of fatigue.

Signs and Symptoms.

Missed menstrual cycle, fatigue, breast tenderness, and nausea are the typical pregnancy signs and symptoms.

Diagnostic Studies.

A urine or serum hCG is diagnostic.

MONONUCLEOSIS

Mononucleosis is a viral infection that typically occurs in adolescence and early adulthood, and is caused by the Epstein-Barr virus. The virus remains in the host for life although reactivation of the virus is usually subclinical.

Signs and Symptoms.

Characterized by fever, sore throat, and lymphadenopathy. Although fatigue and malaise are generally not the presenting symptoms, they can predominate in subclinical infections.

Diagnostic Studies.

A positive mono spot is diagnostic. Patients may also have a mild leukocytosis and a more pronounced lymphocytosis.

FIBROMYALGIA

There is some controversy surrounding the diagnosis of fibromyalgia, and it is, for the most part, a diagnosis of exclusion.

Signs and Symptoms.

Fatigue and malaise are prominent symptoms, along with myalgias and tenderness in the areas of tendon insertions. Subjects may complain of difficulty sleeping, irritable bowel symptoms, anxiety, and depression.

Diagnostic Studies.

As previously mentioned, it is a diagnosis of exclusion, but other connective tissue disease must be ruled out, such as rheumatoid arthritis, polymyalgia rheumatica, polymyositis, and osteoarthritis.

ADDISON'S DISEASE

Addison's disease is a chronic, progressive hypofunctioning of the adrenals caused by atrophy or destruction of the adrenal cortex, usually with an autoimmune origin. Other causes include medications, tuberculosis (TB), amyloidosis, malignancy, or inflammation. It affects both genders equally and can be seen in all ages. The main hormones produced by the adrenal gland are cortisol, aldosterone, and adrenal androgens. Addison's disease is characterized by electrolyte imbalance—there is an increase in Na^+ excretion and a decrease in K^+ excretion that lead to low blood levels of Na^+ and Cl^- and high levels of K^+. This produces volume depletion, dehydration, and hypotension. The cortisol deficiency causes alterations in carbohydrate, fat and protein metabolism, and insulin sensitivity. The metabolic changes lead to hypoglycemia, decreased liver glycogen, and thus fatigue and weakness. The decreased cortisol levels affect melanocyte-stimulating activities, thus producing the characteristic hyperpigmentation of the skin.

The acute form of the disease, termed adrenal crisis, is a more severe and life-threatening form, and is characterized by profound weakness, severe abdominal and back pain, nausea, vomiting, diarrhea, confusion, renal shutdown, and circulatory collapse.

Signs and Symptoms.

Weakness and fatigue are early signs of Addison's disease. The patient may complain of lightheadedness owing to volume depletion, and orthostatic hypotension is found on exam. In most cases, the skin and mucous membranes are hyperpigmented, especially over creases, bony prominences, and nipples. The patient may complain of anorexia, nausea, vomiting, or diarrhea, and weight loss is evident. A complaint of lightheadedness or syncope may lead the practitioner to do an EKG, which shows decreased voltage as a result of a small heart, and prolonged PR and QT intervals.

Diagnostic Studies.

The blood chemistry findings suggestive of Addison's disease include low serum Ca^+, high K^+, elevated BUN, decrease in plasma bicarbonate, and low fasting glucose. The CBC may show an elevated hematocrit owing to volume depletion, a low WBC count, lymphocytosis, and increased eosinophils. Chest x-ray shows a small heart and possibly evidence of TB. Abdominal films may show calcifications in the adrenals and renal TB. More-sophisticated tests can be performed using an adrenocorticotropic hormone challenge to determine its effect on plasma cortisol levels. Other drugs can help to differentiate primary from secondary adrenal insufficiency. Replacement of adrenal hormones results in a good prognosis for these patients.

Weakness

Although many of the above diagnoses for fatigue could also fit into a chief complaint of weakness, this complaint connotes a lack of strength rather than a feeling of lethargy, and it is manifest in many neurological diseases, as well as in adrenal dysfunction, hyperthyroidism, and malignancy.

History

The history should include the type of weakness, whether it is proximal weakness, which might alert you to thyroid disease, malignancy, or adrenal dysfunction, or distal weakness, which would raise an index of suspicion for a neurological cause especially if it was accompanied by paresthesias. Ask the patient when and with what types of activities the weakness is most prominent, and how much it interferes with activities of daily living. Inquire about changes in speech patterns or slurring that might indicate a neurological cause. Ask whether there are any cognitive or personality changes, which are often seen with adrenal dysfunction. The review of systems should include headache, cold or heat intolerance, change in appetite, weight gain or loss, nausea, vomiting or diarrhea, changes in balance or gait, numbness or paresthesia, diplopia or other vision changes, and difficulty with speech or swallowing.

Physical Examination

The physical exam should focus on the neurological and musculoskeletal exams because both are very closely related and will give much information about the type, site, and severity of the weakness. Evaluate muscle mass, strength, and tone; the condition of the joints; and any fasciculations or spasticity. A complete neurological exam should be done, including cranial nerves, mental status, motor and sensory function, and deep tendon reflexes. Assess the skin for any color or texture changes as seen in adrenal or thyroid dysfunction. The head and neck should be assessed particularly for lymphadenopathy or enlarged or nodular thyroid.

Degenerative Neurological Diseases

Although there is a plethora of neurological causes of weakness, the most common diseases include multiple sclerosis, muscular dystrophies, myasthenia gravis, polymyositis/dermatomyositis, amyotrophic lateral sclerosis (ALS), and Guillain-Barré syndrome. Each of these will be discussed briefly in the following.

MULTIPLE SCLEROSIS

Multiple sclerosis (MS) is a degenerative, demyelinating disease that is most often diagnosed in the second to fourth decades of life. It occurs more often in women than in men. The presentation of MS is often vague and transient, with episodic remission and exacerbation. Patients may have remitting or primary progressive MS. The etiology is unknown but it is thought to be autoimmune. A genetic susceptibility is suspected since it is seen more in those of western European lineage who live in temperate zones.

Signs and Symptoms.

Visual disturbances may be the initial presenting symptom, indicating a plaque on the optic nerve. Associated visual disturbances include diplopia, blurred vision, tunnel vision, scotoma, or amaurosis. The visual changes are usually monocular. The patient may complain of intermittent weakness, parasthesias, or numbness of the face or extremities that occurs intermittently, and that may resolve for weeks to months. Patients may report episodes of falling or stumbling, with gait ataxia. Hyperreflexia may be noted, particularly in the lower extremities. Other symptoms include bladder incontinence or retention. Spastic bladder may also occur. In later stages, mental status changes may be noted. Initial symptoms are typically intermittent and the disease may go undiagnosed for months or years.

Diagnostic Studies.

An MRI of the brain and/or spine with and without contrast reveals demyelination of the white matter of the brain, spinal cord, and optic nerves. Lumbar puncture for cerebrospinal fluid analysis may show oligoclonal bands (IgG), protein <55 mg/dL; however, this is not a definitive test for diagnosis.

MUSCULAR DYSTROPHIES

There are seven types of muscular dystrophy, and they are subdivided by chromosomal inheritance, age of onset, and characteristic symptoms.

Signs and Symptoms.

The symptoms, occurring anywhere from a year old to late adulthood, are characterized by progressive muscle weakness and wasting. There may also be mental retardation, skeletal deformities, and cardiac involvement.

Diagnostic Studies.

Diagnosis is made by genetic testing. Creatine phosphokinase is increased in some types. An electromyogram (EMG) may be helpful to distinguish among various muscle diseases.

MYASTHENIA GRAVIS

Myasthenia can occur at any age and may be associated with other autoimmune diseases. It adversely affects the acetylcholine receptors by reducing their number and effectiveness.

Signs and Symptoms.

Limb weakness and fatigability of the affected muscles is a diagnostic sign. The cranial nerves are affected—especially the motor nerves of the face and neck—as manifested by dysphagia, ptosis, and diplopia. Patients may also show signs of respiratory dysfunction.

Diagnostic Studies.

The diagnosis can be made by a Tensilon test. When Tensilon is given intravenously, it improves the strength of the affected muscles within minutes. A serum assay for circulating levels of acetylcholine has a sensitivity of 80%–90% and is widely used. A CT scan can be obtained to rule out thymoma as an underlying cause.

POLYMYOSITIS AND DERMATOMYOSITIS

Polymyositis is a systemic disease of unknown etiology. When rash is present, it is termed dermatomyositis, and, with this form, there is an increased risk of an associated malignancy, particularly ovarian cancer. It is more common in women and in those over 60 years of age.

Signs and Symptoms.

Bilateral proximal muscle weakness is the main symptom and occurs in all cases. Weakness of the legs precedes weakness of the arms, and weakness of the neck flexors may be seen. Symptoms may occur suddenly or be more gradual and insidious in nature. The rash typically has a butterfly pattern on the face with reddish lesions over the eyes and peri-orbital edema. Redness and telangiectasias of the hands and nails is highly suggestive of dermatomyositis, and Raynaud's syndrome may be associated.

Diagnostic Studies.

A muscle biopsy of the affected proximal muscles is the only definitive diagnostic test. Elevated creatine phosphokinase and aldolase levels are common, although not specific. In addition, EMG may be helpful.

AMYOTROPHIC LATERAL SCLEROSIS, OR LOU GEHRIG DISEASE

Amyotrophic lateral sclerosis actually belongs to a group of motor neuron diseases and is characterized by mixed upper and lower motor neuron deficits.

Signs and Symptoms.

Amyotrophic lateral sclerosis is characterized by muscle weakness and atrophy, usually starting in the hands and then progressing randomly and asymmetrically. Other common symptoms include muscle cramps, fasciculations, spasticity, dysarthria, dysphagia, and increased deep tendon reflexes. Over 90% of patients are dead within 3–5 years.

Diagnostic Studies.

An EMG is the most helpful diagnostic test. Muscle biopsy shows histological changes owing to denervation.

GUILLAIN-BARRÉ

Guillain-Barré is an acute, rapidly progressive polyneuropathy that is often preceded by a virus, surgical procedure, or immunization. It is thought to have an immune etiology.

Signs and Symptoms.

Symmetric weakness and paresthesias are the main symptoms. The weakness usually begins in the legs and then proceeds to the arms. Over 50% develop respiratory involvement, which may require mechanical ventilation. Autonomic dysfunction can occur in severe cases and can be fatal. The maximal degree of weakness usually occurs in the first 2–3 weeks.

Diagnostic Studies.

The diagnosis can be made mainly on clinical presentation. Increased protein in the cerebrospinal fluid, and EMG abnormalities assist in confirmation of the diagnosis.

HYPERTHYROIDISM

Although we think of hypothyroidism as causing fatigue, hyperthyroidism can cause symptoms of muscle weakness and lead to difficulty in performing the activities of daily living. Patients have different subjective experiences of their symptoms; therefore, some may describe weakness whereas others may describe fatigue.

Signs and Symptoms.

Common signs and symptoms include muscle weakness, nervousness, insomnia, tachycardia, increased sweating, moist skin, intolerance to heat, exophthalmos, weight loss, hypertension, and hyperreflexia. In the elderly, the presenting symptom may be atrial fibrillation.

Diagnostic Studies. Even though the physical examination may increase suspicions, measuring the thyroid hormones, T_3 and T_4, and TSH confirms the diagnosis. The T_3 and T_4 levels are above normal and the TSH level is below normal, sometimes to the point at which it is barely measurable.

Malignancy

Weakness caused by a malignancy may be associated with the decreased functioning of the organ involved (e.g., lung), or the weakness may be due to a secondary anemia or to weight loss. See individual chapters for specific malignancies.

CUSHING'S DISEASE

Cushing's disease is caused by excess cortisol and corticosteroid hormones, either endogenous or exogenous. Endogenous causes of cortisol hypersecretion include pituitary adenomas; other malignancies, such as small cell lung cancer; and adrenal tumors. Exogenous causes are related to the administration of steroids for the management of other chronic diseases. A thorough medical history will alert the practitioner to chronic diseases or medications that may be causing or contributing to the cushingoid signs and symptoms.

Signs and Symptoms. Although weakness can be profound because of the muscle wasting that occurs, it is generally not the first symptom that will bring the patient to the office. For women, it may be oligomenorrhea or amenorrhea, and hirsutism; for men, impotence. Patients develop a "moon face" and "buffalo hump" with central obesity and thin extremities. Hypertension and osteoporosis develop over time. Purple striae around the thighs, breasts, and abdomen are characteristic of Cushing's; they are prone to easy bruisability, acne, and skin infections with poor wound healing. Patients complain of excessive thirst and polyuria owing to glucose intolerance, and they are prone to renal calculi. Changes in mental health are common and range from mood swings to psychosis.

Diagnostic Studies. The most accurate way to diagnose Cushing's disease is to give intravenous Decadron at bedtime and then check for elevated cortisol levels 8–10 hours later. A 24-hour urine for cortisol and creatinine helps confirm the diagnosis. Glucose tolerance testing shows elevated glucose resulting from insulin resistance. A CBC may show leukocytosis with granulocytosis and lymphopenia.

Fever of Unknown Origin

Fever of unknown origin (FUO) is defined as a temperature of at least 101°F for at least 3 weeks without discovery of the cause (Merck Manual, 2002). In children, over 50% of fevers are due to upper respiratory or viral illness; in adults, one should be more suspicious of malignancy.

History

The history should include the timing and degree of the fever. Recent travel or exposure to illnesses or certain animals is often very helpful. Travel outside the United States can be particularly problematic, and one should consider such diseases as malaria, typhoid, tuberculosis, *Mycobacterium avium* complex, or HIV. Brucellosis and histoplasmosis should be considered if there is animal exposure. Weight loss might indicate a malignant process or might be due to anorexia caused by the fever. As usual, a thorough medicine history, past medical history, and family history might alert the practitioner to a possible cause. Any recent infection should be investigated first because it may not have been adequately treated. A history of frequent infections could raise the index of suspicion regarding an immunocompromised condition, such as HIV, leukemia, or lymphoma. It is important to inquire about sexual practices.

Physical Examination
The physical should include examination of the skin for lesions, redness, increased temperature, or edema, which might indicate infection or an inflammatory process. Examine the lymph nodes. If there is lymphadenopathy in a particular area, it might lead you to the point of infection. If it is generalized, consider lymphoma, leukemia, or HIV. A cardiac assessment is important especially listening for a murmur or friction rub. Pericarditis or endocarditis has a variety of causes and may present as unexplained fever, shortness of breath, precordial pain/tenderness, and tachycardia. The lung assessment is crucial because over 50% of FUO in children are caused by an upper respiratory illness. Observe the skin and nail beds for cyanosis. The abdomen should be palpated for tenderness or masses: smoldering cases of appendicitis, cholecystitis, pancreatitis, or hepatitis might cause a lingering fever.

INFECTION

Any infection, viral or bacterial, can cause prolonged fever. Patients usually have some other complaint that alerts you to the cause of the fever. If bacterial, it can be treated with antibiotics, which should resolve the symptoms. Viral illnesses are more problematic because supportive measures are generally all that can be provided. Be watchful for a secondary bacterial infection to develop with some prolonged viral illnesses.

Signs and Symptoms.

The signs and symptoms are highly variable depending on the source of the infection. Expected are the typical symptoms that accompany a fever, such as headache, malaise, anorexia, and possibly chills. A thorough review of systems is necessary to detect the underlying source of the fever, if not completely obvious by other complaints.

Diagnostic Studies.

Although the diagnostics vary with the underlying cause, ordering a CBC with differential, urinalysis, and chest x-ray is a good place to start with any complaint of FUO. Blood cultures may be necessary as well as cultures of bodily fluids. In babies, a lumbar puncture is recommended to rule out meningitis. Rising antibody titers for typhoid, brucellosis, and other viral infections may be helpful. Ultrasound or CT scan of the abdomen will identify abscesses or other infections in the abdomen, including diverticulitis, peritonitis, cholecystitis, possibly pancreatitis, or appendicitis. A CT scan of the chest can detect cardiac vegetation, which might suggest pericarditis or endocarditis as a cause for the fever.

MALIGNANCY

Many malignancies can cause fever, but lymphoma and leukemia should be at the top of the differential list. Acute leukemia is more common in children, and the chronic leukemias are more common in middle-aged to elderly adults. Hodgkin's lymphoma is more prevalent in children and young adults, whereas non-Hodgkin's lymphoma is more common in middle-aged to elderly adults. Burkitt's lymphoma is more common in HIV patients.

Signs and Symptoms.

With leukemia, common symptoms include unexplained fever, easy bruising or bleeding, fatigue, bone or joint pain, and enlarged liver or spleen. With lymphoma, common symptoms include fatigue, fever, night sweats, lymphadenopathy, and weight loss.

Diagnostic Studies.

A CBC is the first and easiest laboratory test to perform. The abnormalities in the CBC vary some with the type of leukemia—acute or chronic, lymphocytic or myelocytic—but in general there is a proliferation of immature white cells (blasts), anemia, and low platelet count. In lymphoma, there is a leukocytosis, lymphocytopenia, and possibly thrombocytosis. A hypochromic, microcytic anemia is often present. A bone marrow biopsy confirms the diagnosis in both leukemia and lymphoma.

Diffuse Connective Tissue Disorders

The connective tissue disorders include rheumatoid arthritis, Sjögren's syndrome, Behçet's syndrome, vasculitis, systemic and discoid lupus erythematosus, polymyositis, polymyalgia rheumatica, temporal arteritis, and polyarteritis. Although fever can be present in any of the connective tissue disorders, muscle and joint pain are more common presenting symptoms. The specific signs, symptoms, and diagnostics for each of these diseases are beyond the scope of this text.

Immunodeficiency Disorders

Immunodeficiency disorders are numerous and are characterized as primary or secondary, with the secondary being more common than the primary disorders. The primary disorders are classified into B-cell deficiencies (antibody), T-cell deficiencies (cellular), phagocytic disorders, and complement disorders. The secondary immunodeficiencies are classified by cause and include hereditary and metabolic diseases (chromosome abnormalities, uremia, DM, malnutrition, nephritic syndrome, myotonic dystrophy, and sickle cell disease), infectious diseases (rubella; cytomegalovirus; viral exanthemas; mono; and severe bacterial, viral, or fungal infections), infiltrative and hematologic diseases (histocytosis, sarcoidosis, lymphoma, leukemia, myeloma, and aplastic anemia), those caused by surgery and trauma (burns, splenectomy, and anesthesia), and those caused by immunosuppressive agents (radiation, chemotherapy, corticosteroids, and other immunosuppressive drugs). Specific signs, symptoms, and diagnostics are beyond the scope of this text. Some of these are discussed in other chapters.

Drug Reaction

The most likely drugs to cause fever are the chemotherapeutic agents used to treat cancer, mainly as a result of leukopenia. The medical history should be all that is needed, along with a CBC to make this diagnosis. Allergic reactions to any drug, particularly the antibiotics, can cause fever as well as rash. The history is usually all that is necessary to identify the cause of the fever.

Unexplained Weight Loss

History

Malignancy and diabetes should top the list of differential diagnoses for unexplained weight loss. A thorough history and review of systems will alert the practitioner to other complaints that could give clues to the cause, such as cough, hemoptysis, shortness of breath, nausea, vomiting, diarrhea, steatorrhea, hematemesis, melena, fatigue/weakness/lethargy, changing or new moles, persistent pain, enlarged lymph nodes, abnormal menstrual bleeding, breast discharge, and chronic headaches. A thorough medicine history is critical especially in the elderly or those with chronic diseases who are on a multitude of medicines. A psychosocial history is critical, especially in the elderly client who may not be eating due to the inability to shop for groceries because of financial or transportation problems, inability to prepare meals resulting from a functional limitation, poorly fitting dentures or no dentures, or loss of appetite owing to depression or medications. Inquire about smoking and EtOH intake because both of these can increase the risk for both weight loss and malignancies.

Physical Examination
Patients with unexplained weight loss that is due to malignancy may look cachectic, pale, and lethargic or they may look well depending on the amount and cause of the weight loss. Weights over the past year should be plotted out to see how much weight has been lost over a period of time. A slow weight decrease in the elderly is not uncommon and may simply be due to a lack of appetite, to institutional food, or to disinterest in food resulting from a decreased sense of taste and/or smell. A full physical exam is necessary, paying particular attention to any masses, tenderness, swelling, or lymphadenopathy.

MALIGNANCY

Depending on the stage of the malignancy, any are capable of causing weight loss, either as a primary or secondary symptom. However, the most common malignancies to cause weight loss are GI, lung, hematologic, and musculoskeletal.

Signs and Symptoms.

The signs and symptoms will vary with the source of the malignancy, and many are asymptomatic except for the complaint of weight loss.

Diagnostic Studies.

Ordering a CBC and blood chemistries is a good place to start, as well as a chest x-ray and Hemoccult cards, depending on the age and medical history. The results of these and the history should assist the practitioner in narrowing down the search. Other diagnostics such as CT or MRI should be ordered as needed.

Depression and Anxiety
See Chapter 16 for a detailed discussion.

Eating Disorders
See Chapter 16 for a detailed discussion.

FUNCTIONAL AND FINANCIAL MALNUTRITION

Depending on the patient population, malnutrition may be a possibility. It is common in the very poor and in the elderly owing to the inability to purchase, prepare, and consume the proper, varied diet. Eating disorders, depending on the severity, may result in malnutrition. In developing countries, malnutrition is a huge problem, but it is not common in the United States except in the elderly and very poor populations.

Signs and Symptoms.

Aside from the weight loss, other signs of malnutrition include dry skin and hair, pale conjunctivae, cheilosis, glossitis, bruising, lethargy, decreased vibratory sensation, decreased DTRs, bone demineralization, liver or heart enlargement, muscle wasting, lower extremity edema, and growth failure.

Diagnostic Studies.

Malnutrition has a variety of consequences that can involve several body systems. A complete metabolic profile, CBC, and thyroid studies are recommended. Electrolyte imbalance is common especially if the malnutrition is brought on by anorexia or bulimia, and it can be life threatening. Kidney and liver functions may be affected as well. Depending on the chronicity of the problem, dual energy x-ray absorptiometry should be considered because bone health may be at risk. In severe cases, heart failure may ensue and an echocardiogram or more invasive cardiac testing may be needed to evaluate cardiac functioning.

Drug Reaction

There are few drugs that actually cause weight loss (thyroid replacement in greater than therapeutic doses, SSRIs, neuroleptics), but many drugs cause anorexia with weight loss as a secondary side effect. Because drug side effects vary greatly between patients, it is not possible to supply an exhaustive list of drugs that cause anorexia. A few that seem to be most problematic are digitalis, many psychotropic medications, chemotherapeutic agents mostly as a result of nausea, stimulants such as pseudoephedrine or other drugs used to treat obesity, and drugs used to treat attention deficit/hyperactivity disorder.

A complete medication history including over-the-counter medications may allow the practitioner to identify the cause of the weight loss. If a drug is suspected, it should be changed if possible. For patients on multiple drugs, the suspected agents should be discontinued or substituted one at a time in order to determine the offending agent.

MALABSORPTION

Malabsorption falls into two main categories: impaired digestion and impaired absorption, and there are many diseases that fall into each category. Diseases that fall under impaired digestion include gastrectomy, barosurgery, chronic pancreatitis, chronic liver failure, biliary obstruction, lactose intolerance, diverticula, and Zollinger-Ellison syndrome. Diseases that fall into the impaired absorption category include intestinal infections, alcohol, celiac disease, tropical sprue, Whipple's disease, amyloidosis, ischemic or infarcted bowel, Crohn's disease, volvulus, and intussusception.

Signs and Symptoms.

The signs and symptoms vary according to the underlying problem, but common symptoms include weight loss, flatulence, abdominal bloating, edema in the lower extremities resulting from protein deficiency, muscle weakness, possibly diarrhea or steatorrhea, dehydration, glossitis, and bruising. A variety of abnormal findings can be associated with malabsorption syndromes, including iron, folic acid or B_{12} deficiency anemia; calcium deficiency; vitamins A, B, C, and D deficiencies; and niacin deficiency. A combination of weight loss, diarrhea, and anemia should raise the possibility of malabsorption.

Diagnostic Studies.

There are as many diagnostics as there are causes of malabsorption. Measurement of fat in the stool is the most valuable diagnostic for diagnosing malabsorption, and a 3- to 4-day stool collection is advised. Stool specimens for ova and parasites and culture and sensitivity will help to rule out infectious causes. Absorption tests, flat plate of the abdomen, upper GI with small bowel follow-through, endoscopy, and small bowel biopsy may be necessary for definitive diagnosis.

Hyperthyroidism
See p. 388.

 SUGGESTED READINGS

Beers, M., Berkow, R., & Burs, M. (Eds.). (1999). *Merck Manual of Medical Therapeutics* (17th ed). Rahway, NJ: Merck & Co., Inc.
Tierney, L.M., McPhee, S.J., & Papadakis, M.A. (Eds.). (2003). *CURRENT Medical Diagnosis & Treatment*. New York: Lange Medical Books/McGraw Hill.

Chapter 16

Psychiatric Mental Health

Valerie A. Hart
& Patricia Hentz

U nlike other clinical areas discussed in this book, the differential diagnosis of psychiatric conditions can depend *less* on laboratory findings and physical assessment data and *more* on patient's complaints and reports of symptoms. As a result, the art of interviewing and skills of active listening are critical when attempting to rule out conditions with similar symptoms. In addition, the clinician must grapple with the question of whether a presenting symptom is genuine or instead represents factitious behavior or malingering, is related to substance abuse, is a medical condition, or represents one of the overlapping symptoms within one of the categories that will be covered in this chapter.

This chapter will also look at the topic of "medical mimics," or conditions that may easily fall into the category of conditions that are psychiatric in nature but appear to have confusing medical presentations. The authors will focus on common Axis I and Axis II psychiatric disorders and common symptoms or complaints. Since many disorders have overlapping symptoms, critical indicators will be presented as well as examples of focused questions to guide practitioners in determining the differential diagnosis. Owing to practical limitations, this is not intended to be an all-inclusive review but rather a choice of diagnostic areas most likely to be encountered by the advanced practice clinicians in a primary care setting.

Diagnosis of a psychiatric illness requires attention to physical and biological indicators along with a psychiatric evaluation. Psychiatric symptoms may present in response to a medical illness, may be triggered by medications, or may be a very normative response to a stressful life event, such as in the case of grieving a loss. When a psychiatric illness is believed to be the primary problem, a comprehensive psychiatric evaluation is indicated to achieve an accurate diagnosis. For example, when a client presents with complaints of feeling tired, difficulty sleeping, and feeling agitated and anxious, the practitioner would need to rule out a medical illness, determine whether the symptoms are in response to any medications, and explore whether the symptoms are related to a stressful life event. When the above are ruled out, a psychiatric evaluation may be indicated. Conducting a psychiatric evaluation helps to avoid the frequent treatment mistake of focusing on the obvious symptoms of difficulty sleeping, anxiety, or agitation and missing an underlying depression. In such situations, a minor tranquilizer might be prescribed that could actually exacerbate depression by depleting serotonin. The basic disorder may be a depression with coexisting anxiety symptoms.

COMPREHENSIVE PSYCHIATRIC EVALUATION

A comprehensive psychiatric evaluation leads to a diagnosis that encompasses five major axes: clinical disorder (Axis I), personality disorder (Axis II), physical disorders/medical conditions (Axis III), psychosocial and environmental problems/stressors (Axis IV), and the degree of functional impairment (Axis V). Targeted questions in the following areas aid in determining the appropriate psychiatric diagnosis. Although it is not critical to follow this guide in a lockstep manner, attention to the major areas can help in avoiding an inaccurate psychiatric diagnosis. This section provides a brief overview of the psychiatric evaluation. The sections that follow highlight various psychiatric problems and will offer additional guides for assessment.

Problem Identification and Chief Complaint

In the patient's own words, identify the reason for seeking care at this time. Because many common symptoms fall within a variety of psychiatric diagnoses, the practitioner will be looking for specific clusters of symptoms to determine the diagnosis. So, given the chief complaint, "I have been feeling tired recently. I have not been able to sleep well, and I have felt restless during the day and anxious," many more details are necessary to accurately diagnose.

History of Present Illness

A symptom analysis similar to that done for nonpsychiatric complaints is indicated, to determine the history of the specific complaint and to identify any associated problems. This can be integrated in the general assessment. Areas that should be explored include the time line related to symptoms, the relationship of symptoms to life events, any recent conflicts or stressors, any drugs that are used, and how this differs from the client's previous level of functioning. If, at the initial presentation of a complaint, the patient indicates that the problem has existed for some time, the sequence of events leading up to the visit at this particular time may identify important triggers that have either exacerbated the problem or convinced the patient (or family member) that help was needed for the problem.

Pertinent Past Psychiatric History

It is important to determine whether the client has a history of any psychiatric disorders. If so, determine the extent of the illness and all prior and current treatments, medications, and outcomes or responses to the treatments. Ask the patient whether he or she believes that prior treatments were beneficial and how well they were tolerated.

Pertinent Social History

The social history is an essential part of the psychiatric history. It is important to explore questions about education, family relationships, social networks, potential abuse history, and employment. This part of the history should include information on all drug and alcohol abuse because many psychiatric disorders mimic substance abuse. Psychiatric symptoms may actually stem from adverse effects of a prescribed, over-the-counter, or recreational drug. The following sections on specific complaints and problems identify medications that are associated with each of the complaints discussed. Obtaining a history of occupational and recreational activities, as well as the performance of activities of daily living, provides crucial information that is helpful in determining how problems affect an individual's overall life. Finally, the social history is important in determining the disposition of a patient following assessment and diagnosis.

Pertinent Family History

Obtain a family history, including questions about psychiatric history, as well as medical and genetic illnesses.

Medical History and the Review of Symptoms

Many times, psychiatric symptoms are a result of underlying medical conditions. In such cases, the focus for treatment is the medical condition. For example, the following sections identify medical conditions that can cause or exacerbate mental health symptoms, including depression, anxiety, eating disorders, and alterations in thought processes. It is important to identify all allergies or intolerances to both psychotropic and other medications.

Mental Status Examination

The mental status examination comprises five major areas: a) appearance and behavior, b) mood and affect, c) speech and thought processes, d) thought processes and perceptual abnormalities, and e) sensorial, cognitive, and intellectual functioning.

Appearance and Behavior

To assess appearance and behavior, observe gait, dress, grooming, posture, gestures, and facial expressions as the history is performed. Note the patient's apparent nutritional status. Note whether the patient maintains eye contact or exhibits any unusual behaviors during the history. For example, a patient presenting with mania might exhibit psychomotor agitation, distractibility, colorful clothes or bizarre combinations of clothes, excessive makeup, and intrusiveness. The client's behavior may range from entertaining to very irritable.

Mood and Affect

Mood reflects the subjective experience as self-reported. The practitioner should ask the client to describe how he or she feels. For instance, does the patient typically feel well, happy, depressed, anxious, etc. In contrast, affect refers to the practitioner's impression. Note whether your impression is that of a happy, depressed, anxious, flat, or other type of affect.

Speech and Thought Process

The tone, quality, quantity, and rate of speech are important indications of mental status. For instance, in mania, the speech may be pressured, loud, dramatic, and exaggerated; in depression, the speech may be soft and monotone, with little or no spontaneity. In addition to noting speech patterns, consider whether the client's thought processes are clear, logical, and organized. With altered thought processes, a patient's speech may indicate irrelevant information (loose associations), frequent change of topics (flight of ideas), vagueness (circumstantiality), permanent departure from the topic of conversation (tangential thought), halted speech (thought blocking), or other signs of a formal thought disorder.

Thought Content and Perceptual Abnormalities

During the mental status examination, it is important to determine whether the patient is experiencing abnormal content of thought, such as hallucinations or delusions. Ask whether the patient sees things that others cannot see or hears voices that others cannot hear. If so, it is important to explore what type of hallucination is experienced. To assess for delusions, ask the patient whether they have any powers or abilities that others do not have or thoughts that others would consider strange. Determine whether there are obsessions or compulsions, feelings of hopelessness, worthlessness, or guilt.

When patients are experiencing mental health problems, it is vital to assess for suicidal ideation or intent. Sixty percent of depressed clients have suicidal ideations. Patients should be asked whether they have previously performed any acts of self-harm, as well as whether they have any thoughts of harming or killing themselves in the future. Positive responses will require more detailed assessment of current suicidal risk.

The Sensorium, and Cognitive and Intellectual Functioning

Determine each patient's general level of orientation and alertness. Alertness may be affected or blunted by mental health problems such as depression. To assess the level of intelligence, ask about common knowledge issues. Often this can be incorporated as the practitioner explores the client's history, work, and education. Judgment can be assessed in relation to how the client has handled situations in the past as well as any current challenges. Insight may be determined by evaluating the patient's understanding of current health status or living situation.

Assessing for Potential Medical Mimics

Whenever faced with a mental health complaint, it is vital that the differential diagnosis initially include any medical problems that could be correctable. This category includes both nonpsychiatric health problems, as well as the myriad of medications and treatments that may result in complaints that are similar to those of psychiatric problems. Hedeya (1996) provides a set of rules designed to help spot medical mimics (Box 16-1). The mnemonic "THINC MED" is useful when evaluating for underlying medical conditions that present as psychiatric symptoms (See Box 16-2).

Differential Diagnosis of Chief Complaints

Anxiety

Anxiety disorders make up the most common category of psychiatric conditions and are responsible for frequent patient use of the health care system. Anxiety disorders affect approximately 17–19 million American adults a year (Epidemiological Catchment Area and National Comorbidity studies). The U.S. economy loses over $42 billion each year (Greenberg et al., 1999). Both functional impairment and morbidity have been linked to anxiety disorders, and recent studies suggest that chronic anxiety disorders may increase the rate of cardiovascular-related mortality. The etiology of anxiety disorders is a complex

Box 16-1

Rules to Follow for Spotting Medical Mimics

1. Never assume that an emotional symptom has a psychosocial cause until physical causes are fully explored.
2. Always have your patients get a complete physical if they have not had one since the onset of symptoms.
3. Look for a history that does not fit (e.g., a first psychotic break after age 40).
4. Check personal and family history thoroughly.
5. Be suspicious when the onset comes late in life and/or when no stressors are present.
6. Be suspicious of a recent onset of headaches, loss of function, unusual perceptions, visual disturbances, paranormal experiences, or hallucinations.
7. Ask about all drug use, including over the counter and illicit.

dance of genetic predisposition and environmental factors, as in many other psychiatric conditions. It is important to distinguish between *normal* anxiety, which everyone experiences, and anxiety that reaches the level of psychopathology. Anxiety is an unpleasant feeling of apprehension, often accompanied by perspiration, palpitation, stomach discomfort, restlessness, difficulty sitting still, and even tightness in the chest. Anxiety is usually differentiated from *fear* in that when one is fearful, there is an identifiable dreaded object, as opposed to anxiety, in which there is no specific focus. Whereas anxiety is a normal response to stress, pathologic anxiety is distinguished by the intensity, duration, level of impairment to coping it renders, and whether there is an environmental trigger or not.

Anxiety is quite common in the general medical setting. More than 90% of the patients with anxiety present primarily with somatic complaints in primary care and emergency room settings (Stern & Herman, 2000). Patients with anxiety often present in primary care settings with the following symptoms: chest pain (with negative angiogram), irritable bowel, unexplained dizziness, migraine headache, and chronic fatigue. The medical workup for this type of patient relies on both the medical and psychiatric histories, the medication and drug histories, and the physical and neurological exams.

When assessing a patient who may be anxious, the most obvious indicators are those involving the sympathetic nervous system, such as increased heart rate, blood pressure, pal-

Box 16-2

THINC MED

The following represents major categories of medical mimics.

T	Tumors
H	Hormones (thyroid, adrenals, gonadal, insulin)
I	Infections and immune diseases (AIDS, Lyme, mononucleosis, lupus, syphilis)
N	Nutrition (B_{12}, B_1, B_6, manganese, iron overload)
C	Central nervous system (head trauma, MS, seizures, Parkinson's, Huntington's)
M	Miscellaneous (sleep apnea, anemia, CHF)
E	Electrolyte abnormalities and toxins (K^+, NA^+, chemical exposures)
D	Drugs (also include nicotine and caffeine)

lor, dry mouth, increased respiration, and sweating. These familiar signs are representations of the fight or flight response. Patients may also exhibit behavior connected with parasympathetic activity, such as pacing, tapping toes or fingers, and adjusting clothing (displacement activities) (Shea, 1998).

The *DSM-IV–TR* lists twelve anxiety disorders: (a) Panic Disorder with Agoraphobia, (b) Panic Disorder without Agoraphobia, (c) Agoraphobia without History of Panic Disorder, (d) Specific Phobia, (e) Social Phobia, (f) Obsessive-Compulsive Disorder, (g) Posttraumatic Stress Disorder, (h) Acute Stress Disorder, (i) Generalized Anxiety Disorder, (j) Anxiety Disorder Due to a General Medical Condition, (k) Substance-Induced Anxiety Disorder, and (l) Not Otherwise Specified.

Medical Problems and Medications

As with all mental health symptoms, the first step in the differential diagnosis is to rule out any general medical condition (Box 16-3) or medication use (Box 16-4) as the physiological cause of the anxiety. After ruling out a medical condition, the answers to the *initial questions* will determine what follows.

Panic Disorder

Panic disorder is a syndrome characterized by recurrent unexpected panic attacks about which there is persistent concern. Panic attacks are discrete episodes of intense anxiety that peak within 10 minutes and are associated with autonomic arousal (cardiac, pulmonary, gastrointestinal, and neurological symptoms) as well as feelings of depersonalization/derealization and the fear of dying, losing control, or going crazy. After an initial attack, the apprehension of a future attack often occurs and is referred to as anticipatory anxiety. The anticipation is often as distressing (if not more so) to patients than the experience of an actual episode. Questions that should be included in the history in order to assess for panic disorder and panic attack are listed in Box 16-5.

Generalized Anxiety Disorder

Patients with this disorder are worried most of the time about everything. The latest revision of *DSM-IV-TR* requires several events for most days for at least a 6-month period of time as the worry criterion. Patients find this worry impossible to control and usually associated with somatic symptoms, often sleep complaints, muscle pain, bowel function,

---

Box 16-3

Conditions Associated with Anxiety

Hyperthyroid
CHF
Asthma
COPD
Malignancy
Pheochromocytoma
Hyperadrenal
Hypoglycemial DM
Epilepsy
MI

Box 16-4

Medications Causing Anxiety

Caffeine
Thyroid medications
Theophylline
Albuterol

---

mood, or problems at work or in relationships. Questions that should be included in the history to assess for generalized anxiety disorder are listed in Box 16-6.

Social Phobia

Social phobia is characterized by a marked fear of being the center of attention or behaving in a way that will be an embarrassment or humiliation; this phobia is also characterized by the marked avoidance of these situations. The fears are manifested in social situations, such as eating or speaking in public or entering a social gathering, meeting, or classroom. Symptoms of anxiety, such as blushing, and/or fear of vomiting, urgency, micturition, or defecation are also often present. Social phobia can be associated with panic attacks. Social phobia must be differentiated from normal shyness and appropriate fear, as well as from schizophrenia, hypochondriasis, obsessive-compulsive disorder, and paranoid personality disorder. The *content* of the anxiety determines the steps in a decision tree. Formally defined, in Panic Disorder, with or without Agoraphobia, anxiety is related to the fear of having additional episodes and the ramifications of the episodes. Specific Phobia and Social Phobia are related to specific fears. Specific Phobias are divided into the following: Animal type; Nature type; Blood, injection, injury type; Situational type (elevators, tunnels); and Other.

Box 16-5

Questions Related to Panic Disorder and Panic Attack

1. "Have you had episodes when you felt nervous, frightened, anxious, uneasy in situations when most people did not feel that way? "Did the feelings peak within 10 minutes?" (Panic Disorder)
2. "Do you feel nervous in places where you might have a panic attack or when escape might be difficult, such as in a crowd; standing in a line; on a bridge; in a bus, plane, or train?" (Agoraphobia)

Questions Related to Panic Attack

1. "In the past, did these episodes occur unexpectedly?"
   a. "Was your heart racing?"
   b. "Did you have difficulty breathing?"
   c. "Were your hands sweaty?"
   d. "Did you have chest pain?"
   e. "Did you fear that you were dying?"
   f. "Did you feel dizzy or think you were going to faint?"
2. "Have you had an episode and then for a month or more feared having another episode, or attack?"

Box 16-6

Questions Related to Generalized Anxiety Disorder

1. "Have you been worried about many things over the past 6 months?"
2. "Are these worries present most days?"
3. "Do you find it difficult to control your worries?"
4. "Do they interfere with your ability to concentrate on what you are doing?"

Obsessive-Compulsive Disorder

Obsessions (recurring thoughts) and compulsions (recurring actions) over which the patient has little to no control are the hallmark of this condition. They interfere with everyday functioning and cause embarrassment because the sufferer is well aware of the bizarre nature of the behavior. The link to anxiety is that the behavior and thinking is an attempt to control anxiety. The most common obsession is that of "contamination" and washing or avoidance of a particular object that is contaminated. Along with anxiety, patients often experience shame and self-loathing. Another common obsession is self-doubt, such as in checking to see that routine safety chores are done and multiple trips are necessary in order to check and recheck in order to satisfy this doubt. Guilt is a common derivative of this obsession. Intrusive thoughts are another common class of obsessions in which repetitive thoughts of either an aggressive or sexual nature haunt a patient and cause severe distress. The major differentials for obsessive-compulsive disorder include phobias, depressive disorders, schizophrenias and obsessive-compulsive personality disorder, and Tourette's disorder.

Posttraumatic Stress Disorder

This disorder is reserved for symptoms that occur as a result of exposure to stressful or traumatic situations. Related symptoms can be in the form of flashbacks, memories, recurring dreams, or avoidance behavior that was not present before exposure to the stressor. The patient must exhibit either an inability to recall some important aspect of the period of exposure to the stressor (depersonalization, derealization, or Dissociative Amnesia) or show marked anxiety and increased arousal (difficulty sleeping, irritability, the startle response, motor restlessness, hypervigilance, poor concentration). Differential diagnosis includes head injury, substance abuse, other anxiety disorders, mood disorders, dissociative disorders, borderline personality disorder, and malingering.

Mood Disorders

This section will examine several categories of mood disorders, discuss clusters of symptoms, and present the process of continuing assessment. The mood disorders presented will be Major Depressive Disorder, Dysthymic Disorder, Cyclothymic Disorder, Bipolar Disorder, Seasonal Pattern Depression, Postpartum Depression, and Premenstrual Dysphoric Disorder.

Depression can present in a variety of ways and can vary markedly from one individual to the next in regards to the cluster of symptoms. Examples of variations in symptoms include a presentation by one individual who might be experiencing severe sleep disturbance in contrast to another individual who experiences hypersomnia. Some individuals with depression complain of weight gain, whereas others find it hard to eat and lose weight. Whereas avolition is a common presenting feature in depression, some individuals experience restlessness and agitation. Key to treatment is the accurate assessment of presenting symptoms. Based on diagnosis and symptoms, a combination of psychotherapy with medication is often the most effective approach.

The goal in the treatment of depression is remission. The risk of recurrence of depression is 50% after one episode, 70% after two episodes, and 90% after three episodes. Early detection and treatment are critical, as is early intervention when signs and symptoms of recurrence are detected. There is a 5%–11% lifetime prevalence for depression; morbidity is comparable to angina and advanced coronary artery disease, and there is a high mortality from suicide if untreated and undertreated (Stahl, 2000). The ability to accurately diagnose depression is critical. Untreated and undertreated depression significantly increases the risk of suicide as reflected in the following statistics: 1 out of 7 with recurrent depressive illness commits suicide; 70% of suicides have depressive illness; and 70% of suicides see their primary care provider within 6 weeks of suicide. Suicide is the seventh leading cause of death in the United States (Stahl, 2000, p 141).

Symptoms of depression can present as vague physical symptoms, such as fatigue, loss of appetite, and sleep disturbances. In addition, research has shown that up to 30% of individuals who fully meet the criteria for a major depression actually deny being depressed (Shea, 1998). There are helpful tools, such as the Hamilton Rating Scale for Depression to assess for depression; however, they are not a replacement for skillful interviewing.

The assessment of depression includes questions designed to identify whether the person is experiencing a general loss of pleasure in life and whether activities that were once enjoyable are no longer so. It is important to determine whether there is any sense of being sad or a general dysphoric mood and whether any neurovegetative symptoms are evident. Manic and hypomanic symptoms should always be actively sought. As with other mental health assessments, the past psychiatric history should always be elicited, as well as the history of alcohol and/or drug use, as these are commonly associated with depression. What may appear as a major depression may actually be a result of alcohol or street drug use (Shea, 1998).

Medical Problems and Medications
There are several medical conditions (Box 16-7) and numerous medications (Box 16-8) that can be associated with symptoms of depression. If medications are the contributing cause, switching medications may be advised.

Major Depression
To meet the criteria for Major Depressive Episode, an individual must have symptoms over a 2-week period that represent a change from previous functioning, with at least one of the

---

Box 16-7
Medical Problems That Can Present with Symptoms of Depression

Addison's disease, AIDS, anemia, asthma, chronic fatigue syndrome, chronic infection, congestive heart failure, Cushing's disease, diabetes, hyperthyroidism, hypothyroidism, infectious hepatitis, malignancies, menopause, multiple sclerosis, postpartum hormonal changes, premenstrual syndrome, rheumatoid arthritis, systemic lupus, ulcerative colitis, uremia.

Box 16-8

Drugs That Can Cause Depression

Antihypertensives (reserpine, propranolol, methyldopa, guanethidine monosulfate, and clonidine hydrochloride)
Corticosteroids and Hormones (cortisone acetate, estrogen, and progesterone)
Antiparkinsonian drugs (levodopa and carbidopa, amantadine hydrochloride)
Antianxiety drugs (diazepam, chlordiazepoxide)
Accutane
Birth control pills

---

symptoms being a depressed mood or a loss of interest or pleasure (APA, 2000). Five of the nine criteria for Major Depression need to be met.
1. Depressed mood most of the day, nearly every day, as indicated by either subjective report (e.g., feels sad or empty) or observation made by others (e.g., appears tearful). Note: In children and adolescents, can be irritable mood.
2. Markedly diminished interest or pleasure in all, or almost all, activities most of the day, nearly every day (as indicated by either subjective account or observation made by others).
3. Significant weight loss when not dieting or weight gain (e.g., an change of more than 5% of body weight in a month), or a decrease or increase in appetite nearly every day. Note: In children, consider failure to make expected weight gains.
4. Insomnia or hypersomnia nearly every day.
5. Psychomotor agitation or retardation nearly every day (observable by others, not merely subjective feelings of restlessness or being slowed down).
6. Fatigue or loss of energy nearly every day.
7. Feelings of worthlessness or excessive or inappropriate guilt (which may be delusional) nearly every day (not merely self-reproach or guilt about being sick).
8. Diminished ability to think or concentrate, or indecisiveness, nearly every day (either by subjective account or as observed by others).
9. Recurrent thoughts of death (not just fear of dying), recurrent suicidal ideation without a specific plan, or a suicidal attempt or a specific plan for committing suicide.
    In addition to meeting five of the nine criteria, the patient should respond positively to one or both of the following criteria.
- Have you been consistently depressed or down, most of the day, for the past 2 weeks?
- In the past 2 weeks, have you found that you were less interested in most things, less able to enjoy things that you used to find enjoyable?
    If these are met, additional symptoms are assessed that focus on affect, thought process and content, and behavior as seen in the criteria above. Patients should be asked questions inclusive of following areas: appetite changes and weight changes; insomnia or hypersomnia and whether it occurs most days; agitation or retardation that occurs nearly every day; fatigue or loss of energy nearly every day; feeling of worthlessness or guilt; difficulty concentrating or even making simple decisions; and thoughts of harming oneself, feeling one would be better off dead, and suicidal thoughts. The Hamilton Rating Scale for Depression can be used to assess symptoms of patients with depression. The mnemonic "SIGECAPS" is helpful for remembering criteria for depression (see Box 16-9).

Box 16-9

SIGECAPS

S	Sleep	**C**	Concentration
I	Interest	**A**	Appetite
G	Guilt	**P**	Psychomotor
E	Energy	**S**	Suicidality

An individual with major depression may be experiencing difficulty with routine personal care and present as unkempt, unclean, and with a slowness of movement. In contrast, an individual with agitated depression experiences "a nagging need to move" (Shea, 1998). Thought process and content may reflect an inability to plan and make life decisions, what is referred to as "blocking of the future." There is also quite often a marked slowing in thinking as reflected in slowness in responding to questions and long pauses. This change in cognition could be described as if the stream of thought was frozen by an unexpected drop in temperature. In contrast, individuals with agitated depression experience thought process as a stream of thought in a turbulent boil (Shea, 1998). Thought content is often restricted, "ideational caging," the experience of having thoughts trapped within a small network of themes or ruminations.

Dysthymic Disorder

Unlike major depression, individuals with dysthymic disorder are more functional. Dysthymic disorder is marked by a long-standing pervasive mood of feeling sad or depressed most of the time over a period of two years. Individuals will often describe themselves as "this is just the way I always am," Along with the depressed mood, at least two of the following additional symptoms need to be present: poor appetite or overeating, insomnia or hypersomnia, low energy or fatigue, low self-esteem, poor concentration or difficulty making decisions, and feelings of hopelessness. In children, the mood may be irritable rather than depressed, with a minimum duration of 1 year (APA, 2000). Thus, to meet these criteria, this mood must present as stable. Additionally, dysthymic disorder can precede major depression; however, it is important to note that if dysthymic disorder is *not present* before a major depression, the symptoms following treatment of major depression should be viewed as a partial responding rather than as dysthymic disorder. In such cases where the depression is partially relieved, individuals may meet the criteria of apathetic responder. They present with a reduction of depressed mood, continuing anhedonia, lack of motivation, decreased libido, lack of interest, cognitive slowing, and decreased concentration. Anxious responders demonstrate a reduction of depressed mood, continuing anxiety, especially generalized anxiety, worry, insomnia, and somatic complaints (Stahl, 2000). Apathetic responders and anxious responders are often associated with ineffective treatment of the major depression. In such cases, medications need to be adjusted. For a diagnosis of dysthymic disorder after a major depression, the individual must first meet the criteria for a full remission or have been diagnosed with dysthymic disorder prior to the major depression.

Bipolar Disorder

Assessment of depression should always be followed by an assessment of bipolar disorder. Major depressive and bipolar disorders need to be distinguished from episodes of Mood

Disorder due to a Substance-Induced Mood Disorder or those Due to a General Medical Condition (e.g., multiple sclerosis, stroke, and hypothyroidism).

Approximately 10%–15% of adolescents with recurrent major depressive episodes will develop Bipolar I Disorder. Mixed episodes are more prevalent in adolescents and young adults than in older adults. In males, the first episode is more likely to be manic as opposed to females, who present first with depression. Women with Bipolar I Disorder have an increased risk of developing subsequent episodes during the postpartum period (APA, 2000).

Bipolar disorder refers to a cluster of disorders that reflect a marked flux in mood. A manic episode is defined as a distinct period when there is a persistently elevated, expansive, or irritable mood lasting at least 1 week. This mood must coexist with at least three additional symptoms: inflated self-esteem or grandiosity, decreased need for sleep, pressure of speech, flight of ideas, distractibility, increased involvement in goal-directed activities or psychomotor agitation, and excessive involvement in pleasurable activities with a high potential for painful consequences. Hypomanic episodes differ from Manic episodes in the degree of severity. Hypomanic episodes are not usually sufficiently severe to cause marked impairment in social or occupational functioning or to require hospitalization (APA, 2000). They may, however, evolve into fully manic episodes. The mnemonic "DIG FAST" is helpful for remembering the critical criteria for mania (See Box 16-10).

Bipolar I Disorder is characterized by the occurrence of one or more Manic Episodes or Mixed Episodes. Mixed Episodes are characterized by a period of time (lasting at least 1 week) in which the criteria are met both for Manic Episode and for a Major Depressive Episode nearly every day. There is severe impairment of social or occupational functioning as the individual experiences rapidly alternating moods (APA, 2000). Questions that aid in the differential diagnosis for Bipolar I are listed in Box 16-11.

Completed suicides occur in 10%–15% of individuals with Bipolar I Disorder. Suicide ideation and attempts are more likely in the depressive or mixed state (APA, 2000). As such, a suicide risk should always be included in a psychiatric evaluation. Box 16-12 lists several questions that should be addressed to assess suicide risk. If the responses identify a detailed plan for ending life, a lack of hope that things can be better in the future, or an inability to identify reasons for not dying (such as not wanting to leave loved ones), it is considered a psychiatric emergency, requiring immediate intervention.

Bipolar II Disorder is determined when the clinical course includes one or more Major Depressive Episodes and there has been at least one Hypomanic Episode. The symptoms

Box 16-10	
DIG FAST	
D	Distractibility; leaving tasks unfinished
I	Insomnia; decrease need for sleep
G	Grandiosity; increased self-worth
F	Flight of ideas
A	Activity increased; goal directed
S	Speech is pressured; hyperverbal; rapid
T	Thoughtless risk (sex, money)

Box 16-11

Diagnostic Questions for Bipolar Disorder

1. "Have you ever felt up or high, having increased energy, elated mood, needing less sleep, and having rapid thoughts? Were you feeling highly creative, impulsive, or feeling increased productivity that was noticeable to others?"
2. "Have you ever been persistently irritable for several days so that you had arguments or verbal or physical fights or shouted at people?" If yes, determine past or current.

Data from Sheehan et al., 2001.

cause clinically significant distress or impairment in social, occupational, or other important areas of functioning (APA, 2000). To meet the Bipolar II criteria, the individual has not experienced a Manic or Mixed episode.

Cyclothymic Disorder

Cyclothymic Disorder is a chronic, fluctuating mood disturbance including hypomanic and depressive symptoms that do not meet the criteria for Manic Episode. In addition, the depressive symptoms lack the severity, pervasiveness, or duration to meet the criteria for Depressive Episode. To meet the criteria for Cyclothymic Disorder, symptoms need to be present over a 2-year period without a lapse of symptoms longer than 2 months. Many individuals function with minor distress or impairment in social, occupational, or other areas of functioning. Individuals may present as temperamental, moody, unpredictable, inconsistent, or unreliable (APA, 2000).

Mood Disorders with Specifiers
Seasonal Pattern

What differentiates Seasonal Pattern from the other mood disorders is the essential feature of onset and remission that is consistently related to specific times of the year. It may have features similar to those of bipolar or major depression. In most cases, episodes begin in the fall or winter and remit in the spring. A key factor is that the mood is not related to situational stressors or cyclical patterns of work or life demands. Assessment involves tracking symptoms to demonstrate clear evidence of a temporal/seasonal relationship.

Postpartum Onset

There is no simple cluster of symptoms to assess during the postpartum period. Onset may be immediate or as late as 6 months after delivery. Baby blues occurs in up to 70% of

Box 16-12

Questions to Ask for Assessing Suicide Risk

1. "Have you been thinking that you would be better off dead or wish that you were dead?"
2. "Do you have thoughts of harming yourself?"
3. "Have you being thinking about suicide?"
4. "If you have been thinking about suicide, do you have a plan? ... Describe."
5. "Have you attempted suicide?"
6. "In the past, have you thought about or attempted suicide?"

women postpartum. Given the social pressures to "be happy" with the birth of a new baby, women often mask their underlying depression, a phenomenon referred to as smiling depression. Symptoms common in the postpartum onset include fluctuation in mood, mood lability, and preoccupation with the infant's well-being. Severity of symptoms is the key. On a continuum, thoughts can range from focused and realistic regarding the infant's well-being, to obsessive or even delusional. At highest risk are women who have experienced a postpartum episode with psychotic features. Their risk of recurrence is 30%–50%. Women who have had a history of depression are also at greater risk. The Edinburgh Postnatal Depression Scale can be used to help identify postpartum depression. See Figure 16-1 for postpartum mood conditions.

Premenstrual Dysphoric Disorder

Premenstrual dysphoric disorder (PMDD) is characterized by recurrent symptoms that occur during the luteal phase of the menstrual cycle and remit during menstruation. Even though many women express mood changes and other symptoms during the premenstrual phase, 5%–9% fully meet the criteria for PMDD. Differential diagnosis includes bipolar disorder, thyroid dysfunction, premenstrual syndrome, exacerbation of unipolar depression, anxiety disorder, and cyclothymic disorder. Careful tracking of symptoms for at least 2 months is advised to determine a diagnosis of PMDD (Box 16-13).

Substance-Related Disorders

This category includes disorders associated with alcohol and drugs, medication side effects, and mental states that are toxin-induced. Owing to the affect of certain substances on mood, cognition, and perception, as well as behavior, patients may present with a confusing array of symptoms. In the *DSM-IV*, substance-related disorders are cross-referenced in the following disorders: Delirium (Intoxication and Withdrawal); Substance Induced Dementia, Amnesic Disorder, Psychotic Disorder, Mood Disorder, Anxiety Disorder, Sexual Dysfunction, and Sleep Disorder.

Comorbidity with other psychiatric conditions is high with this population. Antisocial Personality Disorder is present in a high percentage (35%–60%) of patients presenting for treatment of substance abuse and dependence. Other psychiatric disorders associated with substance-related disorders include Mood Disorders and Anxiety Disorders.

Prioritizing the differential diagnosis demands ruling out Delirium, Dementia, and Amnesic Disorder. Initial symptoms to be alerted to include a change in cognition, including memory impairment, and disturbed consciousness. If no change of consciousness or memory impairment is present, then look for specific symptoms, which may indicate a substance-induced disorder.

A careful history taking, physical examination for signs of intoxication or withdrawal, and laboratory analysis will determine substance use. If a substance is identified, the clinician needs to consider whether there is a causal relationship between the substance use and the psychiatric symptom. Are the symptoms a direct effect of the substance? Is there a primary psychiatric disorder and the substance use serves to "self-medicate"? Are the psychiatric symptoms and substance abuse independent of one another? Questions related to the timing of the development of psychiatric symptoms and substance use will help determine whether the patient has a primary psychiatric condition or a true substance-abuse disorder. Substance abuse can mimic many common psychiatric symptoms, such as depression, apa-

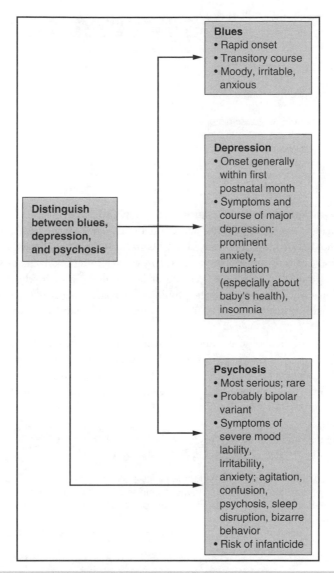

Figure 16-1. ■ Postpartum mood conditions.

thy, agitation, anxiety, panic attacks, thought disturbances, paranoia, and psychosis. Thus, during the assessment of *any* psychiatric illness, the use and possible abuse of substances must be evaluated.

Before reviewing an assessment of substance abuse, there are several terms to clarify. The first is use versus abuse. Sanctioned uses of drugs (e.g., caffeine) have been defined by a culture, vary among cultures, and can change over time. Abuse from a cultural perspective is defined as the self-administration of any drug in a culturally disapproved manner that causes adverse consequences. To the brain, the term use and abuse take on different mean-

---

Box 16-13

Premenstrual Dysphoric Disorder

- Recurring physical, emotional symptoms in late luteal phase, dissipating 1 or 2 days after menses.
- Encourage prospective rating of symptoms.
- Document precipitants.
- Document treatment response history.
- Rule out medical illness with symptoms that mimic PMS.
- Family psychiatric history.
- Note use of stimulants, other mood-altering agents, water-retaining drugs.

---

ings, with a focus on the chemical neurotransmission and the degree of clinically significant impairment or distress. The terms addiction and dependence are frequently confused. Addiction is not defined as a condition in the *DSM-IV*. It refers to a behavioral pattern, as Stahl describes it, of drug abuse characterized by overwhelming involvement with use of a drug (compulsive use) and with the securing of its supply by a high tendency to relapse after discontinuation. Dependence is the physiological state of neuroadaptation necessitating continued administration to prevent the appearance of a withdrawal syndrome (Stahl, 2000).

An assessment of alcohol abuse and dependence and nonalcoholic psychoactive substance use disorders will be reviewed. Box 16-14 presents a set of questions used to determine alcohol dependence. The criteria for *alcohol abuse* relate to use that causes adverse consequences. Box 16-15 presents questions used to determine alcohol abuse.

Box 16-14

Questions to Ask for Determining Alcohol Dependence

1. "In the past 12 months, have you had three or more alcoholic drinks within a 3-hour period on three or more occasions?" If yes, continue with questions 2-8.
2. "Did you need to drink more in order to get the same effect that you got when you first started drinking?"
3. "When you cut down on drinking, did your hands shake, did you sweat, or feel agitated?"
4. "Would you drink to avoid being hung over or to avoid experiencing the above symptoms?"
5. "During the times when you drank alcohol, did you find that you drank more than you had planned?"
6. "Have you tried to reduce or stop drinking?"
7. "On the days that you drank, did you spend substantial time in obtaining alcohol, drinking, or in recovering from the effects of alcohol?"
8. "Did you spend less time is other activities, such as work, hobbies, or being with others because of your drinking?"
9. "Have you continued to drink even though you knew the drinking caused you health or mental problems?"

Data from Sheehan, et al., 2001.

Box 16-15

Questions to Ask for Determining Alcohol Abuse

1. "Have you been intoxicated, high, or hung over more than once when you had responsibilities at school, work, or at home? Did this cause any problems?"
2. "When you were intoxicated in any situation, were you physically at risk, for example, driving a car?"
3. "Did you have any legal problems because of your drinking?"
4. "Did you continue to drink even though your drinking caused problems with your family or other individuals?"

Assessment of drug use, dependence, and abuse follows the questions presented in Boxes 16-14 and 16-15 after determining the drugs used. Question #3 in Box 16-14, referring to symptoms experienced when trying to quit or cut back, can be adapted to be more drug specific regarding withdrawal symptoms. The screening question is, "In the past 12 months, did you take any of the drugs listed below more than once to get high, to feel better, or the change your mood?" (Sheehan et al., 2001). From a list of drugs (See Table 16-1) the patient is then asked to identify any that apply.

Eating Disorders

The world of eating disorders is much more than a list of symptoms. The incidence of eating disorders among young people has increased two to five times since 1955, with anorexia nervosa listed as the third most common chronic illness of adolescence (Stashwick, 1996). According to statistics, it is estimated that 0.5%–1% of girls 14–19 years of age suffer from anorexia nervosa; 1%–5% fit the *DSM-IV* criteria of Bulimia Nervosa; 10%–50 fall under the eating disorder, Not Otherwise Specified (NOS). Although both men and women are affected by cultural norms of physical attractiveness, the impact on self-esteem is greater for women.

Anorexia and bulimia have different profiles even though many symptoms can overlap. For example, about 50% of normal weight individuals with bulimia have a history of

Table 16-1. ■ Abused Substances

Group	Examples
Stimulants	Amphetamines, "speed," crystal meth, "rush," Dexedrine, Ritalin, diet pills
Cocaine	Snorting, IV, freebase, crack, "speedball"
Narcotics	heroin, morphine, Dilaudid, opium, Demerol, methadone, codeine, Percodan, Darvon
Hallucinogens	LSD ("acid"), mescaline, peyote, PCP ("angel dust," "peace pill"), psilocybin, hallucinogenic amphetamines ("STP"), "mushrooms," ecstasy, MDA or MDMA
Inhalants	"Glue," ethyl chloride, nitrous oxide ("laughing gas"), amyl or butyl nitrate ("poppers")
Marijuana	Hashish ("hash"), THC, "pot," "grass," "weed," "reefer"
Tranquilizers	Quaalude, Seconal ("reds"), valium, Xanax, Librium, Ativan, Dalmane, Halcion, barbiturates, Miltown
Miscellaneous	Steroids, nonprescription sleep or diet pills, GHB. Any others?

anorexia and approximately 47% with anorexia exhibit bulimic behaviors. The dominant feature of anorexia is the drive to lose weight. Common patterns include restricting intake and excessive exercising.

Individuals with bulimia are characterized by cycles of binge eating followed by purging with severity of the disorder determined by the frequency of the binge/purge cycles. In severe cases, the bulimia becomes the center of their life with all other aspects of life revolving around the binge/purge cycles.

There are many adolescents and young adults who do not meet the full criteria for anorexia or bulimia but exhibit many of the characteristics. They may fit the diagnosis of Eating Disorder (NOS). As delineated in Schwitzer et al. (2001), "1) perfectionism regarding body image, romantic and other personal relationships, and grades; 2) a fragile sense of self, feelings of inadequacy, and a need to be bolstered by others; 3) self-doubt expressed as sexual intimacy questions and ambivalence about whether one is thin enough to attract a romantic partner and whether one should want to please a partner at all; and 4) a sense of powerlessness in intimate relationships and the world generally." There exists a "high incidence of diagnostically subthreshold problems centering around dissatisfaction with body image. Overall, 35%–45% of adolescent females report difficulties with weight control, regard themselves as too fat, or aspire to become thinner" (Schwitzer et al., 1998).

The aspects that differentiate eating disorders from the "normal" cultural obsessions with weight and thinness are the amount of time and energy involved in the thinking and behaviors associated with an eating disorder and the degree to which it interferes with social functioning.

Anorexia Nervosa

Individuals with anorexia are below 85% of the normal weight for their height that cannot be attributed to a medical condition. It can also be determined by a body mass index equal or below 17.5 kg/m^2 (APA, 2000). Individuals with anorexia do not believe they need to gain weight and have an intense fear of becoming fat even though they are underweight. This fear is not relieved if additional weight is lost. More often weight loss is accomplished through a reduction in total food intake. Over time there is often the pattern of excluding high-caloric foods, leading to a diet that is limited to very few foods.

While the restricting pattern is more common in anorexia, binge–purge behavior may also exist. Although purging may follow a binge episode, purging may also be used even after the consumption of small amounts of food. A significant physical finding in anorexia is an irregular menstrual cycle or amenorrhea. Questions used to screen for anorexia are listed in Box 16-16.

Box 16-16
Questions to Ask When Screening for Anorexia

1. "Do you think that your current weight is normal or excessive?"
2. "Do you think that any part of your body is still too fat?"
3. "Do you have concern or fear about gaining weight even though you are underweight?"

Bulimia Nervosa

Individuals with bulimia are usually within the normal range for weight. The essential features of bulimia nervosa are binge eating and the use of inappropriate compensatory methods to prevent weight gain, such as vomiting or purging. Binge eating is defined as the consumption of a large amount of food a "discrete period of time" (APA, 2000). High-calorie foods are often the ones that are consumed, and binging is associated with the abnormally large amounts of food consumed rather than a relationship to a craving for a specific type of food, such as carbohydrate. A feature of bulimia is an inability to control binges. Individuals with bulimia have a high degree of dissatisfaction with appearance and often, a low self-esteem.

Physical findings may be a noticeable loss of dental enamel on the lingual surfaces of the front teeth as a result of recurrent vomiting. Teeth may become chipped and there may also be an increase in dental cavities. The parotid glands may also be enlarged. Calluses or scars may be noted on the dorsal surface of the hand from inducing vomiting. If the dominant hand is used, calluses or scars may be evident on only that hand. There may be electrolyte imbalances—frequently hypokalemia, hyponatremia, and hypochloremia. Assessment for bulimia nervosa would include the questions listed in Box 16-17.

Eating Disorder not Otherwise Specified

Many individuals present behaviors consistent with some of the features of anorexia and bulimia but do not meet the full criteria for either. In such situations there may be the thinking patterns common to anorexia, such as an extreme fear of gaining weight or a obsessive need to control amount of food or types of foods eaten; however, the individual is not below the 85% mark for weight and may not experience irregular menses or amenorrhea. Individuals may also present with features of bulimia but not fully meet the criteria, such as binge eating and the use of compensatory mechanisms less than twice a week. Other abnormal patterns may include occasions of self-induced vomiting not related to binge eating or a pattern of chewing and spitting out food, not swallowing large amounts of food (APA, 2000). Because there may be no physical indicators associated with these patterns, asking directed questions about eating, weight, and body image is key.

Binge-Eating Disorder

An eating disorder in development is Binge-Eating Disorder. The essential features include recurrent episodes of binge eating with an absence of purging behaviors. There is impaired

---

Box 16-17

Questions to Ask When Screening for Bulimia

1. "In the past 3 months, were there times when you ate very large amounts of food, more than most people would eat, within a short period of time (2 hours)?"
2. "Has this occurred at least twice a week over the last 3 months?"
3. "Did you feel as if you could not stop eating or control what or how much you were eating?"
4. "Have you used any of the following methods to prevent weight gain?"
   a. Purging: self-induced vomiting, laxatives, diuretics, enemas, and other medications
   b. Nonpurging: fasting or excessive exercise

control related to the amount of food consumed and the rate of consumption. It includes the following features: eating is often done alone, eating is not associated with being hungry, it is done to the point of feeling uncomfortably full, and there are feelings of disgust and guilt after overeating. Individuals do present as overweight with marked distress during and after the binge episodes. To meet the criteria for binge-eating disorder, binges average 2 days a week for a period of at least 6 months.

Thought Disorders

Thought disorders are evaluated as they relate to 1) content of thought, 2) form of thought, and 3) perception. In psychiatry, thought disorders are commonly associated with schizophrenia and psychosis. However, the severity and the range of symptoms can vary significantly and often do not result from a primary psychiatric illness. Medical conditions, medications, and medical mimics often present with a clinical picture of a thought disorder.

Assessment of the *content of thought* relates to the client's ability to form an accurate assessment of reality. Major difficulties in this area may include delusions, which involve false beliefs that are held to be true despite proof that they are false or irrational. Examples of delusional thinking include delusions of persecution or of grandeur, somatic delusions, paranoia, and magical thinking.

The second category, *form of thought*, is assessed by listening to how the client presents his or her ideas. Does the client present with looseness of associations? In such situations, the client is unaware that the topics are unconnected. When this is extreme, the practitioner may be unable to understand what the client is talking about. Other difficulties with form of thought include circumstantiality and tangentiality. Circumstantiality is the delay in presenting a point because of numerous unnecessary and tedious details. Tangentiality is the inability to get to the point owing to the introduction of unrelated topics. The degree of circumstantiality and tangentiality can vary significantly. For example, an anxious patient might shift from topic to topic with some awareness of doing so. This would not be considered a thought disorder problem. Serious thought disorder might include neologisms (invented words), word salad (a group of words put together randomly), and clang associations (choice of words based on rhyming).

The third category, *perception*, refers to hallucinations and illusions. Hallucinations are false sensory perceptions that are not associated with external stimuli and may involve any of the five senses. Illusions are misperceptions or misinterpretations of real external stimuli.

Psychotic Disorders

In schizophrenia, psychotic features are evident with two or more of the following characteristics: delusions, hallucinations, disorganized speech, grossly disorganized or catatonic behavior, and negative symptoms. The last of these characteristics, negative symptoms, refers to affective flattening, poverty of speech, avolition, anhedonia, and social isolation. In cases in which the presentation of one of these characteristics is considered very bizarre, only one is needed for a diagnosis of psychosis. Schizophrenia subtypes include Paranoid, Disorganized, Catatonic, Undifferentiated, and Residual. Differential diagnoses include Schizophreniform Disorder, characterized by schizophrenic symptoms of 1–6 months; Schizoaffective Disorder, characterized by a prominent mood component coexisting with the schizophrenic symptoms; Delusional Disorder, characterized by at least 1 month of no bizarre delusions without an active phase of symptoms of schizophrenia; Brief Psychotic Disorder, characterized by symptoms that last more than 1 day but remit by 1 month; Substance-Induced Psychotic Disorder, characterized by symptoms directly related to an abused substance, toxin, or medication; Psychotic Disorder (NOS), characterized by psychotic presentations that do not meet the criteria for any specific psychotic disorder or in situations when inadequate or contradictory information exists; and Psychotic Disorder Due to a General Medical Condition (APA, 2000).

The assessment of psychotic disorders can be guided by the following questions. The patient should also be asked to give an example of each question answered yes to determine the distortion of perception and thought and whether they can be considered "bizarre." In addition, check for evidence of thoughts that are based in reality. For example, if you ask, "Have you ever believed people are out to get you or have been spying on you?" and if, in reality, the person was actually being stalked, it would not be a case of delusional thinking. Delusions are considered "bizarre" when they are absurd, implausible, not understandable, and clearly do not relate to ordinary life experiences (Sheehan et al., 2001). Hallucinations are considered bizarre if a voice comments about the person's thoughts and behaviors or when there are two or more voices conversing with each other (Sheehan et al., 2001).

Box 16-18 lists several questions helpful in assessing for the presence of psychotic disorder. As the questions are answered, consider whether there are signs of schizophrenia, such as disorganized speech, affective flattening, alogia (poverty of speech), or avolition (lack of goal-directed behavior).

Psychotic Disorders Due to General Medical Conditions and Substance-Induced Psychotic Disorder

The nature of hallucinations varies. Understanding the differences may help in determining whether the psychosis has medical origins, is in response to substance abuse, or is psychiatric in nature. A true visual hallucination is a perceptual image that arises from an open space and is not being triggered by an environmental stimulus. Illusions on the other hand are images that are triggered by an actual object or stimulus.

Although it is difficult to present an absolute differentiation of psychosis from schizophrenia or bipolar disorder verses psychosis originating from a general medical process, there are some common categories (Shea, 1998) (see Boxes 16-19 and 16-20). Visual hal-

---

Box 16-18

Diagnostic Questions for Psychotic Disorders

1. "Have you ever believed people are out to get you or have been spying on you?" If yes: "Do you currently believe this?" Example
2. "Have you ever thought that someone could read your mind or that you could read someone's mind?" If yes: "Do you currently believe this?" Example
3. "Have you ever believed that a force outside of you had control over your thoughts or actions?" If yes: "Do you currently believe this?" Example
4. "Have you ever believed you were being sent messages through the TV, radio, or newspaper?" If yes: "Do you currently believe this?" Example
5. "Have you ever heard voices that others around you could not hear?" If yes: "Do you currently hear these?" Example

---

Box 16-19

Common Causes of Delirium

Metabolic

1. Hypoxia, hypercarbia, anemia
2. Electrolyte imbalance, hyperosmolarity
3. Hyperglycemia or hypoglycemia
4. Abnormal levels of magnesium or calcium
5. End-stage liver or kidney disease
6. Vitamin B$_1$ deficiency (Wernicke's encephalopathy secondary to a thiamine deficiency)
7. Endocrine disorders (hyperthyroidism or hypothyroidism, hyperparathyroidism, and adrenal disorders)

Infections

1. Systemic (e.g., pneumonia, septicemia, malaria, and typhoid)
2. Intercranial (e.g., meningitis, encephalitis)

Neurological Disorders

1. Hypertensive crisis, stroke, subarachnoid hemorrhage, vasculitis
2. Seizures
3. Trauma

Drug Withdrawal

1. Alcohol hallucinosis, rum fits, delirium tremens
2. Other withdrawal states (e.g., from barbiturates, as well as acute intoxication with street drugs)

Intoxication

From such agents as digoxin, levodopa, anticholinergics, and street drugs

Postoperative Sequelae

Especially following cardiac surgery

Adapted from Shea, 1998.

---

lucinations in patients whose psychosis is related to delirium differs from the classic psychosis in the following features: 1) more often occurs at night, 2) frequently perceived as moving, 3) briefer in duration, and 4) has no personal significance to the patient. A patient with delirium may see a snake, whereas a patient with schizophrenia may hallucinate about a deceased relative. Asking the client to state the time of day or night when he or she sees the hallucination helps in the differentiation. In medical conditions, hallucinations are often seen at night and when the patient closes his or her eyes. In schizophrenia, visual hallucinations are usually present with auditory hallucinations and occur in an otherwise normal appearing environment and appear somewhat suddenly, as depicted in the movie *A Beautiful Mind*. In a drug-induced psychosis, the environment appears distorted with numerous illusions and hallucinations. With delirium tremens, hallucinations may be pleasant in nature. The term Lilliputian hallucinations are so called because they refer to hallucinations that take the form of little people.

Box 16-20

Organic Causes of Psychosis

Tumors and (Space-Occupying Lesions of the CNS)

Brain abscess (bacterial, fungal, tuberculosis, cysticercosis)
Metastatic carcinoma
Primary cerebral tumors
Subdural hematoma

Cerebral Hypoxia

Anemia
Lowered cardiac output
Pulmonary insufficiency
Toxic (e.g., carbon monoxide)

Neurologic Disorders

Alzheimer's disease
Distant effects of carcinoma
Huntington's chorea
Normal pressure hydrocephalus
Temporal lobe epilepsy
Wilson's disease

Vascular Disorders

Aneurysms
Collagen vascular disease
Hypertensive encephalopathy
Intracranial hemorrhage
Lacunar state

Infections

Brain abscess
Encephalitis and postencephalitic states
Malaria
Meningitis (bacterial, fungal, tubercular)
Subacute bacterial endocarditis
Syphilis
Toxoplasmosis
Typhoid

Metabolic and Endocrine Disorders

Adrenal disease (Addison's and Cushing's diseases)
Calcium-related disorders
Diabetes mellitus
Electrolyte imbalance
Hepatic failure
Homocystinuria
Hypoglycemia and Hyperglycemia
Pituitary insufficiency
Porphyria
Thyroid disease (thyrotoxicosis and myxedema)
Uremia

(Continued on following page)

Box 16-20 *(Continued)*

Nutritional Deficiency

B_{12}
Niacin (pellagra)
Thiamine (Wernicke-Korsakoff syndrome)

Drugs, Medications, and Toxic Substances

Alcohol (intoxication and withdrawal)
Amphetamines
Analgesics (e.g., pentazocine [Talwin], meperidine [Demerol])
Anticholinergic agents
Antiparkinsonian agents
Barbiturates and other sedative-hypnotic agents (intoxication and withdrawal)
Bromides and other heavy metals
Carbon disulfide
Cocaine
Corticosteroids
Cycloserine (Seromycin)
Digitoxin (Crystodigin)
Disulfiram (Antabuse)
Hallucinogens
Isoniazid
L-Dopa (e.g., Larodopa)
Marijuana
Propranolol
Reserpine (Serpasil and others)

Adapted from Shea, 1998.

Substance abuse can produce psychotic episodes. Among the list of common agents are "speed," lysergic acid diethylamide (LSD), hallucinogens, marijuana, cocaine, crack, and phencyclidine (PCP). From a behavioral perspective, psychotic symptoms tend to be very bizarre and can be violent. On physical exam, nystagmus and hypertension may be present. Unlike schizophrenia, drug-induced psychosis usually presents with rapid-onset psychotic symptoms. In addition to street drugs or commonly abused drugs, anticholinergic agents can precipitate delirium, especially in elderly patients. Anticholinergic medications can cause a patient to present with hyperthermia, blurred vision, dry skin, facial flushing, and delirium. The mnemonic "hot as a pepper, blind as a bat, dry as a bone, red as a beet, and mad as a hatter" can be used to describe this toxic state (Shea, 1998). It is important to note that anticholinergic syndrome may be incomplete or hidden by other medications, such as opiates, and not present as a classic anticholinergic syndrome.

ISSUES RELATED TO OLDER ADULTS

The presence of coexisting medical conditions makes accurate psychiatric diagnosis and treatment a complex matter. History-taking and the mental status examination of older adults is similar to those for younger patients, but cognitive impairments make verification from a family member an important difference.

Psychiatric history includes identification (name, sex, marital status), chief complaint, history of present illness, history of previous illnesses, personal and family history, and current medication review. Past history can provide invaluable information in regards to personality organization, coping styles, and defense mechanisms during times of stresses. Family history includes adaptation to old age and the presence of Alzheimer's if known.

Mental disorders of old age include depressive disorders, cognitive disorders, phobias, and substance abuse, particularly alcohol. Psychosocial risk factors that predispose older adults to mental illness include social isolation and the loss of friends, social roles, autonomy, and health.

Other common conditions related to this age group are vertigo, syncope, hearing loss, elder abuse, spousal bereavement, and sleep disorders. The very real possibility for psychiatric symptoms related to either a response to medications or a medical condition is an important concept with elderly patients.

References

APA. (2000). *Diagnostic and Statistical Manual of Mental Disorder* (4th ed.). Text Revision. (*DSM IV-TR*). Washington, DC: American Psychiatric Association.

Greenberg, P.E., Sisitsky, T., Kessler, R.C., Finkelstein, S.N., Berndt, E.R., Davidson, J.R., Ballenger, J.C., & Fyer, A.J. (1999). The economic burden of anxiety disorders in the 1990's. *Journal of Clinical Psychiatry*, 60 (7), 427–435.

Hedeya, R.J. (1996). *Understanding Biological Psychiatry.* New York: W.W. Norton.

Schwitzer, A., Rodriguez, L.E., Thomas, C., & Silimi, L. (2001). The eating disorder NOS diagnostic profile among college women. *Journal of American College Health*, 49, 157–166.

Shea, S.C. (1998). *Psychiatric Interviewing, The Art of Understanding* (2nd ed.) Philadelphia: W.B. Saunders Co.

Sheehan, D.V., Janavs, J., Baker, R., Harnett-Sheehan, K., Knapp, E., & Sheehan, M. (2001). *Mini International Neuropsychiatric Interview*. [Unpublished manuscript].

Stahl, S.M. (2000). *Essential Psychopharmacology* (2ed.) New York: Cambridge University Press.

Stashwick, C. (1996). When you suspect an eating disorder, *Contemporary Pediatrics*, 13, 124.

Stern, T.A., Herman, J.B. (2000). Psychiatry: Update and Board Preparation. New York: McGraw-Hill, 2000.

 SUGGESTED READINGS

First, M., Allen, F., & Pincus, H. (1995) *Handbook of Differential Diagnosis.* Washington D.C: American Psychiatric Press.

Hollander, E. (1999). Anxiety Disturbances. In Hales, R.E., Yudofsky, S.C., & Talbott, J.A. (Eds.). *The American Psychiatric Press Textbook of Psychiatry.* Washington, DC: American Psychiatric Press.

Kessler, R.C. *National Comorbidity Survey, 1990–1992.* [Computer file]. Conducted by University of Michigan, Survey Research Center. 2nd ICPSR ed. Ann Arbor, MI: Inter-University Consortium for Political and Social Research 2002.

Othmer, E., & Othmer, S. (1994). *The Clinical Interview.* Vol. II, Washington, DC: American Psychiatric Press.

Robins, L.N., & Regier, D.A. (Eds.). (1991). *Psychiatric Disorders in America: The Epidemiologic Catchment Area Study.* New York: The Free Press.

PART 3

Assessments and **Differential Diagnosis** with **Special Patient Populations**

Chapter 17
Pediatric Patients

COMMUNICATING WITH INFANTS AND CHILDREN DURING THE PEDIATRIC ASSESSMENT

When assessing infants and children, it is crucial to remember that they are not merely "little adults." Obviously, infants and children have varying communication abilities and interaction skills. Pediatric assessments are more successful when providers take the time to communicate with children in an age-appropriate manner.

Infants

Infants are in the midst of the developmental stage of trust and mistrust, so should be approached slowly. Be prepared for stranger anxiety in an infant of 6–7 months and for separation anxiety in an infant just slightly older. Owing to these normal fears, it is best to conduct most, or all, of your exam with the infant on the parent's lap. During the assessment, integrate use of distraction techniques, such as singing or making funny faces, and/or allow the child to hold onto a familiar security item if present. Rather than a head-to-toe approach, plan your exam in order from noninvasive to invasive, e.g., auscultate the heart and lung sounds first and examine the ears and throat last. Remember to talk in a soothing voice and to avoid sudden movements.

Toddlers

Toddlers are at the height of negativism and are developmentally struggling for independence. They still have fears of parental separation, and they also fear any intrusion to their bodies. Their attention spans are short and they can be strong-willed and uncooperative, especially when tired or ill. Allow toddlers to touch or hold some of your equipment before you begin the physical exam. Demonstrate what you're going to do on a doll or animal or parent before doing it on the child. Use distraction as much as possible and give the child choices when they exist, such as: "Which ear should I look in first?"

Sara F. Barber

Be direct but friendly—tell the child what you are going to do instead of asking permission. At this age, continue to conduct as much of the exam as you can with the child on a parent's lap, working from noninvasive to invasive procedures.

Preschoolers

Preschoolers are magical thinkers and may have fears of pain and body mutilation. They believe that everything is "alive" and may fear unknown equipment or procedures. Involve the child in the exam by describing what you are doing and letting him practice on a doll or stuffed animal first. Move slowly and systematically and explain in simple terms what you're doing. Choose your words carefully as preschoolers are very literal. Allow choices when possible and praise the child frequently for helping and cooperating. A head-to-toe sequence may be possible at this age.

School-Age Children

School-age children generally want to be brave and cooperate—although they still fear pain and the loss of control. They often ask lots of questions and are curious about using your equipment. Allow them to do examine the equipment, and provide concrete answers to their questions, whenever possible, as children at this age become very logical. Teach them the proper names for equipment and body parts. Modesty may begin to appear in this age so be sensitive to this. A head-to-toe sequence is possible for this age.

Adolescents

Adolescents are at the height of trying to fit in and be "normal." They worry about how they stack alongside their peers and may have concerns about their physical appearance, including their height, weight, or the presence of acne. They are striving to be independent and fear the loss of control and possibly even death. Privacy is very important at this age, so plan on examining the child without the parent unless the child prefers it otherwise. Remember to keep body parts covered when you're not examining them. Explain each step of your exam and give the child a chance to ask questions or make choices as you progress. Be very nonjudgmental and talk professionally but casually with them. Teach adolescents about their bodies and stress the normalcy of their features and appearance. Reassure them that others their age feel the same way and try to initiate discussion of sensitive subjects by utilizing this fact, e.g., "Lots of kids your age are faced with tough decisions like whether to try drugs and alcohol. Have you been faced with any situations like that?" Teach self-breast and testicular exams. Give concrete information on sexually transmitted diseases, safe sex, and HIV. Give them an opportunity to ask questions.

PEDIATRIC HISTORY AND PHYSICAL EXAMINATION

Much of the content of earlier chapters regarding the assessment of specific systems is relevant to the pediatric assessment. However, the assessment of infants and children should be based on a knowledge of the anticipated problems of childhood, developmental stages, and the potential risks. The following section summarizes specific questions or examinations that should be considered during pediatric assessment, along with the potential findings that should be considered as "red flags," warranting further assessment or consultation.

Red Flags for the Head Examination

- No growth in head circumference between well visits
- Enlarged head size or excessive growth between well visits

Common Diagnoses for the Head

- Headache
- Head Trauma
- Plagiocephaly

Head

When assessing pediatric patients, remember to ask about head trauma, head growth, and the history of headaches. The head circumference should be measured at all well visits up to 2 years of age, to assess for macro- or microcephaly. Assess the head symmetry and look for plagiocephaly. To accurately assess fontanels, the child should be sitting upright and not crying. Some variants that might be noted in newborns include the following.

- Caput succedaneum—seen at birth, usually following a traumatic vaginal delivery or vacuum-assisted delivery; edema of the soft tissue of the scalp that usually crosses the suture lines; no specific treatment; should resolve in a few days.
- Cephalohematoma—often appears several hours after birth and may increase for the first 24 hours; subperiosteal collection of blood that does not cross the suture lines; may take weeks to months to resolve; watch for hyperbilirubinemia.

Eyes

Ask about vision problems and/or history of eye drainage. The vision portion of the growth and development section of this chapter (see pp. 443-444) provides details on specific vision and screening for children of various ages. Some variations that may be noted in newborns include the presence of "stork bites" (telangiectatic nevi), on the eyelids, nasolabial area, or nape of the neck. Which appear as a purplish-red color and generally diminish and/or disappear by 12 months of age.

Red Flags for the Eye Examination

- Presence of white instead of red reflex may indicate retinoblastoma; an absent red reflex or opacity of the lens may indicate cataracts.
- Dilated and fixed pupils indicate severe brain damage.
- Strabismus requires referral to ophthalmology for further evaluation.

Common Diagnoses for the Eye

- Conjunctivitis
- Allergies
- Corneal abrasion
- Lacrimal duct stenosis
- Strabismus

Ears

Ask about hearing ability and/or difficulties, ear pain, and ear drainage. The general appearance and placement of the ears is important in pediatric assessment. Ears that are set low may indicate genitourinary or chromosomal abnormalities, or a multisystem syndrome such as Turner syndrome; assess for preauricular sinuses.

The otoscopic exam is described in detail in Chapter 5. The otoscopic exam should be saved for last in infants and young children because of the distress it often causes. To examine the inner ear in an infant or young child, pull the pinna down and out. For examination in an older child, pull up and back as you would with an adult. As with adults, the tympanic membranes (TM) should be mobile and intact, and should appear thin, smooth, and pearly gray, with bright light reflexes. The mobility of the TM should be assessed by pneumatic otoscopy if a diagnosis of acute otitis media is expected. Although crying will cause erythema of the TMs, the light reflexes and mobility should remain intact. Diagnosis of acute otitis media should not be based solely on a reddened TM. Also observe for bubbles or an obvious fluid level line behind the TM, which indicates middle ear effusion.

A young child who frequently asks for things to be repeated, seems markedly inattentive, and responds inappropriately to questions should be investigated for hearing deficit. Middle ear effusions and acute OM may cause hearing deficits. The Hearing portion of the growth and development section of this chapter (see pp. 442-443) provides details on hearing screening.

Nose and Sinuses

Ask about nasal drainage, nosebleeds, and breathing interference. Note the characteristics of any drainage. Clear, watery drainage may indicate allergies, especially when coupled with pale, boggy mucosa. Persistent, copious, or purulent drainage may indicate sinusitis.

Red Flags for the Ear Examination

- Pain over the mastoid process, which may indicate mastoiditis
- Foreign bodies, which should be considered if the child complains of strange sounds or sensations in one ear or if there is an obvious blockage or odd color noted on otoscopic exam
- Hearing deficit

Common Diagnoses for the Ear

- Acute otitis media
- Middle ear effusions
- Otitis externa
- Wax impaction
- Foreign body

Unilateral, purulent drainage is seen with foreign bodies. Bloody discharge indicates irritation that may be caused by a foreign body, infection, or excessive nose picking.

Newborns frequently have nasal congestion without other symptoms of illness ("newborn congestion"); this should resolve after 2–3 months. Newborns are obligate nose breathers.

Mouth and Throat

Ask children and/or parents about throat pain, difficulty swallowing, tooth eruption, dental trauma, and brushing habits. Table 17-13 in the growth and development section identifies the typical age of tooth eruption (see p. 449).

Lungs

Ask about breathing patterns, blue spells or apnea, and cough. Children under age 7 are diaphragmatic (abdominal) breathers—this is particularly pronounced in infancy; after age 7, children become more thoracic breathers. Observe the general work of breathing, noting any use of accessory muscles, nasal flaring, and retractions. Breath sounds are heard best by having the child breathe through the mouth. Asking the child to pretend may help with breath sound auscultation; for example, to hear inspiratory sounds, have the child pretend to hold his or her breath as if preparing to go under water . Alternatively, have a child actually blow bubbles, pretend to blow bubbles, or inflate a balloon as you listen to both inspiratory and expiratory sounds.

Red Flags for the Nose and Sinus Examination

- Reports of apnea should be investigated fully and may require hospitalization for monitoring.
- Foreign bodies should be removed as soon as possible, and referral to a specialist should be considered if removal in the office is impossible.

Common Diagnoses for the Nose and Sinuses

- Upper respiratory infection
- Allergic rhinitis
- Foreign body
- Sinusitis

Red Flags for the Mouth and Throat Examination

- An absent suck in a newborn, an obvious communication between the nose and mouth, and/or a bifid uvula should be investigated for cleft palate.
- A unilateral enlarged tonsil should be further evaluated to rule out abscess or lymphoma.

Common Diagnoses for the Mouth and Throat

- Stomatitis
- Oral candidiasis
- Viral pharyngitis/tonsillitis
- Strep pharyngitis
- Dental caries

Heart

Ask about a history of heart murmur, cyanosis, activity intolerance, or syncope. Measure vital signs with blood pressure measurement beginning at age 3. Always assess pulse for rate and rhythm; an apical pulse should be determined in infants.

A common variation of heart rhythm is sinus arrhythmia, in which the heart rate increases with inspiration and decreases with expiration. This fluctuation in rhythm will

Red Flags for the Lung Examination

- Any abnormal breath sounds should be evaluated further with pulse oximeter monitoring and possibly a chest x-ray.
- Cough in the middle of the night or with exertion may indicate asthma, even in a child that does not wheeze.

Common Diagnoses for the Lung

- Asthma
- Upper respiratory infection
- Croup
- Pneumonia
- Bronchitis
- Bronchiolitis
- GERD (may be a cause of cough although not an obvious lung problem)
- Allergies
- Sinusitis

Box 17-1

Characteristics Common to Innocent Murmurs

- Soft, ≤Grade III
- Systolic timing
- Short duration
- Low pitched, vibratory, musical
- Rarely transmitted
- Loudest in left lower sternal border or at 2nd/3rd intercostal space
- Loudest when lying down, during expiration, and/or after exercise
- Sound diminishes with position change from recumbent to sitting
- Intensity and presence may vary over time
- Child has normal growth and development, blood pressure, respiratory rate, and pulses
- No associated thrill or cyanosis

cease if the child is instructed to hold his breath. Assess carefully for murmurs. Up to one half of all children have an innocent (functional) murmur. Box 17-1 includes characteristics that are common to innocent murmurs in general. Table 17-1 identifies characteristics of select innocent murmurs.

In newborns, innocent murmurs are common and are usually systolic, grade I or II, and are not associated with other symptoms. The transition period from fetal to maternal conditions may take 48 hours. Patent ductus arteriosus is a fetal vascular connection that directs blood from the pulmonary artery to the aorta. It typically closes by day 4 following birth. However, if it remains patent, the direction of blood flow is reversed through the ductus owing to the higher pressure in the aorta. Clinical findings in a newborn with a still-patent ductus arteriosus include diaphoresis (especially during feedings) and poor feedings with easy tiring that may result in failure to thrive. Immediately postnatally, the associated murmur is soft and systolic, heard along the left lower sternal border. Soon thereafter, the sound is described as a harsh, rumbling, continuous murmur heard in the left infraclavicular and pulmonic areas. When patent ductus arteriosus is suspected, evaluation by a pediatric cardiologist is essential.

Table 17-1. ■ Types of Innocent Murmurs

Type of Murmur	Characteristics
Still's murmur	Most common; heard most frequently from 3 to 7 years of age; described as vibratory or musical; heard best between lower left sternal border and apex with child supine; probably caused by turbulence in left ventricular outflow tract.
Basal systolic ejection murmur	High-pitched, blowing sounds heard best at the pulmonic area with child supine.
Physiologic peripheral pulmonic stenosis (pulmonary outflow murmur)	Short, systolic; heard best in the axillae and back; usually disappears during infancy.
Venous hum	Humming, continuous murmur; heard best in the supraclavicular areas with the child sitting; can be diminished by having the child lie down, turning the head, or occluding the jugular vessels.

Red Flags for the Heart Examination

- Pathological murmur
- Unequal or absent pulses
- Cyanosis

Common Diagnoses for the Heart

- Innocent murmur

Breasts

Ask about tenderness, nipple discharge, and masses. Asymmetric breast development is normal in an adolescent female. Gynecomastia may be normal in males during puberty. It usually occurs during Tanner Stages II and III and may last up to 2 years. Gynecomastia typically presents as a small, tender, oval mass directly under the areola that may measure up to 2–3 cm. If imaging of adolescent breast tissue is desired, an ultrasound should be chosen over mammogram because of the dense nature of adolescent breast tissue.

Abdomen

Ask about diarrhea, constipation, bowel habits, reflux or spitting up, and stomachaches. A potbellied look is common in early childhood owing to poorly developed muscles. Bowel sounds should be assessed. The liver edge may be palpable 1–2 cm below the right costal margin with deep inspiration and the spleen tip may be palpable 1–2 cm below the left costal margin with deep inspiration. Constipation may cause a palpable fecal mass in the lower left quadrant, and a rectal exam may be indicated if constipation is suspected. To aid in the abdominal assessment of a ticklish child, have the child lie with knees bent or use

Red Flags for the Breast Examination

- Firm, unmovable masses
- Galactorrhea—may indicate hypothyroidism or pituitary tumor

Common Diagnoses for the Breast

- Normal breast bud
- Gynecomastia

Red Flags for the Abdominal Examination

- Failure to pass first meconium stool in first 24 hours of life
- Projectile vomiting
- Blood in stool or emesis
- Chronic diarrhea or constipation
- Severe abdominal pain or guarding
- Abdominal mass

Common Diagnoses for the Abdomen

- Abdominal pain, unknown etiology (possibly related to stress or anxiety)
- Gastroenteritis
- Pyloric stenosis
- Constipation
- Lactose intolerance
- Gas
- GERD

the child's smaller hand under your own to palpate the belly. It is also helpful to engage the child in conversation to provide distraction from what you're doing.

Genitourinary System

Ask about voiding patterns (number of wet diapers in infants, frequency of urination in older children), pain, discharge, and menstrual cycle if applicable. A clean-catch urine sample should be obtained for urinalysis at all well check-ups beginning at age 3, with further testing warranted with abnormal findings.

Female Genitalia

Enlarged labia or mild vaginal bleeding in a female newborn are considered a normal response to maternal hormones. Observe for labial adhesions, which occur mostly in girls 3 months to 6 years of age. No treatment is needed as long as urine and vaginal secretions are not obstructed. Observe the presence and distribution of pubic hair.

Male Genitalia

Observe the location of the urethral meatus. Hypospadias is a congenital defect that causes the meatus to be on the ventral surface of the penis and epispadias results in dorsal placement of the meatus. Palpate the scrotum for the presence of testes; cryptorchidism is the term for an undescended testicle. If the testes are not immediately palpable in the scrotum, but can be "milked" down into the scrotum, consider them descended. If one or both testes are undescended at 1 year of age, referral to a specialist is indicated. Male newborns frequently have an enlarged scrotum as a normal finding.

Red Flags for the Genitourinary System

- Ambiguous genitalia
- Premature puberty
- Hypospadias

Common Diagnoses for the Genitourinary System

- Urinary tract infection
- Enuresis (most common is primary nocturnal enuresis—a child who has never stayed dry through the night)
- Labial adhesion
- Yeast dermatitis
- Diaper dermatitis
- Vaginitis
- Balanitis
- Retractile testes

Musculoskeletal System

Ask about pain or limited movement, joint pain, and history of fractures. Although a comprehensive musculoskeletal assessment should be performed, an emphasis should be placed on specific joints.

Hips

Assessment for hip dislocation is extremely important in all infants and children under 2. Hip dislocation is most common in females and in infants delivered in a breech position (including by Cesarean section). It is more prevalent in whites, Eskimos, and Navajos. There are a variety of specialized maneuvers useful in assessment for hip dislocation. Table 17-2 differentiates between the Barlow's, Ortolani's, and Galeazzi maneuvers.

Although not considered definitively diagnostic of a dislocated hip, the thighs, inguinal area, and gluteal area should be assessed for asymmetric skin folds as potential indications of dislocation. When assessing for hip dislocation or dysplasia, it is essential to differentiate between normal "clicks" and the worrisome "clunk." Normal clicks may be felt when doing some hip manipulation as a result of laxity and movement of ligaments. A definitive clunk is felt when a bone (the femur) actually comes out of its socket. Even though doing these maneuvers is extremely important, it is also important to remember that, as the infant ages, limited abduction becomes an increasingly definitive sign of hip dysplasia. Limited abduction (less than 60%) is also the key sign to look for in bilateral dislocation. If hip dislocation or dysplasia is suspected, radiographic studies are usually done. In an infant under 3 months of age, ultrasound is the usual choice, although this method can still give unreliable results owing to the fact that much of the hip joint is cartilaginous. After 3 months of age, the preferred method of radiologic evaluation is anteroposterior and frog lateral x-rays.

Table 17-2. ■ Special Maneuvers

Barlow's Maneuver

Dislocates a dislocatable hip posteriorly. To do the maneuver: with the infant supine, flex the hip, adduct the thigh, and feel for a palpable dislocation. As the thigh is adducted, the femoral head drops (or can be gently pushed) out of the acetabulum. Do the maneuver gently on an infant who is not crying.

Ortolani's Maneuver

Reduces a posteriorly dislocated hip. To do the maneuver: with the infant supine, place fingers posteriorly over the greater trochanter, flex the hip 90 degrees, abduct the thigh while pushing up with the fingers. Feel for a clunk and palpable jerk as the femur is relocated. Do the maneuver gently on an infant who is not crying.

Galeazzi's Maneuver

Assesses knee height for equality. To do the maneuver: with the infant supine, flex the hips and knees and place the soles of the child's feet on the table near the buttocks. Observe the knees for equal height. The sign is considered positive if the knee heights are unequal. A dislocatable hip will fall out of socket in this position and will cause the knee on the affected side to appear lower.

From American Family Physician website:
www.aafp.org/afp/20000215/1011.html.

Gait

Observe a child's gait during well exam. Toddlers commonly walk with a wide-based gait and a bowlegged (genu varum) appearance. A knock-kneed (genu valgum) appearance is common in preschoolers.

Back

Assessment for scoliosis (a lateral curvature of the spine) should be performed at each well visit starting at age 10. If abnormal findings are present, radiographs should be obtained for confirmation and to guide possible referral. Both the age of the child and the degree of the curve will guide treatment, if any. Scoliosis is more worrisome in a child who is prepubertal because there is more growth to occur and, therefore, more time for a curve to worsen.

Joints

Assess joints by palpating for pain, heat, or deformity. Active range of motion gives information about how muscles and bones are working together for functional movement. Assess active range of motion by engaging a child in games in the exam room. For example, have the child perform jumping jacks, clap, pretend to be a certain animal, and/or walk heel-to-toe on a line on the floor. Passive range of motion gives information about joint mobility and stability and the limits of tendons and muscles. Excessive range of motion may indicate an unstable joint. Assess passive range of motion by flexing and extending the joints through various movements with child relaxed or lying supine.

Elbow

A child's elbow commonly and easily gets dislocated (nursemaid's elbow or toddler's elbow). Dislocation is indicated by refusal to use an arm, especially when accompanied by crying and an appropriate history.

Red Flags for the Musculoskeletal Examination

- Refusal to bear weight or walk
- Refusal to use or bend an arm
- Heat, redness, and/or swelling of a joint(s)
- Hip clunks
- Toe walking—can be a normal phase, and also can be associated with cerebral palsy, tight heel cords, autism, or muscular dystrophy

---

Common Diagnoses for the Musculoskeletal System

- Trauma or injury
- Local sprain or strain
- Torticollis
- Tibial torsion
- Osgood-Schlatter
- Growing pains

Neurological System

Ask about episodes of seizure or loss of consciousness, tremors, or tics. A large part of the assessment of the neurological system in a child can be accomplished by observation during the visit. Watch for symmetry and quality of movement; observe gait, posture, coordination, balance, strength, and tone. Children are generally very active and by watching the way they climb on the exam table, hop around the room, and manipulate objects and toys, you can gain a lot of information. In a newborn or small infant, observe for symmetry of movements, muscle tone, and pitch of the cry. Test deep tendon reflexes. Assess newborn reflexes—absence or persistence past expected age of disappearance may indicate severe central nervous system (CNS) dysfunction and should be investigated fully. Table 17-3 details newborn reflexes.

The pediatric assessment should integrate cranial nerve evaluation. Table 17-4 describes the pediatric assessment of cranial nerves.

During the neurological assessment, assess for developmental milestones. Although children will develop at their own individual speed, any regression in developmental milestones is a major concern. The Denver II is a useful tool when evaluating developmental milestones. See information on developmental milestones elsewhere in this chapter.

Skin

Ask about birthmarks, lesions, and skin conditions. Common birthmarks are listed here.
- Stork bites—commonly appear on eyelids, nasolabial area, or nape of neck; usually disappear by 12 months.

Table 17-3. ■ Newborn Reflexes

	Age Appears	Age Disappears	How to Test	Response	Meaning
Rooting	Birth	3-4 months	With head midline, stroke perioral area	Infant should open mouth and turn head toward stimulated side	Absence indicates CNS disease or depression; sleepy infant may not respond
Sucking	Birth	3-4 months	Place nipple or finger 3-4 cm into mouth, may stroke roof of mouth	Infant should have strong suck	Absence indicates CNS depression; sleepy baby may not respond
Palmar Grasp	Birth	3-6 months	Place finger in infants palm and press gently	Infant should flex all fingers around examiner's finger	Grasp should be strong and symmetrical
Stepping	Birth	6-8 weeks	Hold infant in a standing position with feet against firm surface	Infant should "step" along, raising one foot at a time	Absence indicates paralysis or a depressed infant
Moro	Birth	4-5 months	Make a loud noise or allow infant's head to drop down slightly	Infant's arms should spread, fingers should extend and then flex, then arms should come together; may elicit a cry	Asymmetry may indicate paralysis or a fractured clavicle; absence indicates a brain stem problem

Table 17-4. ■ Pediatric Assessment of the Cranial Nerves

I, Olfactory	Occlude one nostril and offer odors for identification (not frequently tested in the office unless specific concern)
II, Optic	Test visual acuity, visual fields, and examine fundi; test blink reflex in an infant
III, Oculomotor	Test extraocular movements by having child follow a light or a toy in all visual fields, observe infants for tracking abilities; observe for asymmetry of eyelids; pupils should both constrict when light is shined in one eye
IV, Trochlear	Tested in the same way and at the same time as III
V, Trigeminal	For sensory, apply light touch and pressure to points across forehead cheeks and jaw; for motor, have child bite hard on tongue blade or observe an infant chewing on a teething toy
VI, Abducens	Tested in the same way and at the same time as III and IV
VII, Facial	For sensory, observe for eyes tearing, can offer samples for taste; for motor, have child imitate you smiling big, grimacing, puffing out cheeks, and raising eyebrows; observe for facial grimaces in an infant
VIII, Acoustic	Observe balance, do auditory testing as needed, question parents regarding hearing
IX, Glossopharyngeal	Elicit gag reflex or have child say "ah"; observe swallowing
X, Vagus	Tested along with IX
XI, Accessory	Have child shrug shoulders against pressure, turn head against resistance, stick tongue out
XII, Hypoglossal	Have child move tongue back and forth or push against a tongue blade; may just observe this behavior during exam of oropharynx in an infant

- Nevus flammeus (port-wine stain)—pinkish-red color, grows as the child grows.
- Strawberry nevus (raised hemangioma)—may not be present at birth; usually starts out as a grayish white area and later becomes red and raised; most resolve spontaneously by age 10.
- Mongolian spots—usually seen in newborns of African-American, Latin, or Asian descent; generally found in the sacral or gluteal region.

Red Flags for the Neurological Examination

- Absence, or persistence past the expected age, of newborn reflexes
- Spasticity or poor muscle tone
- Unresponsiveness or depressed level of consciousness
- Any loss or regression of developmental milestones
- Abnormal cranial nerve responses

Common Diagnoses for the Neurological System

- Cognitive delay
- Cerebral palsy

Assess all skin for color, texture, and turgor; check for any rashes, lesions, pruritus, or bruising. Observe for skin conditions that may indicate underlying pathology, such as depigmented nevi, café au lait spots, and hemangiomas on the scalp.

GROWTH AND DEVELOPMENT

The growth and development of a child is one of the most important things to consider when assessing and caring for pediatric patients. Parents are very interested in how their child is growing, both physically and developmentally, and assessments of these areas by trained professionals can help indicate possible problems and the need for referral or more intensive evaluation.

Physical Growth

The measurement of a child's weight and height is done at every well visit. If the child is not routinely seen for well visits, this must be incorporated into visits for specific complaints/illness. The head circumference is measured at every well visit from birth to 2 years of age. Each of these measurements is plotted on a growth chart. Other charts have been developed to measure a child's body mass index and/or plot a child's weight versus height. These charts allow for a visual representation that enables practitioners to watch how a child develops in each area over time. Although parents often become interested in what percentile their child "ranks in," providers should stress the importance of watching the growth curves to compare the child against her- or himself, not against others. For example, it is much more worrisome for a child's weight or head size to drop from the 75th to the 25th percentile than it is for a child to continuously grow along the 25th percentile curve. A child whose growth is at the extremes of the growth curves, but whose growth rate is normal and consistent, is likely to be very healthy.

Red Flags for the Skin Examination

- Any mole or lesion that is changing, that has irregular borders, or that is growing should be examined by a dermatologist.

Common Diagnoses for the Skin

- Viral exanthema
- Atopic dermatitis (eczema)
- Contact dermatitis
- Tinea
- Impetigo
- Cellulitis

Trends

The following trends are generalizations that can be used as rules of thumb in assessing pediatric growth and development. An average American newborn weighs around 7 pounds and is 20–21 inches long. The average head circumference of an American newborn is 13–14 inches, with a chest circumference of 2 cm less than that of the head. The head circumference generally increases by $1/2$ inch per month during the first 6 months of life and $1/4$ inch per month during the second 6 months.

Weight

An initial 10% loss of weight occurs in the first 3–4 days of life. This is typically regained by 2 weeks of age. Thereafter, a child's weight typically doubles around 4–6 months, triples at a year, and quadruples around age 2. During the first 6 months of life, a baby gains 5–8 ounces a week. Between 6 and 12 months, this decreases to 3–5 ounces a week. During the second year of life, a child gains 8–9 ounces a month. Toddlers and preschoolers gain $4^{1}/_{2}$ to $6^{1}/_{2}$ pounds a year. A school age child gains 5–6 pounds a year. During the pubertal growth spurt, an average American female gains 38 pounds, and an average male gains 42 pounds.

Length/Height

The length of a child typically increases by 50% at age 12 months, doubles around 4 years of age, and triples by 13 years. The average gain in length in infancy is 1 inch per month during the first 6 months, and then $1/2$ inch per month during the second 6 months. Toddlers, preschoolers, and school age children grow 2–3 inches per year. During the pubertal growth spurt, American girls grow an average of 8–9 inches and reach 95% of their mature height by the onset of menarche or the skeletal age of 13. Boys grow an average of $9^{1}/_{2}$ to 11 inches and reach 95% of their mature height by the skeletal age of 15.

Development by Age

The tables associated with this subsection illustrate age-by-age behaviors and skills that babies and children should develop. Because every child is different, it is impossible to say that these behaviors will occur in all children at the given age. Milestones occur along a wide spectrum, and patterns considered "normal" have wide parameters. The "whole picture" of the child must be taken into effect when comparing a child with a given standard. However, knowledge of the developmental milestones is essential when assessing infants and children. Behavioral observations and/or questions of parents can be used to determine the child's developmental progress.

Newborns/Infants

The term "newborn" is typically applied to babies from birth until 1 month of age. The period from 1 month to 12 months of age is referred to as infancy. The first 12 months of life represent the period of the most rapid change and maturation—both physically and emotionally. See Table 17-5 for infant developmental milestones.

Infant Developmental Red Flags

Because of the importance of early intervention in preventing and/or minimizing long-term consequences of sensory deficits, Table 17-6 is included to provide developmental red flags in infants. As always, there is some parameter for "normal," and the gestational age of the child at birth must certainly be taken into account. However, in terms of early inter-

◢ **Table 17-5.** ■ Newborn/Infant Development Milestones

Time Period	Sensory	Emotional/Behavioral	Motor	Language
Newborn to 1 Month	Sees best at 8-10 inches; cannot focus clearly; startles to loud noises	Cries a lot but responds positively to soft voice and being held	Jerky movements; grasps whatever is placed in hand; turns head	Has varying cries for different needs; may start making gurgling sounds
1-2 Months	May follow some objects with eyes (at least to midline); turns toward some sounds	May smile socially to caregiver; may quiet down in response to human face	Movements become more controlled; lifts chin for a few seconds while on tummy	Makes variety of cooing and gurgling sounds when content
2-4 Months	Focuses better, but no more than 12 inches; follows objects 180 degrees by turning head side to side; prefers bright objects	Crying decreases; displays more emotions	Movements are smoother; discovers hands; may lift chest slightly while prone; may bat at dangling objects	Smiles, gurgles, and coos—especially interactively
4-6 Months	Focuses clearly; fascinated by mirror image; turns purposefully in response to voice	Very active and playful; basks in attention; acknowledges breast or bottle excitedly	Rolls from side to side; holds up chest when prone; supports head well when held in sitting position; no head lag at 6 months	Laughs and giggles; imitates speech sounds
6-9 Months	Begins to recognize sound of own name; puts everything in mouth	May show sharp mood changes; strong attachment to mother; stranger anxiety	Rakes objects; transfers objects from hand to hand; begins to sit alone; crawling motions	Babbles and squeals; repeats sounds over and over; frequently uses syllables such as *ba, da, ka*
9-12 Months	Scrutinizes toys and objects; still puts everything in mouth	May cry when parent leaves; may resist diapering or other things he or she does not want to do; plays peek-a-boo	Refined pincer grasp; goes from sitting to lying; crawls well; may pull self to stand; cruises; may begin to walk	Imitates inflection of conversation; imitates speech sounds; says "mama" and "dada"; may say 2-3 other words; points to objects to indicate wants

vention and evaluation, it is much better to err on the side of caution and refer for further evaluation if any suspicions arise regarding the development of a child.

Toddlers

The period of toddlerhood lasts from the first birthday until the age of three. During this stage the child's rate of physical growth slows down, but the process of moving toward independence continues rapidly as toddlers acquire many new motor, cognitive, and psychosocial skills. Behavioral challenges frequently arise during this period owing to both the toddler's attempts to test limits and his or her own frustration at trying to communicate. See Table 17-7 for toddler developmental milestones.

Table 17-6. ■ Infant Developmental Red Flags

Age	Social/ Emotional	Cognitive/ Visual	Language/ Hearing	Fine Motor	Gross Motor
1 Month	Excessive irritability	Doll's eyes; questionable or no red light reflex; poor alert state	No startle to sound; no quieting to voice	Absent or asymmetrical palmar grasp	Asymmetric movements; increased or decreased tone; asymmetric primitive reflexes
4 Months	Lack of social smile; depressed/ withdrawn affect	No tracking; no ability to fixate on face or object	No turning to voice or sound; no cooing or squeals	No hand-to-mouth activity	Same as above; no attempt to raise head when prone
6 Months	No smiling or response to play	No looking at caregiver; no reaching for objects; no tracking	No babbling; no response to rattles, sounds, or loud noises	No grasping of objects; no holding hands together	No attempt to sit with support; head lag when pulled to a sit; persistence of primitive reflexes
9 Months	No eye contact or interactive play	No reaching for toys; no visual or oral investigation of toys	No response to name or voice; no single or double consonant sounds	No self-feeding; no solids; no picking up of toys with one hand	No sitting (including tripod sit); unequal movements or excessive one-handedness
12 Months	No response to games, books, or interactive play	No visual involvement in environment	No speech imitation	No attempt to self-feed or hold cup; no transfer of objects	No pulling self to stand; no exploring of environment

Table 17-7. ■ Toddler Development Milestones

Age	Cognitive	Emotional/Behavioral	Motor	Language
18 Months	Learns cause and effect; looks for hidden objects; recognizes pictures of familiar people and objects; points to a few body parts	Likes to feed self; likes water play; prefers adults to other children	Likes to throw, roll, push, and pull toys; walks unassisted with wide stance; stoops and recovers; imitates scribbling; makes tower of 3-4 cubes	Adds gestures to speech; likes to imitate activities and speech; uses 10–20 words; may start combining two words; understands "no"
2 Years	Cannot be reasoned with; can picture objects and events mentally; concrete thinking; identifies body parts; matches some colors	"Do-it-myself" stage; may resist bedtime; gets frustrated easily; may respond with "no" constantly; learns to hold up fingers to show age; tries to get adult attention	Runs and climbs; goes up and down stairs alone; scribbling turns into more controlled movements; turns pages one at a time; builds tower of eight cubes	Uses simple sentences; seems to understand most of what is said; increasing use of pronouns; learns songs/rhymes

Preschoolers

The period from age 3 to age 5 is known as the preschool stage of development. Children in this stage are usually very active, energetic, imaginative, inquisitive, and social. They also become increasingly independent with tasks such as self-care. They acquire more language skills and, as a result, can respond more verbally, which often decreases previous behavioral challenges. See Table 17-8 for preschooler developmental milestones.

School-Age Children

The school-age period of development begins with entry into school (around age 5) and lasts until adolescence. This is a period of extensive development. Children become more influenced by peers and groups outside the home, and they are expected to follow certain rules and adhere to some degree of structure in the school setting. Children often remain very imaginative as they learn new things. This is the period when a child develops a sense of self and self-worth, so accomplishment and confidence become important tasks. Refer to Table 17-9 for school-age developmental milestones.

Adolescents

The period of adolescence is the transition from childhood to adulthood. Typically beginning at age 12 or 13, adolescence is a time of change and new responsibilities. With the initiation of puberty, children experience a wide array of physical, emotional, and social changes. The peer group is of utmost importance to an adolescent, and many challenges and temptations arise during this time period. During middle and late adolescence, focus on the future becomes significant and teens gain a sense of morality as they prepare to enter the adult world. Table 17-10 lists adolescent developmental milestones.

Table 17-8. ■ Preschooler Development Milestones

Age	Cognitive	Emotional/Behavioral	Motor	Language
3 Years	Develops more stable sense of self; egocentric thinking; knows names of time components but doesn't understand sequencing; may identify some colors, letters, numbers	Learns to share and take turns; tests limits; seeks approval from adults; likes hearing stories over and over; likes imaginative and imitative play; increased curiosity about bodies	Tiptoes; rides a tricycle; kicks a ball; stands briefly on one foot; undresses self; copies a circle; can brush teeth (although not well)	Speaks about 1000 words; tells simple stories; asks lots of questions; responds to three-part commands; may have a stuttering phase; can consistently produce *m, n, p, f, h, b,* and *w* sounds
4 Years	Uses words to solve problems; begins to understand some concepts of time; knows difference between right and wrong; begins to discern real-life from make-believe; identifies shapes and colors	Has penchant for silliness; shows new fears, which shows awareness of new dangers; likes to help; imitates adults; shares grudgingly; enjoys group activities; fantasy play	Runs, skips, climbs, hops with better skill; uses scissors; dresses self; holds a pencil correctly; draws recognizable shapes; draws a person with 3 parts; catches a large ball	Tells stories; uses four- to five-word sentences; uses prepositions; asks "how" questions; starts using past and future tenses correctly; adds approximately 50 words a month to vocabulary

Table 17-9. ■ School-Age Development Milestones

Age	Cognitive	Emotional/Behavioral	Motor	Language
5 Years	Understands time concepts; recognizes letters and some words; can learn address and phone number; begins to understand opposites; has overall image of self	Likes to please adults; enjoys family activities; embarrasses easily; submits to more rules and shows guilt over misbehavior; can participate in informal games	Displays handedness; can bathe independently; builds elaborate structures; walks downstairs alternating feet; may print name; cuts out simple shapes; copies a square	Speaks in good sentences; uses conjunctions to string thoughts together; has a vocabulary of over 2,000 words and continues to add more; masters most consonant combinations
6 Years	Loses magical thinking; starts to understand concepts of measurement (weight, length, mass); can group things into subgroups based on a common attribute; knows right from left; knows days of the week	Develops better impulse control; may enjoy and succeed at sports and arts & crafts programs; is sensitive to criticism; may resist baths; prefers socializing with same sex	Loves active play; still somewhat uncoordinated; may be reckless; can tie shoes; copies a triangle; very active	Well developed vocabulary with increasingly improved semantics; speaks with good intelligibility; may still distort some sounds/-blends (thr, sk, st, shr, s, z, sh, ch, j)
7 Years	Begins to use simple logic; can tell time; can group objects in ascending order; understands basic addition and subtraction principles	Less egocentric; more cooperative; usually has a best friend of same sex; seeks approval from peers; tends to be critical; tattles on others for not following rules	Has refined hand–eye coordination; rides a bike; swims; printing gets smaller; activity level decreases slightly	Produces all language sounds; uses adultlike grammar; rapid language development
8 Years	Memory span increases; understands causal relationships; can be idealistic	Adheres to simple rules; often idolizes someone; begins to show sense of loyalty; likes secrets and clubs; enjoys projects and collections	Gains better control over small muscles; writes in cursive and draws better; movements are more graceful	Articulation nears adult level; better use of pronouns; understands complex directions; better storytelling skills; likes to tell jokes and enjoys bathroom humor
9–10 Years	Understands explanations; can use reference books and resources; classifies objects	Succumbs more easily to peer pressure; does not want to be different; tends to be self-critical; develops internal standards of right and wrong	Eagerly learns new skills; enjoys team competition; well coordinated with increasing dexterity and eye-hand coordination	Uses language to convey thoughts and looks at another's point of view

(Continued on following page)

Table 17-9. ■ School-Age Development Milestones *(Continued)*

Age	Cognitive	Emotional/Behavioral	Motor	Language
11–12 Years	Begins abstract thinking; increasing spans of attention and concentration	Peer acceptance is very important; critical of parents; acutely aware of opposite sex; vacillates between dependent child and independent preteen	Refines gross and fine motor skills; can do crafts and use tools well	Reading vocabulary of 50,000 words; oral vocabulary of 7200 words; speech is grammatically correct

Hearing/Speech

Whereas the assessment of an infant's hearing is somewhat subjective (unless specific audiological testing is done) it is essential to be aware of the signs of a hearing deficit. Hearing is critical to language development, and the failure to recognize and address a hearing deficit in infancy can be detrimental to a child's development. Basic hearing screenings should be done at each well visit. Parents should be specifically questioned regarding behaviors that indicate normal hearing. Any concerns regarding hearing should be thoroughly addressed. Part of assessing hearing is to assess for any factors that may increase the risk of a hearing deficit. See Box 17-2 regarding the risk factors for hearing deficit.

The development of language skills may provide evidence of intact hearing, and parents can be asked to identify the infant's level of interaction and language development. As long as the child is progressing (and not regressing) in their language skills and there are no physical abnormalities, monitoring and intermittent assessment is acceptable during this

Table 17-10. ■ Adolescent Development Milestones

Age	Cognitive	Emotional/Behavioral	Motor	Language
12–15 Years	Increase in abstract thinking and decrease in concrete thinking; increased ability to relate actions to consequences	Very focused on social life, peer acceptance, physical appearance; grades may suffer; interest in sexuality increases; wide mood swings; values privacy	May enjoy and excel at a specific sport or activity; enjoys video/computer games	Increasing ability to express oneself; may enjoy keeping a journal or diary
15–18 Years	Beginning interest in social problems; may become idealistic and altruistic; inductive and deductive reasoning; may be very introspective; increased creative ability	Risk taking is common; rejection or questioning of parental authority; may experiment with sex, alcohol, or drugs; confusion over self-image may persist	Periods of high energy alternate with periods of lethargy; may enjoy and excel at a specific sport or activity	Language skills at or near adult level

---

Box 17-2

Risk Factors for Hearing Deficit

- An affected family member
- Newborn bilirubin >20 mg/dL
- Congenital cytomegalovirus, herpes, or rubella
- Defects in ear-nose-throat structures
- Birth weight less <1500 g
- Bacterial meningitis
- Use of ototoxic medications
- Intracranial hemorrhage
- Use of mechanical ventilation >48 hr
- Head trauma or temporal bone fracture
- Infections such as mumps/measles associated with sensorineural hearing loss
- Recurrent acute otitis media or middle ear infection

---

stage. However, formal audiometry should be considered if parents express concerns about the child's hearing abilities or there are no recognizable, meaningful sounds or words at 18 months. See Box 17-3 for reasons for referral.

Vision

Vision is the least-developed sense in a newborn, and visual acuity is estimated to be around 20/670 at birth. However, the amazing pace at which visual acuity develops is obvious when watching the overall development of an infant's actions. At 1 month, an infant will stare at large objects. By 2 months, more detail is noticed and babies begin to enjoy gazing at a caregiver's face. As the baby reaches 3–4 months of age, the eyes begin to converge and the infant starts to bring things to the mouth and develop eye–hand coordination. At this age, an infant should be able to track an object 180 degrees. Around 6–7 months of age, a baby can recognize different faces.

Like hearing, it is essential to assess visual acuity at all well checkups. Again, parents are the best evaluators, so they should be questioned in regard to a baby or child's behaviors including tracking ability, response to new and familiar faces, the distance a child sits from a book or television, and the ability to notice details far away. Risk factors for decreased visual acuity should also be assessed (see Box 17-4).

Assessment of the red reflex should be a part of each well visit. Other things that should be assessed in a young infant include the pupillary response to light, the blink reflex, and the ability to fix and follow. An older infant or toddler should also be assessed using the corneal light reflex test and the cover/uncover test. Starting at preschool age, children

---

Box 17-3

Reasons for Audiology Referral

- Hearing threshold levels greater than 20 dB at 500, 1000, 2000, or 4000 Hz
- Presence of middle ear fluid documented for greater than 3 months
- Hearing or language skills seem to regress at any point

Box 17-4
Risk Factors for Decreased Visual Acuity

- Prenatal infections
- Congenital cyanotic heart disease
- Structural malformation
- Family history of vision problems
- Excessive oxygenation in neonatal period
- Hearing problems

should be assessed using visual acuity charts (Allen chart, illiterate E, or Sjögren hand.) The school-age child and adolescent should be assessed using these measures and the Snellen chart for far vision. The Ishihara should be used for color perception. See Box 17-5 for reasons for referral.

Nutrition

Assessing an infant or child's nutrition and diet is an important part of an overall well-child evaluation and requires knowledge of anticipated intake and weight change. For infants, parents should be questioned regarding the frequency of feedings, the type and amount of formula if bottle-fed, and the baby's tolerance of feedings. Once solids are initiated, parents should be asked about what types of foods the baby is taking, how much and at what times of the day, and how much fluid the infant is drinking now that solids have been started. As the child progresses on to more table foods, part of the assessment is determining whether he or she is getting a good variety of foods, is transitioning well to table foods, and is maintaining adequate fluid intake. Table 17-11 includes information that should be used to guide the nutrition questions posed at various ages.

Toddlers and Preschoolers

As a child reaches the toddler stage, her or his appetite naturally starts to decrease as his growth starts to slow down. Toddlers are frequently easily distracted and are picky about what they eat, so mealtimes can be a challenge. Parents should be encouraged to look at their child's diet on a week-by-week basis rather than day-to-day, as toddlers will frequently

Box 17-5
Reasons for Ophthalmology Referral

- Searching nystagmus
- Strabismus (intermittent strabismus is normal until age 4–6 months)
- Absence of blinking to a threat
- Lack of vertical and horizontal following by 2 months of age
- Abnormal or asymmetric red reflex
- Asymmetric corneal light reflex
- Abnormal cover/uncover test
- Visual acuity 20/50 or worse at age 3 years
- Visual acuity of 20/30 or worse at age 5 years
- Difference in score of two lines or more between eyes on visual acuity chart
- Structural abnormality

Table 17-11. ■ Age-Appropriate Nutritional Guidelines

Age	Intake	Anticipated Weight Change
Newborn	110–120 kcal· kg^{-1}· day^{-1}; eats every 1.5 to 3 hr; 20–24 oz/day.	Gains 0.5–1 oz/day
2 months	Eats 6–9 times/day; requires 120–130 kcal· kg^{-1}· day^{-1}; 20-24 oz/day.	Gains 0.5–1 oz/day Or
4 months	Requires 120-130 kcal· kg^{-1}· day^{-1}; eats 24-32 oz/day.	5–8 oz/week
6 months	Requires approx. 100 kcal· kg^{-1}· day^{-1}; Eats 24–32 oz/day. Solids include iron-fortified single-grain cereal mixed with water, formula, or breast milk. Only one new food introduced every 3–7 days. No additives, such as honey, sugar, or seasonings.	Gains 3-5 oz/wk
8-9 months	Requires around 100 kcal· kg^{-1}· day^{-1}; drinks 24–32 oz/day, often with sippy cup. Menu slowly expanded to include tender meats and finger foods. Juice limited to 6 oz/day, diluted with water.	
10-12 months	Drinks 20–32 oz/day. Menu expanding to more table and finger foods. Meal pattern resembles family's (three meal/day + snacks). Whole milk at 12 months. Juice limited to 6 oz/day, diluted with water	Gains 3–5 oz/week. Weight usually triples by 12 months.

have days where they eat very little or eat only 2 or 3 things, and then may make up for it the next day. When assessing toddlers, ask about the child's typical diet, including overall intake and any self-imposed limitations. Preschoolers will frequently go on food jags where they insist on eating the same food over and over. As long as the food is not a high-sugar or empty-calorie item, parents should allow the food choice and remember that the phase usually does not last too long.

School-Age Children

Energy needs for school-age children depend somewhat on the individual's body size, growth pattern, and activity level. Children aged 6–7 years require approximately 90 kcal·kg^{-1}·day^{-1}, 7–10 year olds require approximately 70 kcal·kg^{-1}·day^{-1}, and children 10–12 need 40–55 kcal·kg^{-1}·day^{-1} depending on their size and activity. The school-age period is a time of busy schedules, and children at this age tend to skip meals and snack more often. Also, because children spend a good part of the day away from home, parents become somewhat out of touch with what their child is eating throughout the day. Because of these habits, problems with obesity can begin at this stage. Parents should make an effort to have easy, healthy snacks available. Healthy meals and family mealtime routines should be reinforced at this time period to help prevent obesity.

Adolescents

Like for school-age children, energy requirements for adolescents vary somewhat based on body size and activity level. However, owing to the rapid growth and development during this stage, it is essential that all adolescents are consuming an adequate amount of calories, protein, vitamins, and minerals. Males typically require more kilocalories per day than females based on their larger body mass and prolonged period of growth. Teens involved in athletics also have an increased need for calories. Twelve- to 14-year-old males need approximately 60 kcal·kg^{-1}·day^{-1}, whereas females at this age need 45–50 kcal·kg^{-1}·day^{-1}. At age 15, daily caloric intake decreases to 40–45 kcal·kg^{-1}·day^{-1} for males and 35–40 kcal·kg^{-1}·day^{-1} for females. Daily calcium intake during adolescence should be a minimum of 1300 mg per day.

Because of the teenage lifestyle, healthy eating habits are sometimes difficult to maintain in adolescents. The nutritional history should be considered in the context of overall lifestyle and activity. Because issues of body image and peer influence are at their peak during this age, it is essential to watch for signs of eating disorders and to caution parents on how to carefully discuss the importance of diet with their teen.

In addition to identifying the daily intake of meals and snacks, include questions to identify nutritional supplements and vitamins. Of particular interest is the intake of vitamin D and fluoride. Breast-fed infants who do not receive vitamin D supplementation or adequate exposure to sunlight are at risk for developing rickets. All breast-fed infants should receive a supplement of 200 IU per day of vitamin D unless they are consuming at least 500 mL a day of vitamin D–fortified formula. This practice should begin within the first 2 months of life.

Anticipatory Guidance and Safety

Well checkups are not solely to examine the patient physically, but also to offer advice and insight into upcoming stages and safety issues. A focus of the assessment should include identifying a child's potential risks, in order to be able to appropriately counsel parents.

Create an open dialogue with parents that addresses safety topics by asking about daily practices and home environment. Table 17-12 is an age-by-age list of anticipatory guidance and safety topics, which should be covered at each well child checkup, regarding feeding, sleeping, elimination, safety, and illness. Other issues may certainly arise, and discussion during the visits should be based on parental concerns and questions.

Teething and Tooth Eruption

Assess the child's history of teething and tooth eruption. The primary teeth begin to erupt around 6 months of age. Table 17-13 identifies the typical age of tooth eruption. (The eruption pattern may vary from the expected norm.)

During the assessment of teething and tooth eruption, determine the level of fluoride present in the child's drinking water. It is helpful for providers to know the amount of fluoride in a community's drinking water because any recommendations for supplementation are based on those amounts. Children who do not live in a fluoridated water area but who

Table 17-12. ■ Anticipatory Guidance

Age	Feeding	Sleeping	Elimination	Safety	Illness
Newborn to 1 Month	Feed on demand; ask about duration of feeds (or amount per feeding if on formula); always hold bottle—don't prop	Back to sleep; firm mattress; avoid pillows and blankets; ask about where baby is sleeping and in what position	Breast-fed stool is yellow and pasty; normal bowel frequency varies from after each feeding to every other day; ask about stool frequency and consistency	Do not leave infant alone on high surfaces; set water heater thermostat at 120 degrees; always use a proper rear facing car seat; smoke detectors; sun protection	Call office for rectal temp higher than 100.4; persistent vomiting or diarrhea; refusal to feed, prolonged irritability, bulging fontanel, or yellow tinge to skin or eyes
1–2 Months	Feed on demand; may stretch out time between feeds	Same as above; some routine may slowly develop; may sleep 16–18 hours/day	Babies frequently grunt and strain while stooling, as long as stool is soft then baby is not constipated	Same as above; learn infant/child CPR	Same as above
2–4 Months	Same as above; more routine develops; may slowly increase amount of formula; no solids needed yet; avoid adding cereal to bottle	Same as above	Same as above	Same as above	Same as above
4–6 Months	Night feedings should decrease or stop; may start solids close to 6 months	Should sleep longer stretches at night; routine nap schedule develops; if infant rolls himself to stomach to sleep, it is okay	Same as above	Watch for choking hazards; watch for burns from infant grabbing at hot food or liquids	Call for rectal temp over 101; decreased urination (no wet diaper in 8 hours); prolonged inconsolability; wheezing; cold symptoms (without fever) for over 5–7 days
6–9 Months	Start solids—begin with rice cereal in a soupy consistency; add foods slowly and one at a time (stick with one new food for 3–4 days); night feedings should stop	Establish consistent nighttime rituals, including reading	Stools will change in consistency with addition of solids; rice cereal can be constipating; give diluted juice if constipation is a problem	Make sure house is completely baby-proofed! Lock poisons; cover outlets; pool safety if applicable; choking hazards with new foods; sunscreen	Same as above

(Continued on following page)

Table 17-12. ■ Anticipatory Guidance *(Continued)*

Age	Feeding	Sleeping	Elimination	Safety	Illness
9–12 Months	Increase table/finger foods; offer cup; offer water and diluted juice (no more than 6 ounces of juice/day); establish mealtime routines	Stick with nighttime rituals; security item may help with bedtime	Same as above	Same as above	Same as above

Stage	Feeding	Sleeping	Elimination	Safety
Toddler	Appetite slows; child becomes pickier; offer new foods; avoid battles	Transition to regular bed; consistent nighttime ritual; nightmares may occur; usually one nap during the day	Interest in potty training emerges; most children demonstrate readiness between 24 and 30 months	Always use proper car seat; teach street safety; have a fire escape plan; lock guns away; lock poisons and medications; use sunscreen and bug repellent; caution about burns and falls
Preschooler	Encourage balanced diet; child should use utensils correctly; pickiness may continue	Naps may decrease or stop; bedtime may be moved up when napping ceases; nightmares and terrors may occur	By age 3, 90% of children are bowel trained, 85% are dry during the day, and 60%–70% are dry at night; no interventions if still wetting at night	Same as above; water safety; begin stranger awareness and safety; continue using car or booster seat
School Age	Encourage balanced diet, limiting junk foods; eat as a family; involve child in food preparation	Continue consistent nighttime ritual; average 8-year-old sleeps 9–12 hours a night	Consider interventions (pharmacologic or behavioral) if nocturnal enuresis occurs	Same as above; bike safety; fire safety; child should remain in a booster car seat until age 8 or 80 pounds
Adolescent	Encourage balanced diet and healthy food choices; limit junk and fast food	Erratic sleep patterns; napping may increase; need average of 8–9 hours of sleep per night		Seatbelts; car safety; safe sex; discourage drug and alcohol usage; reinforce sunscreen usage; keep firearms locked

Table 17-13. ■ Patterns of Tooth Eruption

Primary Teeth	Maxillary	Mandibular
Central Incisors	6–8 months	5–7 months
Lateral Incisors	8–11 months	7–10 months
Cuspids/Canines	16–20 months	16–20 months
First Molars	10–16 months	10–16 months
Second Molars	20–30 months	20–30 months
Permanent Teeth	**Maxillary**	**Mandibular**
Central Incisors	7–8 years	6–7 years
Lateral Incisors	8–9 years	7–8 years
Cuspids/Canines	11–12 years	9–11 years
First Premolars	10–11 years	10–12 years
Second Premolars	10–12 years	11–13 years
First Molars	6–7 years	6–7 years
Second Molars	12–13 years	12–13 years
Third Molars	17–22 years	17–22 years

attend school or daycare in such an area (and drink water while at school) may not need additional supplementation. The guidelines in Table 17-14 should be incorporated into the care of pediatric patients.

Table 17-14. ■ Fluoride Concentration in Community Drinking Water

Age	<0.3 ppm	0.3–0.6 ppm	>0.6 ppm
Birth–6 Months	None	None	None
6 Months–3 Years	0.25 mg/day	None	None
3–6 Years	0.50 mg/day	0.25 mg/day	None
6–16 Years	1.0 mg/day	0.5 mg/day	None

Data from U.S. Department of Health and Human Services, Centers for Disease Control and Prevention, www.cdc.gov/mmwr.

 SUGGESTED READINGS

American Academy of Pediatrics. (1997). *Guidelines for Health Supervision* (3rd ed.). Elk Grove Village, IL: American Academy of Pediatrics.

Baker, S., Cochran, W., Flores, C., Georgieff, M., Jacobson, M., Jaksic, T., & Krebs, N. (1999). Calcium requirements of infants, children, and adolescents. *Pediatrics,* 104 (5), 1152–1157. Accessed online at URL www.aap.org/policy/re9904.html on February 16, 2005.

Baker, S., Cochran, W., Greer, F., Heyman, M., Jacobson, M., Jaksic, T., & Krebs, N. (2001). The use and misuse of fruit juice in pediatrics. *Pediatrics,* 107 (5), 1210–1213. Accessed online at URL www.aap.org/policy/re0047.html on February 16, 2005.

Burns, C., Barber, N., Brady, M., & Dunn, A. (1996). *Pediatric Primary Care: A Handbook for Nurse Practitioners.* Philadelphia: W.B. Saunders Company.

Castiglia, P., & Harbin, R. (1992). *Child Health Care: Process and Practice.* Philadelphia: J.B. Lippincott Company.

Ganel, A., Dudkiewicz, I., & Grogan, D. (2003). Pediatric orthopedic physical examination of the infant: A 5-minute assessment. *Journal of Pediatric Health Care,* 17 (1), 39–41.

Gartner, L., & Greer, F. (2003). Prevention of rickets and vitamin D deficiency: New guidelines for vitamin D intake. *Pediatrics,* 111 (4), 908–910. Accessed online at URLwww.aap.org/policy/s010116.html on February 16, 2005.

Graham, M., & Uphold, C. (1994). *Clinical Guidelines in Child Health.* Gainesville, FL: Barmarrae Books.

Legler, J., & Rose, L. (1998). Assessment of abnormal growth curves. *American Family Physician,* 58 (1). Accessed online at URL www.aafp.org/afp/980700ap/legler.html on February 16, 2005.

Millonig, V., & Baroni, M. (1999). *Pediatric Nurse Practitioner Certification Review Guide* (3rd ed.). Potomac, MD: Health Leadership Associates, Inc.

Wong, D., & Wilson, D. (Eds.). (1995). *Nursing Care of Infants and Children* (5th ed.). St. Louis: Mosby.

Chapter 18

Pregnant Patients

*Deborah Blackwell
& James Blackwell*

Pregnancy is considered a wellness condition and not a disease entity. The focus of care during a low-risk pregnancy is therefore on health promotion and maintenance while achieving a healthy outcome for both the woman and child. Advanced practice nurses —specifically, nurse-practitioners—have a strong tradition of delivering wellness care throughout the life span in a cost-effective manner and with a high level of patient satisfaction. Caring for pregnant women is therefore congruent with the advanced practice nursing model.

Pregnancy care from nurse-practitioners should ideally begin with preconception care and continue until 24–28 weeks of pregnancy, when the woman is usually referred to a specialty provider, which typically is either an obstetrician or certified nurse midwife, in preparation for childbirth.

The status of a woman's health directly affects the pregnancy outcome. Preconception care should therefore be used to maximize the woman's physical and psychosocial health and allow her to make informed decisions regarding any potential lifestyle adjustments. Preconception care usually consists of risk factor identification, health behavior advice, substance abuse treatment, chronic illness management, and psychosocial service referrals (Byrd, 2001). Basic prenatal care includes risk assessment, health education and counseling, and management of potential or actual problems.

HISTORY

After pregnancy is confirmed, a complete medical, psychosocial (including the current living situation, and social support and abuse information), family (including genetic), and reproductive history is obtained. This includes a menstrual, contraceptive, gynecologic, sexual, surgical, nutritional (including prepregnancy weight), and medication (including over-the-counter and recreational drug use) history. An estimated date of delivery (EDD) is estimated at this time by using the last menstrual period (LMP). This estimation can be made with either a pregnancy wheel or by applying Naegele's rule of adding 7 days to the first day of the LMP and then subtracting 3 months (Bond, 2004). This method of estimating the EDD depends on the woman having regular menstrual cycles of 28 ± 7 days. If the EDD cannot be accurately estimated by Naegele's rule, an early ultrasound is recommended because of the linkage of specific prenatal interventions with gestational dating of the pregnancy. The EDD should be updated throughout the pregnancy for confirmation of dates by determining when quickening occurs, when fetal heart tones are first auscultated, when the fundal height is at the umbilicus and, most accurately, through an ultrasound estimation at 16–20 weeks.

The reproductive history includes the contraceptive, sexual, and obstetric history. The contraceptive history elicits the last time contraceptives have been used, what types of contraceptives were used, and the dates of any unprotected intercourse. The sexual history helps identify risks for sexually transmitted diseases or ectopic pregnancies. The obstetric history consists of the number of pregnancies and their outcomes using the gravida–para–TPAL nomenclature (Table 18-1). This portion of the history also includes the year of each pregnancy, infant birth weight, gestational age at birth, type of delivery (vaginal or caesarian), length of labor, anesthesia received, and any maternal or fetal complications during the pregnancy.

PHYSICAL EXAMINATION

The initial physical examination is a systematic, complete, head-to-toe examination that is usually performed at the time of the first visit to provide baseline information. The clinical pelvimetry assessment is done at this time to ensure pelvic adequacy for vaginal delivery. Vitals signs, especially blood pressure and weight, are included with each assessment. Subsequent visits are abbreviated in that they focus on the developmental stage of the pregnancy and the overall health of the mother and fetus. Components of these targeted exams (depending on the week of gestation) include fundal height, presentation, fetal heart rate (FHR), fetal movement, the presence or absence of preterm labor signs and symptoms, cervical exam (including dilatation and effacement), urine dipstick, and timing of the next appointment.

Monitoring fetal heart rate is a vital component of fetal surveillance, providing important information on placental function, fetal hypoxia, and whether the intrauterine environment can support and sustain the fetus. The FHR can usually be auscultated at 10–12 weeks with an electronic Doppler and at 18–20 weeks with a fetoscope (Clarke, 2002). A

Table 18-1. ■ Pregnancy Nomenclature		
Letter	Meaning	Definition
G	Gravidity	Total number of pregnancies, regardless of duration or outcome
P	Parity	Number of pregnancies after 20 weeks of gestation
T	Term	Number of pregnancies considered to be 37–40 weeks of gestation
P	Premature/Preterm deliveries	Number of pregnancies between 20 and 37 weeks of gestation
A	Abortions	Number of induced or spontaneous terminations of pregnancy before 20 weeks of gestation
L	Live births	Number of living children who are alive at the time of data collection

normal fetal heart rate is 120–160 beats per minute. A sustained FHR of below 100 beats per minute is indicative of fetal jeopardy. If there is a question of whether the fetal heart rate is being adequately evaluated, the maternal pulse should simultaneously be assessed, to ensure that the FHR and not the maternal heart rate is actually being auscultated. Leopold's maneuvers should be integrated into the prenatal assessment after 28 weeks of gestation in order to locate the most appropriate area for FHR auscultation (Figure 18-1).

Figure 18-1. ■ Leopold's maneuvers. Leopold's maneuvers are a series of four maneuvers designed to provide a systematic approach to determine the orientation of the fetus through abdominal palpation. A, Using two hands and compressing the maternal abdomen, a sense of fetal direction is obtained (vertical or transverse). B, The sides of the uterus are palpated to determine the position of the fetal back and small parts. C, The presenting part (head or butt) is palpated above the symphysis and degree of engagement determined. D, The fetal occipital prominence is determined. (From Beare, PG. Davis's NCLEX-RN Review, 3rd ed. Philadelphia: FA Davis, 2001. Reprinted with permission.)

The provider will document the location of where the fetal heart tones (FHTs) are best heard or the point of maximal intensity. This procedure can reinforce the accuracy of the fetal position as assessed by the examiner through palpation. Fetal heart tones are best auscultated through the fetal back in vertex and breech presentations and toward the mother's flank when the fetus is in a transverse lie. In vertex presentations, FHTs are usually best heard below the mother's umbilicus, in the lower abdomen, whereas, for breech presentations, they are best heard at or slightly above the umbilicus, in the mother's upper abdomen.

Fundal height changes are reflective of fetal growth and correlate closely with the number of weeks of pregnancy after 18 weeks of gestation (Hawkins, 2002). Assessment of fundal height provides an estimation of gestational age in relationship to uterine size. Fundal height is measured by placing the end of a tape measure at the symphysis pubis and extending it to the fundus (Figure 18-2). The uterus is usually palpable above the symphysis at 12 weeks of gestation, midway between the symphysis pubis and umbilicus at 16 weeks, and at the umbilicus at 20 weeks. Small uterine size for dates may be indicative of inaccurate pregnancy dating or intrauterine growth restriction. Large uterine size for dates may be associated inaccurate dates, macrosomia, or multiple gestations (more than one fetus).

LABORATORY STUDIES

Laboratory studies during the initial visit are quite extensive. These screening tests are dependent on the disease prevalence within the screened population (Table 18-2). Laboratory testing throughout the pregnancy is dependent on presenting complaints and the developmental stage of the pregnancy. For example, a glucose screen should be done between 24 and 28 weeks of gestation, whereas an anemia screen (hemoglobin and hematocrit) should be done initially and again at 28–34 weeks. However, if the woman complains of a vaginal discharge later in the pregnancy, a gonorrhea and chlamydia culture could be done even if the initial screen was negative.

PRENATAL EDUCATION

Prenatal education depends on when the visit occurs and any concerns uncovered during the visit, but it usually focuses on preterm labor signs and symptoms, danger signs of preg-

Figure 18-2. ■ Measuring fundal height. (From Dillon, PM. Nursing Health Assessment: A Critical Thinking, Case Studies Approach. Philadelphia: FA Davis, 2003, p. 736.)

Table 18-2. ■ Recommended Pregnancy Screening Tests

Initial Routine Tests for All Pregnant Patients	Additional Tests Depending on the Patient's History	Tests for Subsequent Pregnancy Visits
• CBC • Blood type, Rh, and antibody screen • Urine dipstick (culture and sensitivity if dipstick is positive) • Rubella titer • Serology for syphilis • Hepatitis B surface antigen • Pap smear • Chlamydia/gonorrhea screening	• Sickle cell screen (Sickledex) or hemoglobin electrophoresis for African Americans • Tuberculosis screen • HIV screen • Urine toxicology screen • Diabetes screening • Herpes culture • Serum iron studies • Thyroid studies • Toxoplasmosis titer • KOH/wet prep	• CBC—28 and 36 weeks • Alpha-fetoprotein—15–20 weeks • Diabetes screening—24–26 weeks • Urinalysis—28 weeks • Antibody screen for Rh-neg patients—28 weeks • Retest chlamydia/gonorrhea if positive earlier—34–36 weeks • Group beta strep culture (vaginal/anorectal)—35–37 weeks

nancy, fetal movement awareness, information about prenatal classes, nutrition, exercise, weight goals, teratogens, sexuality, and infant feeding choices. The usual weight gain during pregnancy is $1/_2$–1 pound per week, with a total of 25–35 pounds for the entire pregnancy period. However, the first trimester may exhibit little or no gain, or even a small (2–5 pound) weight loss as a result of nausea and vomiting or inadequate nutritional intake. Rapid weight gain occurs during the second trimester and slows during the third trimester. The usual weight gain pattern is 3–5 pounds during the first trimester, 12–15 pounds during the second, and 12–15 pounds during the third (Bond, 2004). The recommended weight gain for pregnancy is adjusted according to the patient's body mass index (Table 18-3).

Prenatal vitamins are started during the initial visit along with any other medications as indicated by the history or physical exam (e.g., iron or calcium supplementation). For routine pregnancies, prenatal visits are usually scheduled every month or 4 weeks until 32 weeks of gestation. At that time, visits are scheduled every 2 weeks until 36 weeks, at which point the patient is then seen weekly until she goes into labor (Bryd, 2001).

Table 18-3. ■ Recommended Weight Gain After the First Trimester of Pregnancy

Body Mass index	Recommended Rate of Weight Gain	Intervention Suggested	Overall Weight Gain
<19.8 (underweight)	1.1 lb/wk	<2 lb/mo	28–40 lb
19.8–26.0 (normal weight)	1 lb/wk	<2 lb/mo >6.5 lb/mo	25–30 lb
>26.0–29.0 (overweight)	0.66 lb/wk	>3.5 lb/wk <1 lb/wk	15–25 lb
>29.0 (obese)	Individualized	<1 lb/wk >2.5 lb/wk	At least 15 lb

Data from Baxley, E.G. Patient and family education. Section A. Nutrition in pregnancy and lactation. In Ratcliffe, S.D., Baxley, E.G., Byrd, J.E., & Sakornbut, E.L. (Eds.). Family Practice Obstetrics, 2nd ed. Philadelphia: Hanley & Belfus, 2001, pp 57–65.

COMMON CHIEF COMPLAINTS AND DISCOMFORTS OF PREGNANCY
GI Complaints

Gastrointestinal (GI) complaints affect 50%–90% of pregnant women in the United States (Pandolfino & Vanagunas, 2000). These ailments can consist of mild to severe nausea, vomiting, and dyspepsia and are usually caused by increased levels of human chorionic gonadotropin (hCG), by the effects of increased progesterone on smooth muscles in the GI tract, or by uterine displacement of abdominal organs. The practitioner must be able to differentiate normal changes that are associated with pregnancy from more serious disease states and must know which diagnostic tests will not be harmful to either the mother or the fetus.

Heartburn, or gastroesophageal reflex disease (GERD), results from decreased peristalsis of the esophagus, lower esophageal sphincter relaxation, and increased stomach pressure, whereas decreased intestinal motility and bowel compression may contribute to constipation and flatulence. As mentioned, the nausea and vomiting associated with pregnancy are believed to be related to increased levels of hCG and estrogen (Clarke, 2002). Persistent or severe nausea and vomiting, known as hyperemesis gravidarum, may be an early symptom of hyperthyroidism (Baxley, 2001). Beta-hCG has a thyroid-stimulating hormone–like effect on the maternal thyroid, and hyperthyroidism may be evident only by an increase in free T_4 instead of by both the TSH decrease and the free T_4 increase that are usually seen in women who are not pregnant (Turok & Schultz, 2001).

Contributing factors for pregnancy-related nausea and vomiting can include emotional factors and irregular eating habits. An increased incidence of *Helicobacter pylori* has recently been identified in pregnant women with intense nausea compared with those who had never experienced morning sickness (Reymunde, Santiago, & Perez, 2001). Conventional pregnancy-related nausea and vomiting commonly peak at about 10–15 weeks of gestation and resolve at approximately 20 weeks of gestation (Pandolfino & Vanagunas, 2000). Hyperemesis gravidarum only occurs in 0.5 to 10 out of every 1000 pregnancies, but it has an increased incidence rate in multiple gestation and molar pregnancies (Clarke, 2002). More than 50% of patients with hyperemesis gravidarum have elevated aminotransferase levels.

Pregnancy also increases the risk of developing gallstones owing to an increased progesterone level that reduces gallbladder emptying and therefore increases biliary stasis. Subsequent pregnancies exponentially increase the risk of cholelithiasis. However, only 2%–4% of pregnant patients are diagnosed with gallstones and symptomatic disease will occur in just 5–10 of 10,000 deliveries (Pandolfino & Vanagunas, 2000). Upper endoscopy is a safe diagnostic procedure during pregnancy and does not carry an increased risk of preterm labor or other complications (Pandolfino & Vanagunas, 2000). However, as a general rule, any procedures during pregnancy are usually postponed until after delivery unless the risk of the disease outweighs the risk of the procedure and definitive evaluation is needed.

Upper endoscopy may be indicated during pregnancy for significant gastrointestinal bleeding, unresponsive nausea and vomiting, dysphagia, peptic ulcer disease, and severe abdominal pain. Bloody diarrhea, hematochezia, weight loss, and fatigue during pregnancy should initially be evaluated by stool samples for gram stain and culture, ova and parasites, fecal leukocytes, and *Clostridium difficile* toxin. If these tests are negative, a flexible sigmoidoscopy should be done, which does not require conscious sedation and is not associated with any pregnancy complications (Pandolfino & Vanagunas, 2000).

Nausea and Vomiting

SUBJECTIVE

Initial questions regarding pregnancy-induced nausea and vomiting should include whether these symptoms occur more frequently during certain times of the day. Pain should be assessed as to whether it has a gradual or rapid onset and whether eating either alleviates or exacerbates the condition. For example, pain that occurs with eating may indicate an esophagitis, whereas pain that occurs several hours postprandially suggests a duodenal ulcer. Hydration status can be assessed by asking about dark colored urine and excessive thirst. Psychosocial distress also should be evaluated. Worrisome features in the history include fever, abdominal pain, abdominal cramping, diarrhea, jaundice, vaginal bleeding, headaches, neurological signs, projectile vomiting, hematemesis, and melena.

OBJECTIVE

Vital signs should lie within normal limits and not be indicative of dehydration. There should not be any weight loss. The thyroid should be of normal size and shape. Uterine size should be appropriate for dates, and the presence of fetal heart tones (after 12 weeks) is a reassuring sign. A complete blood count (CBC); complete metabolic panel, containing liver enzymes and a calcium level; and a Hemoccult of the stool may eliminate other causes for the nausea and vomiting. Urine ketones and specific gravity should not be indicative of dehydration, and urine dipstick or urinalysis should be negative for infection or hematuria (to rule out renal calculus). Serum titers for *H. pylori* can be drawn.

DIFFERENTIAL DIAGNOSES

Hyperemesis gravidarum, multiple gestation, hydatidiform gestation, molar pregnancy, intestinal obstruction, gastroenteritis, cholecystitis, pancreatitis, hepatitis, diabetes, thyroid dysfunction, migraine, food poisoning, emotional problems, eating disorders.

Dyspepsia

SUBJECTIVE

Heartburn and epigastric/upper abdominal pain are the classic symptoms for dyspepsia, especially after heavy, fatty, fried, spicy, or gas-producing meals. Another symptom may include abdominal bloating or distention. Any psychosocial stressors or depression should be explored. Dyspepsia should be differentiated from dysphagia. Worrisome symptoms include associated chest pain, dyspnea, exercise intolerance, palpitations, diaphoresis, fatty stools, foul-smelling stools, melena, nausea, vomiting, diarrhea or constipation, or fever and chills.

OBJECTIVE

Diagnosis for dyspepsia is usually made on history and physical examination. A CBC, complete metabolic panel, and a Hemoccult for blood in the stool may eliminate other causes for the dyspepsia. Presence of *H. pylori* can be addressed. Dyspepsia occurs at a higher incidence rate in people who are overweight or obese.

DIFFERENTIAL DIAGNOSES

Dyspepsia related to pregnancy, cholecystitis, pancreatitis, cardiac etiology, ulcer, hiatal hernia.

Abdominal Pain

The uterine pressure increases as a result of the growing fetus and placenta, and the increase in amniotic fluid volume. At 12 weeks, the fundus rises above the symphysis. When the pregnant woman is in an upright position, the broad and round ligaments anchor the uterus to the anterior abdominal wall in order to provide uterine stability (Bond, 2004). The weight of the uterus may cause tension on these ligaments, creating inflammation and discomfort. This ligament pain usually resolves when the woman assumes a supine position as the uterus descends backward.

SUBJECTIVE

The woman should be asked whether the abdominal pain can be classified as acute, chronic, or recurrent; whether it has a gradual or rapid onset; and whether the pain has ever occurred before. The severity of the pain (on a scale of 1 to 10) and the progression or resolution of the pain should noted. If there is sharp or dull pain on either or both sides of the abdomen, investigate whether the pain increases in intensity with movement. If there is tightening or pressure in the uterus, ask whether the pressure resolves with position change or with bladder emptying. Inquire about the timing and consistency of the last bowel movement. Worrisome symptoms include regular contractions that do not improve with position change or bladder emptying, nausea, vomiting, diarrhea, melena, hematochezia, hematemesis, fever, anorexia, periumbilical or right lower quadrant pain, one-sided abdominal pain that is constant and increases over time, urinary tract infection (UTI) symptoms, a tender lump in the groin that worsens with prolonged standing, vaginal bleeding or bloody show, or vaginal fluid leaking.

OBJECTIVE

Vital signs and physical examination should be appropriate for the gestational age of the pregnancy. There should be no reproducible tenderness with palpation to the chest wall or pain with deep breathing. There should be no regular contractions felt; no cervical dilatation or effacement; no fluid leakage, possibly indicating rupture of membranes, or bleeding from the os; and no adnexal, abdominal, or pelvic masses or tenderness. Bowel sounds should be normal, and fetal activity should be present. Fetal heart sounds should be heard by Doppler if gestation is over 10–12 weeks. Ultrasonography should show a normal fetal heart motion and no worrisome signs, such as decreased fetal movement, abnormal placenta placement, or abnormal amniotic fluid levels. If the pregnancy is between weeks 4 and 8, the hCG levels should correspond with the gestational age of the fetus and should double every 2–3 days (Raines, 2002).

DIFFERENTIAL DIAGNOSES

Normal fetal activity, ligament pain, Braxton Hicks contractions, preterm or true labor, ectopic pregnancy, abruptio placentae, placenta previa, threatened abortion, complete abortion, missed (incomplete) abortion, premature rupture of membranes, preeclampsia, vaginitis, pelvic inflammatory disease (PID), ovarian cyst rupture, constipation, intestinal obstruction, ulcer, diverticulitis, appendicitis, kidney stone, inguinal hernia, gastroenteritis, UTI, costochondritis.

Musculoskeletal Complaints

Low back pain is a common complaint during pregnancy. The pain may radiate to the legs and may be increase at night. Back pain usually results from the exaggeration of the lumbar spine curvature that balances the woman's center of gravity over the lower extremities in response to the growing uterus. The release of the hormone relaxin causes ligaments in the pubic symphysis and sacroiliac joints to soften in preparation for vaginal delivery. An increased breast size may also result in upper back pain.

Carpal tunnel syndrome results from compression of the median nerve in the carpal tunnel, which results in paresthesias or weakness of the thumb, index, and middle fingers (Viera, 2003). Carpal tunnel syndrome occurs in 20%–60% of pregnant women and often causes these women to awake with burning, numbness, and tingling in the median nerve distribution (Padua, Aprile, Caliandro, et al., 2001; Weimer, Yin, Lovelace, & Gooch, 2002). However, these symptoms usually tend to occur during the last trimester.

Back Pain

SUBJECTIVE

Back pain is reported as a dull, aching pain in the upper or lower back that worsens as the day progresses. Standing or sitting for long periods may aggravate the back pain. The location of the pain is important as well as the information gathered via a "PQRST" report. This inquiry usually provides sufficient diagnostic information and comprises the *precipitating* (P) factors (what aggravates or alleviates the pain, and the symptoms that are associated with the pain), the *quality* (Q) of the pain (achy, burning, cramping, shooting, etc.), the *radiation* (R) of the pain, the *severity* (S) of the pain (typically reported on a 1-to-10 scale and whether it interferes with the usual activities of daily living), and the *timing* (T) of the pain (sudden or gradual onset, duration). Worrisome symptoms include a history of back injuries, problems, or surgeries; UTI or vaginal infection symptoms; bowel changes; uterine contractions; pain, numbness, or tingling that radiates either into the abdomen or down into the legs; and any neurological deficits.

OBJECTIVE

The weight and body mass index of the woman should be noted. Lordosis, gait, paraspinal or costal vertebral angle (CVA) tenderness to palpation, straight leg raises, reflexes, and a neurologic exam should be assessed. A rectal exam should be done to assess for rectal tone and impaction. Urinary tract symptoms, vaginal discharge, or uterine contractions necessitate appropriate evaluation.

DIFFERENTIAL DIAGNOSES

Backache related to pregnancy, muscle sprain or strain, sciatica, arthritis, herniated disc, uterine contractions, vaginal infection, UTI, kidney stone, pancreatitis, gallstones, ulcer.

Muscle Cramps

SUBJECTIVE

The patient experiences calf, thigh, or buttocks cramps, occurring mostly at night or in the early morning. The woman may report excessive exercise or walking. Fluid and calcium intake should be checked through a diet recall. Worrisome symptoms include a history of deep vein thrombosis, a personal or family history of thrombophilic disorders (Table 18-4), recent trauma or surgery, lower back pain or arthritis, or neurologic complaints.

OBJECTIVE

Worrisome symptoms include a positive Homan's sign, unilateral swelling or tenderness, diminished pulses in the lower extremities, redness, abnormal warmth or coldness, numb-

Table 18-4. ■ Thrombophilic States in Pregnancy

Inherited Thrombophilias	Acquired Thrombophilias
Factor V Leiden	Pregnancy/postpartum
Prothrombin A20210	Immobilization
Antithrombin (AT) III	Trauma
Protein C	Postoperative state
Protein S	High estrogen use
Homocysteine	Malignancy
	Nephrotic syndrome
	Heparin-induced thrombocytopenia
	Myeloproliferative disorders
	Paroxysmal nocturnal hematuria
	CHF and atrial fibrillation
	Antiphospholipid antibody syndrome

ness, or pale-appearing calf or leg. Orthostatic blood pressures and pulses should be taken, if indicated. Electrolytes and serum calcium levels may need to be checked.

DIFFERENTIAL DIAGNOSES

Muscle cramps, electrolyte imbalances, thromboembolic disease, varicosities, dehydration, arthritis, sciatica, nerve root compression.

Numbness and/or Tingling in Hand(s)

SUBJECTIVE

The patient reports a dull, achy pain in the wrist, forearm, or hand that may worsen at night. This pain may be associated with paresthesia or weakness in the hand. Edema in the hands or upper extremities may be noted. A history of repetitive activity of the upper extremity may be reported. Sitting, standing, and sleep posture (especially if the woman sleeps with the arm extended against the head) should be investigated.

OBJECTIVE

Tinel's sign and Phalen's test should be performed. Upper extremity, grip, and finger strength should be assessed along with the ability to oppose the thumb to the fingers. An evaluation for thenar atrophy and dry skin on the thumb and index and middle fingers (median nerve distribution) should be completed. The size and shape of joints, skin color, pulses, and capillary refill should be noted.

DIFFERENTIAL DIAGNOSES

Carpal tunnel syndrome, musculoskeletal pain, arthritis, infection, cervical neck injury or disease, nerve damage in the hand, cardiac problems, thoracic outlet syndrome, hyperventilation.

Respiratory Complaints

As the uterus enlarges, it presses against the abdominal organs and diaphragm, and this prevents the lungs from expanding fully. Increased progesterone directly stimulates the central respiratory system to increase tidal volume and decrease blood P_{CO2}. This change is the basis of an increased awareness of breathing or even dyspnea that is experienced during pregnancy (Clarke, 2002). Nasal congestion or stuffiness may result from increased estrogen and progesterone levels, which increase perivascular edema and enlargement of the nasal turbinates. These changes also can lead to episodes of epistaxis.

Dyspnea (Shortness of Breath)

SUBJECTIVE

The pregnant woman may experience labored or heavy breathing, which may be associated with activity. Dizziness or light-headedness may be reported. The woman's smoking history should be obtained. It is crucial to determine the onset (either acute or chronic), the progression, and any past history of dyspnea. Additional investigation should include whether the dyspnea occurred following an episode of eating, drinking, or potential allergen exposure, such as an insect bite. Severe dyspnea and significant oxygen deprivation requires an immediate assessment and referral. History should be negative for fever, cough, trauma, hemoptysis, night sweats, wheezing, chest pain or GI symptoms. Past medical and family history should include assessment for deep vein thrombosis, recent immobilization or prolonged sitting, and thrombophilias such as factor V Leiden, protein C or S deficiency, and antiphospholipid syndrome.

OBJECTIVE

Diagnostic tests are typically not necessary. Vital signs and physical examination, especially of the upper and lower respiratory tracts and cardiac system, should be within normal limits for gestational age. There should be no dependent edema. A CBC should not indicate anemia, and pulse oximetry should be 95% or above. A chest x-ray is not indicated unless absolutely necessary, especially until after 15 weeks of gestation. Ionizing radiation should not exceed a dose of more than 1.5 rads over the entire pregnancy (Wotring, 2004). A chest x-ray generally delivers 8 millirads (1 rad is equal to 1000 millirads) to the ovary without shielding (Stanford & Hobbins, 2001). A risk-versus-benefit assessment should be documented in the provider's note along with documentation that the abdomen had lead shielding and that the lowest exposure technique possible was used.

DIFFERENTIAL DIAGNOSES

Pregnancy-related dyspnea, upper respiratory infection (URI), nasal congestion, asthma, bronchitis, pneumonia, pulmonary embolus, cardiac disease such as congestive heart failure (CHF), anemia, anxiety, hyperventilation, aspiration, anaphylaxis.

Nasal Congestion

SUBJECTIVE

The woman may report nasal stuffiness, rhinorrhea, sneezing, postnasal drip, or cough. History may be positive for epistaxis. Worrisome symptoms include frontal headaches or sensation of fullness or pressure, teeth pain, or fever. Nasal spray and intranasal drug use should be investigated. Past medical history should include inquiries regarding allergic rhinitis, seasonal allergies, sinusitis, nasal or facial trauma, and hypertension.

OBJECTIVE

Vital signs, particularly temperature and blood pressure, should be normal. Nasal turbinates may be pale to red, edematous, and may be either dry or have discharge. Clotted blood may be noted if epistaxis has occurred. Sinuses should be percussed and palpated. There should be no pain with forward head motion. No polyps should be noted and the septum should be intact and not deviated.

DIFFERENTIAL DIAGNOSES

Nasal congestion related to pregnancy, epistaxis, URI, sinusitis, allergic rhinitis, nasal polyps, cocaine or chronic nasal spray use, hypertension, facial trauma.

Fatigue

Fatigue usually occurs during the first and third trimesters of pregnancy. First-trimester fatigue is often associated with the physical and psychosocial pregnancy changes. Fatigue may also be indicative of a more serious physical, emotional, or dietary problem.

SUBJECTIVE

The woman may experience a higher than expected amount of fatigue despite a normal amount of energy expenditure and sleep. Worrisome symptoms include depression, anxiety, anorexia, exercise intolerance that is different from a prepregnancy state, chest pain or discomfort, dyspnea that is unrelated to pregnancy, pica, or other symptoms that may indicate an underlying cause.

OBJECTIVE

Vital signs and physical examination, with attention to the thyroid and cardiac and pulmonary systems, should be normal. Weight gain during the pregnancy should be noted. A CBC and thyroid function tests (TSH and free T_4) are reasonable choices for screening. Other laboratory tests should be conducted as indicated by history or physical exam findings.

DIFFERENTIAL DIAGNOSES

Fatigue due to pregnancy, anemia, thyroid disorder, or other pathological states.

Genitourinary Complaints

Urinary frequency is often at the top of the list of common pregnancy complaints. The kidneys change in size and shape as early as 16 weeks of gestation (Clarke, 2002). Renal enlargement may originally be caused by increased tone and decreased smooth muscle motility, but, after 20 weeks of gestation, it is caused by ureter compression that is the result of a growing uterus. Increases in circulating fluid volume and glomerular filtration rate may contribute to urinary frequency (Hawkins, 2002). During the first trimester, the weight of the growing uterus begins to cause pressure on the bladder. Uterine displacement of the bladder by the end of the second trimester can result in urinary frequency and incontinence. Urinary infections and risk of trauma is greater owing to increased bladder tone relaxation, enlarged bladder capacity, increased bladder pressure, and increased edema of the bladder mucosa.

Urinary Frequency

SUBJECTIVE

The pregnant woman may complain of increased urination or nocturia. Worrisome symptoms include fever, back or flank pain, suprapubic pain, dysuria, urgency, hematuria, dark or cloudy urine, polyuria, polyphagia, or polydipsia.

OBJECTIVE

Vital signs should be normal. An abdominal exam should rule out any uterine contractions or irritability. There should be no CVA or suprapubic tenderness. Complete blood count and glucose levels should be within normal limits. Urine dipstick, urinalysis, and culture and sensitivity tests should be normal.

DIFFERENTIAL DIAGNOSES

Pregnancy-related urinary frequency, UTI, pyelonephritis, kidney stone, diabetes.

Urinary Incontinence

SUBJECTIVE

The main complaint is an involuntary loss of urine that may be associated with coughing, sneezing, or laughing. The increased intraabdominal pressure caused by these actions, along with the enlarging uterus, results in pressure on the bladder, thus leading to incontinence. Multigravidas may experience incontinence more often because of poor perineal muscle tone. Special attention should be given to fluid that does not smell like urine, that increases with lying down, or that gushes with initial standing. These patterns of fluid release may indicate rupture of membranes.

OBJECTIVE

Abdominal exam should rule out any uterine contractions or irritability. Vaginal exam should not reveal any amniotic fluid pooling. Nitrazine and fern tests can differentiate between vaginal discharge and amniotic fluid. A sterile cotton-tipped applicator is used to place vaginal discharge on either nitrazine paper or on a clean microscope slide. If the nitrazine paper changes color and indicates a pH of 7, the discharge may be amniotic fluid. With a fern test, the discharge is allowed to dry on the slide and examined under a microscope. Amniotic fluid forms a fernlike pattern.

DIFFERENTIAL DIAGNOSES

Stress urinary incontinence, rupture of membranes, leukorrhea, vaginitis.

Circulatory Complaints

The initial increase in cardiac output that occurs during pregnancy begins as early as 10 weeks of gestation and peaks at 20–24 weeks. There is an overall increase in blood volume that results in an increased venous pressure below the level of the uterus. This increased pressure can result in varicosities in the legs and perineum (hemorrhoids), especially when the pregnant woman is in an upright position, such as with prolonged sitting or standing. An enlarging uterus compresses the vena cava or pelvic and lower extremity veins leading to venous pooling, which can result in edema, hypotension, dizziness, or even syncope. In order to lessen these complications, the pregnant woman should be instructed not to lie in a supine or recumbent position, but rather in a left lateral tilt. Nasal capillaries may become engorged with blood, leading to nasal congestion or even epistaxis (see also the nasal congestion discussion in this chapter's subsection Respiratory Complaints).

Dizziness or Syncope

SUBJECTIVE

A feeling of dizziness or being faint may be reported when the woman is standing, lying on her back, or changing positions. Information on caloric and fluid intake as well as substance abuse should be elicited. Disorientation to spatial relation (may report either that she feels like she is spinning or that the room is spinning) may be described. The practitioner should ask about precipitating and associated factors, such as micturition, defecation, hyperventilation, coughing, dyspnea, chest pain, palpitations or exposure to a stressful event.

OBJECTIVE

Vital signs with postural (orthostatic) blood pressures, and physical examination, including hydration status and ear, nose, and throat exam, should be normal for gestational age. The CBC should be negative for anemia. Blood glucose, urine specific gravity, and electrolytes should be normal.

DIFFERENTIAL DIAGNOSES

Compression of the vena cava, orthostatic hypotension, dehydration, anemia, hypoglycemia, hyperventilation, psychosocial stress, inner ear or sinus disease, substance abuse, neurological disorders, cardiopulmonary disorders, situational dizziness.

Edema

SUBJECTIVE

Swelling that worsens as the day progresses and that gets better after rest and elevation is generally reported by pregnant women. Edema may be worse during warm weather or after prolonged sitting or standing. The woman should be questioned on the use of any type of constrictive clothing, such as pantyhose, girdles, or tight belts; nutrition, especially sodium and sugar intake; and medication use. There should be no numbness, strength or sensation loss, mental status changes, report of headaches, flashing lights, upper abdominal pain, nausea or vomiting, dyspnea, decreased fetal movement, or decreased urine output.

OBJECTIVE

Vitals signs, especially blood pressure, should be normal for gestational age. Abnormal blood pressure readings that need to be evaluated include 1) 120/75 mm Hg or higher in mid-pregnancy, 2) 130/85 mm Hg in the last trimester, 3) a systolic rise of 30 mmHg or diastolic rise of 15 mmHg over baseline, or 4) a variation of 20 or more in postural (orthostatic) blood pressures (Lindheimer & Akbari, 2000). The woman's weight gain should be noted. An increase of more than 2 pounds per week should be investigated. Cardiac and pulmonary status should be evaluated. Deep tendon reflexes should be normal and urine dipstick should be negative or no greater than a trace for protein. The location, amount, and extent of the edema should be documented. Worrisome symptoms include edema that does not respond to rest and leg elevation, rapidly progressing or generalized edema, hard or painful veins or legs. and temperature changes to the extremities.

DIFFERENTIAL DIAGNOSES

Uncomplicated pregnancy-related lower extremity edema; preeclampsia; hemolysis, elevated liver enzymes, low platelets (HELLP) syndrome; superficial varicosities; phlebitis, renal, or liver disease; local trauma or infection in an extremity; CHF.

PREGNANCY COMPLICATIONS

Anemia

Anemia is not a disease unto itself, but is rather a sign of an underlying disorder. Although the occurrence rate of anemia among pregnant women is not well known, it is thought to be somewhere between 20% and 60% (Yancy, 2004). Anemia can be defined either clinically as a decrease in the oxygen-carrying capacity of the blood or based on laboratory parameters as a decrease in the hemoglobin level or amount of red blood cells (RBCs). The normal hemoglobin for females is 12–16 g/dL. However, this may decrease to 11 g/dL during the first and third trimesters and to 10.5 g/dL in the second trimester (Pagana & Pagana, 1999; CDC] 1990). Anemia during pregnancy is associated with high-output congestive heart failure, premature delivery, low birth weight, and fetal demise.

The first step after evaluating the hemoglobin and identifying the presence of anemia is to evaluate the RBC indices. The mean corpuscular volume (MCV) classifies the average volume, or size, of a single RBC. The MCV can be calculated by dividing the hematocrit by the RBC and multiplying by 10. The mean corpuscular hemoglobin concentration (MCHC) measures the average concentration or percentage of hemoglobin within a single RBC. If this value is not reported within the complete blood count (CBC), it can easily be determined by dividing the hemoglobin by the hematocrit and multiplying this number by 100. The RBC size distribution width (RDW) is an indirect measurement that indicates the degree of homogeneity of the RBC sample. Uniform RBCs will have a normal RDW, whereas a heterogeneous sample of RBCs (i.e., a sample containing some small and some normal RBCs) will have an increased RDW.

The etiology of the anemia can be classified according to the size and color of the RBCs (Table 18-5). The normal MCV is 80–100 fL and determines whether the anemia can be classified as normocytic, microcytic (below 80 fL), or macrocytic (above 100 fL). The normal MCHC is 32%–36% but should validated by a laboratory's normal range, and determines whether the anemia can be categorized as normochromic, hypochromic (under 32%), or hyperchromic (above 36%). The primary purpose of the MCHC is to identify normochromic or hypochromic causes of anemia. Hyperchromic anemia is somewhat unusual and warrants a referral to a hematologist.

The anemias most often diagnosed during pregnancy are folic acid and iron deficiency anemia (IDA). The principle etiologies for these anemias are inadequate nutrition, especially among women in lower socioeconomic groups, and the increased body requirements of pregnancy. The prevalence for IDA is 3.5%–7.4% during the first trimester and may increase to 15%–55% during the last trimester (Mandell, 1999). If IDA is suspected on the basis of a CBC (low hemoglobin and low RBC indices), iron studies should be attained. These iron studies will generally reveal a low serum iron level, decreased serum ferritin,

Table 18-5. ■ Common Causes of Anemia

Normocytic (MCV 80–100 fL) Normochromic (MCHC 32%–36%)	Microcytic (MCV < 80 fL) Hypochromic (MCHC < 32%)	Microcytic (MCV < 80 fL) Normochromic (MCHC 32%–36%)	Macrocytic (MCV > 100 fL) Normochromic (MCHC 32%–36%)
• Iron deficiency (detected early) • Chronic disease • Acute blood loss • Dilutional • Aplastic anemia • Acquired hemolytic anemias (e.g., from prosthetic heart valves) • Dilutional (physiologic) anemia of pregnancy	• Iron deficiency (detected late) • Thalassemia • Lead poisoning • Neoplasms	• Renal disease	• Vitamin B_{12}/folate deficiency • Chemotherapy • Hypothyroidism • Chronic liver disease

increased total iron-binding capacity, and decreased transferrin saturation percentage. Anemia of chronic disease may be confused with IDA when the anemia is microcytic, but will display low serum iron and total iron-binding capacity.

Folate is needed for normal DNA production, but the body stores of folate are limited to a 3-month reserve and may be depleted during high rates of cell turnover, such as during pregnancy. A folate level should be checked if the CBC suggests that a macrocytic anemia (low hemoglobin level and an MCV of >100) is the cause.

SUBJECTIVE

Fatigue, dyspnea on exertion.

OBJECTIVE

Skin pallor, tachycardia, grade II/VI systolic heart murmur, increased respiratory rate, CBC, iron panel, folate level, sickle cell screen or hemoglobin electrophoresis, liver function tests.

DIFFERENTIAL DIAGNOSES

Iron deficiency, folate deficiency, vitamin B_{12} deficiency, sickle cell trait/anemia, thalassemia.

Gestational Diabetes

Diabetes is a group of metabolic disorders that is characterized by hyperglycemia resulting from defects in insulin secretion, insulin action, or both. Gestational diabetes (GDM) involves glucose intolerance that develops or is first discovered during pregnancy and, hence, may include women who have undiagnosed pregestational diabetes. Gestational diabetes complicates 2%–5% of all pregnancies, and women who have GDM are at an estimated 20%–50% increased risk of progression to chronic diabetes later in life (Baxley & Gobbo, 2001; ACOG, 2001).

Screening for gestational diabetes remains controversial. Screening and treatment of gestational diabetes can reduce the rate of fetal macrosomia and fetal mortality but does not appear to reduce other adverse outcomes, such as cesarean delivery rate, birth injury, or the woman's perception of her health. Recommendations vary on whether and to what degree screenings are needed (Table 18-6).

Table 18-6. ■ Gestational Diabetes Screening Recommendations

Universal Screening	Risk Factor-Based Screening	No Recommendation for Screening
• World Health Organization • Third International Conference on Gestational Diabetes	• American Diabetes Association • American College of Obstetricians and Gynecologists • Society of Maternal–Fetal Medicine	• U.S. Preventive Services Task Force • Canadian Task Force on the Periodic Examination

Note: This list is not all inclusive, but rather a sampling of organizations that support each recommendation.

Selective screening of women with risk factors for GDM has a high sensitivity, but low specificity. In other words, it would identify 90% of all pregnant women at increased risk for GDM while falsely identifying others without the condition. Universal screening continues to be widely practiced within the United States between 24 and 28 weeks of gestation with a 50-g 1-hour glucola test using a venous blood sample. An alternative to the glucola is to have the woman eat 18 jelly beans within a 5-minute period (Baxley & Gobbo, 2001). There are two thresholds for an abnormal test: 1) a venous plasma glucose cutoff of 130 mg/dL will identify over 90% of the women who will have a subsequent positive 100-g 3-hour oral glucose tolerance test (OGTT) or 2) a cutoff of 140 mg/dL will detect 80% of women who will have a subsequent abnormal OGTT but will decrease the number of false positives (U.S. PSTF, 1996). A 1-hour screening blood sugar of ≥190 mg/dL may negate the need for a 3-hour OGTT. A fasting blood sugar (FBS) should be checked and if the FBS is elevated (above 95–105 mg/dL), the woman should be considered as having GDM. If the FBS is under 95 mg/dL, a 3-hour OGTT should still be done.

Unfortunately, there remains no universally accepted "gold standard" for diagnosing GDM, and North America and Europe are using different diagnostic test criteria. The measures used in the United States are based on a 100-g 3-hour OGTT. These criteria were originally developed to identify mothers at risk for developing diabetes, but not those women whose newborns were at risk for complications, such as macrosomia. Whereas various expert groups in the United States have proposed different diagnostic values and all predict to some extent newborn complication risk, there is no evidence to date to support any one diagnostic standard (Table 18-7).

The 3-hour OGTT is usually administered after an overnight fast for at least 8, but not more than 14, hours. A fasting blood sugar is obtained, and then a 100-g glucose load is given. Venous blood sugar samples are then obtained at 1, 2, and 3 hours after the glucose load. Either an elevated FBS or two elevated values on the 3-hour OGTT is diagnostic of GDM. If only one value on the OGTT is elevated, the test should be repeated between 32 and 34 weeks of gestation.

SUBJECTIVE

The woman may be asymptomatic throughout the entire pregnancy or may report classic episodes of polyuria, polyphagia, or polydipsia. She may experience more episodes of

Table 18-7. ■ Three-hour OGTT in Pregnancy (Most Common Values Used)

Item	National Diabetes Data Group (1979) (Venous plasma)	Carpenter and Coustan (1982) (Venous plasma)	O'Sullivan and Mahan (1964) (Venous whole blood)
Fasting (mg/dL)	105	95	90
1 hr (mg/dL)	190	180	165
2 hr (mg/dL)	165	155	145
3 hr (mg/dL)	145	140	125

Note: Using a standard 100-g glucose load. Fasting and 2-h levels are most predictive, but diagnosis requires elevation in any two or more values.

UTIs or vaginitis; therefore, recurrent infections should signal an earlier screening for diabetes or at least a random glucose level. Prior obstetric history should be investigated for unexplained stillbirths, spontaneous abortions, unexplained preterm birth, low-birth-weight infant (with undiagnosed preexisting diabetes), newborn weighing 4000 g or more, or a previous incident of major congenital abnormality. Family history should be explored for diabetes, including gestational diabetes.

OBJECTIVE

Maternal age and weight should be noted because major risk factors include an age over 35 years or a pre-pregnancy weight of more than 200 pounds. Excessive weight gain during pregnancy or a fundal height greater than expected is also worrisome. The blood pressure should be noted because diabetics have a predisposition to hypertensive disorders, including preeclampsia. A retinal exam should be completed to assess for retinopathy. A urine dipstick should be evaluated for glycosuria and proteinuria.

DIFFERENTIAL DIAGNOSES

Gestational diabetes mellitus (DM), undiagnosed Type 1 DM or Type 2 DM, hyperglycemia, macrosomia, recurrent UTI or vaginitis (not related to DM).

Hypertension

Hypertensive problems must be identified early and treated promptly during pregnancy to ensure good maternal and neonatal outcomes. Hypertensive disorders occur in 6%–8% of all pregnancies and are the second leading cause of maternal deaths in the United States (NHBPEP, 2000). High blood pressure can occur in pregnancy in one of four ways (Table 18-8). The term "pregnancy-induced hypertension" is no longer used because it does not differentiate between gestational hypertension, which is relatively benign, and the more serious preeclampsia (NHBPEP, 2000). The treatment, prognosis, and effect that elevated blood pressure has on pregnancy has more to do with the underlying pathology than to the actual elevation in pressure (Peters & Flack, 2004).

The diastolic pressure usually drops by an average of 10 mm of Hg below nonpregnant levels by mid-pregnancy and then slowly returns to nonpregnant levels in the third trimester (Poole, 2004). Determination of the woman's nonpregnant blood pressure is important in the evaluation of blood pressure during pregnancy. If the systolic blood pressure increases by more than 30 mm Hg or the diastolic increases by more than 15 mm Hg over baseline, preeclampsia may still occur even if the blood pressure is still within the accepted "normal" range. A certain degree of caution should also be displayed for women with a blood pressure of 120/75 mm Hg or higher in mid-pregnancy or 130/85 mm Hg in later pregnancy (Lindheimer & Akbari, 2000).

SUBJECTIVE

This condition may occur without the woman's awareness. Symptoms may include headache, visual disturbances, edema, heartburn, abdominal pain, and altered mental status.

OBJECTIVE

Evaluation should include the presence of edema, blood pressure measurement, urine dip for proteinuria, reflex testing, retinal changes, hepatomegaly, or right upper quadrant tenderness.

Table 18-8. ■ Blood Pressure Classification in Pregnancy (National High Blood Pressure Education Program, NHBPEP)

NHBPEP Classification	Description
Chronic hypertension	• Hypertension preceding conception, or before the 20th week of gestation. • Usually defined as BP ≥ 140/90 mm Hg.
Preeclampsia–Eclampsia	• A pregnancy-specific systemic syndrome.
Preeclampsia	• Systemic disease with hypertension accompanied by proteinuria after the 20th week of gestation. • May also be diagnosed without proteinuria if there are other systemic symptoms (e.g., visual changes, headache, abdominal pain, abnormal laboratory values).
Eclampsia	• Convulsive stage of the disease; seizures cannot be attributed to other causes.
Preeclampsia superimposed on chronic HTN	• Women who are hypertensive before the 20th week of gestation who develop new-onset proteinuria. • Women with both hypertension and proteinuria before 20 weeks of gestation. • Sudden increase in BP in women who previously had controlled HTN. • Women with thrombocytopenia ($<100,000$ cells/mm^3) and elevated liver enzymes (alanine aminotransferase [ALT] or aspartate aminotransferase [AST]. • Most often associated with the most severe maternal–fetal complications. • Prognosis is much worse than for either condition alone.
Gestational hypertension	• High blood pressure detected for the first time after mid-pregnancy, without proteinuria. • Diagnosis is made postpartum.
Transient HTN	• Elevated blood pressure that occurs without proteinuria late in pregnancy or in the early puerperium, but returns to normal by 12 weeks postpartum.
Chronic gestational HTN	• Blood pressure remains elevated beyond 12 weeks postpartum, but without evidence of preeclampsia.

From National High Blood Pressure Education Program Working Group. Working group report on high blood pressure in pregnancy. (NHBPEP Publication No. 00-3029). Washington, DC: National Heart Lung and Blood Institute, 2000.

DIFFERENTIAL DIAGNOSES

Chronic hypertension (HTN), transient HTN, gestational hypertension, preeclampsia, eclampsia, HELLP syndrome, disseminated intravascular coagulation.

Vaginal Bleeding

Approximately one-fourth of early pregnancies are complicated by vaginal bleeding, and about half of these will end in spontaneous abortion (Deutchman, 2001). Single or serial qualitative hCG levels can be helpful in evaluating vaginal bleeding during early pregnancy because the levels should double every 2–3 days during the fourth to eighth weeks of gestation. In about 30% of all cases, vaginal bleeding that occurs during the second and third trimesters is of unknown etiology. Episodes of bleeding are noted in 10%–20% of all pregnancies and should always be considered serious and potentially life threatening (Poole, 2004).

SUBJECTIVE

Assessment questions should be directed toward any precipitating factors of bleeding (e.g., after sexual intercourse), the amount of vaginal bleeding (saturation of sanitary napkins and frequency with which the napkins must be changed), the quality of the vaginal bleeding (clotted versus flowing), and whether the bleeding is actually coming from the vagina or from the urethral or rectal area. The presence of low back pain, abdominal cramping, foul odor, or any passage of products of conception also should be investigated. Any history of coagulation disorders, recent antiplatelet medication use, and Rh status need to be verified. A screening for intimate partner violence should also be done.

OBJECTIVE

The vital signs should be normal for gestational age. Physical exam should concentrate on uterine size, fetal heart tones, a pelvic exam with cervix visualization, and a digital rectal exam. Other tests that may be useful include a transvaginal ultrasound, hCG level measurement, progesterone level, wet mount, urinalysis, and stool for occult blood. A complete blood count and coagulation studies should be considered.

DIFFERENTIAL DIAGNOSES

Implantation bleeding, placenta previa, abruptio placentae, uterine rupture, threatened abortion, spontaneous abortion, ectopic pregnancy, gestational trophoblastic disease, vaginal infection, foreign body retention, abdominal or vaginal trauma, blood dyscrasias, intimate partner violence.

Vaginal Infections

Observational studies have demonstrated an association between bacterial vaginosis and certain adverse pregnancy outcomes, such as preterm labor, preterm delivery, premature rupture of membranes, and spontaneous abortions. Bacterial vaginosis can be treated with antibiotic therapy, but cure rates are erratic and recurrences are common. There is currently conflicting evidence on whether screening and treatment of asymptomatic bacterial vaginosis in high-risk pregnant women actually reduces the incidence of preterm delivery. The U.S. Preventive Services Task Force (PSTF) therefore neither recommends nor discourages routinely screening these women (U.S. PSTF, 2001). However, the U.S. PSTF does state that treatment is appropriate for symptomatic bacterial vaginosis infections (such as with patient complaints of vaginal discharge). Trichomoniasis is less common than other forms of infectious vaginitis during pregnancy, but vulvovaginal candidiasis occurs in 10% of women during the first trimester and in one-third to one-half of women during the third trimester (Rein & Liang, 1999).

SUBJECTIVE

Inquire whether there have been multiple or new sexual partners, whether sexual activity has recently been resumed, whether there has been any recent douching or antibiotic use, or whether there is a history of abnormal Papanicolaou (Pap) smears. Further assessment should explore the presence of any vaginal discharge, perineal or vaginal sores or lesions, or UTI symptoms. Worrisome symptoms include excessive, malodorous, discolored, itchy, or irritating vaginal discharge; fever; abdominal pain; dysuria; or bleeding or pain after sexual intercourse.

OBJECTIVE

The examination should begin with an inspection of the external genitalia. A pelvic exam should assess for vaginal discharge, signs of vaginal infections (including herpes), and any other vaginal or cervical abnormalities. A normal saline and potassium hydroxide test (wet mount) should be conducted from secretions of the vaginal pool to check for fungal organisms, trichomonas, clue cells, and bacteria. A gonorrhea and chlamydia specimen for culture should be obtained. A nitrazine or fern test should be done to evaluate for rupture of membranes. A Pap smear should be done if it has not been done previously in the initial obstetrical evaluation to assess for dysplasia, carcinoma, or human papillomavirus.

DIFFERENTIAL DIAGNOSES

Leukorrhea, vaginitis, cervicitis, gonorrhea, chlamydia, UTI, rupture of membranes, condyloma acuminatum, genital herpes, or cervical dysplasia or neoplasia.

Urinary Tract Infections

Urinary tract infections consist of either cystitis, an infection in the bladder, or pyelonephritis, an infection in the kidneys. Cystitis occurs in about 1%–2% of the pregnant population, and cultures usually grow out a single pathogen, typically *Escherichia coli* or a species from the genera *Staphylococcus*, *Proteus*, *Klebsiella*, or *Pseudomonas* (Moran, 2004). Untreated UTIs and pyelonephritis may result in preterm labor and delivery, maternal sepsis, or even septic shock and death.

Asymptomatic bacteriuria may be present in 2%–10% of pregnancies and is diagnosed by the growth of 10^5 colonies per milliliter of a single pathogen that is cultured from a clean-voided urinary specimen (Ratcliffe, 2001). This may be indicative of an underlying disorder, such as an anatomic urinary tract abnormality or chronic pyelonephritis. Asymptomatic bacteriuria may lead to pyelonephritis and is associated with an increased risk of preterm labor and low-birth-weight babies.

SUBJECTIVE

Inquiries should be made about the presence of risk factors (frequent/recurrent UTIs, diabetes, urinary tract abnormalities, sexually transmitted diseases). Inquire also about any urgency, frequency, dysuria, suprapubic pain, abnormal urinary flow pattern, discolored or malodorous urine, fever, chills, flank pain. or GI complaints.

OBJECTIVE

Evaluation includes documented fever, clean catch urine, pelvic exam/wet mount (for vaginal infections), costovertebral angle or suprapubic tenderness, urine culture, CBC, and signs of shock (tachycardia, hypotension, and pallor).

DIFFERENTIAL DIAGNOSES

Cystitis, pyelonephritis, asymptomatic bacteriuria, urethritis, vulvovaginitis, sexually transmitted diseases, preterm labor, renal stones.

Size Not Equal to Dates

A fetus may be found to be of a size that is not commensurate with normal growth rates (size not equal to dates) when the uterine size is measured and evaluated during routine prenatal visits. First-trimester uterine sizes are usually determined with bimanual examination, and size–date discrepancies are often not clinically relevant. After 20 weeks of gestation, fundal height measurements begin to correlate (within 2 cm) with gestational age. The fundus should be at the level of the umbilicus at 20 weeks of gestation, and it rises 1 cm per week until 32 weeks of gestation. False small-for-dates presentations may result from inaccurate last menstrual period dates, varying menstrual cycle lengths, improper fundal height measurement, or a fetus in a transverse lie. False large-for-dates presentations may likewise be produced by inaccurate last menstrual period dates and improper fundal height measurement, as well as maternal obesity or short stature.

Small-For-Dates

SUBJECTIVE

No subjective complaints are usually expressed by the pregnant woman; however, she may state that she does not appear as "big" as her gestational age. A 24-hour diet recall should be done.

OBJECTIVE

Weight gain from pre-pregnancy weight should be noted. Fundal height measurements that are 3–4 cm smaller than the estimated gestational age during the 20- to 32-week gestational period require additional follow-up. Serial ultrasound examinations and measurements should be done for body ratios in order to plot growth velocity and to assess amniotic fluid volume.

DIFFERENTIAL DIAGNOSES

Intrauterine growth restriction, which affects about 5% of the general population and as much as 10% of high-risk populations (Table 18-9) (either asymmetric or symmetric), constitutionally small fetus, inaccurate pregnancy dating, improper fundal height measurement, transverse lie of the fetus, oligohydramnios.

Large-For-Dates

SUBJECTIVE

Although no subjective complaints are usually expressed, the fundal height may appear to be increased, especially in pregnant women who are obese or short in stature. The

Table 18-9. ■ High Risk Populations for Intrauterine Growth Restriction

Associated Medical Conditions	Associated Obstetric Conditions
HTN	Pregnancy-induced hypertension
Renal disease	Multiple gestation
Diabetes	Placental abnormalities
Lupus	Intrauterine infections
Sickle cell anemia	Fetal/chromosomal abnormalities
Tobacco use; substance abuse	
Malnutrition	
Maternal heart disorders, especially those with decreased cardiac output	
Thrombophilias	
Chronic lead poisoning	

woman may state that she appears "bigger" than her gestational age or that she is carrying multiple gestations. A 24-hour diet recall should be done.

OBJECTIVE

Weight gain from pre-pregnancy weight should be noted. Fundal height measurements that are 3–4 cm larger than the estimated gestational age during the 20- to 32-week gestational period require additional evaluation. Serial ultrasound examinations and measurements for body ratios should be done in order to plot growth velocity and to assess amniotic fluid volume. A serum glucose and urine dip should be done to evaluate for GDM.

DIFFERENTIAL DIAGNOSES

Inaccurate pregnancy dating, improper fundal height measurement, fetal macrosomia, polyhydramnios, multiple gestation, uterine leiomyoma growth, molar pregnancy, gestational diabetes, maternal obesity.

Preterm Labor

Preterm labor is the onset of labor before 37 completed weeks of gestation. The accurate diagnosis of preterm labor is critical, but often difficult. Fewer than half of the women who have four or more contractions per hour will deliver in 7–14 days of the preterm labor assessment. The diagnosis may be confirmed when there is a cervical dilatation of 3 cm or more in a woman without persistent contractions. Women who are having persistent contractions need a cervical change of at least 1 cm, a dilatation of 2 cm or more, or a positive fetal fibronectin assay for diagnosis (Bernhardt & Dorman, 2004). If the diagnosis is not confirmed, but the index of suspicion remains high, it is entirely reasonable to repeat the cervical examination at a later time. Transabdominal ultrasounds and home uterine activity monitoring have also been used in an effort to identify preterm labor but with mixed results.

SUBJECTIVE

The most common complaint is contractions. The contractions should be evaluated for regularity, consistency, and location. Symptoms of preterm labor include pelvic pressure; a low, dull backache; menstrual-like cramps; a change or increase in vaginal discharge; uterine contractions that occur every 10 minutes or more frequently, with or without pain; intestinal cramping, with or without diarrhea; and contractions that do not resolve with rest and hydration. A history review should concentrate on any previous preterm labor/delivery and a determination of the gestational age. A complete review of systems should be accomplished to screen for precipitating conditions, such as cholecystitis or viral gastroenteritis.

OBJECTIVE

Screening should be done for infection (urinalysis, gonorrhea, chlamydia, syphilis, Group B streptococcus, bacterial vaginosis), urine specific gravity to assess for hydration status, nitrazine testing to assess for rupture of membranes, fetal fibronectin testing (should be done before a digital cervical exam), ultrasound cervical length examination, serial cervical examinations, and drug screening. Fetal fibronectin testing and cervical length evaluation both have a high negative predictive value and are therefore better at predicting when preterm delivery is unlikely to occur as opposed to when delivery will occur (Bernhardt & Dorman, 2004).

DIFFERENTIAL DIAGNOSES

Preterm (true) labor, false labor, maternal dehydration, infectious etiologies (either urinary, vaginal, or sexually transmitted), incompetent cervix, premature rupture of membranes.

Summary

As stated at the beginning of this chapter, pregnancy should be considered a wellness condition and not a disease entity. Advanced practice nurses should tailor their education and interventions to the assessment of the pregnant woman and routinely reassess the clinical situation for any changes. Caring for pregnant women is well within the advanced practice nursing model and advanced practice nurses should know what is needed, what they can provide, and when to refer.

References

ACOG. (2001). Clinical practice guidelines for obstetrician-gynecologists. *Obstetrics and Gynecology* 98 (3), 525–538.

Baxley, E.G. (2001). Patient and family education. Section E. Physiologic changes and common discomforts of pregnancy. In Ratcliffe, S.D., Baxley, E.G., Byrd, J.E., & Sakornbut, E.L. (Eds.), *Family Practice Obstetrics* (2nd ed.). Philadelphia: Hanley & Belfus.

Baxley, E.G., & Gobbo, R. (2001). Complications of pregnancy. Section A. Gestational diabetes. In Ratcliffe, S.D., Baxley, E.G., Byrd, J.E., & Sakornbut, E.L. (Eds.), *Family Practice Obstetrics* (2nd ed.). Philadelphia: Hanley & Belfus.

Bond, L. (2004). Physiology of pregnancy. In S. Mattson & J.E. Smith, (Eds), *Core Curriculum for maternal-newborn nursing* (3rd ed., 96–123). St. Louis: Elsevier Saunders

Bernhardt, J. & Dorman, K. (2004). Pre-term birth risk assessment tools: Exploring fetal fibronectin and cervical length for validating risk. *Lifelines* 8 (1), 38–44.

Byrd, J. (2001). Content of prenatal care. In Ratcliffe, S.D., Baxley, E.G., Byrd, J.E., & Sakornbut, E.L. (Eds.), *Family Practice Obstetrics* (2nd ed.). Philadelphia: Hanley & Belfus.Carpenter, M.W. & Coustan. D.R. (1982). Criteria for screening tests for gestational diabetes. *American Journal of Obstetrics and Gynecology 144*, 768–773.

CDC. (1990). Progress in chronic disease prevention anemia during pregnancy in low-income women—United States, 1987. *MMWR* 39 (5), 73–76,81.

Clarke, K. (2002). Normal pregnancy. In Littleton, L.Y., & Engebretson, J.C. (Eds.), *Maternal, Neonatal, and Women's Health Nursing*. Albany, NY: Delmar.

Deutchman, M. (2001). Diagnosis and management of first-trimester complications. In Ratcliffe, S.D. Baxley, E.G., Byrd, J.E., & Sakornbut, E.L. (Eds.), *Family Practice Obstetrics* (2nd ed., pp. 129–142). Philadelphia: Hanley & Belfus.

Hawkins, C. (2002). Management and nursing care of the pregnant women. In Littleton, L.Y., & Engebretson, J.C. (Eds.), *Maternal, Neonatal, and Women's Health Nursing*. Albany, NY: Delmar.

Lindheimer, M.D., & Akbari, A. (2000). Hypertension in pregnant. In Oparil, S. & Weber, M.A. (Eds.), *Hypertension: A Companion to Brenner and Rector's* The Kidney. Philadelphia: W.B. Saunders.

Mandell, E. (1999). Anemias. In Buttaro, T.H., Trybulski, J. Bailey, P.P., & Sandberg-Cook, J. (Eds.), *Primary Care: A Collaborative Practice*. St. Louis: Mosby.

National Diabetes Data Group (1979). Classification and diagnosis of diaetes mellitus and other categories of glucose intolerance. *Diabetes* 28, 1039–1057.

NHBPEP. (2000). Working group report on high blood pressure in pregnancy. (NHBPEP Publication No. 00–3029). Washington, DC: National Heart, Lung, and Blood Institute.

O'Sullivan, J.B., & Mahan, C.M. (1964). Criteria for the oral glucose tolerance test in pregnancy. *Diabetes* 13, 278–285.

Padua, L., Aprile, I., Caliandro, P., Carboni, T., Meloni, A., Massi, S., Mazza, O., Mondelli, M., Morini, A., Murasecco, D., Romano, M., & Tonali, P. (2001). Symptoms and neurophysiological picture of carpal tunnel syndrome in pregnancy. *Clinical Neurophysiology,* 112(10), 1946–1951.

Pagana, K.D., & Pagana, T.J. (1999). *Mosby's Diagnostic and Laboratory Test Reference* (4th ed.) St. Louis: Mosby.

Pandolfino, J., & Vanagunas, A. (2000). Gastrointestinal complications of pregnancy. *Hospital Physician* 6 (4), 1–14.

Peters, R.M., & Flack, J.M. (2004). Hypertensive disorders of pregnancy. *JOGNN* 33 (2), 209–220.

Poole, J. D. (2004). Hemorrhagic disorders. In Mattson, S., & Smith, J.E. (Eds.), *Core Curriculum for Maternal-Newborn Nursing* (3rd ed., 630–659). St. Louis: Elsevier Saunders.

Rein, M.F., & Liang, B.A. (1999). Diagnosis and treatment of infectious vaginitis. *Hospital Physician,* 35 (10), 46–58.

Raines, D. A. (2002). Evaluation of fetal well-being. In Littleton, L.Y. & Engebretson, J.C. (Eds.), *Maternal, Neonatal, and Women's Health Nursing* (pp. 644–674). Albany, NY: Delmar.

Ratcliffe, S.D. (2001). Commonly encountered medical problems in pregnancy. Section A. Infections in pregnancy. In Ratcliffe, S.D. Baxley, E.G. Byrd, J.E. & Sakornbut, E.L. (Eds.), *Family Practice Obstetrics* (2nd ed., pp. 241–288). Philadelphia: Hanley & Belfus.

Reymunde, A., Santiago, N., & Perez, L. (2001). *Helicobacter pylori* and severe morning sickness. *American Journal of Gastroenterology,* 96(7), 2279–2280.

Turok, D., & Schultz, T. (2001). Chronic medical conditions in pregnancy. Section I. Endocrine problems. In Ratcliffe, S.D., Baxley, E.G., Byrd, J.E., & Sakornbut, E.L. (Eds.), *Family Practice Obstetrics* (2nd ed.). Philadelphia: Hanley & Belfus.

U.S. PSTF. (1996). Screening for gestational diabetes. In *Guide to Clinical Preventive Services* (2nd ed.). Washington, D.C.: Office of Disease Prevention and Health Promotion.

Viera, A. J. (2003). Management of carpal tunnel syndrome. *American Family Physician,* 68 (7), 265–72, 279–280.

Weimer, L.H., Yin, J., Lovelace, R.E., & Gooch, C.L. (2002). Serial studies of carpal tunnel syndrome during and after pregnancy. *Muscle Nerve,* 25 (6), 914–917.

Wotring, R. (2004). Environmental hazards. In Mattson, S. & Smith, J.E. (Eds.), *Core Curriculum for Maternal-Newborn Nursing* (3rd ed., 201–224). St. Louis: Elsevier Saunders.

 # SUGGESTED READINGS

Adams, S.L. (1998). Urinary tract infections in pregnant women. In Collins-Bride, G.M. & Saxe, J.M. (Eds.), *Nurse Practitioner/Physician Collaborative Practice: Clinical Guidelines for Ambulatory Care.* San Francisco: UCSF Nursing Press.

Barron, W.M., & Lindheimer, M.D. (1995). Management of hypertension during pregnancy. In Largh, J.H., & Brenner, B.M. (Eds.), *Hypertension: Pathophysiology, Diagnosis, and Management* (2nd ed.). New York: Raven Press.

Corder-Mabe, J. (1998). Complications of pregnancy. In Youngkin, E.Q., & Davis, M.S. (Eds.), *Women's Health: A Primary Care Clinical Guide* (2nd ed.). Stamford, CN: Appleton & Lange.

Iams, J.D. (2003). Prediction and detection of early preterm labor. *Obstetrics and Gynecology* 101, 402–412.

Mulley, Jr., A.G., & Goroll, A.H. (1995). Screening for anemia. In Goroll, A.H., May, L.A.,

& Mulley, Jr., A.G. (Eds.), *Primary Care Medicine: Office Evaluation and Management of the Adult Patient* (3rd ed.). Philadelphia: Lippincott-Raven.

Remich, M.C. (1998). Promoting a healthy pregnancy. In Youngkin, E.Q., & Davis, M.S. (Eds.), *Women's Health: A Primary Care Clinical Guide* (2nd ed.). Stamford, CN: Appleton & Lange.

Stanford, J.B., & Hobbins, D. (2001). Obstetric risk assessment. Section A. Preconception risk assessment. In Ratcliffe, S.D., Baxley, E.G., Byrd, J.E., & Sakornbut, E.L. (Eds.), *Family Practice Obstetrics* (2nd ed.). Philadelphia: Hanley & Belfus.

U.S. PSTF. (2001). Screening high-risk pregnant women for bacterial vaginosis. In *Guide to Clinical Preventive Services* (2nd ed.). Washington, D.C.: Office of Disease Prevention and Health Promotion.

Zinaman, M.J., Clegg, E., Brown, C.C., O'Connor, J., & Selevan, S.G. (1996). Estimates of human fertility and pregnancy loss. *Fertility & Sterility* 65, 503–509.

Chapter 19

Older Patients

T he comprehensive assessment of elderly individuals requires an understanding of the physiologic changes of normal aging as well as the complex interplay between those changes, disease, and functional status. The process of performing these assessments may need to be adapted based on the frailty of the individual and the setting in which the assessment occurs. Finally, there are some well-recognized "syndromes" that either present in unusual ways or are rarely addressed in the typical clinical encounter that require diligent investigation to prevent functional decline in the elderly. All of these factors contribute to the complexity of the comprehensive geriatric assessment and, furthermore, argue for a multidisciplinary approach in geriatrics.

This chapter addresses these issues by focusing on the concept of functional assessment, from its basic components to highly integrated aspects of role functioning, using the hierarchical model developed by the National Institute on Aging (1993). The model, illustrated in Figure 19-1, provides a holistic view of the individual and provides a guide to management options. Functional assessment is a performance-based approach that explores how disease affects the individual; it is a useful concept in many ways. For example, in the case of elders who have little disease but significant inability to function independently, the clinician is prompted to address management options that provide support to the individual and family in order to maintain as much independence as possible. Conversely, in elders who have significant comorbidities and who have adapted to their disease burden and remain independent, a functional assessment supports management options to allow for continued role functioning.

A functional assessment determines the degree to which an individual is able to perform those activities that enable one to living independently. The basic components are those that produce specific physical movements, for example, the coordination and fine motor control required to grasp a fork or spoon. Specific movements are then required to take the grasping of the spoon to a goal-oriented activity, namely, eating a meal. A higher level of integration of the

Charon Pierson

Figure 19-1. ■ Model of a hierarchy of function (National Institute on Aging, 1993).

physical movements involved in eating with cognitive capability provides the basis for shopping for and preparing a meal or planning a holiday dinner for a larger family (Figure 19-1). Degradation in the ability to perform these tasks results in greater dependence on others and often a change in living circumstances. Dependence among the elderly has implications for society as a whole owing to the demographic shift that has been occurring in most of the developed countries of the world.

THE DEMOGRAPHICS OF AGING

According to U.S. census data, the elderly, aged 65 and older, amounted to 12.3% (35.6 million) of the population in 2002; it is estimated that number will double to about 70 million, or 20% of the population by 2030. The fastest growing group among the elderly are those over 100 years of age. Most of these centenarians are considered to be among the most vulnerable to frailty and disability, which, coupled with the likelihood that they will

Basic Components The basic components of this model are viewed as functional units that form the building blocks of a series of increasingly complex functional tasks. The basic components include strength, balance, coordination, flexibility, and endurance.

Specific Physical Movements These are movement sequences that can be achieved by the integration of two or more basic components. Examples of specific physical movements include carry, reach, bend, stoop, transfer, chair rise, walk.

Task- or Goal-Oriented Activities This level requires all of the physical movements plus varying degrees of cognitive ability to conceptualize the task and follow through to achievement of the goal. Examples of these more complex tasks or activities include the ADLs and IADLs (bathing, grooming, dressing, toileting, shopping, managing money or medications, using the telephone, doing laundry).

Role Function This is the highest level of integration and the most difficult to assess because of its complexity. In the elderly, occupational activities might be replaced by volunteer activities; however, some elderly remain fully engaged in productive occupational activities until they die. This level of integration of functional abilities implies wide-ranging engagement in life, which can occur even in the presence of serious physical disability (e.g., ALS, quadriplegia, MS) in the young as well as the old.

live alone and therefore require support services, such as nursing home care, has caused dire predictions about the failure of the Medicare and Medicaid systems. Current data indicate that only 13% of the elderly population account for 90% of all nursing home expenditures; however, 44% of those who use nursing homes after age 65 start and end as private payers, and 14% spend down their assets to become eligible for Medicaid (http://www.elder-web.com/elderstats/). This increase in the elderly population is occurring worldwide and the projected socioeconomic impact on societies is of great concern to researchers, policymakers, and providers.

As the number of frail and dependent elderly increase, there will certainly be a concomitant rise in the proportion of those who are disabled. The Administration on Aging projects that the percentage of the population with limitations in performing the activities of daily living (ADL) will increase from the current 20% to at least 21.4% using the most optimistic ratios of disability to longevity. Associated with these ADL limitations is the need for home- and community-based or institutional services. The level of services required will largely be determined by psychosocial and economic factors along with medical necessity, all of which should be determined through a comprehensive and perhaps multidisciplinary patient assessment. It is important to remember that aging is a life process that in and of itself does not inevitably produce functional decline.

THE APPROACH TO THE ASSESSMENT OF OLDER INDIVIDUALS

Older individuals are characterized by their heterogeneity; therefore, clinicians must adapt their approaches based on the setting (outpatient, inpatient, or home), on the presenting complaint, and on the capabilities or limitations of the individual. In general, the elderly will have more physical complaints, comorbidities, more medications, and longer medical and surgical histories than a younger person. Information about childhood immunizations may not be relevant, such as for those born before childhood immunizations were developed, and information about family history may not be complete. Certain components of the past history will be more relevant, such as occupational history; military service in wartime; environmental exposures; and functional changes in sensory, physical, or cognitive abilities over time. Lifestyle issues, such as habits, driving ability, nutrition, social support networks, and sleep and elimination patterns require particular attention. Advanced care planning, particularly advanced health care directives and designation of durable power of attorney for health care decisions, should be addressed with regular opportunities for discussion of changing priorities and status of significant members of the family (e.g., death of the spouse, who was the designated decision-maker for health care). Losses, including loss of capability and independence as well as the loss of friends and family, become more frequent with aging. It is important to provide opportunities to discuss and grieve for such losses as frequently as possible during routine health care encounters.

The approach to the physical examination of older adults will not differ greatly from standard examination techniques presented in this text. There are some tests of functional ability that are not routinely considered in the usual examination of the adult; those are presented in the various sections that follow. With older adults who are debilitated, it is important to focus the examination and to reduce extraneous activities and distractions. Whenever possible, begin the examination with maneuvers that can be accomplished with the patient in his or her current position. For example, when the patient arrives to the examination seated in a wheelchair, check vital signs, heart rate, extremities, or anything else that can be done in the seated position first. If a patient's ability to transfer from the wheelchair is in question, observe the transfer before the patient becomes fatigued. The exertion of getting on the examination table could fatigue an individual enough to preclude optimal performance. Likewise, perform all supine or standing examinations together to preserve the patient's stamina. A reordering of the sequence of the examination should be done in a logical and thoughtful manner.

Attend to the safety of the elder person by removing obstructing objects, providing adequate lighting, and standing in close proximity to the individual to prevent falls. Turn off background music or television if possible and speak clearly, facing the elder person, to facilitate good communication. Be aware that glare off windows and other shiny surfaces can cause discomfort as well as compromise vision during interviewing and testing.

THE PHYSIOLOGY OF AGING

A common adage indicates that aging changes consist of about one-third disease, plus one-third disuse, plus one-third normal aging. The relationships among these three factors are important but often difficult to define. Although chronological aging does produce change in biochemical processes, actual function is remarkably well maintained in humans. Most of the impact of the changes relates to a decrease in physiologic reserve, and very little of the impairment seen among elderly populations is due to actual physiologic changes in the human organism. It is probably more helpful to view aging as a continuum upon which physiological and pathological processes seem to vary infinitely within a given population.

Table 19-1 lists the major physiological changes associated with aging and the known or postulated impacts those changes have on functional or disease states. Some of these

Table 19-1. ■ Physiologic Changes of Aging and Their Impacts

Physiologic Change	Functional and Clinical Impact
Thinning of dermis and epidermis; decreased epidermal proliferation and collagen flexibility; changes in elastic fiber network	Increased skin fragility and cell irregularity; increased vulnerability to trauma and irritant dermatitis; susceptible to infection with break in epidermis; decreased elasticity; increased wrinkling and dryness; uneven pigmentation
Decreased amount of subcutaneous fat; decreased size of fat pads	Sagging of skin; decreased fat pads on soles of feet may change gait or ability to ambulate
Decreased sebaceous and eccrine gland activity; loss of hair pigment	Decreased rate of nail and hair growth; decreased sweating ability may lead to hyperthermia; thinning and graying of hair; increased susceptibility to infection
Increased threshold for pressure and touch; decreased vibratory sense in toes; decreased thermal sensitivity	Potential for injury and burns due to decreased sensation
Increased translucency and flattening of cornea; thickening and rigidity of choroid and iris; decreased production of aqueous humor; decreased mass of ciliary muscle; decreased number of rods, cones, and ganglion cells; increased yellowing and density and decreased elasticity of lens; liquefaction of vitreous body	Decreased accommodation to light intensity; impaired color discrimination; decreased night vision acuity; blurring and changes in visual acuity; pupils less reactive to light; floaters and light flashes increase; presbyopia; increased dryness; vulnerable to infection
Tympanic membrane thinner, less resilient; sclerotic changes to tympanic membrane; ossicles become calcified; pinna widens, elongates, and stiffens	Some degree of impaired auditory function; decreased sensitivity to high-frequency tones (presbycusis); ears may look larger
Decreased salivation, number of olfactory cells, and thirst	Decreased sensitivity to taste and smell; increased tendency to dehydration and undernutrition
Enlargement of alveolar duct; decreased elastic recoil; increased closing volume; loss of cilia, increased size and stiffening of trachea and bronchi; calcification of chest wall; decreased cough reflex, forced vital capacity, forced expiratory volume per second, and forced expiratory flow; increased residual volume, functional residual capacity, and residual volume/total lung capacity	Altered pulmonary function; decreased sensitivity to changes in levels of oxygen and carbon dioxide; loss of alveoli; decreased ability to clear infectious or environmental material
Increased weight of heart and vessels; left ventricular posterior wall and aortic thickness; decreased early diastolic closure rates of mitral valve; valves become more sclerotic; decreased response to beta-adrenergic stimulation	Decreased cardiac output and heart rate at rest and exercise, myocardial contractile efficiency, maximal oxygen uptake, and responsiveness to catecholamines; increased systolic pressure, left ventricular ejection time, and preejection period, stroke volume with progressive exercise, and ectopic activity; murmurs, S_4 heart sounds, and orthostatic blood pressure changes may occur

(Continued on following page)

Table 19-1. ■ Physiologic Changes of Aging and Their Impacts *(Continued)*

Physiologic Change	Functional and Clinical Impact
Decreased production of saliva, gastric juices (including intrinsic factor, peptic and hydrochloric acids); decreased gastric motility; mucosal and muscle atrophy; decreased size and activity of liver, hepatocytes, secretory acini and islets of Langerhans; decreased splenic blood flow	Decreased protection of teeth and tongue from bacteria, taste sensation, vitamins B_{12} and D, and carbohydrate absorption; protein, iron, and folic acid digestion; difficulty talking and chewing; delayed gastric emptying and maldigestion; impaired fat absorption; decreased drug metabolism and hepatic protein synthesis; decline in glucose tolerance
Decreased number of glomeruli, filtration of blood, and glomerular filtration rate as much as 30%–40%; thickened tubular membranes and fatty degeneration; stiffening and narrowing of renal vasculature; decreased expandability and compressibility of detrusor; decreased bladder sensation	Decreased clearance of medications and other waste products; decreased urine concentrating capacity; BUN and creatinine do not generally change; decreased creatinine clearance; decreased bladder capacity; increased urinary frequency and postvoid residual volume
Decreased secretion TSH and T_4, insulin, rennin, aldosterone, ACTH, growth hormone; decreased response to TRH, ACTH,	Laboratory values may change and must be interpreted carefully; stress response is not as robust
Decreased bone mass, size and number of muscle fibers; lean body mass replaced by fat	Increased incidence of microfractures, decreased lean body mass and total body water; more vulnerable to fractures, balance, and gait problems
Decreased sleep efficiency; possible decreased total sleep time; increased sleep latency; more arousal during night; decreased REM latency and total REM sleep	Increased time to fall asleep; more time in bed waiting to fall asleep; earlier awakening; more daytime napping; no increase in daytime sleepiness

Data from Blair, 1990; Cotter & Strumpf, 2002; and Alessi, 2000.

changes are easily detected, such as the age-related attrition of oocytes in the ovaries that leads to the loss of female reproductive ability. Other changes are much less obvious, such as the loss of nephrons in the kidney that may affect the ability to excrete drug metabolites. The former, loss of female reproductive ability, is inevitable after a certain age, whereas the latter, loss of nephrons, is much more complex and variable. Although the loss of nephrons may be a given, the effect of that loss on an individual's function may vary considerably based on other factors, such as disease states (e.g., hypertension) and other physiologic variables (e.g., intracellular fluid volume). Interactive effects from physiologic changes, such as the effect of declining levels of estrogen production following menopause on bone remodeling, complicate the picture. Thus, geriatric assessment is most effective when it is focused on functional impact rather than on disease states. Functional assessment allows the variability that occurs with the complex relationships among disease, disuse, and physiology to remain secondary to the development and implementation of a treatment plan.

FUNCTIONAL ASSESSMENT

Within the context of health assessment, functional assessment provides an alternative perspective on the health status of an individual. In the traditional model of health assessment taught in nurse practitioner programs, the focus is on the clinical diagnosis and the development of sound diagnostic reasoning. This medical model approach assumes that a reason for the client's presenting symptoms can be uncovered and an intervention can be instituted to cure the problem. Although some conditions are reversible in the elderly, many are not; thus, the focus of the assessment needs to be on maximizing the elderly client's function and maintaining or improving well-being.

In clinical trials, the effects of interventions on functional ability are frequently measured and reported as indicators of the quality of life. The domains of quality-of-life indicators encompass physical, emotional, spiritual, and psychosocial measures; many instruments have been developed for the purpose of measuring various indicators (Gerety, 2000). Many of these measures are self-reported; however, with elderly clients, caregiver reports and direct observations are commonly used. Moreover, measured domains frequently overlap, and it may be difficult to separate the effects that emotional or intellectual functions have on physical function. One way to overcome some of these measurement dilemmas is to use standardized performance-based measures that integrate basic components of a movement and provide the opportunity to observe a client perform a task or a goal-oriented function. This is the basis for the hierarchical model of function depicted in Figure 19-1.

Measures of Function

Two scales are commonly used to measure functional ability: the Physical Activities of Daily Living (Box 19-1) and the Instrumental Activities of Daily Living (IADL) (Box 19-2). Although both scales are relatively crude, they have been largely accepted as adequate for determining the need for assistive services and for classifying the level of care required for institutional services. Both instruments are scored based on the level of independence in performance of the task, and they both provide snapshots of a person's ability to live independently. Most health professionals accept the goal-oriented activities depicted in Figure 19-1 as minimal criteria for independent functioning in the modern world.

For the well elderly, the 10-Minute Screener for Geriatric Conditions has been recommended (American Geriatrics Society, 2003). This brief screening tool (Table 19-2) addresses vision, hearing, leg mobility, urinary incontinence, nutrition and weight loss, memory, depression, and physical disability. Using a combination of subjective and objective measures, the 10-Minute Screener covers all the basic ADL and IADL functions in a manner that fits well within the outpatient examination. A positive screen requires further evaluation, in some cases by a specialist or a geriatric specialist.

Measures of Cognitive Function

Cognitive impairment is not synonymous with dementia; therefore, a positive screen on the Mini-Cog (Box 19-3) requires a more thorough evaluation. The most commonly used screening tool for the next step in the evaluation of cognitive function, which measures more than just short- and long-term memory, is the Mini-Mental State Examination

Box 19-1

Physical Self-Maintenance Scale (Activities of Daily Living, or ADLs)

In each category, circle the item that most closely describes the person's highest level of functioning and record the score assigned to that level (either 1 or 0) in the blank at the beginning of the category.

A. Toilet
1. Care for self at toilet completely; no incontinence — 1
2. Needs to be reminded, or needs help in cleaning self, or has rare (weekly at most) accidents — 0
3. Soiling or wetting while asleep more than once a week — 0
4. Soiling or wetting while awake more than once a week — 0
5. No control of bowels or bladder — 0

B. Feeding
1. Eats without assistance — 1
2. Eats with minor assistance at meal times and/or with special preparation of food, or help in cleaning up after meals — 0
3. Feeds self with moderate assistance and is untidy — 0
4. Requires extensive assistance for all meals — 0
5. Does not feed self at all and resists efforts of others to feed him or her — 0

C. Dressing
1. Dresses, undresses, and selects clothes from own wardrobe — 1
2. Dresses and undresses self, with minor assistance — 0
3. Needs moderate assistance in dressing and selection of clothes. — 0
4. Needs major assistance in dressing, but cooperates with efforts of others to help — 0
5. Completely unable to dress self and resists efforts of others to help — 0

D. Grooming (neatness, hair, nails, hands, face, clothing)
1. Always neatly dressed, well-groomed, without assistance — 1
2. Grooms self adequately with occasional minor assistance, eg, with shaving — 0
3. Needs moderate and regular assistance or supervision with grooming — 0
4. Needs total grooming care, but can remain well-groomed after help from others — 0
5. Actively negates all efforts of others to maintain grooming — 0

E. Physical Ambulation
1. Goes about grounds or city — 1
2. Ambulates within residence on or about one block distant — 0
3. Ambulates with assistance of (check one)
   a ( ) another person, b ( ) railing, c ( ) cane, d ( ) walker, e ( ) wheelchair — 0
   1.__Gets in and out without help. 2.__Needs help getting in and out
4. Sits unsupported in chair or wheelchair, but cannot propel self without help — 0
5. Bedridden more than half the time — 0

F. Bathing
1. Bathes self (tub, shower, sponge bath) without help. — 1
2. Bathes self with help getting in and out of tub. — 0
3. Washes face and hands only, but cannot bathe rest of body — 0
4. Does not wash self, but is cooperative with those who bathe him or her. — 0
5. Does not try to wash self and resists efforts to keep him or her clean. — 0

For scoring interpretation and source, see note following the next instrument.
Scoring Interpretation: For ADLs, the total score ranges from 0 to 6, and for IADLs, from 0 to 8. In some categories, only the highest level of function receives a 1; in others, two or more levels have scores of 1 because each describes competence that represents some minimal level of function. These screens are useful for indicating specifically how a person is performing at the present time. When they are also used over time, they serve as documentation of a person's functional improvement or deterioration.

Republished with permission from Lawton MA, Brody EM. Assessment of older people: self-maintaining and instrumental activities of daily living. Gerontologist 1969, 9:179–186. Copyright © The Gerontological Society of America. Reproduced by permission of the publisher.

Box 19-2

Instrumental Activities of Daily Living (IADLs) Scale

In each category, circle the item that most closely describes the person's highest level of functioning and record the score assigned to that level (either 1 or 0) in the blank at the beginning of the category.

A. Ability to Use Telephone
1. Operates telephone on own initiative; looks up and dials numbers.   1
2. Dials a few well-known numbers.   1
3. Answers telephone, but does not dial.   1
4. Does not use telephone at all.   0

B. Shopping
1. Takes care of all shopping needs independently.   1
2. Shops independently for small purchases.   0
3. Needs to be accompanied on any shopping trip.   0
4. Completely unable to shop.   0

C. Food Preparation
1. Plans, prepares, and serves adequate meals independently.   1
2. Prepares adequate meals if supplied with ingredients.   0
3. Heats and serves prepared meals or prepares meals, but does not
   maintain adequate diet.   0
4. Needs to have meals prepared and served.   0

D. Housekeeping
1. Maintains house alone or with occasional assistance (eg, heavy-
   work domestic help).   1
2. Performs light daily tasks such as dishwashing, bedmaking.   1
3. Performs light daily tasks, but cannot maintain acceptable level of
   cleanliness.   1
4. Needs help with all home maintenance tasks.   1
5. Does not participate in any housekeeping tasks.   0

E. Laundry
1. Does personal laundry completely.   1
2. Launders small items; rinses socks, stockings, etc.   1
3. All laundry must be done by others.   0

F. Mode of Transportation
1. Travels independently on public transportation or drives own car.   1
2. Arranges own travel via taxi, but does not otherwise use public
   transportation.   1
3. Travels on public transportation when assisted or accompanied by
   another.   1
4. Travel limited to taxi or automobile with assistance of another.   0
5. Does not travel at all.   0

G. Responsibility for Own Medications
1. Is responsible for taking medication in correct dosages at correct time.   1
2. Takes responsibility if medication is prepared in advance in separate
   dosages.   0
3. Is not capable of dispensing own medication.   0

H. Ability to Handle Finances
1. Manages financial matters independently (budgets, writes checks,
   pays rent and bills, goes to bank); collects and keeps track of income.   1
2. Manages day-to-day purchases, but needs help with banking,
   major purchases, etc.   1
3. Incapable of handling money.   0

(Continued on following page)

Box 19-2 *(Continued)*

Scoring Interpretation: For ADLs, the total score ranges from 0 to 6, and for IADLs, from 0 to 8. In some categories, only the highest level of function receives a 1; in others, two or more levels have scores of 1 because each describes competence that represents some minimal level of function. These screens are useful for indicating specifically how a person is performing at the present time. When they are also used over time, they serve as documentation of a person's functional improvement or deterioration.

Republished with permission from Lawton MA, Brody EM. Assessment of older people: self-maintaining and instrumental activities of daily living. Gerontologist 1969, 9:179–186. Copyright © The Gerontological Society of America. Reproduced by permission of the publisher.

Table 19-2. ■ 10-Minute Screener for Geriatric Conditions

Problem	Screening Measure	Positive Screen
Vision	Two parts: Ask: "Do you have difficulty driving or watching television or reading or doing any of your daily activities because of your eyesight?" If yes, then: Test each eye with Snellen chart while patient wears corrective lenses (if applicable)	Yes to question and inability to read > 20/40 on Snellen chart
Hearing	Use audioscope set at 40 dB; test hearing using 1000 and 2000 Hz	Inability to hear 1000 or 2000 Hz in both ears, or inability to hear frequencies in either ear
Leg mobility	Time the patient after asking: "Rise from the chair. Walk 20 feet briskly, turn, walk back to the chair, and sit down."	Unable to complete task in 15 sec
Urinary incontinence	Two parts: Ask: "In the past year, have you ever lost your urine and gotten wet?" If yes, then ask: "Have you lost urine on at least 6 separate days?"	Yes to both questions
Nutrition, weight loss	Two parts Ask: "Have you lost 10 lb over the past 6 months without trying to do so?" Weigh the patient	Yes to the question or weight < 100 lb
Memory	Three-item recall	Unable to recall all items after 1 min
Depression	Ask: "Do you often feel sad or depressed?"	Yes to the question

(Continued on following page)

Problem	Screening Measure	Positive Screen
Physical disability	Six questions: "Are you able to..." "...do strenuous activities like fast walking or bicycling?" "...do heavy work around the house, like washing windows, walls, or floors?" "...go shopping for groceries or clothes?" "...get to places out of walking distance?" "...bathe, either a sponge bath, tub bath, or shower?" "...dress, like putting on a shirt, buttoning and zipping, or putting on shoes?"	No to any of the questions

Reprinted from Am J Med, Vol. 100, Moore AA, et al. Screening for common problems in ambulatory elderly: clinical confirmation of a screen instrument, 440, Copyright 1998, with permission from Excerpta Medica, Inc.

Box 19-3

Mini-Cog Assessment Instrument for Dementia

The Mini-Cog assessment instrument combines an uncued 3-item recall test with a clock-drawing test (CDT). The Mini-Cog can be administered in about 3 minutes, requires no special equipment, and is relatively uninfluenced by level of education or language variations.

Administration

The test is administered as follows:

1. Instruct the patient to listen carefully to and remember 3 unrelated words and then to repeat the words.
2. Instruct the patient to draw the face of a clock, either on a blank sheet of paper, or on a sheet with the clock circle already drawn on the page. After the patient puts the numbers on the clock face, ask him or her to draw the hands of the clock to read a specific time, such as 11:20. These instructions can be repeated, but no additional instructions should be given. Give the patient as much time as needed to complete the task. The CDT serves as the recall distractor.
3. Ask the patient to repeat the 3 previously presented words.

Scoring

Give 1 point for each recalled word after the CDT distractor. Score 1–3.
- A score of 0 indicates positive screen for dementia.
- A score of 1 or 2 with an abnormal CDT indicates positive screen for dementia.
- A score of 1 or 2 with a normal CDT indicates negative screen for dementia.
- A score of 3 indicates negative screen for dementia.

The CDT is considered normal if all numbers are present in the correct sequence and position, and the hands readably display the requested time.

Source: Borson S, Scanlan J, Brush M, Vitaliano P, Dokmak A. The mini-cog: a cognitive "vital signs" measure for dementia screening in multi-lingual elderly. Int J Geriatr Psychiatry 2000; 15(11): 1021–1027.

(MMSE). Domains measured by the MMSE include orientation to time and place, registration, attention and calculation, recall, naming, repetition, comprehension, reading, writing, and drawing. Testing with the MMSE takes approximately 10 minutes and must be administered in a standard manner to obtain valid results. The total possible score is 30 points; however, scores are highly correlated with age and educational level of the individual (Ashla, 2000). Scores on the MMSE will not differentiate between delirium and dementia, although both conditions will cause scores below the cutoff of 24 (Francis, 2000). Comprehensive information on the development, reliability and validity testing, and scoring of the MMSE can be found online (http://www.minimental.com). The MMSE is only available for purchase to qualified health care professionals through Psychological Assessment Resources (telephone 813-968-3003). A description of the qualifications for purchase can be found at http://www.parinc.com.

Whenever there is a question of cognitive impairment, a screen for depression is warranted because depression and dementia commonly coexist. The most commonly used instrument is the Geriatric Depression Scale (GDS) (Box 19-4). Originally, the GDS contained 30 items; a brief 15-item version is as reliable for screening. The presentation of

---

Box 19-4

Geriatric Depression Scale (GDS, Short Form)

Choose the best answer for how you felt over the past week.

1. Are you basically satisfied with your life?	yes/**no**
2. Have you dropped many of your activities and interests?	**yes**/no
3. Do you feel that your life is empty?	**yes**/no
4. Do you often get bored?	**yes**/no
5. Are you in good spirits most of the time?	yes/**no**
6. Are you afraid that something bad is going to happen to you?	**yes**/no
7. Do you feel happy most of the time?	yes/**no**
8. Do you often feel helpless?	**yes**/no
9. Do you prefer to stay at home, rather than going out and doing new things?	**yes**/no
10. Do you feel you have more problems with memory than most?	**yes**/no
11. Do you think it is wonderful to be alive now?	yes/**no**
12. Do you feel pretty worthless the way you are now?	**yes**/no
13. Do you feel full of energy?	yes/**no**
14. Do you feel that your situation is hopeless?	**yes**/no
15. Do you think that most people are better off than you are?	**yes**/no

Score 1 point for each bolded answer. Cut-off: normal (0–5), above 5 suggests depression.

Source: Courtesy of Jerome A. Yesavage, MD. For 30 translations of the GDS, see http://www.stanford.edu/?yesavage/GDS.html

For additional information on administration and scoring refer to the following references:

1. Sheikh JI, Yesavage JA. Geriatric Depression Scale: recent evidence and development of a shorter version. *Clin Gerontol.* 1986;5:165–172.

2. Feher EP, Larrabee GJ, Crook TH 3rd. Factors attenuating the validity of the Geriatric Depression Scale in a dementia population. *J Am Geriatr Soc.* 1992;40:906–909.

3. Yesavage JA, Brink TL, Rose TL, et al. Development and validation of a geriatric depression rating scale: a preliminary report. *J Psychiatr Res.* 1983;17:27.

Decision Support Box

When there is a suspicion of delirium as a cause of cognitive impairment, the Confusion Assessment Method (CAM) is the most widely used and accurate algorithm, with a sensitivity of 46%–100% and specificity of 90%–95% when applied by trained health care professionals (Francis, 2000). Delirium is present if there is an acute onset and fluctuating course, plus inattention, plus either disorganized thinking or altered level of consciousness. The findings of inattention, disorganized thinking, and altered level of consciousness can be demonstrated by the MMSE plus a trained caregiver's or professional's observations.

depression in the elderly may be atypical, with fatigue and somatic symptoms predominating; therefore, traditional criteria (DSM-IV) for diagnosis of depression may not apply. Because depression is so difficult to detect and the suicide rate is so high in the elderly, routine screening has been suggested (Lesser & Banyas, 2000).

THE ATYPICAL PRESENTATION OF COMMON CONDITIONS

The atypical presentation of common illnesses is a hallmark of geriatric care. Among the most common symptoms that may herald the onset of infection are cognitive changes, changes in the level of ADL or IADL abilities, decreased appetite, or sudden onset of urinary incontinence. Even those clients who are already debilitated may exhibit a measurable decline in function from baseline. The following two case studies compare the presentations of illness for a simple urinary tract infection in two females, one aged 23 years old and the other 83 years old. The cases contrast the clinical reasoning processes used to arrive at a diagnosis.

CASE 1: Linda M. is a 23-year-old single female, gravida 0, who presents with a 24-hour history of severe dysuria, frequency, and urgency. Her symptoms began approximately 8 hours after sexual intercourse with her long-time male partner, with whom she has had a monogamous relationship for the past 2 years. She denies fever, flank pain, anorexia, or malaise. Last normal menstrual period began 2 weeks ago. She has been on a triphasic oral contraceptive for the past 4 years and has regular menstrual cycles every 28 days lasting 2 to 3 days without intermenstrual spotting or discharge. She denies vaginal discharge, odor, itching, or irritation. Although she has never had similar symptoms in the past, her sister has a long history of cystitis, so Linda attributes these symptoms to a urinary tract infection. She is otherwise in good health, does not smoke, drink alcohol, or take other drugs, and takes no medications other than her oral contraceptives and an occasional ibuprofen for headaches.

Physical signs include normal vital signs, mild suprapubic tenderness, and sensation of increased urgency with palpation over the bladder. There is no costovertebral angle tenderness. A clean-voided midstream urine sample reveals clear, straw-colored urine without obvious blood; dipstick analysis is positive for leukocyte esterase and nitrites.

CASE 2: Mrs. T. is an 83-year-old woman who has resided in a long-term care facility for the past 12 months. She has mild dementia of the Alzheimer's type; osteoporosis with a history of right femoral neck fracture status post–internal fixation and pinning 1 year ago; stage C congestive heart failure well controlled on a diuretic and a beta blocker; osteoarthritis of hands, knees, and low back; and a history of stage I breast cancer treated 10 years ago with lumpectomy and radiation. Functionally at baseline, Mrs. T. requires assistance with ADLs and IADLs and supervision for medications; she uses a walker and requires assistance to ambulate outside her room, but in her room she is able to get to the toilet or her chair by herself with her walker; she is normally continent of urine and stool with an occasional episode of enuresis; she requires assistance with bathing and grooming; her appetite is good and she feeds herself and eats with others in the dining room; her mental status score on the Folstein mini-mental is 20/30, and she is alert, pleasant, and participates in many activities in the facility.

The nurse practitioner was called to the facility to see Mrs. T. for a sudden change in her condition, which began approximately 12 hours earlier. The nursing assistant on the evening shift reported that Mrs. T. did not eat any of her dinner and seemed more confused than usual. During the night, she was incontinent of urine three times, soaking the bed each time. When the charge nurse assessed her on rounds in the morning, Mrs. T. was very lethargic, did not know her name or where she was, could not respond appropriately to any questions, and became quite agitated when the nurse attempted to auscultate her heart and lungs. There had been no recent change in her medication regimen. Her vital signs were normal and she was afebrile. There had been no change in her weekly weights, and her bowel movements had been regular. By the time the nurse practitioner arrived to examine her, Mrs. T. was very agitated, shouting and crying out for her dead husband; she was trying to get out of her bed; she had been put in adult diapers, which were saturated with urine and stool. Her skin was warm and dry without any obvious lesions or erythema, her color was pale, and she was inconsolable and unable to respond coherently to any questions. Although the cardiac auscultation was less than ideal, the nurse practitioner did not appreciate any extra sounds or murmurs. Lung sounds were somewhat diminished at the bases bilaterally, although again, the examination was hampered by Mrs. T.'s agitation. The abdominal examination was also unremarkable.

Case Analysis

Nurse practitioners can feel comfortable treating a client such as Linda M. with a telephone consultation (University of Michigan Health System, 1999). Her symptoms do not suggest any complicating factors, and, although the urine dipstick for leukocyte esterase is cost effective with good sensitivity (75%–96%) and specificity (94%–98%), treatment without an examination or urinalysis is an acceptable option (Gonzales & Kutner, 2003). In contrast, when faced with the situation of Mrs. T., the nurse practitioner must perform a more extensive examination, including at least a urinalysis and possibly a culture and sensitivity on a catheterized urine specimen, a complete blood count with differential, pulse oximetry if available, and possibly even a chest radiograph; blood cultures are rarely useful except in situations in which acute fulminant bacteremia is suspected (Bentley et al., 2001).

The differential diagnosis for an older client with a sudden change in condition includes infectious processes, most commonly involving the lungs, skin, and gastrointestinal or urinary tracts; cardiac decompensation; drug toxicity; fecal impaction; and occult trauma from an undocumented fall or injury. With such a varied differential, a comprehensive examination is essential and a thorough knowledge of the client and the environment is more likely to guide the process of clinical reasoning. In the case of Mrs. T., the nurse practitioner examined the skin for obvious cellulitis; reviewed the record for changes in medication, weight, and stool pattern; and examined the heart, lungs, and abdomen for obvious signs of cardiac decompensation and pain. Armed with knowledge of the client's previous level of function and the meager clinical findings, the nurse practitioner will prioritize the differential diagnoses with the following considerations.

Although Mrs. T. has Alzheimer's disease, a sudden worsening of cognitive status or level of consciousness is not characteristic of the progression of dementia and usually indicates what is commonly called delirium. Delirium is a reversible condition frequently caused by infection (Table 19-3). According to the nurse practitioner's chart review, Mrs. T. is not on any new medications or any medications likely to cause toxicity; there is a fairly stable record of normal bowel movements, so impaction or gastroenteritis are not the likely culprits; there was no recent weight gain, which is common in worsening congestive heart failure, although another weight should be obtained to compare with the most recent one. When a client resides in an institution, the environment is a strong consideration in the analysis of the problem. In this case, there had been no recent outbreak of upper respira-

Table 19-3. ■ Differentiating Dementia, Depression, and Delirium in the Elderly

Characteristic	Dementia	Depression	Delirium
Onset	insidious	insidious or precipitated by an event	acute
Duration	months–years	months–years	hours–days
Fluctuations	no or occasional due to stress	some, may feel worse in the morning	prominent with abnormal day/night cycles
Affect	labile	flat	variable
Alertness	normal or lethargic	normal or lethargic	highly variable from lethargy to agitation
Attention	normal to progressively abnormal inattention	normal to mildly distracted	prominently abnormal, fluctuates
Orientation	impaired but may be close to correct	normal	usually abnormal, may fluctuate
Memory	abnormal	normal	normal when registers
Speech/ Language	anomic or worse	normal to slightly slowed	dysarthric/misnaming
Speech Content	empty or sparse	normal	confused or incoherent
Perceptual	normal to moderately abnormal	normal	hallucinations common

tory infection or influenza in the facility, so pneumonia is less likely to be the cause. Tachypnea of >25 breaths per minute, not seen in the case of Mrs. T., is one of the few physical findings with a positive predictive value (90%) for pneumonia, although pulse oximetry is helpful in absolutely ruling out pneumonia as a source of infection (Bentley et al., 2001). The physical examination did not reveal any other possible sources of sepsis, such as skin infections. The sudden onset of complete incontinence in a client who has been mostly continent could be due to either the cognitive changes attendant to delirium, or an infection in the urinary tract. Several urinary pathogens, most notably some of the strains of *E. coli*, have a direct irritative effect on bladder mucosa and can cause incontinence.

Clinical and laboratory findings that lend support to a diagnosis of urinary tract infection would include an elevated WBC count of >14,000/mm^3 and/or a left shift; pyuria on the microscopic urinalysis of >10 WBCs per high-power field; and/or a positive leukocyte esterase test. The absence of pyuria is equally significant in that it provides a negative predictive value approaching 100% and is therefore more useful in excluding the diagnosis of urinary tract infection (Bentley et al., 2001). Additionally, clinical practice guidelines suggest that in 77% of episodes of functional decline in long-term care residents, infection is the cause and the most frequent site of such infection is the urinary tract (55%). Taking all of this into consideration, urinary tract infection is the most likely diagnosis for Mrs. T. at this point.

It is clear from this case analysis that a simple urinary tract infection can cause widespread and rapid physical decline in frail elders, particularly those who are institutionalized. The assessment process is much more involved and less focused when there is an atypical presentation, which is common among the elderly regardless of whether they reside in long-term care or present to the emergency room from home. Adequate treatment of the underlying infection should resolve the delirium and the patient should return to baseline functioning.

GERIATRIC SYNDROMES

There is no commonly accepted definition or list of "geriatric syndromes." There is, however, some agreement about their common characteristics. Geriatric syndromes tend to be multifactorial in nature, have vague or atypical presentations, progress and result in frailty, and they are often interrelated and display some degree of iatrogenesis or medical error. In short, they are often precipitated by a convergence of events that causes a cascade of further problems and ends in a serious change of health status. Case 2 in the preceding section is an example of the geriatric syndrome of delirium, which is precipitated by a urinary tract infection and also leads to urinary incontinence. It is not unusual for such a situation to progress rapidly to additional adverse events: a fall as the patient attempts to climb out of bed, malnutrition and dehydration owing to the loss of appetite and the presence of infection, and skin breakdown resulting from the constant presence of urine on the perineal and coccygeal areas. Many of the geriatric syndromes are adverse events that occur as a result of immobility and hospitalization or inappropriate prescribing of medications; such syndromes require systems interventions to improve or change outcomes. Among these syndromes are four—falls, delirium, pressure ulcers, and underfeeding—that have been labeled as "medical errors" because they are largely preventable in hospitalized elders (Tsilimingras, Rosen, & Berlowitz, 2003).

It is important that nurse practitioners have a basic understanding of the risk factors, causes, and clinical presentations of geriatric syndromes and routinely assess for factors that may be amenable to intervention beyond the medical issues. Prevention is particularly important in managing geriatric syndromes both in the hospitalized and in the community-residing elder. For example, falls in the home can be prevented with a thorough evaluation of any senior who reports a single fall or who demonstrates an unsteady gait; an appropriate intervention should be instituted for any problems detected.

Details of the fall provide direction for further investigation. Not only are the date, time, and location of the fall important, but also as much detail about what the patient was experiencing before the fall can provide important clues. Ask about the presence of dizziness, blurred vision, weakness, palpitations, and a sensation of faintness preceding the fall and an awareness or lack thereof of the sensation of falling in an effort to uncover possible medical reasons for the fall. The Get Up and Go test is a simple screening measure that takes only minutes and can be conducted by trained staff. Instruct the patient to stand up from a seated position without using his or her arms or the chair arms for support, walk a few feet away, turn around and return to the chair, and sit down again without using any support. If the examiner observes any instability or difficulty with this test, further evaluation of gait and balance is required.

Using the example of falls again, a home safety evaluation that includes questions about lighting, clutter on floors, footwear, bathroom configuration, stairways, sidewalks, and the availability of help in the case of a fall can focus attention on areas where safety can be improved to prevent falls. A useful tool that can be completed by patients or their families is available on line at the Merck Institute of Aging & Health in their Falls Toolkit (http://www.miahonline.org/tools/falls/content/Falls_tool_04.html). In the case of patients who have fallen frequently, a home visit by a nurse or physical therapist is very helpful to determine what risk factors are modifiable. When patients fall in hospitals or long-term care facilities, similar attention to environmental and other system factors that increase risk has been shown to reduce falls by as much as 30% (Tsilimingras, Rosen, & Berlowitz, 2003). Owing to the multifactorial nature of the risk of falling, interventions are most successful when they go beyond a simple plan to treat medical risk factors. A multidisciplinary approach that includes patient and family education, training in gait and balance, strengthening exercises, nutrition counseling, behavior modification, and elimination of environmental hazards has been found to be most successful.

Pressure ulcers are another common condition that is preventable both in the home and in institutional settings. Tissue trauma occurs when soft tissue is compressed between a bony prominence and a hard or rough surface or when shearing of the skin occurs with movement. The trauma produces visible change of the skin, ranging from a mild erythema or discoloration to deep ulceration down to bone. The important point to remember when assessing individuals who are immobile and dependent in ADLs and being cared for at home is to include the caregivers in the process. Ask about caregivers' knowledge of the importance of keeping skin clean and dry and their ability to move, transfer, and position the patient. Support for caregivers is a crucial part of geriatric care and one that is often forgotten in clinical practice. Provide links to aging services, such as respite care, caregiver support groups, and educational classes to help families cope with the burden of caregiving.

THE ASSESSMENT OF DRIVING SAFETY

Most people rely on the automobile as the most convenient and efficient mode of transportation for obtaining medical services, groceries, and other necessities of life, as well as for maintaining social contacts with friends, families, and organizations, such as a church or place of employment. The need to drive might be related to a lack of public transportation as well as a sense of independence that seniors are reluctant to relinquish. The ability of an older individual to drive safely is dependent on a number of factors, which need to be considered in a comprehensive assessment of that individual. Drivers 65 years and older will account for at least 16% of all motor-vehicle crashes and 25% of all fatal crashes, making unsafe driving among the elderly a significant and growing public health problem (American Medical Association, 2003).

General History

At least one or two questions about driving should be included in the comprehensive history of any older adult. Questions might be as simple as "Do you drive an automobile"? "Have you changed your driving patterns recently"? "Are there any situations in which you feel uncomfortable driving"? Many seniors voluntarily restrict their driving when they recognize a feeling of discomfort with, for example, driving after dark or driving on high-speed highways. In addition, families might express concerns about the ability of a senior to drive safely with such comments as "He's had a couple of 'near misses' with the car recently" or "No one will ride with her anymore because it's too scary." Comments from family members should always be addressed both with the family and the client. It is important to remember that increasing chronological age is not an indicator of an inability to drive safely.

Focused History

Another option is to give all older clients the questionnaire *Am I a Safe Driver?* (available on-line at http://www.ama-assn.org/ama1/pub/upload/mm/433/appendixb.pdf). Positive responses can provide a starting point for a more comprehensive evaluation of driving safety. The American Medical Association (AMA) resource on safe driving contains other useful resources for practice to ensure that this issue is addressed.

Certain medical conditions or medications should be "red flags" to the nurse practitioner as areas for exploration of medically impaired driving. Obvious acute events include myocardial infarction, stroke, brain injury, syncope, vertigo, seizures, delirium, or recent surgery. Other chronic conditions include those that affect vision, cognition, strength, mobility, and uncontrolled diabetes mellitus. The most common offending medications are listed in Box 19-5. Any new medication has the potential to affect driving ability temporarily; thus, clients should be cautioned to restrict driving at least temporarily until the response to the new medication is known.

Box 19-5

Medications That Might Affect Driving Ability

1. Alcohol
2. Anticholinergics
3. Anticonvulsants
4. Antidepressants
   a. Bupropion
   b. Mirtazapine
   c. Monoamine oxidase (MAO) inhibitors
   d. Selective serotonin reuptake inhibitors (SSRIs)
   e. Tricyclic antidepressants (TCAs)
5. Antiemetics
6. Antihistamines
7. Antihypertensives
8. Antiparkinsonians
9. Antipsychotics
10. Benzodiazepines and other sedatives/anxiolytics
11. Muscle relaxants
12. Narcotic analgesics
13. Nonsteroidal antiinflammatory drugs (NSAIDs)
14. Stimulants

Habits

Alcohol consumption is known to impair driving ability in any driver and may be an even greater concern among the elderly. Ask specifically about the type, quantity, and timing of drinking behavior, and verify with an independent observer if possible.

Physical Examination

The AMA guidelines provide useful information on appropriate physical examination techniques to validate medical recommendations about driving ability; however, the report cautions that there are currently no tests that predict crash risk. These tests focus on vision, cognition, and motor function and can be integrated into the routine examination. Begin with a general observation of the client, including appearance, gait, interactive ability, looking specifically for signs of depression, dementia, delirium, motor instability, or generalized weakness. Vision is responsible for 95% of driving-related inputs (American Medical Association, 2003), and vision testing should at least include tests for acuity and visual fields. Although contrast sensitivity is an important factor in the ability to distinguish objects against a background, currently there are no validated clinical measures for this dimension of vision. Decreased accommodation also contributes to comfort with driving at night and is easily tested but not easily quantified.

Cognition is the most complex variable to test in the driving safety assessment. The ability to drive the car and navigate from one point to another requires many complex cognitive skills: crystallized and working memory, selective and divided attention, visual perception and processing as well as visuospatial skills, and executive skills (American Medical Association, 2003). These skills are not adequately tested on the MMSE; therefore, supplemental tests specific to the higher executive functions are suggested, such as the clock-drawing test and the trail-making test (available at http://www.ama-assn.org/ama/pub/category/10791.html). There are specific criteria for scoring each of these additional tests as well as clear directions for their administration. Research has demonstrated that the Trail-Making, part B test is a reasonable predictor of "at-fault" crashes in older drivers (Staplin, Lococo, Gish, & Decina, 2003). It is possible that a client with mild dementia on the MMSE could still score well enough on these supplemental tests to continue driving. The problem arises when the dementia progresses and those afflicted fail to recognize that they have become unsafe drivers. This usually results in a family situation where family members are forced to take away the driving privilege and request the assistance of the nurse practitioner or other professionals.

Motor ability testing involves testing range of motion in the neck, motor strength in both upper limbs and the right lower limb, and trunk stability and balance. Adequate range of motion of the neck without excessive pain or hesitation is essential for checking behind and to the sides of the car. Often a client with a lack of central vision owing to macular degeneration can still drive safely if the peripheral vision is intact and the ability to turn the head quickly allows adequate scanning of the street and traffic situations. Although adequate range of motion is difficult to quantify, it is rarely the sole reason for restriction of driving. Upper limb strength is essential for steering and the lower right limb is usually the one used for acceleration and braking. Strength should be graded on a scale of 0–5, with 4–5 signifying adequate strength against at least some resistance. Adaptive technologies in some automobiles may compensate for less than adequate strength in one or more areas. The rapid pace walk is specifically suggested (American Medical Association, 2003) as a good predictor of driving safety. The client is timed walking as swiftly as possible along a 10-foot path marked on the floor both away from and toward the examiner. A cane can be used, but this should be noted on the chart. A completion time of greater than 9 seconds indicates a possible need for intervention.

Resources

Many states now have safe-driving programs for at-risk drivers that provide further testing and driver rehabilitation. Testing might include on-road tests or simulations of driving situations in a computer-monitored setting. Some vision problems can be corrected with lenses or other medical interventions, although a referral might be needed to an ophthalmologist or low-vision specialist. Automobiles that are easier to drive, have controls in more convenient locations, have better visibility, and are fully automatic rather than manual may compensate for restricted movement and strength, allowing an elder to continue driving. Restricting driving to familiar locations, daylight hours, low-traffic situations, and good weather may also suffice in some situations. The AMA (2003) strongly recommends against the use of a "co-pilot" to allow unsafe drivers to continue driving, although this practice has been accepted by some state driver-licensing agencies. Even the best and most observant co-pilots might not have time to alert the driver to a potential hazard, and the driver might not respond quickly enough to avoid a crash.

Addressing client and family concerns about safe driving for an elderly person is one of the most common issues in clinical practice. It is incumbent on nurse practitioners to know

---

Box 19-6

Resources for Safe Driving

AARP 55 ALIVE Driver Safety Program
1 888 227–7669

American Automobile Association (AAA)
Foundation for Traffic Safety
1 800 993–7222
www.aaafoundation.org

AAA Safe Driving for Mature
Operators Program
Call your local AAA club to find a class near you.

National Safety Council Defensive
Driving Course
1 800 621–7619

Driving School Association of the
Americas, Inc.
1 800 270–3722

---

the laws in the state where they practice regarding reporting medically unsafe drivers; reporting guidelines vary across the country. Besides reporting or referring questionably safe drivers for further evaluation, it is important to help clients and their families plan for a transition to a nondriving status because everyone who drives will stop driving one day. Make available resources, both local and national, for clients who are in this dilemma (Box 19-6). Open the dialogue at every opportunity with clients and their families to monitor changes and the need for further interventions. Incorporate an awareness of the need for and an ability to accomplish an evaluation of an older person for safe driving.

HEAD, EYES, EARS, NOSE, AND MOUTH

Specific attention should be directed toward those organs that affect functional ability: the eyes, ears, and mouth directly affect one's ability to see, hear, and eat. There are some particular points to remember when assessing these systems.

- An examination of the eyes should always include measuring ocular pressure to rule out glaucoma, which is a serious cause of blindness and is more common with aging; screening for close and distance vision, particularly when there are questions related to driving or medication-taking ability; dilating the pupil to examine the retina for macular degeneration, a common cause of blindness in the elderly; and screening for cataracts, also increasingly common with age. Referral to an optometrist or an ophthalmologist is ideal and may be covered by Medicare and other insurance depending on the diagnosis.
- Examination of the ears should include carefully inspecting and removing cerumen impactions, which are a common cause of hearing loss. In addition to the Whisper Test,

screening with an audioscope at 40 dB and testing both ears using 1000 and 2000 Hz provides reasonable sensitivity (94%) and specificity (72%) in community-dwelling populations (American Geriatric Society, 2003). Referral to an audiologist is ideal; however, many seniors do not have the ability to pay for hearing aids and in some cases hearing aids do not help with speech discrimination.

- Examination of the mouth should include a through inspection of the teeth. Ill-fitting or missing dentures and loose teeth can severely affect the ability to chew and eat sufficient food to maintain nutrition. Referral to a dentist is ideal; however, many seniors without dental insurance do not have the ability to pay for dental services or replacement dentures.

NEUROMUSCULAR SYSTEM

Specific attention should be directed toward gait and mobility, which greatly affect functional ability and predict risk of falling. Beyond the usual examination of range of motion and strength, there are several specific tests to measure performance that can be incorporated into an examination.

- The Timed Get Up and Go Test should be administered to all clients who have experienced a fall or who report difficulty with strenuous activities, such as fast walking, heavy housework, shopping, or climbing stairs. It is easy to perform and takes very little additional time during the examination. Place a chair in an unobstructed location and instruct client to rise from the seated position, walk 20 feet, turn, walk back to the chair, and sit down. Time this activity with a stopwatch. In populations that cannot complete the task in 15 seconds or less, research has shown a strong correlation (0.6–0.8) with other measures of gait and balance (Gerety, 2000).

- Contributors to pathologic gait include foot or joint pain, weakness, sensory impairment, bone and joint abnormalities, and an impaired neurological system. The Tinetti Performance-Oriented Mobility Assessment (POMA) scale is a more sensitive and specific test of gait, balance, and mobility (Box 19-7). The gait and mobility components of the POMA include opportunities to evaluate the initiation of gait, adequacy of step length and height, step and path symmetry and continuity, and ability to turn and pick up speed. Balance is tested by observing immediate standing balance, balance during tandem, one-leg, heel, and toe standing, and a nudge to the sternum or tug from behind. The POMA is sensitive and reproducible and can be used to measure improvement over time; thus, it is often used in clinical trials of exercise interventions.

- The Functional Reach Test is another useful test for upper extremity function that correlates well with an increased risk for falls and dependence (Behrman et al., 2002). Give the client the following instructions: stand with your feet hip-width apart and your right (dominant) side next to but not touching a wall. Extend your right arm (or whichever is closest to the wall) parallel to the floor at shoulder height with your fingers extended. Now reach forward as far as you can, bending at the waist but do not lift your heels off the floor. The examiner measures the distance in centimeters from the back of the shoulder to the tip of the middle finger in the "normal reach" position and again in the "forward reach" position. Differences greater than 25 cm are a significant predictor of falls and increased dependence in ADLs and IADLs.

Box 19-7

Tinetti Balance and Gait Evaluation

Tinetti Balance and Gait Evaluation

BALANCE

Instructions: Seat the subject in a hard armless chair. Test the following maneuvers. Select one number that best describes the subject's performance in each text, and add up the scores at the end.

1. Sitting balance
   Leans or slides in chair   =0
   Steady, safe   =1_____
2. Arising
   Unstable without help   =0
   Able but uses arms to help   =1
   Able without use of arms   =2_____
3. Attempt to arise
   Unable without help   =0
   Able but requires more than one attempt   =1
   Able to arise with one attempt   =2_____
4. Immediate standing balance (first 5 seconds)
   Unsteady (staggers, moves fee, marked trunk sway)   =0
   Steady but uses walker or cane or grabs other objects for support   =1
   Steady without walker, cane, or other support   =2_____
5. Standing balance
   Unsteady   =0
   Steady but wide stance (medial heels more than 4 inches apart) or
   uses cane, walker, or other support   =1
   Narrow stance without support   =2_____
6. Nudging (with subject's feet as close together as possible, push
   lightly on the sternum with palm of hand three times)
   Begins to fall   =0
   Staggers and grabs, but catches self   =1
   Steady   =2_____
7. Eyes closed (at same position in No. 6)
   Unsteady   =0
   Steady   =1_____
8. Turning 360 degrees
   Discontinuous steps   =0
   Continuous steps   =1_____
   Unsteady (grabs and staggers)   =0
   Steady   =1_____
9. Sitting down
   Unsafe (misjudges distance, falls into chair)   =0
   Uses arms or lacks smooth motion   =1
   Safe, smooth motion   =2_____

GAIT

Instructions: The subject stands with the examiner, and then walks down the hallway or across the room, first at the usual pace and then back at a rapid but safe pace, using a cane or walker if accustomed to one.

  10. Initiation of gait (immediately after being told to go)
    Any hesitancy or several attempts to start   =0
    No hesitancy   =1_____

(Continued on following page)

Box 19-7 *(Continued)*

11. Step length and height
   Right swing foot:
       Fails to pass left stance foot with step   0
       Passes left stance foot   1_____
       Fails to clear floor completely with step   0
       Completely clears floor   1_____
   Left swing foot:
       Fails to pass right stance foot with step   =0
       Passes right stance foot   =1_____
       Fails to clear floor completely with step   =0
       Completely clears floor   =1_____
12. Step symmetry
   Right and left step length unequal   =0
   Right and left step equal   =1_____
13. Step continuity
   Stopping or discontinuity between steps   =0
   Steps appear continuous   =1_____
14 Path (observe excursion of either left or right foot
   over about 10 feet of the course)
   Marked deviation   =0
   Mild to moderate deviation or uses walking aid   =1
   Walks straight without aid   =2_____
15. Trunk
   Marked sway or uses walking aid   =0
   No sway but flexion of knees or back or spreads
   arms out while walking   =1
   No sway, flexion, use of arms, or use of walking aid   =2_____
16. Walking stance
   Heels apart   =0
   Heels almost touching while walking   =1_____
   Balance score _____ 16   Gait score: _____ 12
             Total score: _____ 28

*Modified from M Tinetti. Performance-Oriented Assessment of Mobility Problems in Elderly Patients. *Journal of the American Geriatric Society,* Vol. 34, pp. 119-126, 1986. Lippincott Williams & Wilkins.

NUTRITIONAL ASSESSMENT

Nutritional deficiencies are a prevalent problem among the elderly, ranging from 15% among community-dwelling elderly to as much as 65% among hospitalized patients. Undernourishment among institutionalized elders increases mortality rates as well as places discharged individuals at risk for serious malnutrition; malnutrition then predisposes the elder to frailty, dependence, and long-term care placement.

One of the key factors in tracking malnutrition is measuring and recording clients' heights and weights. Most adults overestimate their height and underestimate their weight on self-report; height is a particular problem because adults tend to lose 1 inch of height every 20 years after age 35–40. Measurement of standing height is difficult if there is any degree of kyphosis (underestimates the actual height). The following are some tips to ensure accurate height and weight measures in difficult situations.

- Ask the client to stand with his or her head flat against the wall; the lower border of the eye should be aligned with the upper opening of the auditory canal (the Frankfurt plane). If the head does not touch wall, measure and record that distance to estimate the degree of kyphosis.
- Estimates of actual adult height can be made with either a wingspan or knee-to-heel measurements. For the wingspan method, measure from the center of the sternum to the tip of the middle finger with the arm extended straight and supported at a 90 degree angle from the body. Take two measurements and use the average if there is a difference. To measure knee height, have the client seated on a straight chair, with hips, knees, and ankles at a 90 degree angle, which you can check with a goniometer if necessary. Measure (in centimeters) from the top of the knee to the bottom of the heel with a rigid tape measure or large wooden calipers, if available. Trunk-to-limb proportion varies by gender, ethnicity, and race; however, the following formulas for whites have been validated with larger northern Europeans as well as smaller southern Europeans.

$$\text{Males} = (2.02 \times \text{knee ht.}) - (0.04 \times \text{age}) + 64.19$$

$$\text{Females} = (1.83 \times \text{knee ht.}) - (0.24 \times \text{age}) + 84.88$$

- Obtain an accurate weight, and make sure the scale is calibrated. For residents of long-term care facilities, always use the same scale for the same patient and, if there is a change in scale, make sure to note that beside the weight. Document what the patient is wearing and always weigh in that same state. Significant weight loss is a quality indicator measure and a pattern of weight loss in any facility will trigger an investigation by state and federal regulatory agencies. Ask the patient's usual body weight if possible. Calculate ideal body weight using the same formula as for any other population.
- Once you have obtained an accurate height and weight, calculate the body mass index (BMI). For amputees, add the following percentages of the weight obtained on the scale prior to calculating the BMI: below knee 6%, at knee 9%, above knee 15%, arm 6.5%, arm below elbow 3.6%. The formula for calculating BMI is the same for the elderly as for any other population. A BMI of <21 or a total body weight of <100 pounds is an indicator of a high risk for protein–energy malnutrition.
- Useful laboratory measures that indicate protein–energy malnutrition or potentially poor outcomes in hospitalized elders include a serum albumin level below 3.4 g/dL and total cholesterol below 160 mg/dL.
- Nutrition screening can be accomplished by asking clients to complete diet records or food frequency questionnaires or by screening for other risk factors, such as those in the Nutrition Screening Initiative (Box 19-8). The Nutrition Screening Initiative is appropriately used with well elderly and provides an appropriate screening tool with support documentation available online (http://www.cdhcf.org/nsi/). For residents in long-term care facilities, the Mini Nutritional Assessment is the best validated instrument for screening; it is available online at http://www.ltcnutrition.org, along with supporting documentation.
- Although a lot of attention is devoted to undernutrition, obesity, defined as a BMI of >30, or 20% greater than ideal body weight, is also an independent risk factor for func-

Box 19-8

Nutritional Screening Tool

The Warning Signs of poor nutritional health are often overlooked. Use this Checklist to find out if you or someone you know is at nutritional risk.

Read the statements below. Circle the number in the "Yes" column for those that apply to you or someone you know. For each "yes" answer, score the number in the box. Total your nutritional score.

DETERMINE YOUR NUTRITIONAL HEALTH

	YES
I have an illness or condition that made me change the kind and/or amount of food I eat.	2
I eat fewer than 2 meals per day.	3
I eat few fruits or vegetables or milk products.	2
I have 3 or more drinks of beer, liquor or wine almost every day.	2
I have tooth or mouth problems that make it hard for me to eat.	2
I don't always have enough money to buy the food I need.	4
I eat alone most of the time.	1
I take 3 or more different prescribed or over-the-counter drugs a day.	1
Without wanting to, I have lost or gained 10 pounds in the last 6 months.	2
I am not always physically able to shop, cook and/or feed myself.	2
	TOTAL

Total Your Nutritional Score. If it's –

0–2   **Good! Recheck** your nutritional score in 6 months.

3–5   **You are at moderate nutritional risk.** See what can be done to improve your eating habits and lifestyle. Your office on aging, senior nutrition program, senior citizens center or health department can help. Recheck your nutritional score in 3 months.

6 or more   **You are at high nutritional risk**. Bring this Checklist the next time you see your doctor, dietitian or other qualified health or social service professional. Talk with them about any problems you may have. Ask for help to improve your nutritional health.

Remember that Warning Signs suggest risk, but do not represent a diagnosis of any condition. Turn the page to learn more about the Warnings Signs of poor nutritional health.

These materials are developed and distributed by the Nutrition Screening Initiative, a project of:

- AMERICAN ACADEMY OF FAMILY PHYSICIANS
- THE AMERICAN DIETETIC ASSOCIATION
- THE NATIONAL COUNCIL ON THE AGING, INC.

The Nutrition Screening Initiative ¥ 1010 Wisconsin Avenue, NW • Suite 800 • Washington, DC 20007

The Nutrition Screening Initiative is funded in part by a grant from Ross Products Division of Abbott Laboratories. Inc.

tional decline in the elderly. Women have a higher prevalence of functional decline than men at the upper end of the BMI categories (three times greater risk at a BMI of >35), independent of the usual factors, such as depression and polypharmacy (Jensen & Friedmann, 2002).

- Dehydration is common in the elderly and has serious consequences. The average fluid intake for community-dwelling elderly persons is less than 1,000 mL per day. Thirst is not a reliable indicator of the need for fluids, and most elderly individuals need reminders to drink fluids. The best method for monitoring hydration status is with the BUN/creatinine ratio; anything greater than 20:1 is highly suggestive of dehydration.

- The prevalence of constipation is about 30% among the elderly regardless of their state of health. The type and amount of food and fluids strongly influences the occurrence of constipation among the elderly. Additionally, the elderly are very likely to take laxatives; routine laxative use occurs with more than 50% of residents of long-term care facilities. With a decrease in gastrointestinal motility and fluid intake, a tendency to eat easily digestible foods (i.e., less fibrous), and the common use of medications that are constipating, special attention should be directed toward the prevention of constipation. Besides causing great discomfort, constipation can lead to fecal impaction, which can be life-threatening.

ADVANCE CARE PLANNING

Discussions about clients' preferences for limits on medical intervention should be initiated long before clients become incapable of making their wishes known; such discussions should also be a routine part of primary care practice (Agency for Healthcare Research and Quality, 2003). All states recognize and provide guidelines for some type of official document that outlines an individual's care preferences. Nurse practitioners should become familiar with these documents and make them available to their clients or provide referrals to a service that can facilitate this process. Most of the time, clients make these decisions with their family members; however, it is not uncommon for families to disagree over the details of a plan. For nurse practitioners who care for residents of long-term care facilities, family discussions and case conferences are a useful way to resolve issues of disagreement.

Decision Support Box

Murphy and colleagues (1994) interviewed 287 elderly patients (mean age, 77 years) in a geriatrics practice about their wishes to undergo CPR following a cardiac arrest during an acute illness. Before learning the facts about the probability of survival to discharge for elderly patients, 41% opted for CPR. After learning the probability of survival (10%–17%), only 22% opted for CPR; of that number, only 6% over age 85 would choose to undergo CPR in the same conditions. Using a scenario of having a chronic illness and choosing CPR when there was a life expectancy of 1 year or less, only 11% opted for CPR before learning the probability of survival to discharge after CPR declines to 0%–5%; after the discussion, the number decreased to 5%. Prognostic information, when given during a discussion of decisions related to end-of-life choices, has a significant influence on elders' decisions.

In order to make good decisions, clients need to feel comfortable asking questions about death, dying, and medical interventions. They also need to be assured that having an advance care directive does not mean they will be abandoned by the health care team. Decisions reached at any point are never irreversible; in fact, advance care decisions should be revisited at least annually and whenever a significant change in the client's or the family's condition has occurred. Nurse practitioners can play a significant role in educating clients and their families about the realities of cardiopulmonary resuscitation, tube feedings, artificial ventilation, and other invasive procedures by giving factual and unhurried explanations. Most people have only seen optimal outcomes after heroic efforts at resuscitation portrayed in the media; the realities of likely or average outcomes need to be addressed in order for individuals to make decisions consonant with their own values and wishes.

CONCLUSION

The assessment of older individuals requires a thorough understanding of physiology, awareness of the client's environment, good communication skills, avoidance of ageist thinking, and good critical thinking ability—plus time and patience. It is often the lack of time that leads to problems. Sufficient time to perform some of the additional tests of functional ability, as well as time to talk with family and caregivers, is optimal. Ideally, home assessments can be made in cases of a concern about safety and the ability to function independently. A multidisciplinary team approach facilitates management of complex situations and affords families and their elders the best opportunities for maximizing health and quality of life.

References

Agency for Healthcare Research and Quality. (2003). *Advance Care Planning: Preferences for Care at the End of Life*. Research in Action, Issue 12. AHRQ Publication Number 03–0018. Accessed online at URL http://www.ahrq.gov/research/endliferia/endria.htm on February 23, 2005.

Alessi, C. (2000). Sleep. In *Comprehensive Geriatric Assessment*. Osterweil, D., Brummel-Smith, K., & Beck, J. (Eds.). New York: McGraw-Hill.

American Geriatrics Society. (2003). *Geriatrics at Your Fingertips*. Accessed online at URL http://www.geriatricsatyourfingertips.org/ on February 23, 2005.

American Medical Association. (2003). *Physician's Guide to Assessing and Counseling Older Drivers*. Accessed online at URL http://www.ama-assn.org/ama/pub/category/10791.html on February 23, 2005.

Ashla, M. (2000). Cognitive function, mood, and behavior assessments. In *Comprehensive Geriatric Assessment*. Osterweil, D., Brummel-Smith, K., & Beck, J. (Eds.). New York: McGraw-Hill.

Behrman, A., Light, K., Flynn, S., & Thigpen, M. (2002). Is the functional reach test useful for identifying falls risk among individuals with Parkinson's disease? *Archives of Physical Medicine and Rehabilitation*, 83 (4), 538–542.

Bentley, D., Bradley, S., High, K., Schoenbaum, S., Taler, G., & Yoshikawa, T. (2001). Practice guideline for evaluation of fever and infection in long-term care facilities. *Journal of the American Medical Directors Association*, September/October, 246–258.

Blair, K. (1990). Aging: Physiological aspects and clinical implications. *Nurse Practitioner*, 15 (2), 14–16, 18, 23, 26–28.

Cotter, V. & Strumpf, N. (2002). *Advanced Practice Nursing with Older Adults: Clinical Guidelines*. New York: McGraw-Hill.

Francis, J. (2000). Delirium. In *Comprehensive Geriatric Assessment*. Osterweil, D., Brummel-Smith, K., & Beck, J. (Eds.). New York: McGraw-Hill.

Gerety, M. (2000). Health status and physical capacity. In *Comprehensive Geriatric Assessment*. Osterweil, D., Brummel-Smith, K., & Beck, J. (Eds.). New York: McGraw-Hill.Gonzales, R., & Kutner, J. (2003). *Current Practice Guidelines in Primary Care*. New York: Lange Medical Books.

Jensen, G., & Friedmann, J. (2002). Obesity is associated with functional decline in community-dwelling rural older persons. *Journal of the American Geriatrics Society*, 50, 918–923.

Lesser, I., & Banyas, C. (2000). Depression. In *Comprehensive Geriatric Assessment*. Osterweil, D., Brummel-Smith, K., & Beck, J. (Eds.). New York: McGraw-Hill.

Merck Institute of Aging & Health. (2003). Toolkits. Accessed online at URL http://www.miahonline.org/index.html on February 23, 2005.

Murphy, D., Burrows, D., Santilli, S., Kemp, A., Tenner, S., Kreling, B., et al. (1994). The influence of the probability of survival on patients' preferences regarding cardiopulmonary resuscitation. *New England Journal of Medicine*, 330 (8), 545–549.

Nutrition Screening Initiative. (N.D.) Accessed online at URL http://www.cdhcf.org/nsi/ on February 23, 2005.

Staplin, L., Lococo, K., Gish, K., & Decina, L. (2003). *Model Driver Screening and Evaluation Program: Final Technical Report Volume II: Maryland Pilot Older Driver Study*. Department of Transportation and Highway Safety, Document # 809 583. Accessed online at URL http://www.nhtsa.dot.gov/people/injury/olddrive/modeldriver/2_chap_4a.htm on February 23, 2005.

Tsilimingras, D., Rosen, A., & Berlowitz, D. (2003). Patient safety in geriatrics: A call for action. *Journals of Gerontology: Medical Sciences*, 58A (9), 813–819.

University of Michigan Health System. (1999). *UTI in adult women: Diagnosis and management*. Accessed online at URL http://www.guidelines.gov on February 23, 2005.

Index